T0199369

Behavioral
Neurology
in the Elderly

Behavioral Neurology *in the* Elderly

Edited by
José León-Carrión
Margaret J. Giannini

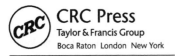

CRC Press
Taylor & Francis Group
Boca Raton London New York

CRC Press is an imprint of the
Taylor & Francis Group, an **informa** business

CRC Press
Taylor & Francis Group
6000 Broken Sound Parkway NW, Suite 300
Boca Raton, FL 33487-2742

© 2001 by Taylor & Francis Group, LLC
CRC Press is an imprint of Taylor & Francis Group, an Informa business

First issued in paperback 2019

No claim to original U.S. Government works

ISBN-13: 978-0-367-45519-4 (pbk)
ISBN-13: 978-0-8493-2066-8 (hbk)

Visit the Taylor & Francis Web site at
http://www.taylorandfrancis.com

and the CRC Press Web site at
http://www.crcpress.com

Library of Congress Card Number 2001025749

Library of Congress Cataloging-in-Publication Data

Behavioral neurology in the elderly / edited by José León-Carrión and Margaret J. Giannini.
    p. cm.
Includes bibliographical references and index.
ISBN 0-8493-2066-6 (alk. paper)
1. Geriatric neuropsychiatry. 2. Clinical neuropsychology. I. León-Carrión, José. II. Giannini, Margaret Joan, 1921-
[DNLM: 1. Aging—psychology. 2. Behavior—Aged. 3. Brain Diseases—prevention & control—Aged. 4. Cognition—Aged. 5. Neuropsychology—Aged. WT 145 B419 2001]
RC451.4.A5 B43 2001
618.97'689—dc21
                                                   2001025749
                                                      CIP

To my father and the memory of my mother

J.L.C.

Preface

Major developments in science, technology, and health care now offer an unprecedented longevity to individuals living in modern society. Whereas at the beginning of the 20th century the average life span did not extend much longer than a person's 40th decade, today, on average, we can expect to live well into our 70s. Reaching the age of 80 is no longer as much of a feat as it used to be. Now, there is an ever-larger older adult population made up of men and women with almost double the life expectancy their ancestors had no more than 100 years ago. This is a fact. We live longer than we used to, and this obviously means there has been an increase in the *quantity* of life. However, our modern society, which has made such great progress in so many areas, is no longer content with quantity. Society now demands increasing *quality* of life for the older adult population.

The aim of this book is to help achieve this goal: greater quality of life for the oldest members of our society. Once we are assured of a longer life, we want to make sure that the time spent living it will be spent in the best physical and mental states possible. *Behavioral Neurology in the Elderly* seeks to provide a close look at the current knowledge regarding the neurobiological foundations of human behavior, specifically focused on older adults. Quality of life directly depends on the functioning of the adult brain and the way in which cognition, emotions, and behavior emerge from these brain functions. How can we place this quantity of life if we lack memory of our experience? And what if we cannot reason? What happens to our emotions and feelings as we age? What if we must physically depend upon others to fulfill our needs and desires? We hope to answer these and other questions within these pages, offering solutions and guidance regarding treatment, where necessary, and prevention, when timely.

Neuropsychologists, neurologists, neuropsychiatrists, and neuroscientists in general have much to offer in the quest to further improve mental health in the elderly adult population. Ongoing research continues working toward achieving this important objective. *Behavioral Neurology in the Elderly* has been conceived in the hope that it can be useful to all those who work with older adults, to those people who are more concerned with improving the quality of life rather than simply maintaining life or just providing care. We must go beyond. Old age should not be a time of illness or a time of idleness or boredom. Healthy old age today is a time of gratification and joy during which the fullness of knowledge and emotion that the older adult offers blends into the creative flow and prosperity of our society.

It is our hope that this book contributes to this goal and can be useful to all those who strive to give the best of themselves in their commitments to maintain the knowledge and wisdom generated by a healthy adult brain integrated within our society.

José León-Carrión
Margaret J. Giannini

Since the times of Clausius, physics has had to deal with two different concepts of time: that of time as a repetition and that of time as a decline. However, it is obvious that we must go beyond this duality. Neither repetition (negation of time) nor decadence (time understood as decline) can do justice to the complexity of the physical world. We must therefore secure a third concept of time which embraces positive and constructive aspects as well.

— Ilya Prigogine
Nobel Prize Winner in Chemistry

Irreversible processes play a fundamental role in structuring the physical world.

— Albert Einstein

Editors

José León-Carrión, Ph.D., is Professor of Neuropsychology and Director of the Human Neuropsychology Laboratory at the University of Seville, Spain. He is involved with several rehabilitation programs, including the Center for Brain Injury Rehabilitation (C.RE.CER) in Seville, an interdisciplinary center for neurorehabilitation. He is also Vice President of the International Brain Injury Association (IBIA) and President of the Academy for the Advancement of Brain Injury Rehabilitation.

Professor León-Carrión is a member of the Euroacademy for Multidisciplinary Neurotraumatology and the European Brain Injury Society. He has served as President and Chair of the Second World Congress on Brain Injury and has participated in conferences worldwide. He is also the Executive Director of the Revista Española de Neuropsicología.

Professor León-Carrión is a member of several journal editorial boards. He is recognized for international books and articles related to assessment and rehabilitation of brain injury and for textbooks in neuropsychology.

Margaret J. Giannini, M.D., F.A.A.P., is the immediate past Deputy Assistant Chief Medical Director for Rehabilitation and Prosthetics, Department of Veterans Affairs, Washington, D.C. In 1979, President Jimmy Carter appointed Dr. Giannini as the first Director of the National Institute of Handicapped Research, now known as the National Institute of Disability and Rehabilitation Research. Dr. Giannini was a founder and director of the Mental Retardation Institute of New York Medical College, the first and largest facility for the mentally retarded and the developmentally disabled of all ages and etiologies in the United States and the world. She established one of the first university-affiliated facilities at New York Medical College.

Dr. Giannini is a Diplomate of the American Board of Pediatrics, a Fellow of the American Academy of Pediatrics, and a member of the Institute of Medicine of the National Academy of Sciences. She is the recipient of many national and international awards in recognition of her professional and humanitarian services and achievements. She has chaired more than 35 international conferences on rehabilitation and developmental disabilities in many countries, including Israel, Spain, China, Russia, Argentina, India, and Egypt. She has published extensively and she lectures nationally and internationally. She is Chairman of the Board of Trustees, The American University of Rome, Italy.

Contributors

Juan Manuel Barroso y Martín, Ph.D.
Department of Experimental
  Psychology
School of Psychology
University of Seville
Seville, Spain

Antonio Benetó-Pascual, M.D.
Sleep Unit
Clinical Neurophysiology Service
"La Fé" University Hospital
Valencia, Spain

Linas A. Bieliauskas, Ph.D.
Associate Professor of Psychology
Medical Center and University of
  Michigan Health System
Ann Arbor, Michigan
U.S.A

G. Kim Bigley, M.D.
Clinical Associate Professor
School of Medicine
University of Nevada
Reno, Nevada
U.S.A.
and
Medical Director
Multiple Sclerosis Center
Washoe Institute for Neurosciences
Reno, Nevada
U.S.A.

Jack Burks, M.D.
Clinical Professor
School of Medicine
University of Nevada
Reno, Nevada
U.S.A.
and
Medical Director
Washoe Institute for Neurosciences
Reno, Nevada
U.S.A.
and
President
Multiple Sclerosis Alliance
Englewood, Colorado
U.S.A.

Robert N. Butler, M.D.
President and CEO
International Longevity Center
  U.S.A., Ltd.
and
Professor, Department of Geriatrics
  and Adult Development
Mount Sinai School of Medicine
New York, New York
U.S.A.

Helio Carpintero, Ph.D.
School of Psychology
Complutense University
Madrid, Spain

Amaya Castela, M.D.
Department of Neurology
Virgen de Valme University Hospital
Seville, Spain

Salvador Chacón Moscoso, Ph.D.
Department of Experimental
  Psychology
School of Psychology
University of Seville
Seville, Spain

Cristoforo Comi, M.D.
Department of Neurology
University "Amedeo Abogador"
Novora, Italy

Eva Cuartero, M.D.
Department of Neurology
Virgen de Valme University Hospital
Seville, Spain

**María Rosario Domínguez-Morales,
M.D.**
Director
Center for Brain Injury Rehabilitation
  (C.RE.CER)
Seville, Spain

Luis Fornazzari, M.D., FRCPC
Clinical Director
Neuropsychiatry Program
Centre for Addiction and Mental Health
University of Toronto
Ontario, Canada

Ingrid C. Friesen, Ph.D.
Private Practice
Vancouver, British Columbia
Canada

Javier García Orza, Ph.D.
Department of Basic Psychology
School of Psychology
University of Malaga
Malaga, Spain

Margaret J. Giannini, M.D., F.A.A.P.
Chairman, Board of Trustees
The American University of Rome
Rome, Italy

José M. González Infantes, M.D.
Department of Psychiatry
School of Medicine
University of Cadiz
Cadiz, Spain

Victor Herbert, M.D., J.D., M.A.C.P.
Professor of Medicine
The Mount Sinai–NYU Health System
New York, New York
U.S.A.

Haydon Hill, M.D.
Clinical Associate Professor
School of Medicine
University of Nevada
Reno, Nevada
U.S.A.
and
Medical Director
Rehabilitation Services
Washoe Institute for Neurosciences
Reno, Nevada
U.S.A.

Francisco Pablo Holgado Tello, Psych.
Department of Experimental
  Psychology
School of Psychology
University of Seville
Seville, Spain

Luis M. Iriarte, M.D.
Associate Professor of Neurology
Department of Neurology
Virgen de Valme University Hospital
Seville, Spain

María Dolores Jiménez, M.D.
Department of Neurology
Virgen de Valme University Hospital
Seville, Spain

José León-Carrión, Ph.D
Department of Experimental Psychology
School of Psychology
University of Seville
Seville, Spain
and
Center for Brain Injury Rehabilitation
  (C.RE.CER)
Seville, Spain

Javier Márquez-Rivas, M.D.
Department of Neurosurgery
Virgen de Rocío Traumatology Hospital
Seville, Spain

Catherine A. Mateer, Ph.D.
Department of Psychology
University of Victoria
Victoria, British Columbia
Canada

Francesco Monaco, M.D.
Department of Neurology
University "Amedeo Abogador"
Novora, Italy

Inés Monguió, Ph.D.
Private Practice
Ventura, California
U.S.A.

Jorge Moreno, Psych.
Department of Neurology
Virgen de Valme University Hospital
Seville, Spain

Pilar Moya Corral, M.D.
Department of Psychiatry
School of Medicine
University of Cadiz
Cadiz, Spain

María J. Mozaz, Ph.D.
School of Psychology
University of the Basque Country
San Sebastián
Gipuzkoa, Spain

Manuel Murga Sierra, M.D.
Department of Neurosurgery
School of Medicine
University of Seville
Seville, Spain

José Antonio Pérez-Gil, Ph.D.
School of Psychology
Department of Experimental
  Psychology
University of Seville
Seville, Spain

Eliana A. Quintero-Gallego, Psych.
Bosque University
Bogota, Colombia

José I. Ramírez Benítez, M.D.
Department of Psychiatry
School of Medicine
University of Cadiz
Cadiz, Spain

María José Ramos-Platón, Ph.D.
Department of Psychobiology
Complutense University
Madrid, Spain

José Miguel Rodríguez Santos, Ph.D.
Department of Basic Psychology
School of Psychology
University of Malaga
Malaga, Spain

Héctor Salgado, M.D.
Department of Neurosurgery
Virgen de Rocío Traumatology
  Hospital
Seville, Spain

Dolores Torrecillas, M.D.
Department of Neurology
Virgen de Valme University Hospital
Seville, Spain

Table of Contents

PART I Fundamentals

Chapter 1
The Psychology of Aging in Historical Perspective..3
Helio Carpintero

Chapter 2
Gerontology as a Specialty of Medicine...23
Robert N. Butler

Chapter 3
Neurobehavioral Epidemiology of Aging...35
José León-Carrión, Eliana A. Quintero-Gallego, and Margaret J. Giannini

Chapter 4
Neuroanatomy of the Functional Aging Brain 67
*José León-Carrión, Héctor Salgado, Manuel Murga Sierra,
Javier Márquez-Rivas, and María Rosario Domínguez-Morales*

PART II Cognition and Behavior in Elderly People

Chapter 5
General Cognitive Changes with Aging..85
Linas A. Bieliauskas

Chapter 6
Memory and Executive Dysfunction in Elderly People:
The Role of the Frontal Lobes 109
Ingrid C. Friesen and Catherine A. Mateer

Chapter 7
Motor Functions and Praxis in Elderly People......................................125
María J. Mozaz and Inés Monguió

Chapter 8
Normal and Pathological Language in Elderly People...151
José Miguel Rodríguez Santos and Javier García Orza

Chapter 9
Emotional Disorders in the Neurologically Deteriorating Older Adult 183
Inés Monguió

Chapter 10
Aging, Sleep, and Neuropsychological Functioning Outcomes.........................203
María José Ramos-Platón and Antonio Benetó-Pascual

PART III Neurobehavioral Assessment

Chapter 11
Neuropsychological Assessment in Elderly People...243
José León-Carrión and Juan Manuel Barroso y Martín

Chapter 12
Minimal Cognitive Impairment..279
Luis Fornazzari

Chapter 13
Evaluation of Intervention Programs for Elderly People: Enhancing Validity 287
*Salvador Chacón Moscoso, José Antonio Pérez-Gil,
and Francisco Pablo Holgado Tello*

PART IV Advances in Treatment

Chapter 14
Neuropharmacology for Older Adults...311
*José León-Carrión, María Rosario Domínguez-Morales,
and Manuel Murga Sierra*

Chapter 15
Dementia in Primary Care..323
Luis M. Iriarte, Amaya Castela, and Dolores Torrecillas

Chapter 16
Neurobehavioral Syndromes in Patients with Cerebrovascular Pathology 337
María Dolores Jiménez, Eva Cuartero, and Jorge Moreno

Chapter 17
Treating Depression in Elderly People 363
José M. González Infantes, José I. Ramírez-Benítez, and Pilar Moya Corral

Chapter 18
Advances in the Prevention and Treatment of Age-Related
Organic Memory Disorders 379
*José León-Carrión, Mariá Rosario Domínguez-Morales,
and Juan Manuel Barroso y Martín*

Chapter 19
Anticonvulsant Drugs and Cognitive Functions in Elderly Patients
with Epilepsy 403
Francesco Monaco and Cristoforo Comi

Chapter 20
Multiple Sclerosis: Impact on Elderly People 411
Jack Burks, G. Kim Bigley, and Haydon Hill

Chapter 21
Vitamin, Mineral, Antioxidant, and Herbal Supplements: Facts and Fictions..... 425
Victor Herbert

Index 441

Part I

Fundamentals

1 The Psychology of Aging in Historical Perspective

Helio Carpintero

CONTENTS

1.1   Introduction 3
1.2   Old Age through the Ages 4
    1.2.1   Greece...4
    1.2.2   Rome 5
    1.2.3   The Middle Ages...6
    1.2.4   The Modern Age 8
    1.2.5   The 19th Century: Cabanis, Quételet 11
1.3   Hall's *Senescence* (1922) 14
1.4   Some Analytic Perspectives on Aging..15
    1.4.1   Charlotte Bühler's "Course of Life"..16
    1.4.2   Erikson's Views on Aging..17
1.5   Some Modern Developments..18
1.8   Coming into the Present 20
References...21

1.1   INTRODUCTION

Scientific psychology first emerged as a study of the relationship between the mind and the biological structures of an organism. As William James put it, scientific psychology is the science of mental states and their antecedent and consequent physiological processes.[1] Further, according to Wilhelm Wundt, this science focuses on the adult mind, in which all intervening elements and forces are operating according to general laws.

Evolutionary theory, as conceived by Charles Darwin, introduced new and important considerations. The theory focused on mental processes as instruments for adaptation, with new developments and variations deeply affecting all mental activities. Because the human mind had evolved from more primitive structures through adaptation and toward greater control, only through a developmental approach could it be fully understood. Such a view stressed the relevance of the

0-8493-2066-/01/$0.00+$1.50
© 2001 by CRC Press LLC

study of child psychology as a means to obtain a deeper understanding of those processes from which the adult mind is formed. The study of developmental psychology soon followed the Wundtian steps toward the construction of the new science of mind. Notwithstanding, the main focus of study was placed on the early years of life, when habits, feelings, and learning receive a lasting impact and an acquired structure.

Little by little, attention was directed to other age levels, as new adaptive problems and social needs appeared and demanded the intervention of psychologists. In addition, social changes had taken place in Western societies, among them a substantial increase in life expectancy for both men and women. As a result, substantial variations have appeared in the social structure. Different age groups, for example, tend to interact more exclusively among themselves. As a consequence of these changes, elderly people are confronted with the challenge of adapting to today's very different living conditions. The social adaptation of the elderly population is beginning to rely more and more on scientific knowledge and new resources emerging from new technologies.

Humans are historical beings, and all of the different human dimensions are of a historical nature.[2] All these dimensions must be viewed in a certain historical context, within which they are to be interpreted and evaluated. Age is no exception to the rule. It has been noted that "a form of collective life is, among other things, a particular way of spending one's allotted time." This fits in quite well with the different views of old age described as follows: "old age sometimes functions as an empty wait for death, while in other societies it is an age of positive attributes, sure of itself, perhaps even proud and hopeful."[2] The meaning of old age is based on each society's general outlook regarding old age. A valuable aspect of life, it has at times been deemed positive, at times negative. The following overview of the different ways in which old age has been valued through the annals of time emphasizes the historical, and not purely biological, nature of aging.

1.2 OLD AGE THROUGH THE AGES

In classical times, elderly people, scarce in number, were often valued as living receptacles of wisdom. Positive considerations, however, have not always prevailed. As Sumner put it, "older people are generally the possessors of power and authority, but they lose physical power, skill and efficiency in action."[3] The dual nature of this attitude toward old age underlies the two morally opposite ways in which societies treat their aged: one of conventional respect and consideration, and one of physical suppression, as some sort of social liberation.

1.2.1 GREECE

In classical Greece, old age was largely viewed as a declining stage of human life. In the Homeric poems, youth symbolized strength and power, whereas elderly people were limited to giving counsel and advice. Going one step farther, Greek comedy treated elderly people as objects of ridicule. Sparta alone put the political direction of the city-state in the hands of the *Gerusia,* the Council of Elders, in what appears to have been an exception among the Greek cities.[4]

According to historical data it is the philosophers who seem to have been most interested in the peculiar quality of the various stages of life. Pythagoras presents a broad view of the different stages of life, each stage comprising 20 years, and characterizing old age as the fourth period (which spanned from 60 to 80 years of age).[4]

Plato (427–347 B.C.) is generally known as having maintained a positive view of old age. In his *Republic*, he stressed the relevance of the knowledge and experience of the elders to governing the city. This was based on the transmission of good habits and manners from the aged to the young, and in the establishment of an order dominating the whole. When Socrates queried one of his older friends about his experience of life, as a person well advanced in life's path, he was told that, while for a few, the proximity of death was felt as a liberation, for others it was a source of anxiety and fear, impelling them to believe in the fables about life after death in Hades. The fables held that each would experience in the afterlife what was merited from the present life. However, for wise men and philosophers, the real wisdom was to leave this world of sensation behind and to return to the world of ideas, the world of reality and truth. The aged were closer to such a desired end (*Republic*, 329 e sqq.).

In contrast, Aristotle (384–322 B.C.) offered a view critical of the aged. In *Rhetoric,* he presents a vividly negative image of elderly people. This Aristotelian idea of old age would reappear many times in the centuries to follow. The image of elderly people was that of doubtful, spiteful, stingy, cowardly persons, their temperaments having become cold, their strength and warmth lost. They are portrayed as having minds that could only be captivated by thoughts of their own profit. The philosopher argues that most experience in life is that of failure, and that the aged have learned that gain is a difficult task, while loss is easy. He maintains that elderly people experience weak passions, and that their minds are turned toward the past instead of looking into the future (*Rhetoric*, 1389 b 13 sqq.). He sees weakness, egocentrism, and concentration on past life as the main traits of this stage of life. While Plato conceived of elderly people as approaching the highest human goals in life after death, Aristotle took a much more worldly and empirical stance in viewing old age as full of limitations and problems. The respective and contrasting philosophies of the two philosophers clearly represent the dual face of aging.

1.2.2 ROME

The Romans have been characterized as a pragmatic, nontheoretic society, interested in human affairs and in dominating the world. Notwithstanding, their roots were in the home and the family was revered. Ancestors were honored above all, and old age was mainly viewed as a stage of wisdom to be honored. Such a view seemed to decline as the Empire supplanted the old Republic, and military power supplanted democracy.

In early Roman times, elderly people were seen as vessels of tradition and virtue. In *De Senectute,* Cicero (106–43 B.C.) raised his voice in praise of the aged. In parallel with the Platonic model, he stressed that the negative view of aging was mainly due to four factors: the loss of control of business, the weakening of the body, the tendency of life's pleasures to disappear, and the approach of death.[5] Cicero discarded these factors as unacceptable, arguing that many aged people lead an active life[5] and that, although the strength and force of their youth have been lost, they are able to endure. The aged, he argued, continue to experience the pleasures of friendship and philosophy; while the burning desires of youth vanish, the mind achieves freedom and calm. Cicero maintained that death is a natural process, not to be feared or viewed as an ending if a new life awaits beyond. Cicero's outlook was based on the idea that nature is both the fate and cause of real processes. Hence, the assumption that aging and death are natural processes inspired him to regard both as propitious, driving him to raise his voice in praise (*laudatio*). The arguments set forth by Cicero would endure for centuries, reappearing in one form or another up to the present, where they can be found as recurring themes in literature on the subject of aging.

Later, under the Empire, there is a contrasting view of age, where an old man, "after losing his family and political power, ... is left alone, retaining only his aches, ugliness and weakness."[3]

Still, the earlier position persists, and praise of old age may be found in the famous *Letters to Lucilius* from Seneca (4 B.C.–A.D. 65), a man of the Stoa, a Stoic. Stoicism relies on the acceptance of nature, the ultimate reality from which everything flows and to which everything returns. Age is considered a natural condition affecting the body and soul differently. With age, the body feels tired (*lassum*), or, toward the end, more than tired, decrepit (*decrepitum*). The soul, however, is regarded as full of power (*viget*) and as experiencing the pleasures of thinking and being alive. Life is an expectation of its end, and wisdom is coincident with nature. When that which must disappear has vanished, it is right and must be felt as right, in keeping with the ordinance of nature. The wise man must say: "*accipio conditionem*"; i.e., I accept the rule, that is the law of nature.[6] Seneca offers a positive view, old age signifying nearing the end, the end signifying freedom from body and the return to nature. Such a doctrine, although Stoic in origin, was readily accepted by religious groups that also believed in a life after death and facing the Supreme Being. Stoicism has had a long-lasting influence, through medieval and up to modern times. This philosophy, which regards old age as a time to prepare oneself for the end of this life, has been an important contribution toward a positive outlook on old age.

1.2.3 THE MIDDLE AGES

In Western civilization, medieval times were defined by the interactions between Roman civilization, which emerged and developed in the Mediterranean, and northern peoples, such as the Germans, whose mentality was based on totally different grounds. The elements of the ancient culture were lost, and a period of Dark Ages spread over the known world. Christianity spread and with it the view of the world as a temporary stage for humans, and a means to obtain final "salvation."

St. Isidore of Seville (c. 560–636), a bishop and theologian from the Visigoth Kingdom of Spain, set forth one of the first compilations of knowledge during the Middle Ages. His *Etymologiae* is an encyclopedia that offers a synthesis of classical culture, in which he expounds through the analysis of terms viewed from an etymological perspective. It includes information regarding the "six ages of man," the last of which is termed "senium," the sixth age, the age of the elderly. According to St. Isidore, the sixth age begins at 70 and has no fixed age to end, as it is the final age, ending with death.

Within the pages of the *Etymologiae,* it is suggested that the term *senes* (old man) would come from the "loss of senses." The mind becomes clumsier, and as the blood cools, elderly people become more and more imprudent. This is a clear instance of galenic humoral theory, which equated wisdom with heat.

St. Isidore considered that old age was a combination of both good and bad aspects. Freedom from passions, weakness of sexual desires, growth of wisdom, and wide experience are deemed positive values, whereas on the negative side are illnesses, weakness of body, loss of love, and sadness.[7] The Aristotelian model is clearly maintained in these pages. No special consideration seems to be forthcoming from the religious beliefs of the author.

It has been said that the Black Death that assailed Europe beginning in late 1348 destroyed one fifth of the population. This introduced important demographic changes, an important effect of which was greater power in the hands of the older population. In Venice, not only the *doges* but the whole political system relied on aged members of the great families. Similar regimes dominated Italy in pre-Renaissance times.[4]

In her general view of senescence, Simone de Beauvoir[8] affirms that historical considerations on this topic have mainly focused upon men, neglecting women. True, women have remained largely unheeded and marginalized in historic treatises until recent times, but medieval literature does offer a few examples with a positive appreciation of elderly women. For example, two masterpieces of Spanish literature present two elderly female main characters. The first is found in the 14th century *Libro de Buen Amor* (Book of Good Love) by Juan Ruiz, a book of joyful stories and love poems. An elderly go-between in love intrigues, "Trotaconventos," is portrayed, qualified by some as "the first great character in Spanish literature." Given that she is worldly in the affairs of love, Trotaconventos' assistance is called upon by young lovers in need of aid. Experience and cunning, psychological insight, and social ability are blended in this character, who later serves as a model for the second one, "Celestina." Also a procuress, Celestina is the main character in the Renaissance novel *Tragicomedia de Calixto y Melibea* (1499) by Fernando de Rojas. Able in her art to the point of being reprehensible, Celestina uses her deep knowledge of the human condition to meddle in ways that did not fit moral standards. Nonetheless, owing to her ingenuity and skills, Celestina became established as a symbol of sorts in the ways of human affairs. Old age has its own set of values and virtues: this would seem to be the lesson to be learned from these literary creations.

1.2.4 THE MODERN AGE

In modern times, little by little references to religious beliefs began to disappear, and man and woman became more and more centered upon this world and less focused on the next. Adaptation and control of worldly affairs became the up-and-coming values, and the weaknesses and infirmities of old age became serious handicaps against true worth.

Some essential traits have been captured by William Shakespeare (1564–1616) in *As You Like It* (II, vii), in his famous monologue on the seven ages of man:

> All the world's a stage,
> And all the men and women merely players:
> They have their exits and their entrances;
> And one man in his time plays many parts,
> His acts being seven ages

which ends with these lines:

> The sixth age shifts
> Into the lean and slipper'd pantaloon,
> With spectacles on nose, and pouch on side,
> His youthful hose, well sav'd, a world too wide
> For his shrunk shank, and his big manly voice,
> Turning again toward childish treble, pipes
> And whistles in his sound. Last scene of all,
> That ends this strange eventful history,
> Is second childishness, and mere oblivion,
> Sans teeth, sans eyes, sans taste, sans every thing

Here old age is signified as the loss of everything, mind and reason included, and the return to childishness and oblivion. The empiricism found in the work of Aristotle many centuries before once again appears, bringing to the fore this negative image of the last age of man.

During the 17th and 18th centuries this negative picture did not change. Neither the economic powers nor the Church were interested in the problem. Exceptions were the English and American Puritan societies, where a kind of gerontocracy of parents and ministers exalted the value of elderly people.

In the medical world, a fledgling European gerontology began to appear, first with some Renaissance books by Gabriele Zerbi and Marsilio Ficino (both printed in 1489). These ideas were later developed in the work of Girolamo Brisianus (*Geraeologia*, 1583), Luigi Cornaro (1558), Georg Pictorius von Villingen (1549), and, in Portugal, E. Madeyra Arraes. In addition, the work of the Spanish hygienist Cristobal Mendez (1553) should be distinguished in this area, as he pointed out exercises that would help aged people maintain a good state of health.[9]

Sir Francis Bacon's *The History of Life and Death* (1626), one of his last published works, has at times been considered the foundation of modern gerontology.

In this work, Bacon (1561–1626), pioneer of British Empiricism, examines the physical conditions of life and the life cycle in natural terms, as simple effects of the natural constituents of the individual. Bacon differentiated between the body and the soul, and described the body as being of two different types: the living, material body and the supernatural body. He considered the living body the result of the mixture of elements, while God "blew" the supernatural body into a man. According to the book, everything contains a "spirit or pneumatic body,"[10] but living beings have a second body, "a living spirit"[10] permeating the whole body but essentially concentrated in the brain. Living bodies are fatty ones and undergo self-change and renovation, while inanimate bodies are hard and cannot change or renovate themselves. Bacon describes life as a process that implies activity and movement. In its early stages, movement and activity is that of growth, which later stops. Gradually then, this inherent activity and movement becomes a conspiracy of sorts between the active principle or *spiritus,* and the external air. A dryness and wasting of the body is produced, causing it to deteriorate and leading finally to its end. *Spirits,* combined with external air, dry up the fats of the body, leading to a natural process of "consumption." Here is where Bacon places the roots of aging, considering it a universal process, encompassing both inanimate objects and living entities, among which he includes human nature. This aging process implies desiccation, a drying up that deteriorates the body and causes a loss or *depredatio,*[10] which becomes irreversible as senescense begins. Bacon examines two principal processes of life: the deterioration of the body (*consumptio*) and its repair (*reparatio*), both governed by natural laws. To intervene or cause any change in these processes, he maintains that one must be familiar with these natural laws. Intervention is considered possible in at least three ways: the prevention of consumption, the perfection of repair, and the renovation of that which is already old (*prohibitio consumptionis, perfectio reparationis, renovatio veterationis*).[10,11] Such ideas imply that, by taking into account the laws of the process, there is a real possibility of strengthening and prolonging life. To increase well-being, destructive risk factors must be controlled or reduced. Longevity is a multicausal process related not only to situation variables, such as the time period, climate, and place, but also to such factors as heredity, the habits of bodily functions and physical constitution, birthday (according to astrology), living habits and diet, the quality of the living conditions and the home, and psychological characteristics such as affections (*affectus*), motivations (*studia*), and occasional events (*accidentia*).[11]

The empirical approach to the problem of senescence found in these pages is noteworthy. For example, a large part is devoted to different types of nourishment, and attention is also paid to eating habits: the precept "eating before being hungry and drinking before being thirsty" is referred to here as the key recommendation for an elderly person wishing to live a long life.[11] Annotated records of very aged historical figures, such as Moses, Abraham, Solomon, and many others, are included; geographic areas favoring aging are also mentioned (not only countries with cold climates, but also islands such as Japan and the Canary Islands were seen to stimulate longevity among their inhabitants).[11] He also summed up those signs announcing death even in a healthy state, before illness appears.

Bacon considered healthy habits more important than rare potions and elixirs of eternal youth. He wrote in the "De Augmentis Scientiarum:"[11]

> It is far more probable that a man who knows well the nature of arefaction and the depredations of the spirits upon the solid parts of the body, and clearly understands the nature of assimilation and of alimentation, whether more or less perfect, and has likewise observed the nature of the spirits, and the flame as it were of the body, whose office is sometimes to consume and sometimes to restore, shall by diets, bathings, anointings, proper medicines, suitable exercises, and the like, prolong life, or in some degree renew the vigour of youth, than that it can be done by a few drops or scruples of a precious liquor or essence.

Bacon goes on to say, "Life under religious rules, or devoted to studies of philosophy and humanities seems to lengthen; diet and moderate exercise, do the same also; contrarywise, fatigue activates spirits, with subsequent destruction of body. Psychological moods deeply influence body states. Passions are not without consequence on lengthening or shortening life." "Great fears shorten life ...; anger indulged ... is beneficial," but not "suppressed anger," which activates destructive spirits; great shame is pernicious, as is also envy, while "hope is ... the most useful" of all feelings."[10] He considers that in a comparison between younger and older persons, neither the body nor mind of the latter would surpass those of the former; the defects of old minds would parallel those of the body.[10] Bacon shows himself in the end alienated from those favoring the superiority of youth, but at the same time, offered advice on how to keep oneself at one's best, by adapting life to natural laws and conditions. Another singular trait of his personality can be found in his defense of active euthanasia, which he considered a special task to be performed by physicians, who were not only charged with the restoration of health, but also with those actions that serve "only to make a fair and easy passage from life" for people suffering illnesses, "all hope of recovery being gone."[11]

This book on "life and death" seems to have been highly appreciated among the physicians from the Baroque period as it has been noted that the great physician Boerhaave was deeply influenced by Bacon's work.

Aside from empirical considerations such as Bacon's, the stereotype of poor, limited, weak old age was strong enough to remain in force during the Enlightenment. For example, an 18th-century Spanish physician, Andres Piquer,[12] held an opinion of senescence wholly based on those put forth by Aristotle, Hippocrates, and Horace. He remarked on the obvious validity of such observations and how they coincidenced with his own medical experience. Piquer considered education and mortification as the best means to govern the mind during life.

Not far removed are the reflections on man's life by the Frenchman Georges Louis Leclerc, Comte de Buffon (1707–1788). Buffon, one of the greatest naturalists of his time, wrote a natural history of man, from a developmental perspective. Built upon the Cartesian mind/body dualism, he considered it best to analyze the mind from a natural point of view. According to Buffon, body constituents are growing during the first stages of development, but they soon begin to multiply and accumulate without real growth: humors and organs begin to lose their flexibility. He wrote that the onset of the process of senility clearly commences at the age of 70 and that senescence would end at the age of 80 or 100 years.[13] "As age grows ... body is dying little by little and part after part ... death is nothing except the last stage of such a series of steps, the last facet of life." Buffon considered death only an aspect of the entire process of life.

As growth is followed by destruction, he was inclined to accept a rather mechanical view of development, that could only be affected by too much nourishment or excessive diet; neither race nor climate nor lifestyle would change the duration of life in a meaningful way.[13]

Buffon also offered some interesting figures on life expectancy. For a newborn baby, he estimated life expectancy to be 8 years, while at age 70, it was over 6 years, and only 3 years for all ages over 77.[13] With such figures, death became something quantitative and well defined, that would lose its menacing face. The age of reason was "cleaning up" the image of the final act of the play of life.

1.2.5 THE 19TH CENTURY: CABANIS, QUÉTELET

Empiricism proved that the contents of the human mind were dependent upon the natural conditions of the body. The French philosopher Étienne Bonnot de Condillac (1715–1780) and the heirs of John Locke conceived the formation of the mind as a process closely related with experience and age, and largely based on feelings and emotions. Organic development was seen as a biological process paralleled or followed by a similar evolution taking place in the mind. Old age should not be taken as a destructive stage, but as the final scene of the natural process of the development of the mind. Given the multiple variations of individuals arriving at the last age, a normal evolution was supposed to be operating. Quantitative and qualitative changes would indicate the active causes intervening in the process. Those degenerative processes that could appear in senescence had to be viewed as mental conditions, instead of mere organic damage.

Pierre Jean Georges Cabanis (1757–1808), an enlightened French thinker deeply interested in the study of the human mind and its dependence on organic conditions,[14] wrote on the subject of age and mental faculties. His writings seem to have been largely influenced by Bacon, as he considers that young bodies are more flexible than older ones, the latter having become filled up with materials. Faculties are stronger at early stages of development, and as the individual becomes older, "the action of life begins to find strong resistance, fluid movements are harder, and the feeling of strength and well-being ... decreases day after day, in a notable way."[14] The same is true for "moral happiness," which is identical to well-being,[14] and which begins to fade as the feelings of unrest and uneasiness gradually appear. The upper limit for the mature age is placed between 49 and 56 years of age, and implies "a true climactic age"[14] for both sexes in that it constitutes the threshold of senescence. Body changes are followed by changes in ideas and feelings; sometimes, the melancholic mood diminishes; and other times anxiety appears as an effect of bad circulation.[14] "As age progresses, mind operations become day after day slower and hesitant; character becomes, little by little, shy, suspicious, opposed to any haphazardous project. The difficulty of being grows continuously; the feelings of life are not openly exteriorized, and a fatal need forces the old man to retreat upon himself: should not such an egoism, by which he is usually condemned, be viewed contrariwise as an immediate effect of nature?"[14]

Age also brings with it the loss of recent memory and, at the same time, more vivid recall of childhood memories. At an early age, the impressions received by the brain are stronger, but receptivity would diminish along with age, and interference would also deteriorate the quality of contents. Long before the enunciation of Ribot's law of regression, Cabanis noted that "it may be seen ... that memories disappear in an inverse order to that under which impressions were received, beginning with the more recent and weak ones, and progressing toward the older and more durable ones."[14]

Step by step, the study of mind from a physiological and natural point of view was advancing along with the century. The Belgian social researcher Adolphe Quételet (1796–1874) demanded an emphasis on more detailed and quantitative knowledge. His book, *Sur l'homme et le développement de ses facultés, ou Essai de physique sociale* (1835), has been viewed as "the first effort to apply mathematical analysis to the study of the human being, not only of his body, but also his behavior, morals, mind and soul."[15] In these pages, the names of Gall, Lavater, Pinel, and Esquirol are frequently cited. Quételet also took into account many quantitative anthropological studies, on crime, marriage, and so forth. Interested at first in phrenology and its achievements, he later became critical of it and maintained the need to "study man through his *actions,* and to ascend from effects to causes,"[16] always placing individuals within society, and societies within the whole of humanity.

Humans, as natural beings, are subject to a development according to laws of largely unknown physical and moral dimensions. There are some constant values in different dimensions of being, but there are also variations due to accidental causes, and these differences are all around the average value. Such variations are "regulated with such harmony and precision that can be classified" and quantified, but they cancel each other out when large numbers of subjects are considered.[16] Instead of concentrating upon individuals as such, Quételet stressed the need for statistical studies to clarify the "general facts" and to remove meaningless peculiarities.[16] He was in search of social laws, not immutable laws as in the physical sciences, but laws that change in accordance with social changes that are essential in societies. He wanted to study the "average man," status determined by statistical procedures. "Man, I consider here, in his society, to be the equivalent of the gravitational center in a physical body; he is the average around which all the social elements oscillate."[17] Individuals are free beings, but "free will disappears and is without visible effects when observations are made upon a large number of individuals."[16] Statistics would cast light on the essential traits of the human being.

Some social phenomena are related to age. For example, marriage, mortality, and life expectancy are age-related phenomena. Physical body traits also correlate with the body's developmental level. Mental faculties seem equally affected by age, but correlations here are less defined, and quantification is reduced to quasi-nominal scales. For example, courage varies among individuals, and individuals may be compared in this domain, but an "absolute degree" of courage would be meaning-less,[16] as no courage unit could be employed to measure it.

Using statistical arguments, Quételet noted that psychopathological disturbances correlated with age levels; feeble-mindedness was related to childhood, and insanity to senescence.[16] He made more concrete comparisons: "In Norway, only 1/8 of the demented population is over 60, while in Paris, they represent 1/6 of the total."[16] Suicide was analyzed, and data from Berlin (from the 1818–1824 period) showed 12% of people over 70 years old committed suicide, while data from Paris showed 14.5% in the same age range.[16] He did the same with marriage, and the figures impelled him to affirm that strong laws seem to govern such behavior.

Quételet showed that moral and physical phenomena of elderly people had to be considered from social and historical perspectives, and not only from a physical perspective. He maintained the need for a detailed developmental study of human faculties.[17] Faculties would develop in an orderly way, memory first, then imagi-nation, and last reason.[16] In addition, while the natural faculties of the "physical man" would appear as stable, those related to the "intellectual man" seem to be in continuous progress, owing to scientific advancements.[17] As knowledge spreads out through society, variations tend to diminish and to concentrate toward the mean.[17] Civilization would equate to normalization, in physical, moral, and psy-chological phenomena.

In his approach, Quételet established the basis for a quantitative study of human behavior that reconciled the physical, intellectual, and moral dimensions of the "average man," which could represent innumerable variations.

Variations also became central to biological evolutionism as conceived by Charles Darwin (1809–1882) in *On the Origin of Species* (1859). Darwin as well stressed the relevance of physical and mental qualities in the common task of adapting the organism to its environment. Usefulness for survival became the ulti-mate reason for maintaining such qualities along the hereditary process. Adaptation becomes maximized when qualities endlessly change and can confront nearly all types of situations. As Darwin's cousin, Sir Francis Galton, a man of genius, wrote, "the moral and intellectual wealth of a nation largely consists in the multifarious variety of the gifts of the men who compose it."[18] Study of the subject occupied him for a good part of his life. In 1883, at the International Exhibition of London, he carried out mass observations and tested a large number of people on sensory and mental qualities. There he saw how average measures, representing the "average man," showed steady deterioration with age.

Interest in the study of psychological abilities soon concentrated on the early part of life, childhood. Physical training, school activities, and mental and moral education demanded such an approach. But it is no surprise that one of the pioneers of child psychology, the well-known American researcher Granville Stanley Hall, became interested toward the end of his life in the study of the final years of the course of human life. His work became a milestone in the field.

1.3 HALL'S *SENESCENCE* (1922)

Granville Stanley Hall, one of the pioneers of the new psychology in the United States, is the author of *Senescence*, which is usually considered the founding block of the psychological study of aging. The author considered himself a "genetic psychologist."[19] He had explored the early part of life at length in his book *Adolescence* (1904), later condensed in *Youth* (1907). As he grew older, he turned his attention toward his new stage. Although he found it a "depressing theme,"[19] he saw it as an introduction to the authentic life for himself. Some indications suggest that the experience of World War I may have influenced the author's mature view.

According to Hall, senescence represents the fourth life period, beginning in the 40s, and culminating in "senecritude," which ends with death. It "has its own feelings, thoughts, and will, as well as its own physiology, and their regimen is important, as well as that of the body."[19] Most important, this age must accomplish a task in modern societies that has not yet been recognized. Such a task is this: "intelligent and well-conserved senectitude has very important social and anthropological functions in the modern world ...; the chief of these is ... synthesis, ... in our very complex age of distracting specializations."[19] Hall states that "age is in quest of first principles,"[19] in quest of real wisdom that should be offered to societies in need of it. Old age cannot be merely "contemplative,"[19] but has to achieve some goals, perhaps summed up in the old precept: "old men for counsel."[19] This is a basic need for modern societies: an impartial and broadly general world view, a characteristic quality of the knowledge that an elderly person has accumulated and that is missing among younger minds.

His picture includes data on creativity and production in science and art of both the under- and over-40 populations, offering a balanced result; vital statistics, which show a slow lengthening of life from the 19th to the 20th century, and countless opinions and stories related to old age.

Great attention is paid here to the objective aspects of the problem. In fact, Hall explored many institutions and social care services for elderly and poor people. Here he detected "the growing magnitude of the economic problem of old age."[19] Another interesting point is his review of literature dealing with medical and health care devoted to this life period, epitomized in a cumulative way without further integration. He was clearly against a mere hereditary explanation for longevity; instead, he maintained that senescence is "a state of mind"[19] and that it depends on knowledge and control of the conditions of such a state. Hall considers mental attitude to be the crucial factor; as a matter of fact, the 70th birthday is viewed as "the saddest" of all, and "the most dangerous milestone."[19] The meaning is that feelings and interpretations about life play a role as basic as biological factors might. All scientific data are interpreted by the mind and, based on these grounds, "psychology must henceforth have a place here second only to biology in formulating conclusions."[19]

The book also covered those theories that at that time were dealing with the problem of prolonging life, such as Weismann's immortality of germ plasma and Metchnikoff's ways of furthering senescence, endocrinology, and rejuvenation, among others. Nonetheless, in the end, he focused his hopes on psychology. Life, according to Hall, depends on motivation and on those forces that make up the conditions of human life. These are mainly related to endocrine functions, which set the stage for a unified functioning of biological activities, psychological moods and feelings, and genetic processes.[19]

Egocentrism, demand for others' attention, "patheticism," erotic decline, the tendency to alternate moods, irritability, sleep disturbances, capriciousness, loss of attention to personal care, and the dulling of sensations are frequently accompanied by mental starvation, as sources for stimulation are diminished. According to Hall, all these phenomena indicate that "the old need a higher kind and degree of self-knowledge."[19] He is against the view of old age as a second childhood, as "there is nothing rejuvenative about it,"[19] although it is true that is a "stage of postmaturity that involves … the transvaluation of all values,"[19] and especially all those related to menopause and the loss of beauty and attractiveness in women. For men, the loss of generative potency would be in many cases their "very most psychalgic experience."[19] While sex declines, love is subject to sublimation or evolves to friendship.

The picture that emerges from these pages is mostly descriptive and largely based on self-analysis and qualitative expositions of life in old age. All these traits should be viewed as materials to be used in favor of Hall's project: the defense of an image of an old man as an active being in a crusade against ignorance and in search of objectivity.[19] The image of Nietzschean Zarathustra seems to symbolize his ideal.[19] In fact, he proposed to complement youthful virtues with those of the aged person,[19] as, in other aspects, he was inclined to combine the viewpoints of different psychological schools, to get "a sound knowledge of man."[19]

Hall included a chapter with long citations and comments on some answers he received from distinguished people to a questionnaire sent by him, dealing with their experiences on age and its more salient traits. He also added an ending in which he deals with attitudes toward death, viewed as the total end of life, although he tried to reconcile such a view with some feelings of acceptance and satisfaction for the life that has been lived.

The final pages are an exhortation to further the knowledge of aging, which he considered an unexplored topic among psychologists. However, although the book was frequently cited in later works, its lack of methodology and its over-abundance of occasional and erudite information made it an oddity, without serious scientific consequences.

1.4 SOME ANALYTIC PERSPECTIVES ON AGING

During the first half of the 20th century, many different schools of psychological thought aimed at obtaining supremacy in the field. Strongly influenced by evolutionism and the ever-growing knowledge of biological structures governing animal and human behavior, most focused on early life as the period in which the structure develops that will explain mature life and adaptations.

Psychoanalysis on the one hand and behaviorism on the other have viewed human childhood as the stage in which habits, knowledge, and sources for action are acquired by the subjects, and such elements would allow explanations of behavior.

This does not mean that no reflection on aging might be found in the classic works of other representative authors. For example, well-known psychodynamic theorists such as Carl G. Jung and Alfred Adler outlined drafts of the psychology of old age that are not without interest.

Jung (1875–1961), in a well-known paper on "The decline of life,"[20] considered old age a period of life full of problems, as instincts have lost control of behavior, and imagination has given up, while the subject is confronted by the limitations of everyday reality. Moreover, Jung lamented that there was no school at all for those entering into this last part of their lives, wholly "unprepared" for the approaching tasks.[20] In his view, some changes usually bring less tolerance and a degree of fanaticism. It would be desirable to prepare people for departure from life, as the main religions have taught for centuries. The teachings would present certain images and symbols, which could be employed to adapt the mind to the coming experience. This would not be a question of faith, but of reconciliation between conscious thought and unconscious protoimages, in search of mental calm.[20]

Adler (1870–1937), on the other hand, offered a vivid picture of old age in accordance with his basic teachings. He had taught that the normal person relies psychologically on a sense of self-worth and power, whereas neurotics view themselves as faulty or inferior people when compared with others. The elderly person, under normal circumstances, might be considered a sort of functional neurotic: with feelings of uselessness, unworthiness, and of being slighted, which can generate a hostile attitude toward the world.[21]

Both pictures deal with deep motivations, mostly rooted at an unconscious level, guiding the life of elderly people, and causing most of the difficulties usually associated with that period of life.

New understanding has come from longitudinal studies on intelligence and child development. Here is found increased interest in adult and later life, combined with a growing preoccupation with the underlying sources that govern cognitive abilities and their laws. Some representative works are considered below.

1.4.1 CHARLOTTE BÜHLER'S "COURSE OF LIFE"

Charlotte Bühler (1883–1974) was deeply influenced by her husband, Karl, and together in the 1930s they represented the pinnacle of the German school of developmental psychology. This school of thought was centered in Vienna and oriented closely with, but independent of, Gestalt psychology. Charlotte Bühler soon became interested in longitudinal studies of life careers, and through them she eventually became devoted to humanistic studies of human life, especially after the couple was exiled to the United States as the Nazis seized power in Germany and Austria.

Her book on the human course of life as a psychological problem (*Der menschliche Lebenslauf als psychologisches Problem*) is, without doubt, a milestone in the field. It is focused on human life as a goal-oriented activity, and strives to understand its structure and developmental laws.

Old age here represents the second part of the life curve, a period characterized not by "expansion," which corresponds to youth and mature age, but by "restriction"[22] or diminishment of reproductive possibilities and functional activities (from the 50th year on). The basic proposition of the book is related to the dual nature of the life course: there is a line that represents vitality, and another that represents personal achievements; and these lines do not run strictly parallel. Climax in the former precedes climax in the latter. When an individual creates an objective work, this may develop at its own pace, enlarging and reinforcing from outside the life course of its author.[22] Cultural creatures would help their creators maintain youthfulness of spirit. And childhood and youth should be viewed as a draft and projection of what life will be later in its definite form.[22]

Charlotte Bühler combined sociobiographical data with subjective declarations and information and objective production and works.[22] Her study greatly benefited from information from applied psychology and concrete research on job performance and age. However, Charlotte Bühler also added interesting analyses of life careers from well-known people in the arts and culture, and stressed the importance of having a global view of biographical achievements to evaluate each of its parts.

Such a global view of the life course has also been the focus of the reflections on human development by another dynamic theorist, Erik Erikson.

1.4.2 ERIKSON'S VIEWS ON AGING

Erik Erikson (1902–1994), psychoanalyst, was born and raised in Germany and later emigrated to the United States. He was attracted to the study of children in Vienna under the direction of Anna Freud. There, he was also influenced by the Bühlers' work, and he continued these studies after settling in the 1930s in Boston, where he became very influential. Nevertheless, he was not entirely free from suspicion and restrictions during the McCarthy period.

Whereas Freudian psychoanalysis had concentrated upon childhood as the source of all determinations of later life, Erikson wanted to take the life cycle as a whole, conceiving it as a succession of stages. Each stage was characterized by certain traits and delimited *a parte ante* and *a parte post* by a crisis, whose results would influence the course of the following periods. He also added new periods to the classical ones, covering the whole life span, and revised the dynamics that are in force during each stage with leeway for cultural and social factors.

Human life is characterized by a sense of identity, which does not imply an absence of change, but the building of a dimension of sameness throughout the variations. Identity emerges through experiences during childhood and youth, facing an opposite tendency toward confusion and lack of life goals. The earlier crises have already been resolved in previous steps. The first crisis, related to "basic trust versus basic mistrust" (the first 2 years of life), creates a basic feeling toward the world, depending on interpersonal experiences. Next comes the second crisis, "autonomy versus shame and doubt" (the 2-year-old), resulting from early explorations that include the child's own body and sexual organs and raise early prohibitions. This crisis is followed by "initiative versus guilt" (3 to 5 years), characterized by the so-called Oedipus conflict, and the fourth crisis, "industry versus inferiority" (during the elementary-school years). After adolescence, when the sense of values leads to a personal identity, life is experienced as a project that reaches toward certain concrete goals. This is followed in early adulthood by the conflict between "intimacy versus isolation," when the search for love and intimacy is balanced by the fear of rejection and the need for solitude. Finally, there is the tension between "generativity versus stagnation" in later adulthood, devoting oneself to others or choosing an egoistic lifestyle.

It is precisely the next level that is dedicated to old age, and defined by an opposition between "ego integrity versus despair." The former trait is found in those who accept "one's one and only life cycle as something that had to be and that, by necessity, permitted no substitutions."[23] This reflects what sort of life is built, and is, quoting the Spanish Golden Age dramatist Calderon de la Barca, the "patrimony of the soul."[23] Despair, on the contrary, arises from the proximity of death and the fear of losing valued people and achievements. If integrity surpasses despair, one acquires wisdom, the virtue *par excellence* of old age. It implies emotional integrity and self-acceptance, and represents the positive end of all the previous crises through which the individual has built his or her personality.

This developmental approach to the life cycle as a whole clearly empathizes with themes and questions raised by theoreticians interested in viewing human psychology without losing the flavor of existence and self-actualization. Many psychiatrists and psychologists stressed, as an alternative "third force" to mere naturalistic considerations based on simple learning theories, the need to look at human life from the perspective of self-construction.[24,25] This trend was largely influenced by the contemporary existentialism of Heidegger and Sartre, as well as the philosophy of human life of José Ortega y Gasset, both rooted in the phenomenology of Husserl.

As one of the best-known representatives of this school of thought, Abraham Maslow (1908–1970), put it, life guided by values has sense and becomes ordered, and its structure is submitted to a motivational hierarchy dominated at the top by self-actualization needs. He analyzed such values and their effects on older people coming from different cultures. As their concrete content is of a sociohistorical nature, they all must be seen in definite here-and-now coordinates.[26] Aging is, then, primarily, a question of self-fulfillment in a historical context.

1.5 SOME MODERN DEVELOPMENTS

It is easy to see that in recent times, under the influence of such a vast variety of different points of view regarding human life (i.e., phenomenological, developmental, humanistic, and so forth), aging became a central topic in psychology, with inspiration coming from sources other than mere biological and naturalistic views.

Psychology began to pay greater attention to aging when stimuli from several fronts converged in the need for a global consideration of aging and its psychosocial characteristics and demands. It seems that, following World War II, life expectancy lengthened rapidly everywhere, and in some places, the need for a supplementary workforce and difficult economic conditions were conducive to older people staying on at certain types of jobs, lengthening the working period of life. The rapid growth of the over-60s population, in Western societies, and its increasing political weight in democracies, have also been decisive factors in bringing the study of the psychology of the elderly population to the fore. Nonetheless, the social demands for early retirement have, in many cases, caused an increase in the population that gives up work and has much more leisure time.

Two books that blend empirical research with philosophical reflections will be considered here: B. F. Skinner and M. Vaughan's *Enjoy Old Age*[27] and E. Mira y Lopez's *Hacia una vejez joven (Towards a Young Old Age)*.[26] Both represent a positive view of aging and highlight the need for a constructive attitude in facing life.

B. F. Skinner (1904–1993), the great theorist of behaviorism, and perhaps a frustrated man of letters, in collaboration with the gerontologist Margaret Vaughan, produced a book on aging offering advice and suggestions to elderly people who wanted help from experts. The book covers the usual topics in this sort of work. The need to keep oneself active, to have a good temper, to maintain adequate levels of stimulation, and to employ tricks and aids to enhance memory, social contacts, and life enjoyment are stressed. The interesting aspect is that, in concert with his theoretical position as a behaviorist, Skinner maintains that behavior is mainly under the control of the environment, mostly governed by its effects. Certain consequences arise from such principles: first, the problems of aged people should be treated as questions that need environmental changes and improvements, instead of mental accommodation of concepts and ideas. Taking notes, improving lighting, or changing furniture will improve the surroundings of aged people and, as a consequence, will afford them greater satisfaction and confidence. The second point is closely related to the first; it is necessary to reexamine all personal activities to discover those that will strengthen the individual, those that are felt to be satisfying, and then guiding life according to these real values instead of maintaining old prejudices and past life habits. Changing the world, and changing the repertoire of habits, will permit new adaptation to the new situation. And new satisfactions are to be obtained through these changes.[29]

Another positive perspective on aging may be found in the book *Toward a Young Old Age* by E. Mira y Lopez. Mira (1896–1964) was a well-known Spanish psychologist who, following his exile to Latin America, did most of his work in Brazil where he advocated applied psychology.[30] He created an interesting panoramic vision of aging, taking as points of reference the enormous numbers of aged people in modern societies and the generally good conditions for living an active life experienced by a large segment of these people.

According to his view, old age is not a simple phenomenon, but a complex one, with various dimensions. "A perceptual aging may be easily differentiated from an intellectual one, sentimental aging from volitional aging …, It is of no interest … to qualify someone as old or young, but to say exactly in what aspects one is old and in what other aspects one is young, or, better yet, *how* is he young or old."[28] He suggested the need for a new life project that would be suitable to an individual's psychophysical condition, and the introduction of those changes that would readapt the environment to the new parameters.[28] Instead of defending a remedial attitude in the face of the new problems, Mira adopted a rather creative and active resolution, to favor the adoption of new programs ensuring a feeling of well-being, efficacy, and adjustment. He maintained that past, present, and future should recombine in

the life of the elderly, in a balanced integration that would assume the essential part
played by the future, ideals, and projects in human life.

1.8 COMING INTO THE PRESENT

There have been many advances since the 1950s. Although forward movement had
begun before, World War II slowed development for a time, and new efforts were
commenced shortly following its end. In the United States, the American Psychological Association Division of Maturity and Aging was created in 1945, the National
Institute of Mental Health incorporated a section on aging in 1953, and congresses
and publications on the specialty began to appear. The most widely cited journal,
Journal of Gerontology, was founded in 1946, and studies and publications dealing
with this topic multiplied between 1955 and 1965.[31,32] Taking into account many
bibliographic indicators, it has been noted that "a coherence of the field developed
about 1960."[33] Some aspects became permanent and well-defined dimensions for
research in the field: cognitive abilities, learning and memory, motivation, sexuality,
personality, psychobiological processes, prevention, and intervention.

Some insights can be gained from the analysis of the titles of some specialized
handbooks.[34,35] For example, it may be noted that, when the first one-volume handbook on the behavioral aspects of aging was edited by James E. Birren (*Handbook
of Aging and the Individual*) in 1959,[36] the aging process was related directly to the
question of individuality. A step farther was taken in 1977, when the editorial
program of a comprehensive handbook included three different volumes, one on the
Biology of Aging,[37] a second on the *Psychology of Aging*,[38] and a third on *Aging and
the Social Sciences*.[39] This throws some light on the growing complexity of research
in the field, and on the three main divisions into which the field is becoming
organized — biology, psychology, and social sciences. (A more recent view of the
field may be found in Birren;[40] here the state, the process, and the subject who
endures these changes have been clearly differentiated.)

It has been said that the psychology of aging is still in its infancy and has only
recently begun to emerge as a field with clearly specified research programs.[41] Within
the so-called cognitive revolution, cognitive aspects as well as emotions have
regained the first place in psychological study. Both are essential dimensions in the
complex process of aging. From both inside the field and out, interest in the psychology of aging is rising constantly. Many suggestions are still latent in a long
tradition of experiences, reflections, and analysis, which have been only briefly
delineated in these pages. The time approaches in which aging will display all its
theoretical potentialities, to reveal new dimensions of the complexity of human life.

The continuous growth of life expectancy in Western societies will demand a
new global evaluation of the meaning it may have in the social dynamics of the so-
called third age. Hall was right in considering that there is a broad life program for
people arriving at this age, but he interpreted it, in a peculiar way, as the devotion
to wisdom. Now, the historical present is giving way to a large number of fully
active and healthy older adults, who need to find new concrete goals and tasks aside
from the professional areas covered by adults. A new "third age culture" is needed.

Only with the cooperation of all the human sciences can this problem be confronted and resolved.

REFERENCES

1. James, W., *Principles of Psychology*, Dover, New York, 1890 (reprint, 1950).
2. Marías, J., *The Structure of Society*, The University of Alabama Press, Tuscaloosa, 1987.
3. Summer, W. G., *Folkways*, Dover, New York, 1959.
4. Minois, G., Historia de la vejez, *De la Antigüedad al Renacimiento*, Nerea, Madrid, 1989.
5. Cicero, *Caton L'ancien-De la Vieillisse; Lelius-De l'Amitiè; Desd Devoirs*, Garnier, Paris, undated.
6. Seneca, *Obras Completas*, Aguilar, Madrid, 1957.
7. Isidoro de Sevilla, S., *Etimologías*, Biblioteca de Autores Cristianos, Madrid, 1951.
8. Beauvoir, S. de, *La Vejez*, Edhasa, Barcelona, 1983.
9. Granjel, L. S., Historia de la vejez, in *Gerontología, Gerocultura, Geriatría*, Universidad de Salamanca, Salamanca, 1991.
10. Bacon, F., Historia Vitae et Mortis, in *The Works of Francis Bacon*, Spedding, J., Ellis, R. L., and Heath, D. D., Eds., Longman, London, 1861, 207.
11. Bacon, F., *Opera Omnia*, J. B. Schonwetter, Frankfurt, 1665.
12. Piquer, A., *Philosophia Moral para la Juventud Española*, Ibarra, Madrid, 1755.
13. Buffon, C., De l'homme," in *Oeuvres* I, F. Didot, Paris, 1843.
14. Cabanis, P. G., *Rapports du physique et du moral de l'homme*, Imp. Crapelet, Paris, 1805.
15. Sarton, G., *Ensayos de Historia de la Ciencia*, Uthea, Mexico, 1968.
16. Quételet, A., *Sur l'homme et le développment de ses facultés, ou Essai de physique sociale*, Bachelier, Paris, 1835.
17. Quételet, A., *Du système social et des lois que le régissent*, Guillaumin, Paris, 1848.
18. Galton, F., *Inquiries into Human Faculty and Its Development*, Macmillan, London, 1883.
19. Hall, G. S., *Senescence. The Last Half of Life*, Appleton, New York, 1922.
20. Jung, C. G., *La Psique y sus Problemas Actuales*, Poblet, Madrid, 1932.
21. Adler, A., *The Individual Psychology of Alfred Adler*, Harper, New York, 1964.
22. Bühler, C., *El Curso de la Vida como Problema Psicológico*, Espasa, Madrid, 1943.
23. Erikson, E., *Childhood and Society*, Norton, New York, 1978.
24. Spiegelberg, H., *Phenomenology in Psychology and Psychiatry, a Historical Introduction*, Northwestern University Press, Evanston, IL, 1972.
25. Carpintero, H., *Esbozo de una Psicologia Según la Razon Vital*, Real Academia de Ciencias Morales y Politicas, Madrid, 2000.
26. Maslow, A., Self-actualization and beyond, in *Challenges of Humanistic Psychology*, Bugental, J. T., Ed., McGraw-Hill, New York, 1967, 279.
27. Skinner, B. F. and Vaughan, M. E., *Disfrutar la Vejez*, Martinez Roca, Barcelona, 1986 (orig. *Enjoy Old Age*, Norton, New York, 1983).
28. Mira y Lopez, E., *Hacia una Vejez Joven*, Kapelusz, Buenos Aires, 1961.
29. Skinner, B. F., Intellectual self-management in old age, *Am. Psychol.*, 38, 239, 1983.
30. Carpintero, H., *Historia de las Ideas Psicológicas*, Pirámide, Madrid, 1996.
31. Brumer, S., Some documentation for the history of psychological gerontology, in *Handbook of the Psychology of Aging*, Birren, J. E. and Schaie, K. W., Eds., Van Nostrand Reinhold, New York, 1977.

32. Dosil, A., La psicogerontología como disciplina científica: visión diacrónica y situación actual, in *Tratado de Psicogerontologia*, Saez, N., Rubio, R., and Dosil, A., Eds., Promolibro, Valencia, 1996.

33. Birren, J. E., Cunningham, W.R., and Yamamoto, K., Psychology of adult development and aging, *Annu. Rev. Psychol.*, 34, 543, 1983.

34. Birren, J. E., *Handbook of Aging and the Individual: Psychological and Biological Aspects*, Chicago University Press, Chicago, 1959.

35. Riegel, K., History of psychological gerontology, in *Handbook of the Psychology of Aging*, Birren, J. E. and Schaie, K. W., Eds., Van Nostrand Reinhold, New York, 1977.

36. Baltes, P. B., Reese, H. W., and Lipsitt, L. P., Life-span developmental psychology, *Annu. Rev. Psychol.*, 31, 65, 1980.

37. Birren, J. E., *Encyclopedia of Gerontology. Age, Aging and the Aged*, Academic Press, San Diego, CA, 1996.

38. Finch, C. E. and Hayflick, L., *Handbook of the Biology of Aging*, Van Nostrand Reinhold, New York, 1977.

39. Birren, J. E. and Schaie, K. W., *Handbook of the Psychology of Aging*, Van Nostrand Reinhold, New York, 1977.

40. Binstock, R. H. and Shanas, E., *Handbook of Aging and the Social Sciences*, Van Nostrand Reinhold, New York, 1976.

41. Fernandez-Ballesteros, R., *Psicologia del Envejecimiento: Crecimiento y Declive*, Universidad Autónoma de Madrid, Madrid, 1996.

2 Gerontology as a Specialty of Medicine

Robert N. Butler

CONTENTS

2.1 Introduction 23
2.2 History of Geriatrics 24
2.3 The Field of Geriatrics..26
2.4 Health Promotion and Disease Prevention 28
2.5 Caring for the Older Patient 29
2.6 Expanding the Field..30
2.7 Antiaging Interventions..31
2.8 Conclusion...32
References..33

2.1 INTRODUCTION

We have seen a massive increase in the absolute number and relative proportion of older persons. Although many enjoy healthy lives, we are also witnessing the rise of a significant minority of frail aging persons. Clearly, the disorders of longevity present new challenges to both the field of medicine and to society as a whole.

As disabled and chronically sick persons grow older, they are joined by a large number of older persons who have become sick and disabled for the first time. Around the world, the costly and socially devastating escalation in the number of bedridden and frail aged — especially those over 85 — raises the question, "Can we afford "longevity?" Already, the rising costs of technology used to treat diseases and prolong life have been major forces driving the transformation of health care. Enormous changes are occurring in traditional physician- and hospital-based medicine, with the concomitant development of a continuum of long-term services, from home-care, day care centers, and assisted living facilities, to end-of-life and hospice care.

If costs are not contained, research is not successful, and more efficient systems of care not put in place, caring for the aging population will become increasingly expensive in the 21st century. Can we afford longevity? If we are to answer in the

0-8493-2066-/01/$0.00+$1.50
© 2001 by CRC Press LLC

affirmative, we must support the development of the still nascent field of geriatrics and its integration into all fields of medicine.

2.2 HISTORY OF GERIATRICS

Geriatrics is the medicine of the 21st century. It is a capacious field, interdisciplinary and action oriented, requiring the application of gerontology, the study of biological, social, and behavioral aspects of aging. Geriatrics is influenced by specialties such as psychiatry and rehabilitation medicine and is strongly dependent upon an interdisciplinary team. Indeed, in its historical development, geriatrics is especially indebted to the fields of social work, nursing, clinical pharmacy, and psychiatry. Psychiatrists have played a seminal role in the development of geriatrics in the United States and, of course, have helped create geriatric psychiatry as well. Today, geriatric psychiatry is the second largest branch of geriatrics, following geriatric medicine.

The modern history of geriatrics began over 100 years ago, when Jean Charcot, a French neurologist living in the 19th century, predicted the coming establishment of geriatrics. He said:

> The importance of a special study of the diseases of old age would not be contested at the present time.... If the pathology of childhood requires clinical consideration of a special kind which is indispensable to be practically acquainted with, senile pathology too has its difficulties which can only be surmounted by long experience and a profound knowledge of its peculiar character.

The term *geriatrics* was introduced in 1909 by an American physician, Ignatz Leo Nascher, who worked at Mount Sinai Hospital in New York. In 1935, Marjorie Warren, a British physician who treated patients in a workhouse infirmary, helped create modern geriatrics. Warren is considered the mother of British geriatrics. However, despite the creation of the American Geriatrics Society and the Gerontological Society of America in the 1940s, geriatrics did not begin to become established in the United States until the 1970s.

On the other hand, the new or modern gerontology began in the 1950s, when, for the first time, longitudinal studies began replacing cross-sectional data. Better sampling was achieved by studying healthy older persons who lived in the community rather than in nursing homes. Primarily, these studies were conducted in the United States at Duke University under the direction of Ewald Busse and, simultaneously, at the National Institute of Mental Health (NIMH) under the direction of an interdisciplinary team. Principal investigators were James E. Birren, Samuel W. Greenhouse, Louis Sokoloff, Marian Radke-Yarrow (who brought her special knowledge of childhood development), and this author. Later, the National Heart Institute organized the Baltimore Longitudinal Study on Aging (BLSA) under the direction of Nathan Shock.

Some critics claimed that these study samples of healthier older persons were an unrepresentative cohort of "super aged." However, the studies enabled researchers to differentiate between the fundamental aging process and the concomitants of aging. The healthy cohorts in these studies were predecessors to the "successful aging" populations later studied by John W. Rowe and others.

Exciting scientific discoveries about the nature of aging came to light as a result. For example, between 1955 and 1966, the NIMH studies concluded that senility (the popular term for dementia) in old age was not inevitable and that cerebral physiological status (as measured by total cerebral blood flow, oxygen and glucose consumption) declined with disease, not age, as had been previously believed. This work was confirmed in the late 1970s by Stanley Rapoport who used positron emission tomography (PET) to provide a precise and quantitative measure of cerebral functions. There are other examples:

> The NIMH study found that much that was attributed to aging was not inevitable, but due instead to disease, social factors, and even personality.
> The Duke University and NIMH studies demonstrated continuing sexuality in old age.
> The Baltimore Longitudinal Study on Aging found that cardiac output, even under stress, does not automatically decline as a consequence of age.

In Gothenburg, Sweden, Alvar Svanborg discovered that fast-reacting muscle fibers can be retrained in individuals in their 80s. More recently, María Fiatarone of Harvard University reported similar findings, and advanced resistance training has become a major treatment modality as well as a preventive measure.

The first residency program in geriatrics in the United States was established in 1968, under the direction of Leslie S. Libow. Until the 1980s, neither geriatrics nor gerontology were treated as serious topics, either in the preclinical or clinical level of medical training. A study by the American Association of Medical Colleges noted that, of 126 medical schools, only 45 offered electives in geriatrics. Even worse was the finding, upon careful questioning, that a little over 2% of medical students actually enrolled in the electives.

In 1975, the National Institute on Aging (NIA) came into being. The NIA contracted with the Institute of Medicine of the National Academy of Sciences to make recommendations about bringing the field of geriatrics into the mainstream of medical education. The committee, under the leadership of Paul Beeson, a distinguished internist, developed the influential report, "Aging and Medical Education."

In 1982, the nation's first medical school department of geriatrics was established at the Mount Sinai School of Medicine. It fulfilled its stated mission by creating the conventional triad of an academic medical school department: (1) undergraduate, postgraduate, and continuing medical education; (2) multisite clinical services; and (3) basic and clinical research. In addition, it developed studies in health and aging policies.

In the 1970s and 1980s Anthony Cerami at Rockefeller University demonstrated that glucose played a role in aging. His work suggested that the nonenzymatic glycosylation of DNA may contribute to some of the abnormalities observed with diabetes and with aging, including increased chromosomal breakage, decreased DNA repair and synthesis, and increases in DNA–protein cross-links.

Building on the pioneering work of Hans Selye with the role of the adrenocortical secretion of glucocorticoid in adaptation to stress, Robert M. Sapolsky studied the relationship of the adrenal cortical system with aging. Because the adrenocortical system helps mediate an individual's response to stress, there is a sensitive relationship to the outer world, which also must reflect some of the interrelationships between intrinsic and extrinsic phenomena. Sapolsky's studies attempted to discover if adrenocortical secretion accounts for individual differences in "successful" or "unsuccessful" aging.

Another important body of work, led by Carl W. Cotman of the University of California at Irvine, is related to synaptic plasticity and neurotrophic factors. Cotman's work demonstrates that aged brains in rodents have the capacity to maintain and repair their circuitry. The underlying mechanisms for such compensatory activities are becoming amenable to molecular analysis. Even in the presence of Alzheimer's disease, it has been found that the brain is capable of growing new fibers and forming new connections. Cotman's work indicates that age-related neurodegenerative diseases do not destroy the brain's plasticity. In 1998, Fred H. Gage discovered that brain cells continued to regenerate in persons 70 years old. Thus, the new gerontology not only concerns discovery of what biological functions may be maintained, but how to improve or restore function.

Another example of the new gerontology is exemplified by the widely influential work of Leonard Hayflick, whose name is associated with the so-called biological clock — that is, the limitation in the number of doublings of cells in glass (the Hayflick limit), noted in 1961.

The elucidation of underlying mechanisms has led to major revisions in the interpretation of aging, with the hopeful prospects and realities of both preventive and therapeutic interventions.

2.3 THE FIELD OF GERIATRICS

Geriatrics is the overarching specialty that involves all medical fields. It is concerned with identifying, preventing, diagnosing, and treating both the medical and psychosocial conditions of late life.

Geriatric medicine is neither chronic disease medicine nor long-term care medicine, although attention to both chronic disease and long-term care is required. The focus is placed on the prevention, diagnosis, care, and treatment of both the medical and psychosocial conditions of late life. The geriatrician is both interventionist and care coordinator.

Geriatric medicine is oriented toward the two great building blocks of medical practice, the history and physical examination. If the patient's history is complete, a physician can make a correct diagnosis 85% of the time; 10% of the time a physical examination will confirm or uncover the answer; and diagnostic tests are useful tools in 5%. The "geriatric assessment" also comprises a comprehensive study of social, environmental, and personal factors.

The medicine of youth is relatively simple; it usually involves one disease. The medicine of old age provides many more complex diagnostic and treatment challenges. It is intellectually exciting. Medical schools teach "Occam's Razor"

(William of Occam, 1280–1349), which asks doctors to find a single diagnosis to account for symptoms. "What can be done with fewer [assumptions] is done in vain with more." But this rule is not applicable to old age because there is usually more than one diagnosis.

The field of geriatrics espouses an interventionist approach in which patient care is interdisciplinary. Overall assessment and treatment programs are linked with individualized care plans and long-term disease management. Rather than focusing on a specific organ or system, geriatricians are concerned with the overall functional status of their patients. A geriatrician takes into account the patient's special characteristics and the conditions that intensify with age-related changes. They understand that aging per se is a risk factor; patient assessment must incorporate identification of risks, establishment of plans to control them, and efforts to predict the future. For example, work and family history are explored in greater detail than they are in younger patients.

At the same time, geriatricians must be alert to emergencies in this population. A change in mental status may reflect significant underlying and potentially fatal conditions such as heart attack or acute dehydration following diarrhea. Syncope, heat stroke, acute infections such as pneumonia, and gastrointestinal bleeding require immediate attention.

Clinically, emphasis is placed on modifying problems as well as finding solutions. However, of equal importance is the geriatrician's need to avoid harm and preserve the quality of life of the patient. The geriatrician needs to know when not to treat, when to wait, which is more relevant in geriatrics than it is with care of younger patients. Invasive diagnostic and therapeutic procedures cannot be undertaken casually. Older patients are particularly susceptible to nosocomial infections, and physicians must carefully evaluate the necessity for routine hospital procedures. For example, catheterization can increase the risk of urinary tract infections. Surgery with anesthesia may result in fixed confusional symptoms. Frequently, one sees older patients who have been "successfully" treated in hospitals lose their functional capacity because health-care workers have ignored their physical fitness, nutrition, emotional state, and social circumstances. Frightened and depressed older patients can lose morale; with loss of appetite, they lose weight; without physical exercise, they lose bone and muscle. Their home environment frequently lacks the resources they need to recover properly. Geriatricians must employ a multidisciplinary approach to address the many challenges facing older people when they become ill.

It is important for physicians who care for older patients to understand both the possibilities and the limits of reserve or homeostasis. The fragility or progressively lowered reserve of the aging person is strikingly revealed in the body's sensitivity to changes in ambient temperature, resulting in more fatalities of older persons during summer heat waves and from deadly hypothermia in the winter cold. The body's thermoregulatory control and its adaptiveness to temperature changes are reduced with aging. Tranquilizers and alcohol increase the risk.

After age 75, and especially after 85, the characteristic geriatric patient emerges with multiple, complex, interacting, often simultaneous acute and chronic physical and psychosocial conditions. It is common for many doctors to be involved in the care of one patient, and for each to prescribe a variety of medications. Necessary polypharmacy may lead to adverse drug reactions when communication breaks down between a patient and doctors, and between the doctors themselves. Geriatricians must also be alert to drug dosage in older persons, who metabolize drugs differently than younger persons. For example, diazepam remains in the body of an 80-year-old from 5 to 8 days, compared with 24 h in a 22-year-old.

Communication and empathy can be lost in modern high-tech medicine and bottom-line-based managed care. Geriatricians discuss topics that are often neglected by other doctors. Oftentimes, because of their own embarrassment or discomfort, physicians cannot be candid when their patients ask questions about sex, or about dying and death. A doctor's inability to respond openly to aging patients on these issues may do damage to the doctor–patient relationship. The assessment of function in the older patient not only delineates the past and immediate situation but projects into the future and deals with the ultimate passage: dying and death.

Older persons need to be listened to and touched. The laying on of hands is one of the secrets of geriatrics. The physician must shake hands (gently when shaking arthritic hands), touch shoulders, feel the pulse, and manually examine any part that hurts. The physician must listen and learn from older patients, and allow them to relate their life stories. Generally, an older patient will articulate the problem and lead a doctor who listens carefully to the diagnosis. A geriatrician must be sensitive to grief, depression, and anxiety in late life, and observant of panic attacks. Sometimes, these are characterized by apprehension when night falls, bringing an impending sense of death. Such episodes may occur by themselves or be associated with attacks of asthma, congestive heart failure, and other lung and heart conditions. Special attention must be directed to the possibility of suicide, especially in men in their 80s, who are the number one suicide group.

2.4 HEALTH PROMOTION AND DISEASE PREVENTION

In the *Guide for the Perplexed*, begun in 1176 at age 41 and completed in 1190 when he was 55, Moses Maimonides (1135–1204), Spanish Jewish physician and philosopher, wrote, "Among a thousand persons only one dies a natural death; the rest succumb early in life owing to ignorant or irregular behavior."

Geriatricians can have a great impact on helping the older patient to live a longer and healthier life. A prescription for longevity that includes a healthful diet, a sound lifestyle, and an exercise program tailored to the individual can help promote health and prevent unnecessary disabilities.

Sarcopenia (the deterioration of 30 to 40% of muscle power) accompanying old age is not inevitable. It is largely the consequence of inactivity. Exercise can lead to well-preserved lean body mass and increased vital capacity of the lung. For ambulatory older persons, walking is an excellent exercise. It is inexpensive and accessible. For the nonambulatory patient, Maria Fiatarone has proved that it is possible for older people to regain muscle function. In an 8-week study, she engaged frail 86- to 94-year-old men and women in weight-lifting exercises for 45 min three times a week. Fiatarone found that it was possible for older people to "pump-iron" and regain function. Muscle strengthening can help the frail older individual overcome instability that can result in falls and possible bone fracture.

With regard to preservation of brain function, scientists have found that normal age-related intellectual decline occurs later in the healthy brain than had been previously thought, with provable recircuitry of neural pathways and the continued capacity to learn. Biologist Marian Diamond found an increased number of dendrites in laboratory rats who aged in enriched environments compared with controls. Neurobiologist Carl Cotman observed, "Alzheimer's disease is not a disease of sudden failure, but one where regeneration and degeneration coexist in a kind of struggle for cellular survival. Regenerative growth appears to help preserve function in the wake of neuronal degeneration and is an example of functional adaptive plasticity."

Geriatricians play an important role in helping older patients maintain mental acuity by exercising caution when prescribing medications that can affect balance and memory; being sensitive to signs of alcohol abuse, especially in older women; encouraging older patients to continue to work for pay or on a voluntary basis; and controlling high blood pressure, to reduce the possibilities of stroke and multi-infarct dementia.

2.5 CARING FOR THE OLDER PATIENT

Older patients require greater individuation of diagnosis and care than do younger patients, as there is greater standard deviation from the mean of physiological and psychological measures. Specific host factors as well as the general physiological aspects of aging influence the development of the disorders of longevity and alter the clinical presentation of diseases.

Conditions unique to old age include normal pressure hydrocephalus (a dementia that can be confused with Alzheimer's disease), polymyalgia rheumatica, and the gammopathies, including multiple myeloma. Some presentations that are "unusual" in young patients become "usual" in older patients, such as apathetic hyperthyroidism, where a patient who presents as hyperactive at a young age is apathetic in old age. Jean Martin Charcot, who wrote a pioneering text on the diseases of old age, noted, "In the aged the greatest disorders manifest themselves by slightly marked symptoms and they may even pass unnoticed."

Although age and disease are separate, chronological age is still a powerful determinant of the incidence of diseases that are believed to be the diseases of aging and/or longevity. The relationship of aging to disease constitutes a "gray area." With age there is a steady increase in systolic blood pressure, a growing intolerance to glucose, and declining bone density. At a threshold these apparent aging phenomena become diseases or conditions, e.g., high blood pressure, type II or postmaturity diabetes, and osteoporosis, respectively.

Sir Ferguson Anderson, pioneering geriatrician of Scotland, originally described the characteristic tendency of older persons to underreport medical conditions. Physicians, too, commonly write off potentially treatable conditions, such as memory loss, congestive heart failure, and erectile dysfunction, and dismiss the symptoms as inevitable consequences of aging.

Certainly, the practice of everyday medicine and surgery has made clear since the 1950s that, in general, older persons can tolerate most operative procedures. Following an attempt on the life of then-President Ronald Reagan, journalists expressed amazement that an older man could tolerate a thoracotomy. In fact, Reagan's response was characteristic of the capability of older persons to survive surgical procedures.

It is controversial whether aging is always fatal. The German pathologist Ludwig Aschoff always found diseases to explain an older person's death and concluded that no one lives long enough to die of old age.

The concepts of complexity, multiplicity, and homeostatic dysregulation cannot be overemphasized when treating an older patient. Profound and rapid changes may occur. A sudden change in mental status may augur a change in physical status. Older persons may go in and out of frailty and confusion. "Failure to thrive" is a common geriatric syndrome. Howard Fillit has described the phenomenon of a "frailty identity crisis," when frailty becomes fixed. It represents a critical turning point in the life of the patient and in the attitude of the physician. The final outcome may involve multiple organ or system failure, which may come about precipitously in a cascade of debilitating events or in downward stair-step fashion. Ultimately, everything shuts down. Death results from an aggregate of problems that can be precisely determined only after an autopsy has been performed.

Unfortunately, autopsies are performed in a small fraction of cases, and it has become standard practice to assign death to one convenient diagnosis or mechanism of death on the death certificate. In the United States, Medicare does not pay for autopsies to be performed. Perhaps allowing a random sampling of 20% of all cadavers to be autopsied would enable the medical community, and future patients, to continue to benefit from this final peer review.

2.6 EXPANDING THE FIELD

Why is it so difficult to attract physicians to geriatrics? In the United States the fields suffers from the absence of role models, low financial compensation compared with other high-tech fields of medicine, the decline of primary care medicine, and the lack of funded departments, department-equivalents, and other programs. Moreover, the development of geriatrics has been deterred by the opposition of practitioners of traditional internal medicine and even of family medicine.

Another critical issue is the cost of medical education. In 1994, the average U.S. medical school graduate had incurred a debt of between $53,000 and $77,000, according to the Association of American Medical Colleges. Such debt makes high-fee procedure-based and surgical specialties especially attractive. However, underlying all the rational reasons given is an uneasiness about aging and the psychological issues of denial.

Some internists object to the field of geriatrics on the grounds that they "see older patients and do a good job. What's all the fuss?" This conventional argument is answerable by the following quasi-syllogism: Internists and other physicians see patients, all of whom have hearts. This does not make them cardiologists.

There are now 80 accredited specialties and subspecialties in medicine. Internists express the fear that medicine will become even more fragmented, "dividing up the body for profit." However, specialization has brought great benefits, as can be seen in the contributions of cardiology, critical care medicine, hand surgery, and proctology, to mention only a few. In fact, since geriatrics is oriented to treating the whole person, it actually supports the integration of medicine.

We do not need to develop another expensive practice specialty; rather, we need to integrate geriatrics within all primary and specialty medicine. Geriatrics should primarily be a consultative, management, and academic specialty, with geriatricians assuming academic responsibilities of leadership, teaching, research, and service innovation in all medical schools.

The government is the only source of sufficient funding to provide the necessary support for geriatrics with funds for curricular development, creation of a cadre of academic geriatricians, including physician-scientists and nurses, and the building of the necessary infrastructure for teaching, such as clinics, teaching nursing homes, inpatient units, home care and hospice programs. However, it must also be noted that foundations and individual philanthropy have played a significant role in helping to build the field.

2.7 ANTIAGING INTERVENTIONS

Humankind has gained over 30 years of life since the turn of the century in the developed world. Today, scientists are trying to discover genetic and chemical interventions that will enable us to live even longer.

At least 700 genes are involved in the aging process, and it is extremely unlikely that a single intervention will increase the life span of the species. Furthermore, scientists believe that some of the changes that come about with aging may be protective and that intervention may be injurious. Nonetheless, it is possible that specific interventions may one day slow down or even reverse specific changes that come about as a result of the aging process. For example, recent studies strongly suggest that poor immune function may play an important role in disease and death in older persons. Interventions aimed at improving the body's ability to withstand diseases could have a significant effect on longevity. However, despite extensive media attention, substances such as dehydroepiandrosterone (DHEA) and N-acetyl-5-methoxytryptamine (melatonin) have thus far failed to demonstrate efficacy in retarding the aging process.

A variety of "antiaging medicines" have gained popularity and are receiving widespread attention in the media. It should be understood that such theories are distinct from geriatric medicine. "Age reversal" is not an established specialty and has yet to prove itself.

More promising are studies that link free radical damage to several age-related diseases, such as Alzheimer's disease, Parkinson's disease, osteoarthritis, cataracts, arteriosclerosis, and many cancers. There is evidence to suggest that vitamin C and

E supplements to a well-balanced diet may boost the body's ability to reduce free radical damage.

Finally, studies are under way to determine how dietary restrictions can extend life. Since the 1930s, restricted diets in rodents have been found to delay most late-life diseases, including neoplastic and degenerative diseases as well as several age-dependent changes in biochemical, anatomical, and physiological processes.

2.8 CONCLUSION

The rapidity with which geriatrics integrates within American medicine will be a measure of the commitment of resources by our nation's political leadership, the power of patient advocacy, and the willingness of private philanthropy to support its development by endowing professorships and programs. It will also be a measure of the receptivity of traditional, academic medicine, especially internal medicine, whose academic practitioners have often fought the development of geriatrics. Finally, it will reflect the level of recruitment of medical students into general internal medicine and family practice. There is still little financial support, few role models, and the persistent uneasiness of doctors-to-be, graduate doctors, and the public to confront the frightening aspects of aging.

In the United States, health reforms emphasize the production of primary care physicians to build toward a ratio of 50% primary care doctors to 50% specialists found in most industrialized countries. Residency quotas are being applied. This will take a long time. If every resident were to become a primary care physician, it would be 2004 before the goal of 50–50 is achieved, assuming the clock started running in 1993.

Geriatrics may be helped by reforms in the financing of postgraduate medical education. However, contemporary policy emphasis upon increasing the numbers of primary care doctors should not deemphasize specialized medicine per se, which at its best has done so much to make American medicine the envy of much of the world.

Part of the social transformation of health assessment, care, and treatment will also follow from increasing attention to public education, health promotion and disease prevention, occupational safety and health, and new forms of education for health providers, including physicians, nurses, medical technologists, and social workers. A necessary intersection of geriatrics with occupational and environmental medicine will evolve. Work history and environmental exposure determine a significant portion of the status of older persons, and yet our history-taking and physical examinations have not focused sufficiently on these critical parameters. Moreover, the family (genetic) history has not been adequately pursued. This will become increasingly important because of the human genome project.

Because of changing demography and cost-containment strategies, patients with various diseases are not in hospitals as long as they used to be. Although this may be advantageous for the exchequer and even for patients, since hospitals can be dangerous places, short hospitalizations preclude adequate opportunity by medical students to observe and follow the natural course of diseases or to know patients and their families. This serious challenge to the education of physicians and nurses can be compensated for by teaching at multiple sites, the inpatient and outpatient units of hospitals, community health centers, and long-term care settings, encompassing home care, assisted living and nursing home care, as well as hospices. Nursing homes and homes for the aging provide opportunities to follow the course of various infectious disorders, for example, pneumonia. Moreover, there is a lot to learn about many obscure and unrecognized conditions in old age that are frequently seen in nursing homes. The concept of the teaching nursing home is growing.

It could be concluded that geriatrics is simply fine medical care — the way all care for all persons with all conditions should be ideally treated — with full attention to the patient as a whole, working in tandem with other health providers and the family. But geriatrics also requires a specific body of knowledge, finely honed skills, and a positive attitude toward old age. Perhaps soon, geriatrics will also have much more to offer in the way of specific treatments derived from research on aging and longevity: antioxidants, growth factors, applications of caloric restriction, hormones, immune adjuvants, as well as major transformations of diet and exercise and the creation of more effective systems of assessment and optimal functional care.

Where does geriatrics fit in this era of industrializing medicine? It has been said that geriatricians are not cost-effective because they (1) uncover problems that do not need to be addressed, (2) take more time compared with other doctors, and (3) "promote a sickness bias in patient referral patterns." However, as Christine Casual maintains, geriatric patients remain the most difficult patients to manage in a coordinated and cost-effective program. The growth of the frail aged population will represent the greater challenge to both managed care models and fee-for-service medicine.

REFERENCES

Butler, R. N., The future of geriatrics: a call to action, in *Healthy Aging: Challenges and Solutions*, Dychtwald, K., Ed., Aspen Publishers, Gaithersburg, MD, 1999, 113–119.

Butler, R. N., The teaching nursing home, *JAMA*, 245, 1435–1437, 1981.

Fillit, H. M. and Picariello, G., *Practical Geriatric Assessment*, Greenwich Medical Media Ltd., London, 1998.

Moses, S. A., Long-term care choice: a simple, cost-free solution to the financing puzzle, in *Healthy Aging: Challenges and Solutions*, Dychtwald, K., Ed., Aspen Publishers, Gaithersburg, MD, 1999, 285–303.

Schneider, E. L. and Miller, A. R., Anti-aging interventions, in *Textbook of Geriatric Medicine and Gerontology*, 5th ed., Brocklehurst, J. C., Tallis, R., and Fillit, H. M., Eds, Churchill Livingstone, London, 1998, 1445–1459.

3 Neurobehavioral Epidemiology of Aging

José León-Carrión, Eliana A. Quintero-Gallego, and Margaret J. Giannini

CONTENTS

3.1 Introduction 36
3.2 The Demography of Aging in the World 37
3.3 General Demographic Data 38
3.4 The Epidemiology of Aging in the World..40
3.5 Aging and Neuropharmacology...41
3.6 Neurological Epidemiology of Aging 42
    3.6.1 Dementia 42
        3.6.1.1 Incidence 43
        3.6.1.2 Prevalence 44
        3.6.1.3 Risk Factors 45
3.7 Behavior and Affective Epidemiology in Aging 46
    3.7.1 Depression...46
3.8 Comorbidity: Two Sides of the Same Coin 48
    3.8.1 Manic Syndromes and Dementia..48
    3.8.2 Depression and Dementia 48
3.9 Concluding Remarks...49
3.10 Summary 51
References...53
Appendix A: Internet Addresses..55
Appendix B: Epidemiological Studies in Dementia, 1995 to 2000.......................56

0-8493-2066-/01/$0.00+$1.50

La vejez (tal es el nombre que los otros le dan)
puede ser el tiempo de nuestra dicha.
El animal ha muerto o casi ha muerto.
Quedan el hombre y su alma.
Vivo entre formas luminosas y vagas
que no son aún la tiniebla.

— Jorge Luis Borges

Old age (such is the name that others have given it)
Can be the time of our happiness.
The animal has died, or has almost died.
Left behind is the man and his souls.
Alive amongst luminous and vague forms
That are not yet darkness.

3.1 INTRODUCTION

Elderly people and the problems that they face have become a focus of great interest for scientists and international health organizations alike. This new focus is reflected in the priority that issues that affect older persons have been given in social policy making. The volume of research on aging is growing every day as can be seen in specialized databases. A search on MedLine will reveal a plethora of citations related to aging, genetics, and epidemiology. There is an abundance of recent studies by epidemiological units as well as research by university groups, all of which offer clinical, social, economic, and health solutions for the challenges society faces because of our "aging population."

The National Institute on Aging (NIA), for example, has sponsored outstanding research that addresses the special needs of older Americans and promotes improvements in scientific understanding of the aging process.[1] Among its principal research objectives are (1) understanding what constitutes a healthy aging process; (2) maintaining and enhancing brain function, cognition, and other behaviors in elderly people; and (3) reducing health disparities among older persons and populations.

In October 1992, the General Assembly of the United Nations in resolution 47/5 decided to proclaim the year 1999 as "The International Year of the Elderly."[1,2] It was decided that research would be focused on the aging process and on the genetic map from which researchers would try to discover information that explains the deterioration of the immune system, the characteristics of the genetic programming of the biological clock, and the probability of developing chronic illnesses and disabilities such as heart disease, cancer, or senility. The World Health Organization (WHO) would conduct research and develop global strategies to help countries formulate national policies to tackle the public health impact that large numbers of people reaching senior years entails.

Both the organizations and the scientific community, including biochemists, geneticists, neuroscientists, and behavioral scientists, are working conjointly to understand the human life span, the aging process, and the pathologies that affect elderly people. The goal of this work is to offer better pharmacological, cognitive, surgical, and psychological treatment to increase quality of life and, in some cases, to prolong life. Yet, there are still many unanswered questions that challenge biology, behavioral sciences, and medicine.

This chapter discusses some of the epidemiological studies conducted in elderly populations. These studies are divided into two categories. The first represents the focus that researchers took in the past decade given that, until recently, researchers were primarily concerned with the brain. The second category reflects the principal interests that concern researchers of this decade, the main focus of which is behavior. In concordance with this, the affective disorders and the neurological diseases that affect older people will be presented. Mainly, epidemiological data related to dementia and depression will be described as examples of the most common problems in elderly people.

The hope for this chapter is that the reader find it easy to read, useful and, pleasant. It is hoped that the epidemiology described here will serve as a valuable basis for identifying risks and discovering protective factors for preventing disease in the population that will eventually inherit the Earth — the elderly.

3.2 THE DEMOGRAPHY OF AGING IN THE WORLD

In the past, little attention was given to elderly people. With the average person living to be only 25 years old,[3] there were simply not enough old people for old age to be considered an issue. However, a gradual increase in life expectancy has been witnessed throughout the history of Western civilization. In ancient Greece and Rome the average life expectancy was between 18 and 25 years. In 17th-century Europe, people normally lived to the age of 28 to 30. In the 18th century, the life span increased and the average person could expect to live around 30 to 45 years.[4]

Because of improvements in medical diagnosis, pharmacology, microsurgery, organ transplants, genetics, nutrition, and other sciences, life expectancy has been prolonged to levels that were unthinkable in previous centuries. For example, by the year 2020 it is projected that women will live, on average, until age 88 and men will live to be approximately 83 years old.[3–5]

There is some difference in life expectancy statistics when comparing developing countries and developed countries. This discrepancy is possibly caused by factors related to life conditions involving such aspects as access to medical care or health policy. Despite these differences, there is still a tendency in these countries toward an increase in the number of people who will reach advanced ages. In 1960 the life expectancy for both sexes in underdeveloped countries was 45.6 years, whereas in developed countries it was 69.8 years. By the year 2025, it will be 68.9 in underdeveloped countries and 77.2 in developed countries.[6] The consequences of this increment in life expectancy is that there is a greater number of people with the potential to reach advanced ages. This increase in longevity also serves to postpone the arrival of old age, which will consequently generate a redefinition of the limits of the different stages of life. Years ago one could consider a person who was over the age of 30 as old; however, in the year 2020 men and women will not be considered old until the age of 80. Some authors suggest that a redrawing of the limits of the stages of life is necessary. Dychtwald[3] proposes that a person from 18 to 25 should be considered a "youth." When a person reaches age 25 and until the age of 40 this period of life should be contemplated as "youth adulthood." (The concept of youth would thus be extended.) People from the age of 40 to 60 would be considered as being in a period of their lives coined "middlescense" (this is a new stage). From age 60 to 80 one would be in late adulthood (this is a concept that has been postponed and extended somewhat). People 80 to 100 years old would have entered the stage of "old age" (a concept that has been postponed and extended considerably). Finally, a person who is 100 or more would be considered as having reached the stage of "very old age." (Again, this is a concept that has also been postponed.)

3.3   GENERAL DEMOGRAPHIC DATA

The world's population doubled in the last half of the 20th century. In 1950, there were $2\frac{1}{2}$ billion people in the world. By 1960, there were 3 billion. In 1975, there were 4 billion and by the 1980s there were 5 billion. It is expected that in a few years' time the population will continue to grow, especially in underdeveloped countries.[7] It is predicted that Asia will contribute some 2 billion people to the world population in the next three decades; Africa will contribute 1.3 billion people to the world population; and Latin America and the Caribbean will, in comparison, have only a very moderate population increase of some 334 million between 1995 and 2050.

More concretely, the following ten countries, listed in order from the highest population growth to the lowest, will experience the highest birthrates over the next 30 years: India, China, Pakistan, Nigeria, Ethiopia, Indonesia, the United States, Bangladesh, Zaire, and Iran. In regard to other countries, specifically in Europe, there is the expectation that the birthrate will drop and that population growth will slow. It is predicted that Europe's population will decline by 27 million over the next 30 years and by another 64 million between the years 2025 and 2050.

Thus, one must expect a dramatic change in the global balance of population. A much larger share of the world's people will live in Africa, south of the Sahara. In 50 years Western Africa will have the same population as all of Europe. Eastern Africa will have many more people than all the countries of South America, the Caribbean, and Oceania combined (Table 3.1).[7]

In 1950, there were only 131 million people aged 65 or older. In 1995, their number had almost tripled and was estimated at 371 million people (6% of the world population). Between the present time and the year 2025, the number of people 65 and older will increase to more than 1.4 billion elderly people worldwide. Thus, the percentage of elderly people increased from 5.2% in 1950 to 6.2% in 1995. And the growth continues. By 2050 one out of ten people worldwide will be over the age of 65.[8]

The most rapid change is occurring in developing countries, but the highest number of elderly people is still found in developed countries.[6–9] The percentage of the population constituted by elderly people is 14% in Europe and 13% in North America, whereas in developing countries in Asia and Africa the percentage of

TABLE 3.1
World Population

	Total Population (in 1000)				Percentage of Total Population			
	1950	1995	2025	2050	1950	1995	2025	2050
World Total	2,523,878	5,687,113	8,039,130	9,366,724	100	100	100	100
Africa	223,974	719,495	1,453,899	2,046,401	8.9	12.7	18.1	21.8
Latin America and Caribbean	166,337	476,637	689,618	810,433	6.6	8.4	8.6	8.7
North America	171,617	296,645	369,016	384,054	6.8	5.2	4.6	4.1
Asia	1,402,021	3,437,787	4,784,833	5,442,567	55.6	60.4	59.5	58.1
Europe	547,318	728,244	701,077	637,585	21.7	12.8	8.7	6.8
Oceania	12,612	28,305	40,687	45,684	0.5	0.5	0.5	0.5
Least developed countries	197,572	579,035	1,159,255	1,631,820	7.8	10.2	14.4	17.4

Source: Data from www.nasa.ac.at/Research/LOC/Papers/gkm/chap1.htm.

elderly people is 5 and 3%, respectively. In developing countries the growth of the population is 21% and the fraction that corresponds to older people is 54%, whereas in developed countries the growth of the population is 88%, anticipating an accelerated growth (123%) of older people. This accelerated growth rate explains why these countries give so much attention to elderly people (on the level of public health, social security, etc.).[6]

Specifically for the European Economic Community[10] the average for people older than 80 by the year 2020 will be as follows: total for the European Union, 57%; Spain, 5.6%; Denmark, 4%; the United Kingdom, 4.8%; France, 6.1%; Italy, 7.1%; and Germany, 6.1%. In Spain there is a particular concern about the increase in the number of elderly people accompanied by a decrease in the birthrate. There are more than 5 million people over the age of 65. In many regions, this population is greater than the population of those under the age of 15.

With respect to the United States, people 65 years or older numbered 34.4 million in 1998, representing 12.7% of the U.S. population. The number of older Americans has increased by 3.2 million or 10.1% since 1990, compared with an increase of 8.1% for the under-65 population. Another phenomenon is that the older population itself is getting older. In 1998, the 65- to 74-year-old group (18.4 million) was eight times larger than it was in 1900, but the 75- to 84-age group (12.0 million) was 16 times larger and the 85 or older group (4.0 million) was 33 times larger.[11]

The world population has increased notoriously in recent years and so has the elderly population, even though there are some differences in developed countries when compared with underdeveloped countries. However, is there a collective consciousness among those who are affected by the aging of the population? Have public health policies of a primary preventive nature been established or is society waiting until the problem is upon it to develop tertiary means of prevention and treatment? The world is facing what some authors call "the Gray Revolution," which is a movement toward a world in which there are more elderly people. The world is "going gray" because fertility rates are low and so are death rates. This is a situation that will affect our parents and in a few years it will affect us. Is the current generation ready to assume responsibility for the care of elderly people? And when it is our turn, who will take care of us? It is possible that the predictions for the year 2020 will come true and that the future will belong to elderly people.

3.4 THE EPIDEMIOLOGY OF AGING IN THE WORLD

The demographic transition that is taking place because of the decrease in the percentage of children, the reduction of the mortality rate, and the aging of the population necessitates some changes in the profile of disease and in health policies and services.

Developing countries are characterized by an epidemiological transition with the coexistence of communicable diseases, the growing role of chronic disease, the reappearance of problems that had disappeared (such as cholera) or that had been controlled (such as malaria, tuberculosis, and dengue), the appearance of new problems (AIDS), and the growing problem of trauma caused by violence or accidents.

The developed countries, for their part, face the pathologies that are endemic to development and civilization, such as degenerative cardiovascular illnesses and problems with mental health and accidents, originating from a mixture of agents such as lifestyle and environmental factors.[12]

The aging of the population in developed countries as well as underdeveloped countries generates a series of pathologies associated with age that were not seen years ago. Thus, it is imperative today and in the coming years to act on the illnesses related to aging, differentiating the primary processes of growing old from the secondary ones, and identifying risk factors and protective factors on environmental, cultural, economic, and personal levels. Diagnoses must consider the factors of genetics, personal clinical history, family and social relations, consumption of psychoactive substances, lifestyles, behavior, etc. to develop strategies and/or therapies that can slow down the aging process and generate a better quality of life for older people.[1]

It seems that a large part of the elderly population (at least three out of four people) dies as a result of one of the following three chronic illnesses: cardiovascular illnesses, cerebrovascular illnesses, or neoplasias. Cardiovascular illnesses (coronary pathologies, alterations in heartbeat, high blood pressure, and arterial pathologies) are responsible for 50% of all deaths in individuals aged 65 and older, and represent 65% of the total of illnesses for which patients seek primary care.[6] Other common illnesses in this population are locomotive, respiratory (bronchitis, EPOC), and digestive (problems involving mastication, hernias, gastric hyposecretion, constipation, and fecal incontinence).

3.5 AGING AND NEUROPHARMACOLOGY

People aged 65 and older consume more medications than any other age group. This group sustains situations of inappropriate use, and in many cases problems of overmedication or undermedication. On average, 95% of older people take 5 to 12 medications per day. This presents the problem that many senior citizens may mix psychotropic and neurological medication with other drugs,[43] which may be prescribed or nonprescribed. Salzman[44] states that treating older people with psychotropic drugs is a less precise process than their therapeutic classification, and predicting the therapeutic effect is not always possible in aged people. At the same time, the high comorbidity in elderly people makes it more difficult to know the exact desired and nondesired clinical effects of psychotropic and neurological drugs.

Another factor that stands out when considering the consumption of medication by elderly people is that the aging process can alter the pharmacokinetics and the pharmacodynamics of drugs. Psychotropic medication seems not to produce age-related changes in the gastrointestinal tract in the absence of gastrointestinal pathology, but when used at the same time as other drugs that are commonly consumed by elderly people these may affect absorption (for example, anticholinergic drugs), which results in a delay of clinical effects. Distribution of drugs to the central nervous system can also be affected by aging, mainly because total body water decreases as one gets older, while body fat and body mass increase. The metabolism and excretion of drugs depend on a number of factors, including the type of drug, the state of the liver, the renal blood flow, the size of the kidneys, the tubular excretory capacity, and glomerular filtration.

Altered sensitivity to psychotropic and neurological drugs was once thought to be related to pharmacodynamics changes. Now it is considered that these changes seem to be related to pharmacokinetic alterations or to diminished homeostatic responses.[45]

The effects of neuroleptic drugs can be influenced by aging. Higher active blood levels can be produced; thus, the effects of the drugs are prolonged. This makes older people more vulnerable to the side effects of these kinds of drugs. Older people taking neuroleptics often experience sedation, extrapyramidal symptoms, orthostatic hypotension, and anticholinergic reactions.

Because of the frequency of anxiety and insomnia among this population, benzodiazepines are very commonly prescribed to elderly people. Caution must be taken when prescribing these drugs to elderly people because they normally produce a short-term benefit but their beneficial effect is lost when used for prolonged periods of time. Some researchers have even pointed out that patients taking benzodiazepines can present symptoms that resemble dementia because these drugs can produce cognitive impairments similar to those seen in dementia. Another problem with these types of drugs is that they easily create dependency, and produce withdrawal effects (tremors, agitation, seizures, etc.) when patients try to give them up. The interaction that benzodiazepines could have when taken with other drugs must also be considered.

Among the anti-Parkinson medications, the combination of levodopa with carbidopa seems to be the best treatment option because it produces the fewest side effects. Anticholinergic drugs may produce cardiovascular, ocular, gastrointestinal, urologic, and/or psychiatric side effects in older people.

3.6 NEUROLOGICAL EPIDEMIOLOGY OF AGING

One of the most intriguing epidemiological trends observed in developed nations over recent decades is the increasing occurrence of neurological diseases in elderly people, such as Alzheimer dementia (AD), vascular dementia (VaD), primary malignant brain tumor, Parkinson's disease, and amyotrophic lateral sclerosis (ALS).[13]

3.6.1 DEMENTIA

Dementia in accordance with the operational definition by Cummings and Benson[14] is an acquired syndrome involving intellectual disturbances that are characterized by persistent alterations in at least one area of mental activity, such as memory, language abilities, visual-spatial abilities, personality, or mood and cognition. Dementia typically progresses through phases that are rated as mild, moderate, and severe. Eventually dementia leads to death.

In mild dementia, patients can maintain judgment, live alone, and take care of their own personal hygiene habits. When the next phase approaches, greater difficulties emerge, and to perform daily activities a certain level of supervision is required. Finally, in severe dementia, there is so much cognitive and physical decline that constant supervision is mandated.[15]

Every type of dementia leads to the same fateful end; however, there are differences in the way the cognitive aspects are affected and the course that the deterioration takes. Nevertheless, dementia in its different modalities has been considered the most common and most disabling late-life mental disorder.

In recent years there has been considerable advancement in the understanding of the epidemiology of dementia (cortical, subcortical, and mixed). Different studies have been centered on the main types of dementia that most affect this age group, which are AD and VaD.[8]

Many studies have been done on the rate of incidence, that is, on the number of new cases of the disease that have been reported in a determined period of time within a specific population, and on the rate of prevalence, which refers to the number of people affected in a period of time within a community. These studies are conducted principally in developed countries and show little geographic variation between countries and regions.[8]

Even though many of the results of the studies can appear contradictory, it is a fact that dementia is an important problem for people 65 and older and that it has a great impact on public health.[16] Notwithstanding, there is still a need for studies that permit valid comparisons to be made and that use diagnostic criteria that are precise and standardized.[17]

3.6.1.1 Incidence

There are fewer studies on the incidence of dementia than there are on its prevalence. One of the authors who has studied this topic extensively is Jorm. He reconsidered and analyzed work done in this area taking into account criteria such as methodology, size of the population sample, age, and results. Despite finding clear methodological differences, he takes as an approximate datum 1% of the population above 65 years old.[17]

One aspect that clearly emerges when looking at the diverse studies is that the incidence of AD as well as VaD rises after age 60.[8] In a meta-analysis, Gao et al.[18] examined the articles identified through a MedLine search on "incidence of dementia" and "incidence of Alzheimer's disease" and found that dementia is associated with a significant quadratic age effect. In fact, 5% of people over the age of 65 will develop some form of dementia, and this figure increases to 20% in people over the age of 80. There is a good deal of controversy when considering people in their 90s. One view is that all people will develop dementia if they live long enough, but there is an opposing view that holds that the risk of developing dementia levels out, and may even decline in extreme old age. Little is known about dementia in the "oldest of the old," but it is important to consider this to clarify whether dementia is an inevitable consequence of aging or if it is simply a disorder that occurs within a specific age range.[19]

The incidence of VaD has been studied much less extensively. Among the few data available, substantial variations in the incidence rates have been observed, possibly because of methodological discrepancies. Leys et al.,[20] in a community-based study, identified the incidence rates of VaD. It was found that 20 to 40 people out of 100,000 in the age group of 60 to 69 years old suffered from VaD. This figure increases to 200 to 700 per 100,000 when considering people over the age of 80.[20]

3.6.1.2 Prevalence

AD is one of the most common dementia conditions, and it accounts for more than 40 to 90% cases of dementia among elderly patients.[21,22] Its prevalence is approximately twice that of VaD.[22]

Some studies indicate that the prevalence estimates in developed countries have been remarkably stable. The average rate for European countries for people with dementia who are older than 65 is between 5.7 and 15.4%. Of these, between 3.4 and 13% are moderate cases, while between 0.6 and 5.6% correspond to serious cases.[23] The studies from developing parts of the world have reported unusually low prevalence rates for dementia. However, more studies are needed in these regions because there are variables that should be examined to identify clues about these conditions.[19]

Until a few years ago, the studies on the prevalence of VaD were not very precise, given that the diagnostic criteria were not clear. Nevertheless, in recent years, more standardized definitions of VaD are beginning to be used. The European Community Concerted Action on Epidemiology and Prevention of Dementia carried out an analysis of the available information on the prevalence of VaD in Europe. It analyzed 23 reports; however, of these only five met the criteria for inclusion. Of these five, two of the investigations mixed the entities of Alzheimer's disease vascular (AdV) and VaD in such a way that the data reported are combined. It was found that the prevalence of VaD increases with age, in every country. In the 70 to 79 age group, it is generally higher in men, in the range of 3.2 to 4.8%, as compared with women, who have a prevalence rate of 2.2 to 2.9%. In one group of older people, studies showed more differences for men than for women. Similarly, between the ages of 80 and 89 the prevalence in men is from 3.5 to 16.3% and in women it is from 2.8 to 2.9%.[22]

In non-European countries, studies on prevalence are scarce. In an American study the prevalence of VaD in people approximately 65 years old was 2.8%.[22] On the other hand, about 1 in every 10 people over age 65 is diagnosed with AD, and it is believed that over 4 million Americans have AD.[19,24]

To explain why Japanese people have so much of a lesser predisposition toward developing AD, Graves et al.[25] suggest that lifestyle may decrease the risk of expressing cognitive decline over a 2-year follow-up period. Other aspects that may be influential are the greater social support characteristic of Japanese culture as well as the role that Japanese language and culture may play in neural connectivity during brain development and/or in mental stimulation in adult life.[25]

However, Eefsting et al.[26] have shown that the rate of VaD has decreased and senile dementia of the Alzheimer's type is now the major cause of dementia.

Chandra et al.[27] conducted a study on the prevalence of AD and other dementias in rural sectors. They found that the overall prevalence rate for AD was 0.62 in the population aged 55 or older and 1.07% in the population aged 65 or older. Greater age was significantly associated with higher prevalence of both AD and all dementias, but neither gender nor literacy was associated with prevalence. The possible explanations include low overall life expectancy, short survival with the disease, and low

specific incidence, potentially as a result of differences in the underlying distribution of risk and protective factors compared with populations with higher prevalence.[27]

Despite the different methodologies that are presented in the studies, the following conclusions have been drawn:

1. The prevalence of dementia depends on age and its rate doubles every 5 years.
2. There is a difference regarding gender such that VaD is more frequent in men than in women, whereas it appears that there is a slightly higher prevalence rate of AD in women.[28]
3. There is a difference between nations such that VaD is more frequent in Japan, China, and Russia, whereas AD is more frequent in Europe and the United States. Similarly, it seems that the numbers are higher in rural than in urban communities.[17–22]

3.6.1.3 Risk Factors

In longitudinal studies, diverse factors have been identified as environmental risk factors for AD. In a large study conducted by Launer et al.[28] the risk of AD associated with diverse factors (family history, sex, educational level, smoking, cranial traumatism) was examined. The authors made an analysis consisting of four prospective population studies, which were conducted in Europe on individuals aged 65 or older, with 528 cases of incidental dementia. In this study, it was observed that the consumption of cigarettes did not appear to protect against the development of AD. Additionally, the antecedents of traumatism without loss of consciousness are not associated with the development of the illness. Another interesting risk factor that is not completely explained is the association between low levels of education and the increase of risk for developing AD, especially in women.[28]

Epidemiological studies on VaD are limited by diagnostic uncertainties due to the lack of common diagnostic criteria. However, it is generally assumed that in addition to arterial hypertension other factors are associated with an increased risk of VaD. These factors are low education level, alcohol abuse, heart disease, occupational exposure to pesticides and herbicides, and liquid plastic or rubber exposure. Another associated factor is the use or not of aspirin, but this finding may be an artifact due to the longer life expectancy of patients who take aspirin. However, additional epidemiological studies are necessary to identify risk factors for VaD and to evaluate whether risk factors for VaD differ according to the subtype of VaD: multi-infarct dementia, strategic single infarct dementia, small vessel disease with dementia, hypoperfusion dementia, hemorrhagic dementia, and other mechanisms.[22]

Heart attack is one of the risk factors for developing VaD and AD alike. Heart attack in and of itself constitutes an important health problem. It is the third leading cause of death in developed countries and is, as well, a source of physical and psychological disabilities.[29] Different studies have shown that heart attack notably increases the risk for dementia. In a study in Japan, the frequency of dementia was 27.2% in patients with a history of heart attack and 3.4% in control groups. Another study conducted in New York shows that the prevalence of dementia increases 3 months after the occurrence of a heart attack in patients 60 and older by more than 26.3%. Kokhen conducted a long-term study of 25 years. He found that the incidence of dementia increased from 7% in the first year to 48% in the last year of the study.[22]

Other factors that appear to be associated with both types of dementia are the presence of the apolipoprotein E gene on chromosome 19[30] and episodes of delirium, which *appear* to increase the risk of dementia over a median 32.5 months in elderly patients. Two possibilities for the association of delirium with the risk for dementia have been pointed out: first, delirium may give rise to brain injury, which results in predisposition to dementia and, second, delirium may serve as a marker of a sub-clinical dementing process.[31]

3.7 BEHAVIOR AND AFFECTIVE EPIDEMIOLOGY IN AGING

Epidemiological predictions indicate that there is a high probability that the incidence of "mental" illnesses will be on the rise in the future. This is due, on the one hand, to the increase of life expectancy of people who suffer disturbances or mental disabilities and, on the other hand, to the increase in numbers of people who reach ages in which the chances of acquiring certain illnesses are greater.[17]

There are few epidemiological studies on these problems given that (1) there is not much clarity in regard to the concepts that are studied or the forms of measurements or diagnosis; and (2) the behavioral and affective alterations show up in the majority of cases, mixed with other pathologies.

The behavioral alterations that are most typically found in elderly people include paranoid schizophrenia, alcoholism, affective disorders, and depression.[32] This last affliction is the most frequent in the elderly population. Depression is seen in its pure form or accompanied by other physical and/or neurological disorders.

3.7.1 DEPRESSION

The common symptoms of depression are dysphoric moods, loss of interest, and anxiety, among others. Additionally, physical symptoms appear such as altered sleep patterns, loss of appetite, lack of energy, and fatigue. As well, there may be flaws in memory related to attention difficulty and concentration. Depressive symptoms in elderly people are very similar to those in young people. Depression may be brought on by feelings of helplessness and dependence caused by physical and/or mental illness, loss of productive capacity, feelings of loneliness due to the loss of one's spouse or one's social support network (friends and family). In many cases institutionalization can be a factor for bringing on depression. Risk factors for depression that also have been widely studied and about which there is considerable literature include the importance of remaining sexually active, and the negative effects of being single, having a poor social support network, or suffering from physical or neurological diseases.

Casado et al.[33] analyzed diverse factors that play an important role in the appearance of depressive symptoms in elderly hospitalized patients. In the patients examined there was a common background of depression and chronic illness. The motivating factor behind the hospitalization was illness and a lack of family and social support.[33] When gender difference in depressive symptomology is taken into account, the results reported among elderly patients in Spain are the same as those predicted by the literature. Prevalence of depression is higher in females than in males; the prevalence in women is 46% and in men 19.6%. Even so, other factors such as little emotional support from children, lack of a confidant, few social activities, and a sense of losing control[34] were associated with depression in both sexes. However, gender is not a variable that clearly explains the differences in symptomology. In fact, in another study done with people over 85 in Finland, it was found that the prevalence was greater, in major disturbances as well as minor ones, in men.[35]

Because depression in elderly people can appear combined with other physical or neurological illnesses, it is sometimes difficult to distinguish its symptoms. Therefore, when making a diagnosis, it is necessary to be cautious and consider more defined criteria, which permit the therapist to make early differential diagnoses (dementia vs. pseudodementia vs. depression) and to develop the respective therapeutic measures. Some of the characteristics that have been mentioned as peculiar to depression as it affects the elderly are as follows:

1. The episodes are longer and more frequent and are more resistant to pharmacological treatment.
2. Episodes are accompanied by delirium and hallucinations.
3. There is a greater risk for suicide.
4. The episodes are accompanied by psychomotor agitation and disturbed sleep patterns.[32]

The rates of prevalence in the community that are reported in different studies vary, but it is clear that this is a syndrome that is common among elderly people. It is possible that the differences reflected in the studies are due to the methods of evaluation or the periods of time used. Nevertheless, what has been indicated is that the symptoms of depression decline with age (contrary to what happens with dementia). One study conducted with a population sample of 2725 individuals between the ages of 18 and 79, administering two inventories to measure symptoms of depression and anxiety, showed that symptoms of depression diminish with age, in men as well as in women.[36]

Another aspect that deserves attention is a study that examined the relationship between depression and mortality. This was a community-based cohort study with a French population sample that found that social relations did not significantly modify the depression–mortality associations for either men or women, although the depression–mortality effect was reduced by 12.8% in men.[37] The association between depression and mortality in elderly people is still not resolved. Penninx et al.[38] studied 3056 men and women in the Netherlands between the ages of 55 and 85 during a 4-year period. The study found that men with minor depression had a 1.80-fold higher risk of death than men without depression, while in the women, minor depression did not significantly increase the risk of death. Major depression was associated with a 1.83-fold higher mortality risk, in both genders.[38]

Despite all the studies related to risk factors for developing depressive symptomology, the studies on the relationship of depression with physical illnesses and death, and studies on protective factors, the magnitude of the increasing duration of life demands that more epidemiological studies on depression be conducted in the elderly population.

3.8 COMORBIDITY: TWO SIDES OF THE SAME COIN

The common message that the different studies communicate is that there is a high association (comorbidity) between psychological disorders — depression, anxiety, hallucinations, etc. — and neurological illnesses. Some studies indeed show that these kinds of disorders frequently co-occur. For example, the National Co-morbidity Study revealed that about 80% of all psychiatric disorders diagnosed in the U.S. population involved co-morbid disorders.[39]

3.8.1 MANIC SYNDROMES AND DEMENTIA

On many occasions it is difficult to diagnose manic syndromes because of the high prevalence of comorbidity, especially with neurological disorders.[40] Some authors have even tried to explain the increase of the incidence of manic syndromes in old age by suggesting that it has to do with a manifestation of a demential process. However, other authors do not find support for these assertions. What does appear to be true is that the associations between manic syndromes and neurological illnesses could help elucidate the cerebral components of these syndromes.[40]

It is difficult, therefore, to establish when a manic syndrome is a direct consequence and when it is a comorbid condition. As Shulman indicates "manic syndromes in old age represent three broad groupings: (1) middle-age onset of depressives who convert to bipolarity after a latency of many years and frequent depressive episodes, (2) a group of mixed-age bipolar patients who have continued to cycle a heterogeneous group of neurologic, or (3) those with central nervous system disorders."

The main neurological illnesses associated with manic syndromes appear to be cerebrovascular diseases. However, there are other neurological conditions comorbid with manic syndromes that include brain stem tumors, central nervous system tumors, normal-pressure hydrocephalus, neurosyphilis, hyperthyroidism, and hemodialysis. In regard to the compromised structures, these are located in the right hemisphere, specifically in the orbitofrontal circuit involving the cortex, limbic system, and subcortical nuclei.

3.8.2 DEPRESSION AND DEMENTIA

A widely studied problem is the relationship between dementia and depression. Some authors indicate that the depressive disorders are associated with mild cognitive impairment, while others consider that any degree of impairment can increase the probability of depressive symptoms.[33] It is clear that symptoms of depression exist in patients with dementia and depression and dementia are not entities that exclude one another. Additionally, patients with depression as well as ones suffering dementia show evidence of cognitive alterations when administered objective tests whose execution, besides the results in themselves, could give indications for a diagnostic differential. Hofman et al.[41] conducted a study using a battery of psychometric tests to differentiate patients with AD from patients with depression and healthy older people. The test used was successful at differentiating healthy patients from those that showed signs of dementia and depression; however, it was not sensitive enough to differentiate patients with dementia from those with depression. In fact, both groups showed deficits in basic executive operations, slowed information processing, and attention deficits.[41]

There are many studies in which researchers try to clarify the relationship between dementia and depression or cognitive deterioration and depression. Furthermore, there is an attempt to identify the frequency of each one of these alterations in elderly populations. Shulman et al.[42] conducted a study on bipolar disorders in old age with a special focus on neurological comorbidity, high mortality, and management. Some of the conclusions were that these disorders are associated with late-onset neurological disorders (cerebrovascular disease) involving the right hemisphere and orbitofrontal cortex.[42]

3.9 CONCLUDING REMARKS

In old age there is a decrease in cognitive, perceptual, and physical functioning. Additionally, there is a greater propensity toward suffering certain illnesses. Subjective experience of these illnesses is modified, and in many cases the symptoms appear mixed in such a manner that those that can be observed constitute the tip of the iceberg; that is, the symptoms are not necessarily manifestations of the illness that elderly people most frequently suffer from.

The most significant changes that occur, whether the cause is old age or illness, are those that affect the functions of the muscular-skeletal system, cognition, and aerobic and neurological capacities. The elderly person shows changes in his or her physical appearance: the hair changes its pigmentation and it falls out; the skin becomes more flaccid, dry, and thin; there are changes in the heart and a decrease in the maximum heart rate; there are respiratory difficulties due to the rigidity of the thorax cavity; and there are sensory-receptive, emotional, and cognitive changes.

The decrease in cognitive functions is associated with loss in cortical volume (cortical atrophy), the decline in the sulci of the brain, and biochemical changes that occur at a cellular level. The areas of the brain that are affected by age are the frontal, the parietal, and the temporal lobes, which produce the associated behavioral changes. Elderly people have difficulties in remembering the time sequence of events and the circumstances in which information was learned (source amnesia). As well, there is a decline in constructive and visual-motor tasks and there is greater difficulty in recalling information that has been recently learned, as well as mistakes in the generation of strategies when searching for information contained in the semantic memory.

In synthesis, as one ages, deficits in cognitive flexibility, in fluency, and in judgment occur. Subsequently, individuals begin to exhibit problems in memory tasks or tasks related to impairments at the temporal medial cortex. It seems that a protective factor against this decrease is the educational and cultural level that the person has achieved, given that this facilitates the quantity of neuronal connections that could compensate for the losses, thus making the decrease in cognitive capacity less noticeable.

The increase in longevity accompanied by the decline in fertility is the universal cause of the aging of the population. This affects society in general and people in particular. The social repercussions are numerous; some of the most important are the effects this has on rates of production, consumption, savings and investment, conditions of the labor market, the types of services that are necessary, and the patterns of public spending.

Because of the increase in the elderly population in the future, there will be more people at risk for suffering dementia. Dementia is the progressive and irreversible decay of the cognitive functions that affects everyday life and independence. It is very common to find individuals with dementia who are bedridden, unable to control their sphincters, incapable of moving themselves, unable to reason, to remember, to learn, and, in synthesis, with a diminished quality of life. The cause of death of these patients may be the dementia itself or it may be any other type of common age-related illness (respiratory failure, digestive infections, etc.).

The consequences of this progressive degeneration are such that dementia could be considered as "the epidemic of the 21st century." This affects three groups:

1. Elderly people, who experience the effects of this illness at the same time as they witness their social circles become smaller and their personal influence and acquisitive power become reduced to levels of insignificance. The suffering reaches the point where one more day of life loses its meaning.

2. The family, who must assume the social and economic responsibility of this person, at the same time generating mechanisms of attention and care for its elderly relative, as well as ways for coping with the stress created by the situation.

3. Society, which has the responsibility for encouraging the production of care settings with adequate conditions, developing health policies, preventive care, creating strategies of training health-care professionals and social workers, and generating areas of action at the level of health-care services, law protection, support for the family, investigation with the goal of facing the consequences of this problem in such a way that it constitutes a priority.

Epidemiological studies, such as those described in this chapter, produce data on the incidence and prevalence of dementia, the relationships with alterations in behavior and emotions (for example, depression), the environmental (geographic), social (cultural), and lifestyle (physical activity, eating habits, etc.) factors that have potential positive effects on the aging process, and the severity and the course that illnesses take. The studies are equally useful in the investigative sense and in the practical sense. In these studies can be found the answers to the questions of what is normal and what is pathological in the aging process, and they orient the public health and educational policies, as well.

The priority of this century should be the comparative investigation between cultural and economic groups (using standardized methodologies and unique diagnostic criteria) with the goal of detecting environmental risk factors as well as populations at high risk for developing dementia. These studies should include the cost of health services, which include the social economic impact that illness has on the patients and on the family. As well, studying people who reach advanced ages (people who live to be 100 years old or more) in good health could give valuable information about what should be considered normal (nonpathological) aging. It is clear that the better the mechanisms underlying these pathologies are understood, the greater possibility there is of designing resources that respond to the needs of the affected population.

Dementia and depression are important problems in the elderly population. In fact, between 15 and 20% of elderly people suffer from significant depressive symptoms and at least 45% of the people 85 years of age or older suffer from dementia. In addition, there are other conditions that exist but that are not studied, such as anxiety disorder, alcohol abuse, and inadequate prescriptive medicines, among others.

> El deber de los jóvenes es gritar para que no se duerman los antiguos,
> y deber de los viejos es avisar, para que los jóvenes no se precipiten
> por el despeñadero de las imprudencias.
>
> **— Sneider**

> The duty of the young is to shout so that their elders do not sleep,
> And the duty of the old is to warn the young so that they do not
> rush over the cliff of imprudence.

3.10 SUMMARY

Changes produced in most recent years: *Important statistical information:*

Changes produced in most recent years:		Important statistical information:
Decline in the birthrate	1950	200 million people >65 years
Decline in the mortality rate	2020	1 billion people >65 years
Increase in the world population	2025	1.2 billion people >65 years
Increase in people >65 years old	Today	61% of elderly people live in developed countries; today 1 in 5 people is elderly.
	2025	70% of elderly people live in developing countries.
		55% of elderly people are women

Main illnesses that affect the elderly population:

Cardiovascular diseases

Cerebrovascular illnesses

Neoplasias

Health and epidemic priority 21st century: Dementia (AD and VaD)

Most important emotional alteration: Depression

The prevalence of dementia increases with age: 65–69, 1.4%; 70–74, 2.8%; 75–79, 5.6%; 80–84, 11.1%; 85 or older, 23.6%.

AD is more frequent than VaD, even though there are also geographic and gender differences.

In developed countries, the number of dementia cases is projected to increase from 7.4 million to 10.2 million. In developing countries, as well, there is an expected increase in the cases of dementia.

15–20% of the elderly population suffers from depression.

The risk factors for developing dementia as well as depression are still not clear.

Consequences of demographic and epidemiological changes:

1. Changes in the rates of production and consumption
2. Changes in the job market
3. Changes in productivity
4. Changes in health services

Necessary measures:

1. Aging with good health (OMS)
2. Raising awareness about the changes produced by aging
3. Detecting and acting on the causes of death
4. Guaranteeing elderly people access to health care
5. Generating means of health promotion: behavioral diagnosis of the health situation of elderly people, identifying more effective strategies to encourage behavior that promotes health, designing and implementing community programs and health policies
6. Intervening on the level of primary care and prevention (evaluating lifestyles, social support, coping styles, social demographic variables)

Problems with the epidemiological studies:

There is a lack of uniformity in the methodology used and in the diagnostic criteria.

There are few comparative studies (between regions, countries).

In the elderly population illnesses appear combined with other illnesses, and it is difficult to differentiate the contribution of each illness to the observed behavior.

REFERENCES

1. Hodes, R., available at http://www.nih.gov/strat-plan/2001-2005/1.htm.
2. Available at http://www.portaltercera.com.ar/aniointernacional.htm.
3. Dychtwald, K., Speculations on the future of aging, *21 Century Online Mag.*
4. Kirkwood, T., Human senescence, *BioEssays*, 18, 1009–1015, 1996.
5. Xavier, F. A., *Transformações nos padroes de mortalidade por idade e causas*, Fundação Joao Pinheiro, São Luis, Brazil, 1992.
6. Available at http://www.nasa.ac.at/Research/LOC/Papers/gkm/chap1.htm.
7. Available at http://www.nasa.ac.at/Research/LOC/Papers/gkm/chap1.htm.
8. *The Prevalence of Dementia; Alzheimer's Dis. Int.*, 3, April, 1999.
9. Available at http://www.un.org/esa/socdeu/age4res2.htm.
10. Fernández, J. N., personal communication, 2000.
11. Available at http://www.aoa.dhhs,gov/stats/profile/default.htm.
12. Sheridan, C. and Radmacher, S., *Health Psychology Challenging the Biomedical Model*, Wiley, New York, 1992.
13. Riggs, J., Changing demographics and neurologic disease in the elderly, *Neuroepidemiology*, 14, 477–485, 1996.
14. Cummings, J. L. and Benson, F., *Dementia, a Clinical Approach*, Plenum Press, New York, 1992.
15. Banich, M., *Neuropsychology. The neural bases of mental function*, Houghton Mifflin, Boston, 1997.
16. Ostrosky-Solís, F., Ardila, A., and Chayo-Dichy, R., *Rehabilitación Neuropsicológica*, Planeta, Mexico City, Mexico, 1996.
17. Henderson, A. S., *Demencia: Epidemiología de los Trastornos Mentales y de los Problemas Psicosociales*, Meditor, Madrid, 1994.
18. Gao, S., Hendrie, H. C., and Hall, K. S., The relationships between age, sex and the incidence of dementia and Alzheimer's disease: a meta-analysis, *Arch. Gen. Psychiatr.*, 55, 809–815, 1998.
19. Jorm, A. F., Cross-national comparisons of the occurrence of Alzheimer's and vascular dementias, *Eur. Arch. Psychiatr. Clin. Neurosc.*, 240, 218–222, 1991.
20. Leys, D., Erkinjuntti, T., Desmond, D., Schmidt, R., Englund, E., Pasquier, F., Parnetti, L., Ghika, J., Kalaria, R., Chabriat, H., Scheltens, P., and Bogousslavsky, J., Vascular dementia: the role of cerebral infarcts; *Alzheimer Dis. Assoc. Disorders*, 13, S38–S48, 1999.
21. Gavrilova, S. I. and Bratsun, A. L., Epidemiology and risk factors of Alzheimer's disease, *Vestn. Ross. Akad. Med. Nauk*, 1, 39–46, 1999.
22. Leys, D., Pasquier, F., and Parnetti, L., Epidemiology of vascular dementia, *Haemostasis*, 3–4, 134–150, 1998.
23. Abengózar, Ma. C., *Envejecimiento Normal y Patológico*, Promolibro, Valencia, 1997.
24. Hendrie, H. C., Epidemiology of dementia and Alzheimer's disease, *Am. J. Geriatr. Psychiatr.*, 6(2 Suppl. 1), S3–S18, 1998.
25. Graves, A. B., Rajaram, L., Bowen, J. D., McCornick, W. C., McCurry, S. M., and Larson, E. B., Cognitive decline and Japanese culture in a cohort of older Japanese Americans in King Country. Wan the Kame project, *J. Gerontol. B Psychol. Sci. Soc.*, 54, S154–161, 1999.
26. Eefsting, J. A., Boersma, F., Van den Brink, W., and Van Tilburg, W., Differences in prevalence of dementia based on community survey and general practitioner recognition, *Psychol. Med.*, 6, 1223–1230, 1996.

27. Chandra, V., Ganguli, M., Pondar, R., Johnstan, J., Belle, S., and Dekosky, S. T., Prevalence of Alzheimer's disease and other dementias in rural areas: the Indo US Study, *Neurology*, 51, 1000–1008, 1998.

28. Launer, L. J., Andersen, K., Dewey, M. E. et al., Rates and risk factors for dementia and Alzheimer's disease. Results from the EURODEM pooled analyses, *Neurology*, 52, 78–84, 1999.

29. Reitsma, J., Limburg, M., Kleifmen, J., Bonsel, G., and Tijssen, J., Epidemiology in the Netherlands from 1972 to 1994: the end of the decline in stroke mortality. *Neuroepidemiology*, 17, 121–131, 1998.

30. Espert, R., Bertolín, J. M., Navarro, J. F., and González, A., Epidemiology and risk factors of Alzheimer's disease, *Rev. Neurol.*, 119, 70–76, 1995.

31. Rockwood, K., Cosway, S., Carver, D., Jarrett, P., Stadnyk, K., and Fisk, J., The risk of dementia and death after delirium, *Age Aging*, 28, 551–556, 1999.

32. Carstensen, L. and Edelstein, B., *El envejecimiento y sus trastornos*, Martínez Roca, Barcelona, 1987.

33. Casado, Ma. A., Jáuregui, J., Rubio, G., Álvarez, S., Martínez, M. L., Pérez, P., Marín, J., and Santo-Domingo, J., The prevalence of depressive symptoms and cognitive impairment in patients older than 65 years admitted to a general hospital, *Eur. J. Psychiatr.*, 12, 19–25, 1998.

34. Zunzunegui, M. V., Béland, F., Llácer, A., and León, V., Gender differences in depressive symptoms among Spanish elderly, *Soc. Psychiatr. Psychiatr. Epidemiol.*, 33, 195–205, 1998.

35. Palvarinta, A., Verkkoniemi, A., Ninesto, L., Kivela, S. L., and Sulkava, R., *Soc. Psychiatr. Psychiatr. Epidemiol.*, 34, 352–359, 1999.

36. Henderson, A. S., Korten, A. E., Levings, C., Jorm, A. F., Christensen, H., Jacomb, P. A., and Rodgers, B., Psychotic symptoms in the elderly: a prospective study in a population sample, *Int. J. Geriatr. Psychiatr.*, 7, 484–492, 1998.

37. Fuhrer, R., Dufourl, C., Antonucer, T. C., Shipley, M. J., Helmer, C., and Dortiguez, J. F., Psychological disorder and mortality in French older adults: do social relations modify the association, *Am. J. Epidemiol.*, 149, 116–126, 1999.

38. Penninx, B. W., Geerlings, S. W., Deeg, D. J., van Eijk, J. T., van Tilburg, W., and Beekman, A. T., Minor and major depression and the risk of death in older persons, *Arch. Gen. Psychiatr.*, 56(10), 889–895, 1999.

39. Van Balkom, A. J. L. M., Beekman, A. T. F., de Beurs, E., Deeg, D. J. H., van Dyck, R., and van Tilburg, W., Comorbidity of the anxiety disorders in a community-based older population in the Netherlands, *Acta Psychiatr. Scand.*, 101, 37–45, 2000.

40. Shulman, K. and Herrmann, N., The nature and management of mania in old age, *Psych. Clin. North Am.*, 22, 649–665, 1999.

41. Hofman, M., Hampel, H., Neugebauer, A., Muller, S., and Pahn, F., Alzheimer's disease, depression and normal aging: merit of simple psychomotor and visuospatial tasks, *Int. J. Geriatr. Psychiatr.*, 15, 31–39, 2000.

42. Shulman, K. I., Tohen, M., Satlin, A., Mallya, G., and Kalunian, D., Mania compared with unipolar depression in old age, *Am. J. Psychiatr.*, 149, 341–345, 1992.

43. Cadiex, R. J., Drug interactions in the elderly: how multiple drug use increases risk exponentially, *Postgrad. Med.*, 86, 179–186, 1988.

44. Salzman, C., Neuropsychopharmacology, in *Principles of Geriatric Neurology*, Katzman, R. and Rowe, J. W., Eds., Davis, Philadelphia, 1992, 32–45.

45. Irwin, R. P. and Nutt, J. G., Principles of neuropharmacology: I. Pharmacokinetics and pharmacodynamics, in Klawans, H. L., Goetz, C. G., and Tanner, C. M., Eds., *Textbook of Clinical Neuropharmacology and Therapeutics*, 2nd ed., Raven Press, New York, 1992, 1–14.

APPENDIX A

Internet Addresses

http://www.aging.unc.edu/ The Institute on Aging works to enhance the well-being of older North Carolinians.

http://www.mcs.net/~grossman/macareso.htm Internet Resources for the Aging connecting to government information sources, associations, organizations, and educational and support services.

http://www.neuropat.dote.hu/idos/inea.htm Links to other international sites, organizations, government sites, medical sites, institutions, journals, professional information, Web resources, nonprofit organizations, and information for elderly people.

http://www.apa.org/pi/aging/otherlinks.html Links to a sites, such as APA Division 20 (Adult development and aging), National Council on the Aging, Inc., American Association of Retired Persons, Gerontological Society of America, U.S Senate Special Committee on Aging, Administration on Aging, National Institute on Aging, American Federation for Aging Research, American Geriatric Society, Association for Gerontology in Higher Education.

http://marcopolo.ncl.ac.uk/APE/ The aim of this site is to provide a focus for gerontological research in Europe by maintaining an up-to-date database of researchers, institutions, meetings, training opportunities, and other resources.

http://www.aoa.dhhs.gov/aoa/stats/statpage.html Statistics concerning population growth.

http://www.iiasa.ac.at/Research/LUC/Papers/gkh1/ Papers related to aging.

http://www.eclac.org/Celade-Esp/bol66/DE_SitDemBD66.html Information on Latin America population.

http://www.aoa.dhhs.gov/siteindex.html Addresses of institutions and organizations related to aging, alphabetically ordered.

http://www.who.int/ World Health Organization.

http://www.nih.gov/ National Institutes of Health.

http://www.socenne.com.br/links.htm Information on neurological illnesses.

APPENDIX B

EPIDEMIOLOGICAL STUDIES IN DEMENTIA, 1995 TO 2000

Authors	Year	Country	Journal	Sample	Prevalence	Tools
Eefsting, J.A.; Boersma, F.; Van den Brink, W.; Van Tilburg, W.	1996	The Netherlands	*Psychol. Med.*	Noninstitutionalized group	Prevalence according to the GP was 2.2%, and based on the epidemiological approach 5.2%	Assessed both by the GP and with the epidemiological test battery (MMSE, CAMDEX)
Shaji, S.; Promodu, K.; Abraham, T.; Roy, K.J.; Verghese, A.	1996	India	*Br. J. Psychiatr.*	Rural population in India	Prevalence: 31.9% 58%: VaD, 41% AD	A door-to-door survey, adaptation of the MMSE, CAMDEX-Section B and CAMDEX-Section H
Leys, D.; Pasquier, F.; Parnetti, L.	1998	France	*Haemostasis*		Prevalence of VaD ranges from 2.2% in 70- to 79-year-old women, to 16.3% in men >80 years	Community-based studies
Riedel Heller, S.G.; Schork, A.; Matschinger, H.; Angermeyer, M.C.	2000	Germany	*Neuroepidemiology*	N: 1692 Aged 75+	Face-to-face interviews prevalence of moderate and severe dementia was 5.3% When including information on respondents by proxy and institutionalized individuals, the prevalence rate increased to 6.3 and 10.5%, respectively	Face-to-face interviews using SIDAM and proxy interviews with relatives of fragile and functionally dependent individuals
Lin, R.T.; Lai, C.L.; Tai, C.T.; Liu, C.K; Yen, Y.Y.; Howng, S.L.	1998	Taiwan	*J. Neurol. Sci.*	N: 2915 Aged 65 and over	Prevalence was 3.7%, increasing from 1.3% in people 65–69 years old to 16.5% in people 85 years old and older. AD (58 cases, 53.7%), VaD (25 cases, 23.1%), and mixed dementia (eight cases, 7.4%)	MMSE, CERAD, neuropsychological battery, neurobehavioral examination; criteria of ICD-10NA, NINCDS-ADRDA, and NINDS-AIREN

Authors	Year	Country	Journal	Sample	Results	Methods
White, L.; Petrovitch, H.; Ross, G.W.; Masaki, K.H.; Abbott, R.D.; Teng, E.L.; Rodriguez, B.L.; Blanchette, P.L.; Havlik, R.J.; Wergowske, G.; Chiu, D.; Foley, D.J.; Murdaugh, C.; Curb, J.D.	1996	United States	JAMA	N: 3734 Aged 71 through 93	Prevalence ranged from 2.1% in men aged 71 through 74 years to 33.4% in men aged 85 through 93 years; 5.4% for AD and 4.2% for VaD	Cognitive performance was assessed using standardized methods, instruments, and diagnostic criteria
Ferini Strambi, L.; Marcone, A.; Garancini, P.; Danelon, F.; Zamboni, M.; Massussi, P.; Tedesi, B.; Smirne, S.	1997	Italy	Eur. J. Epidemiol.	N: 673 Aged: over 59 years of age	Prevalence of all types was 9.8% above age 59; AD 5.2% and VaD 2.7%	Hodkinson abbreviated mental test
Graves, A.B.; Larson, E.B.; Edland, S.D.; Bowen, J.D.; McCormick, W.C.; McCurry, S.M.; Rice, M.M.; Wenzlow, A.; Uomoto, J.M.	1996	United States	Am. J. Epidemiol.	N: 3045	Prevalence rate for all dementias was 6.3% Prevalence rates for dementia increased continuously with age and were 30, 50, and 74% for participants aged 85–89, 90–94, and ≥95 years, respectively; for AD: 14, 36, and 58% for these three age groups	
Lyketsos, C.G.; Steinberg, M.; Tschanz, J.T.; Norton, M.C.; Steffens, D.C.; Breitner, J.C.	2000	United States	Am. J. Psychiatr.	N: 5,092 Aged: 65 years old or older	329 participants with dementia, 214 (65%) had AD, 62 (19%) VaD, and 53 (16%) had another DSM-IV dementia diagnosis; depression (27%), apathy (27%), and agitation/aggression (24%) were the most common in participants with dementia	Neuropsychiatric Inventory

APPENDIX B (CONTINUED)

EPIDEMIOLOGICAL STUDIES IN DEMENTIA, 1995 TO 2000

Authors	Year	Country	Journal	Sample	Prevalence	Tools
Lyketsos, C.G.; Sheppard, J.M.; Rabins, P.V.	2000	United States	Am. J. Psychiatr.	N: 21,251 Aged 60 and older	The prevalence of dementia was 3.9% (N = 823); it was dependent on age (age 60–64, prevalence = 2.6%; age 85 and older, prevalence = 8.9%)	Data from the hospital database
Liu, H.C.; Lin, K.N.; Teng, E.L.; Wang, S.J.; Fuh, J.L.; Guo, N.W.; Chou, P.; Hu, H.H.; Chiang, B.N.	1999	China	J. Am. Geriatr. Soc.	N: 2753 men and 2544 women Aged 41 to 88 years	31 cases of dementia were identified by the DSM-III-R criteria; 18 cases of Alzheimer's disease, 10 cases of vascular dementia, and three cases of other dementias; the prevalence rate in individuals aged 65 and over was 2.0%	Chinese version of the MMSE, the MMSE-T1 assessment for dementia by neurologists
Nakajima, K.; Ueda, Y.; Kono, I.; Tanaka, N.; Mizuno, T.; Makino, M.; Iwamoto, K.; Mori, S.; Takanashi	1998	Japan	Nippon Ronen Igakkai Zasshi	N: 12,931 Aged 65 years or older	Prevalence: 4.8%	Questionnaire, examined by neurologists, Hachinski ischemic score (HIS)
Boersma, F.; Eefsting, J.A.; van den Brink, W.; Koeter, M.; van Tilburg, W.	1998	The Netherlands	J. Clin. Epidemiol.	Aged 65 and over	Prevalence: 6.5%	DSM-III-R, CAMDEX MMSE

Authors	Year	Country	Journal	Sample	Findings	Assessment
Andersen, K.; Lolk, A.; Nielsen, H.; Andersen, J.; Olsen, C.; Krogh Sørensen, P.	1997	Denmark	Acta Neurol. Scand.	N: 3346 Aged 65–84 years	Prevalence: 7.1%, including the very mildly demented; the prevalence rate of very mild dementia was 2.8%	CAMCOG, the cognitive section of The Cambridge Examination for Mental Disorders of the Elderly, seven neuro-psychological tests, medical examination, and CT scan; the severity of dementia was assessed by the CDR (Clinical Dementia Rating)
Walstra, G.J.; Teunisse, S.; van Gool, W.A.; van Crevel, H.	1997	The Netherlands	J. Neurol.	N: 200 patients Aged 65 years	Of the patients, 170 (mean age 79.2 years) were demented; 31 were treated for potentially reversible causes. Prevalence of reversible dementia is of the order of 1%	CAMDEX
D'Alessandro, R.; Pandolfo, G.; Azzimondi, G.; Feruglio, F.S.	1996	Italy	Eur. J. Epidemiol.	N: 365 Aged over 74	Prevalence of dementia was 21.9% (21.9% men, 21.8% women)	Neurological and neuropsychological assessment
Liu, C.K.; Lin, R.T.; Chen, Y.F.; Tai, C.T.; Yen, Y.Y.; Howng, S.L.	1998	China	J. Formos. Med. Assoc.	N: 1016	Prevalence of dementia was 4.4% (3.2% in men and 5.8% in women): 2.0% for those 65 to 74 years old; 8.3% for those 75 to 84 and 24.4% for those ≥85 years; 6.0% for those who were illiterate; AD (22 cases, 48.9%), VaD (11 cases, 24.4%), mixed dementia (MIX: 5 cases, 11.1%)	Chinese Mini-Mental Status Examination (CMMSE), Blessed Dementia Rating Scale, a comprehensive neurobehavioral examination, and neuropsychological tests
Hendrie, H.C.; Osuntokun, B.O.; Hall, K.S.; Ogunniyi, A.O.; Hui, S.L.; Unverzagt, F.W.; Gureje, O.; Rodenberg, C.A.; Baiyewu, O.; Musick, B.S.	1996	United States	Am. J. Psychiatr.	N: 4706 Aged 65 years and older	Prevalence rates of dementia (2.29%) and Alzheimer's disease (1.41%)	Screening stage followed by a clinical assessment

APPENDIX B (CONTINUED)

EPIDEMIOLOGICAL STUDIES IN DEMENTIA, 1995 TO 2000

Authors	Year	Country	Journal	Sample	Prevalence	Tools
Gurland, B.J.; Wilder, D.E.; Lantigua, R.; Stern, Y.; Chen, J.; Killeffer, E.H.; Mayeux, R.	1999	United States	Int. J. Geriatr. Psychiatr.	Randomly selected elderly persons	Prevalence of dementia was found to be higher in Latinos and African-Americans than in non-Latino whites	Screening stage followed by a clinical assessment with regard to functioning in daily tasks and other measures of quality of life
López Pousa, S.; Llinás Regla, J.; Vilalta Franch, J.; Lozano Fernández de Pinedo, L.	1995	Spain	Neurologia	N: 244 people Aged over 65 years	Prevalence: 13.93 ± 4.34% 41.18% AD and VaD, 17.64%	Spanish version of the MMSE, CAMDEX
Lobo, A.; Saz, P.; Marcos, G.; Día, J.L.; De la Cámara, C.	1995	Spain	Arch. Gen. Psychiatr.	N: 1080	5.5% of the elderly were considered to have a dementing disorder; AD: 4.3%, and VaD: 0.6%; depressive disorders were found in 4.8% of the elderly	Spanish versions of the MMSE, the Geriatric Mental State Schedule-Automated, Geriatric Examination for Computer Assisted Taxonomy package
von Strauss, E.; Viitanen. M.; De Ronchi, D.; Winblad, B.; Fratiglioni, L.	1999	Sweden	Arch. Neurol.	N: 1848	AD: 76.5%, VaD: 17.9%; the prevalence of dementia increases from 13% in the 77- to 84-year-old subjects to 48% among persons 95 years and older	Clinical exams by physicians, psychologists, and interviewed by nurses

Authors	Year	Country	Journal	Sample	Results	Method
Farrag, A.; Farwiz, H.M.; Khedr, E.H.; Mahfouz, R.M.; Omran, S.M.	1998	Egypt	*Dement. Geriatr. Cogn. Disord.*	N: 2000 subjects	Prevalence ratio of 4.5. 2.2 for AD, 0.95 for VaD, 0.55 for MIX, and 0.45 for secondary dementias; age-specific prevalence tends to be doubled every 5 years	MMSE test
Azzimondi, G.; D'Alessandro, R.; Pandolfo, G.; Feruglio, F.S.	1998	Italy	*Neuroepidemiology*	Aged over 74 years N: 773	Prevalence was 21.9% (21% men, 21.9% women)	MMSE
Fillenbaum, G.G.; Heyman, A.; Huber, M.S.; Woodbury, M.A.; Leiss, J.; Schmader, K.E.; Bohannon, A.; Trapp Moen, B.	1998	United States	*J. Clin. Epidemiol.*	Aged 65 and older	Prevalence of dementia for persons ≥68 years was 0.070; prevalence of dementia increased through age 84; neither race nor gender differences were significant; incidence increased through age 84	Self- and informant report on health history, functional status, and memory; Consortium to Establish a Registry for Alzheimer's Disease (CERAD), Neuropsychology Battery administered to all subjects, and CERAD Clinical Battery to those with impaired memory; clinical consensus to determine presence and type of dementia
Vilalta Franch, J.; López Pousa, S.; Llinàs Reglà, J.	1998	Spain	*Rev. Neurol.*	Aged over 69 years	The prevalence of depression (depressive disorders plus pseudo-dementia) was 9.1%; in the group of patients with dementia, the frequency of depression was 28.15% while in the group with no dementia it was 5.4%; no differences were seen in the prevalence of depression between patients with Alzheimer-type dementia (ATD) and those with vascular dementia (VD)	CAMDEX

APPENDIX B (CONTINUED)

EPIDEMIOLOGICAL STUDIES IN DEMENTIA, 1995 TO 2000

Authors	Year	Country	Journal	Sample	Prevalence	Tools
McCracken, C.F.; Boneham, M.A.; Copeland, J.R.; Williams, K.E.; Wilson, K.; Scott, A.; McKibbin, P.; Cleave, N.	1997	England	*Br. J. Psychiatr.*	418 people were interviewed with a high percentage (55%) of young elderly (65–74) men	The prevalence of dementia ranged from 2 to 9% and of depression from 5 to 19%, and there were no significant differences in levels between English-speaking ethnic groups and the indigenous population	Geriatric Mental State Examination, AGECAT, and ethnically matched interviewers
Gabryelewicz, T.	1999	Poland	*Psychiatr. Pol.*	Aged 65–84 years *N*: 1000	Prevalences of dementia were found in the age groups 65–69, 70–74, 75–79, 80–84: 1.9, 5.8, 8.6, and 16.5%, respectively; rates for vascular dementia (2.7) were higher than those for dementia of the Alzheimer's type (2.3), mixed dementia (0.5), and secondary dementia (0.2%); in the younger subgroups (65–74 years), vascular dementia was the most frequent and in the older subgroups (75–84 years) the most frequent was Alzheimer's type	MMSE, Cambridge Mental Disorders of the Elderly Examination

Authors	Year	Country	Journal	Sample	Findings	Instrument
Ott, A.; Breteler, M.M.; van Harskamp, F.; Claus, J.J.; van der Cammen, T.J.; Grobbee, D.E.; Hofman, A.	1995	The Netherlands	Br. Med. J.	N: 7528, Aged 55–106 years	Prevalence of 6.3%; prevalence ranged from 0.4% at age 55–59 years to 43.2% at 95 years and over; Alzheimer's disease was the main subdiagnosis (339 cases; 72%); the relative proportion of vascular dementia (76 cases; 16%), Parkinson's disease dementia (30; 6%), and other dementias (24; 5%) decreased with age	MMSE, CERAD battery
Obadia, Y.; Rotily, M.; Degrand Guillaud, A.; Guelain, J.; Ceccaldi, M.; Severo, C.; Poncet, M.; Alperovitch, A.	1997	France	Eur. J. Epidemiol.	N: 1062, Aged 70 years and over	177 cases of dementia (9.2%), including 82 cases of AD (5.5%); prevalence of AD increased significantly with age and was higher among women (OR: 4.24) and persons with no formal educational level (OR: 2.47)	
Woo, J.I.; Lee, J.H.; Yoo, K.Y.; Kim, C.Y.; Kim, Y.I.; Shin, Y.S.	1998	Korea	J. Am. Geriatr. Soc.	N: 2171, Aged 65 years and over	The prevalence of total dementia was 8.8% for men and 9.9% for women; the prevalence of Alzheimer's disease was 3.2% for men and 5.3% for women and that of vascular dementia 3.1 and 2.1%, respectively	Korean version of the Mini-Mental State Examination (MMSE-K)
Rajkumar, S.; Kumar, S.; Thara, R.	1997	India	Int. J. Geriat. Psychiat.	N: 750, Aged 60 years and older	The prevalence of dementia was 3.5%, the percentage increasing with age; these rural prevalence estimates were higher than in urban settings	Geriatric Mental State schedule (GMS)

APPENDIX B (CONTINUED)

EPIDEMIOLOGICAL STUDIES IN DEMENTIA, 1995 TO 2000

Authors	Year	Country	Journal	Sample	Prevalence	Tools
Copeland, J.R.; McCracken, C.F.; Dewey, M.E.; Wilson, K.C.; Doran, M.; Gilmore, C.; Scott, A.; Larkin, B.A.	1999	England	*Br. J. Psychiatr.*	5222 individuals aged ≥65 years	Incidence rates of the dementias increase with age; the patterns are similar between AD and VaD; in England and Wales the dementia cases expected each year are: 39,437 AD, 20,515 VaD, and 155,169 Undifferentiated	Geriatric Mental State/History and Aetiology Schedule
Gussekloo, J.; Heeren, T.J.; Izaks, G.J.; Ligthart, G.J.; Rooijmans, H.G.	1995	The Netherlands	*J. Neurol. Neurosurg. Psychiatr.*	Aged 85 years and over	The overall incidence of dementia was 6.9 per 100 person-years at risk; the incidence was significantly higher for women than for men, respectively, 8.9 vs. 2.7 per 100 person-years at risk; in the fastest growing age group 7 out of 100 persons develop dementia each year	MMSE followed in a stratified sample by the geriatric mental state schedule (A3)/AGECAT

Authors	Year	Country	Journal	Sample	Findings	Methods
Liu, C.K.; Lai, C.L.; Tai, C.T.; Lin, R.T.; Yen, Y.Y.; Howng, S.L.	1998	Taiwan	*Neurology*	N: 2915 community inhabitants Aged 65 years and older	The annual incidence for total dementia was 1.28%, which increased with age from 0.77% for 65- to 74-year-olds to 6.19% for persons aged 85 years or older; AD (25 cases, 41.7%, IR = 0.54%) was the most common cause of dementia, followed by VaD (19 cases, 31.7%, IR = 0.41%) and mixed dementia (9 cases, 15.0%)	MMSE
Zhang, M.; Katzman, R.; Yu, E.; Liu, W.; Xiao, S.F.; Yan, H.	1998	China	*Psychiatr. Clin. Neurosci.*	N: 1970 subjects Aged 65 or older	The total incidence of dementia was 1.15% annually, 0.98% for males and 1.27% for females	MMSE, medical history and physical examination, a neurological examination and an intensive neuropsychiatric interview and testings
Kiyohara, Y.	1999	Japan	*Rinsho Shinkeigaku*	Elderly persons from a Japanese community of Hisayama	Among the 58 cases of dementia, the frequency of vascular dementia (VD) was 43%: the rate was 2 times higher than that for Alzheimer's disease (AD); in the subjects of VD, the most frequent type of stroke was due to small-artery disease, which caused multiple lacunar infarction (40%) and Binswanger's disease (12%)	MMSE

4 Neuroanatomy of the Functional Aging Brain

José León-Carrión, Héctor Salgado,
Manuel Murga Sierra, Javier Márquez-Rivas,
and María Rosario Domínguez-Morales

CONTENTS

4.1 Introduction 67
4.2 Cerebral Atrophy in Elderly People 68
4.3 White and Gray Matter 70
4.4 Cerebral Ventricles 71
4.5 Corpus Callosum 74
4.6 Limbic Structures 76
4.7 Frontal Lobe 77
4.8 Basal Ganglia and Cerebellum 78
4.9 Other Structures 79
4.10 Concluding Remarks 79
References 79

4.1 INTRODUCTION

Does the brain really age? It seems that accumulated experience clearly indicates that throughout a lifetime cognitive, emotional, and behavioral functions regulated by the brain tend to decline, some more than others and more severely in certain people. It seems probable that the neuropsychological decline is closely associated with the appearance of diseases that affect the brain. As early as 1951, Vogt and Vogt[1] proposed the term *pathoclisis* to refer to the vulnerability of brain tissue to time. They affirmed that some gray matter structures exhibited a higher susceptibility to pathogens.

The recent appearance of modern techniques of neuroimaging is allowing scientists to study different cerebral structures and their functioning noninvasively. This can be done in sick people as well as healthy people, young and old. Thanks to these recent advances, this chapter reviews some of the latest discoveries about the aging of the functional brain.

0-8493-2066-/01/$0.00+$1.50
© 2001 by CRC Press LLC

4.2   CEREBRAL ATROPHY IN ELDERLY PEOPLE

Findings obtained from studies of age-related changes in brain morphology and behavior of mice have demonstrated age-dependent cerebral atrophy and cognitive dysfunction. Shimada[2] followed the apparently normal development of mice and found that mice developed brain atrophy with advancing age. The neocortex was diffusely atrophic in aged mice, with the frontal cortex the most affected. The enthorinal cortex, amygdala, and nucleus accumbens were also atrophic. Other subcortical structures were mildly atrophic, but the hippocampus was not atrophic. Mild to moderate hypertrophic astrocytosis was observed in the atrophied regions but no Alzheimer-type pathology was seen. The cortical atrophy was due to both loss of neurons and shrinkage. Brain atrophy was not remarkable in normal aging control mice. Because of the morphological changes observed, cognitive impairment was observed with advancing age. All these features of mice were inherited (Figure 4.1).

The cerebral hemisphere becomes atrophic with age. Oguro et al.[3] studied cerebral structures in 152 normal subjects older than 40 using magnetic resonance imaging (MRI). They observed that men showed significant age-associated atrophy in the tegmentum and pretectum of the midbrain and the base of the pons. In women, only the pretectum of the midbrain showed significant aging effects after the age of 50, and thereafter remained rather constant. They found that only men had significant age-related reduction in the cerebellar vermis area after the age of 70. Both men and women showed supratentorial brain atrophy that progressed by decades. In men, correlation between supratentorial brain atrophy and the diameter of the ventral midbrain, pretectum, and base of the pons was also found. In women, correlation was found between brain atrophy and the diameter of the fourth ventricle.

Using MRI-based planimetry, Woo et al.[4] measured cortical and ventricular atrophy in patients with Alzheimer's disease (AD). They found that patients with AD exhibited greater cerebral atrophy than control subjects. Cerebral atrophy was significantly correlated with age in healthy volunteers but not in patients with AD. In patients with AD, age of onset was negatively correlated with the estimated rate of disease-attributed cerebral degeneration. Age, age of onset, and their interaction successfully explained cerebral and cortical atrophy in patients with probable AD. Woo et al. concluded that age of onset may be a strong predictor of the rate of cerebral degeneration in AD, so the control of age and the age of onset are essential in the quantitative study of AD.

Significant sex differences in the aging of brain were found by Murphy et al.[5] They found, in the magnetic resonance imaging study, that age-related volume loss was greater in men than in women in whole brain as well as frontal and temporal lobes, whereas it was greater in women than men in hippocampus and parietal lobes. They also found that, in the positron emission tomography (PET) study, significant sex differences existed in the effect of age on regional brain metabolism, and asymmetry of metabolism in the temporal and parietal lobes, Broca's area, thalamus, and hippocampus.

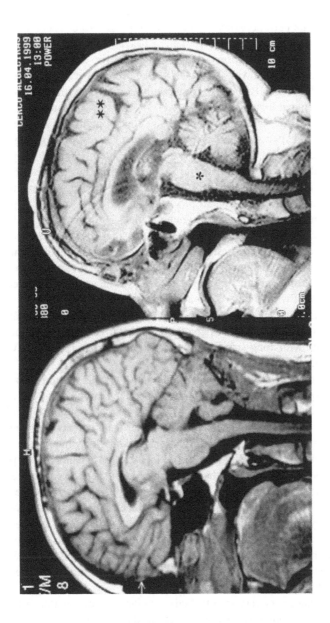

FIGURE 4.1 Cerebral atrophy: Base of the pons (*) and supratentorial giral atrophy (**). 70 years (right) – 25 years (left).

4.3 WHITE AND GRAY MATTER

In the transmission of information within the brain and between the central nervous system (CNS) and the periphery, myelin plays an important role related to velocity and reliability. Normally, when a demyelinating disease appears, neurobehavioral and cognitive deficits can be observed. Normal cognitive development requires normal myelination of the pathways of the CNS. One of the most frequent and easily observed abnormalities in MRI images is the well-known white matter hyperintensities (WMH) or leukoaraiosis (see Figure 4.1). A study by Salonen et al.[6] found that signal intensity of the white matter increased concomitantly with widening of the cerebrospinal fluid spaces while basal ganglia remained stable. High-signal foci in white matter increased in number and size after the age of 50, and the periventricular high-signal foci were constant after the age of 65. They suggest that their visual impression of a decrease in signal intensity of the central gray matter with age seems to be mistaken. Pathological processes should be suspected if periventricular foci are found in middle-aged or young subjects.

It is widely accepted that when WMH appear in the MRI images, the actual neuropathological changes in the brain are shown. Nevertheless, the originally proposed link between this phenomenon and cerebrovascular disease is somewhat tenuous; although cerebrovascular risks play a role in producing WMH, age emerges as the best predictor of white matter lesions.[7] An equal frequency of WMH has been observed in normal aged people and in matched patients with stroke and AD, although the severity of the lesion was greater in the latter patients.[8,9] The incidence of WMH increases with long-standing hypertension,[10] and it is unclear whether diabetes is a risk factor in elderly people.[11,12]

A study by Bronge et al.[13] found that white matter lesions in patients with AD are influenced by apolipoprotein E (APOE) genotype. They examined 60 AD patients with MRI and observed that patients with the APOE genotype sygma4/4 had more extensive white matter lesions in the deep white matter than patients with genotypes sygma3/3 and sygma3/4. There was a correlation with age for white matter lesions in the deep white matter in patients with the APOE sygma3/3 genotype. In patients carrying at least one sygma4 allele, the white matter lesions showed no age correlation. The authors conclude that in APOE allele sygma4 carriers, white matter lesions represent a pathological process related to the etiology of the disease.

It has been hypothesized that the pathology underlying most of the WMH emerges in a chain of events that starts with age-related neuron loss, which results in axonal degeneration and subsequent invasion of the cerebrospinal fluid (CSF) into perivascular spaces. So, leukoaraiosis is related to water content of the white matter, which increases dramatically with advancing age.[7]

On the other hand, it is very rare to find variations in gray matter in the aged brain. Hence, when hypointense spots are found in the gray matter, they should be interpreted as clear signs of specific brain damage.

4.4 CEREBRAL VENTRICLES

Wen et al.[14] conducted a study of Biondi ring tangles (BRTs) in the choroid plexus (CP) of AD and normal aging brains. The CP produces up to 90% (450 to 1000 ml/day) of CSF to nourish and to protect the brain in the CSF suspension. The CP also acts as a selective barrier between blood and CSF to regulate ions and other essential molecules. The accumulation of intracellular inclusions called BRTs in CP cells of AD and aging brains may affect the vital function of the CP of producing the CSF. Therefore, these authors suggested that BRTs might represent a significant and measurable biomarker for AD.

In aging people an important cause of dementia is idiopathic normal pressure hydrocephalus (NPH). Usually, it is difficult to differentiate between normal aging and vascular dementias in which brain atrophy with ventricular dilatation (hydrocephalus exvacuo or central atrophy) is present. A study was conducted by Kitagaki et al.[15] to elucidate the distinctive features of the distribution of CSF in idiopathic NPH. They used MRI to investigate the morphological features and volume of CSF space in patients with idiopathic NPH compared with those with other dementias. Results showed that patients with idiopathic NPH had significantly increased CSF volume in the ventricles and decreased volume in the superior convexity and medial subaracnoid spaces as compared with patients presenting with other dementias. The Sylvian CSF volume in patients with idiopathic NPH was significantly greater than in patients with AD. The volume of the basal cistern was comparable among the three groups. In several patients with idiopathic NPH, focally dilated sulci were observed over the convexity or medial surface of the hemisphere. They concluded by indicating that their findings of enlarged basal cisterns and Sylvian fissures and of focally dilated sulci support, rather than exclude, the diagnosis of shunt-responsive idiopathic NPH and suggest that this condition is caused by a suprasylvian subaracnoid block (Figure 4.2).

Another study, by Foundas et al.,[16] investigated the age-related changes of the insular cortex and lateral ventricles using conventional MRI volumetric measures. Significant age-related changes were found in the lateral ventricles and in the CSF insular space. Increasing age accounted for a significant amount of the variance for the lateral ventricle, but not for the insula. They also observed that, although there was a continuous linear increase in lateral ventricular volume with age, the CSF insular space increased linearly until the fourth decade, then plateaued until the seventh decade, with a linear increase thereafter. The authors suggest that age-related changes occur in the region of the insular cortex, but differ from age-related changes of the lateral ventricles.

Bakshi et al.[7] performed an analysis of 100 consecutive normal studies of intraventricular CSF pulsation artifact (VCSFA) on fast fluid-attenuated inversion recovery (FLAIR) MRI. Results showed that 72 subjects had VCSFA in at least one ventricular cavity. The fourth ventricle was the most common site of VCSFA, followed by the third ventricle, and the lateral ventricles. VCSFA was usually severe

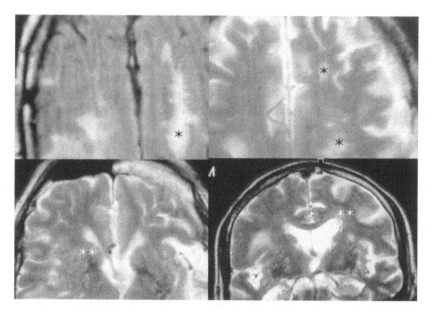

FIGURE 4.2   Cerebral leukoaraiosis. Axial and coronal MRI images. Periventricular **
and semiovale centrum lesions *.

in the third and fourth ventricles. Fourth ventricular VCSFA was significantly associated with third ventricular VCSFA. Increasing third ventricular size and, to a lesser
extent, increasing age, were significantly associated with VCSFA. Ghost pulsation
of VCSFA occurred across the brain parenchyma in the phase encoding direction.
The authors concluded that VCSFA on axial FLAIR images represented artifact
inflows caused by inversion delay and ghosting effects. VCSFA might obscure or
mimic intraventricular lesions, especially in the third and fourth ventricles. Although
common in adults of all ages, VCSFA is associated with advancing age and increasing ventricular size. Thus, altered CSF flow dynamics that occur with ventriculom-
egaly and aging contribute to VCSFA on axial FLAIR MRI images (Figure 4.3).

Berardi et al.[18] have studied the effect of ventricular size on cognition. They
studied the discrepancy between face–word memory compared with right–left asymmetry of lateral ventricle size in right-handed young and elderly subjects. Results
showed that older subjects differed significantly from young subjects in face but
not word memory. Old subjects had significantly larger lateral ventricles and more
lateral ventricle asymmetry than did young subjects. They did not observe any group
trend toward disproportionate age-related enlargement of the right ventricle relative
to the left. In older people, lateral ventricle asymmetry is correlated with face–word
memory discrepancies in the expected direction. Worse word than face memory was
associated with disproportionate enlargement of the left lateral ventricle. Those
correlations were not significant in young subjects. The authors concluded by suggesting that the group trend toward disproportionate nonverbal/visual, as opposed
to verbal age-related memory differences, was not associated with a group trend
toward disproportionate enlargement of the right ventricle. Individual deviations

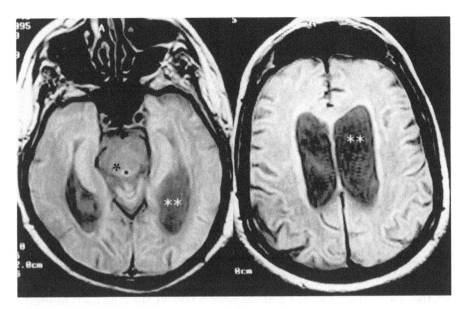

FIGURE 4.3   Normal pressure hydrocephalus: Ventricular dilatation (**) and cerebral aqueduct with fluid-attenuated inversion (*).

from the normative pattern of age-related ventricle enlargement, however, are associated with different patterns of material-specific memory changes.

There is a significant enlargement of the maximum width of the interhemispheric fissure in males and females. There is also a significant enlargement of the ventricular system that is more severe in men than in women in aged schizophrenics as seen in computed tomography (CT) compared with normal controls.[19] Based upon the relation between the third ventricle enlargement and the positive and depressive symptoms in all patients, it is suggested that the advanced third ventricle enlargement may decrease these symptoms in aged schizophrenics. In the same way, Garver et al.[20] suggest that the atrophic psychosis identified by progressive ventricular enlargement throughout adult illness, exhibiting delayed response of positive symptoms during neuroleptic treatment, may also proceed to a praecox dementia in later life. In contrast, in a putative neurodevelopmental psychosis associated with static ventricles during the course of adult illness, conventional neuroleptics appear to have little effect (except sedation) on positive symptoms, but do appear to induce negative symptomatology and partial disengagement from the burden of persistent psychotic thought processes in such static ventricle psychosis (Figure 4.4).

Studies on age-related changes of diffusional anisotropy in the cerebral white matter in normal subjects were conducted by Hanyu et al.[21] The anisotropic rotations (ARs) are the apparent diffusion coefficients perpendicular to the nerve fibers to those parallel to the nerve fibers. They found that ARs were significantly higher in elderly than in young subjects in the anterior and posterior white matter surrounding the lateral ventricle. Significant correlation between age and AR was found in the anterior white matter. The ventricular index was significantly higher as an indicator of brain atrophy in elderly than in younger subjects, and significantly correlated

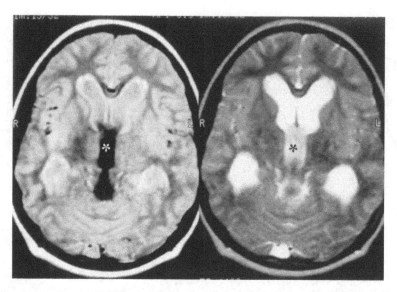

FIGURE 4.4   Altered CSF flow dynamics patent in MRI. VCSFA in the third ventricle (*).

with AR in the anterior white matter. The ventricular index also showed the highest correlation for AR. No significant correlation among ARs, the corpus callosum (CC), and age was observed.

4.5 CORPUS CALLOSUM

Different authors have studied the possibility of age-related differences in the anatomy of the CC. Silver et al.[22] conducted a study of the magnetization transfer ratio (MTR) of normal brain white matter. They observed the highest values in the CC. No significant sex differences were found for any region studied. Small but significant age-related reductions in MTR were noted in the CC. These small but significant differences related to age have to be considered when evaluating MTR in pathological states.

A study was conducted by Salat et al.[23] using MRI to examine sex differences in CC atrophy in 76 healthy elderly subjects. They used the cerebellum and pons as noncortical control structures, and also related CC and its subregions to cognition. Results showed that women had a slightly larger posterior sector of the CC than men did. Age-related atrophy of the anterior and middle sectors of the CC but not the posterior sector was observed in women but not in men. They also found that cerebellum and pons size were similar in men and women not showing age-related atrophy. Visual memory was related to CC area in women but not in men; they did not find other significant structures related to cognition. This finding suggests that selective age-related atrophy of the CC differs in men and woman late in life.

A study by Davatzikos and Resnick,[24] using a new image analysis technique to investigate local variability in brain morphology, found a robust sex difference in the splenium of the CC. They observed a greater interhemispheric connectivity in women in the MRI images from 114 individuals. In addition, they found that bulbosity of the CC obtained a good correlation with a better cognitive performance in women but not in men. These findings also suggest that the degree of interhemispheric connectivity has different implications for men and women.

Neuroimaging research on AD has revealed some particularities of the CC, suggesting a loss of metabolic functional interactions between different cortical regions. Atrophy of CC as the major tract of intracortical connective fibers may reflect decreased cortical functional integration. Teipel et al.[25] investigated if regional atrophy of the CC is correlated with regional reductions of cortical glucose metabolism, and whether primary white matter degeneration is a possible cofactor of CC atrophy in AD. They found that the total cross-sectional area of CC was significantly reduced in patients with AD, with the most prominent changes in the rostrum and splenium and relative sparing of the body of the CC. Frontal and parietal lobe metabolism was correlated with the truncal area of the CC in AD. White matter hyperintensities did not correlate with CC atrophy in the patients with AD.

A study by Hampel et al.[26] evaluated the CC as an *in vivo* marker for cortical neuronal loss. They observed that the total callosal area was significantly reduced in the patients with AD, with the greatest changes in the rostrum and splenium and relative sparing of the callosal body. Regional callosal atrophy correlated significantly with cognitive impairment in patients with AD, but not with age or the white matter hyperintensities score. They concluded that callosal atrophy in patients with AD with only minimal white matter changes may indicate loss of callosal efferent neurons in corresponding regions of the cortex. Because these neurons are a subset of corticocortical projecting neurons, region-specific callosal atrophy may serve as a marker of progressive neocortical disconnection in AD (Figure 4.5).

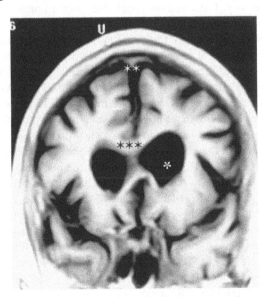

FIGURE 4.5   Cognitive deterioration in the elderly: Ventricular enlargement (*), enlargement of interhemispheric fissure (**) and corpus callosum atrophy (***).

Thompson et al.[27] observed a midsagittal loss of 24.5% at the CC posterior midbody of the CC that matched with increases in structural variability in corresponding temporoparietal projection areas. Confidence limits on three-dimensional (3D) cortical variation, visualized in 3D, exhibited severe increases in AD from 2 to 4 mm at the callosum to a peak of 19.6 mm at the posterior left Sylvian fissure. Normal Sylvian fissure asymmetries (right higher than left) were accentuated in AD and were greater in patients with AD than in controls. The author suggested that severe AD-related increases in 3D variability and asymmetry may reflect disease-related disruption of the commissural system connecting bilateral temporal and parietal cortical zones, regions known to be at risk of early metabolic dysfunction, perfusion deficits, and selective neuronal loss in AD.

4.6 LIMBIC STRUCTURES

Surprisingly, age-related shrinkage is minimal in the limbic-diencephalic areas. A study by Raz et al.[28] found in the hippocampal formation only a weak trend toward age-related shortening of the gray matter T1. They also found no correlation between age and the volume of the two other limbic regions, the parahippocampal gyrus (a part of the entorhinal cortex) and the anterior cingulate gyrus. Contrary to their hypothesis, in the examined age range the volume of limbic structures was unrelated to any of the cognitive functions; verbal working memory, verbal explicit memory, and verbal priming were independent of cortical volumes. Nevertheless, among the participants older than 60, reduction in the volume of the limbic structures predicted declines in explicit memory. Chronological age adversely influenced all cognitive indices, although its effect on priming was only indirect, mediated by declines in verbal working memory. These authors concluded that the limbic-diencephalic areas are relatively stable with age.

The frequency of hippocampal formation atrophy (HA) in normal aging and AD was evaluated by Santi et al.[29] They observed HA in 29% of the normal elderly group, strongly related to increasing age: 15% of normal people between 60 and 75 years had HA, and 48% of subjects 76 to 90 years old had HA. Among the groups of patients, the frequency of HA ranged from 78% in those with memory and cognitive impairments to 96% in the advanced AD groups. Unlike the normal elderly group, percentages were not related to age. A disproportionate number of males having HA was found in the normal elderly group and in the cognitive impairment group when compared with females. The results demonstrate that hippocampal formation atrophy is related to memory and cognitive impairments.

A study by Mu et al.[30] evaluated the normal age-specific values for the hippocampal formation, the amygdala, and the temporal horn of the lateral ventricle by age group, ranging from 40 to 90 years of age. They found significant differences in standardized volumes of the hippocampal formation, the amygdala, and the temporal horn among the 61- to 70-year-old, 71- to 80-year-old, and 81- to 90-year-old groups. They were not significant between the 40- to 50-year-old and 51- to 60-year-old groups. The authors did not find significant differences in side or sex among the age groups for any of the structures. They concluded that age has to be considered when evaluating neuroimages, especially in patients in the early stages of AD.

4.7 FRONTAL LOBE

A study by Raz et al.[31] found that shrinkage of the prefrontal cortex mediates age-related increases in perseveration. Levine et al.[32] evaluated the hypothesis that age cognitive decline is related to frontal dysfunction. They used conditional associative learning (CAL) including inhibitory processing as a measure of frontal function. Results show that older adults and focal frontal patients showed impaired CAL performance, but the deficit was greater in the latter group, where it was specific to participants with dorsolateral prefrontal cortical lesions. The deficits were attributable to strategic rather than basic associative processes. Data suggest that age-related decline in inhibitory processes is due to dorsolateral prefrontal dysfunction.

A study using PET to explore the neurophysiological changes related to cognitive disability in aging with a focus on frontal lobe was conducted by Esposito et al.,[33] in people between 18 to 80 years old, using the Wisconsin Card Sorting Test (WCST) and Raven's Progressive Matrices (RPM). They observed task-specific reductions of regional cerebral blood flow (rCBF) activation with age in the dorsolateral prefrontal cortex during the WCST and in portions of the inferolateral temporal cortex involved in visuospatial processing during the RPM. They also found reduced ability to suppress rCBF in the right hippocampal region during WCST and in mesial and polar portions of the prefrontal cortex during the execution of the two tests. Task-dependent alterations with age in the relationship between the dorsolateral prefrontal cortex and the hippocampus were also documented. The authors indicate that, despite some cognitive overlap between the two tests and the age-related cognitive decline in both, many of the changes in rCBF activation with age were task-specific, reflecting functional alteration of the different neural circuits involved in the performance of WCST by young people. Reduced activation of areas critical for the execution of the tests in conjunction with the inability to suppress areas normally not involved in the performance of the two tests suggest that, overall, reduced ability to focus neural activity may be impaired in older subjects. The authors indicated that the context dependencies of the age-related changes are most consistent with system failure and disordered connectivity.

An interesting study was performed by Pfefferbaum et al.[34] reporting on structural brain changes during a 5-year period in healthy control and alcoholic men. They obtained MRI scanning images during treatment and 5 years later, and compared images with those from a control group. Results showed that the cortical gray matter diminished in volume over time in control subjects, most prominently in the prefrontal cortex, while the lateral and third ventricle enlarged. The alcoholic patients showed similar age-related changes with a greater rate of gray matter volume loss than the control subjects in the anterior superior temporal lobe. The amount of alcohol consumed during follow-up predicted the rate of cortical gray matter volume loss, as well as sulcal expansion. The rate of ventricular enlargement in alcoholic patients who maintained virtual sobriety was comparable with that in the control subjects. The authors concluded that during a 5-year period, brain volume shrinkage is exaggerated in the prefrontal cortex in normal aging with additional loss in the anterior superior temporal cortex in alcoholism. The association of cortical gray matter volume reduction with alcohol consumption over time suggests that continued alcohol abuse results in progressive brain tissue volume shrinkage.

Brennan et al.[35] investigated the possibility of changes in executive functioning associated with the prefrontal zone of the brain. They employed the Tower of Hanoi task. Analysis of results showed similar executive capacities among the young adult group and the older group in the three-disk task (the easiest task to do). On the four-disk task, where problem-solving complexity increased, young adult participants showed superior performance than either young elderly or older elderly participants. These findings are consistent with the hypothesis of age differences in executive functioning.

Kramer et al.[36] reported similar conclusions in a series of three studies examining age-related differences in executive control processes and more specifically in the executive control processes that underlie performance in the task-switching paradigm. First, they observed that large, age-related differences in switch costs were found early in the practice. Second, and most surprising for them, after relatively modest amounts of practice old and young adult switch costs were equivalent. Older adults showed large practice effects on switch trials. Third, age-equivalent switch costs were maintained across a 2-month retention period. Finally, the main constraint on whether age equivalence was observed in task-switching performance was memory load. Older adults were unable to capitalize on practice under high memory loads.

Clinical and pathological evidence for a variant of AD was observed by Johnson et al.[37] They identified a subgroup of patients with pathological confirmed AD who presented disproportionate impairments on frontal lobe functioning tests and had a higher-than-expected degree of neurofibrilary tangle pathology in the frontal lobe during the early stages of dementia. These findings suggest the existence of a frontal variant of AD that has distinctive clinical and pathological features.

A review of the theories of the frontal lobe[38] related to cognitive aging suggests that the prefrontal cortex has a general function of temporal integration supported by four specific processes: prospective memory, retrospective memory, interference control, and inhibition of strong responses. The frontal lobe theories seem to perform well for aging, with the exception of an inability to account for age-related declines in item recall and recognition memory, possibly as a result of age-related declines in medial temporal function.

4.8 BASAL GANGLIA AND CEREBELLUM

It is well known that motor activity is not the same across the life span, and changes with normal aging. Basal ganglia has been associated with planning, execution, and control of movements.[39] Age-dependent loss of neurons in the putamen and in the caudate nucleus, as well as a reduction of the volume of the caudate and the lentiform nuclei, have been documented in postmortem investigations by Raz et al.[40] Age-related iron accumulation in the globus pallidus produces areas of hypointensity that may distort volume estimates. The extent of the hypodense spots in this zone is related to the aging brain.[41]

Autopsy of brains has revealed an age-related shrinkage of cerebellum, a reduction in the cerebellar weight, and an attrition of the cells of Purkinje in the cerebellar hemispheres and in the vermis.[42,43]

4.9 OTHER STRUCTURES

Some cerebral structures maintain their size throughout the lifetime, as is the case of those in the brain stem: the pons and medulla.[44] The same occurs with the tectum.[45] Volumetrically, the ventral pons and medulla remain stable across the life span.[46,47]

4.10 CONCLUDING REMARKS

The data reviewed here clearly indicate that with time, the morphology and functioning of the brain change. This change is not the same for the whole brain, and it appears there are structures that remain more stable across the life span (hippocampus, parahippocampal and cingulate gyrus, and insula, pons, medulla, tectum). Other areas are areas prone to be affected (frontal and prefrontal lobe, basal ganglia, cerebellum, cerebral ventricles, corpus callosum) by aging. The causes and mechanisms of such selective aging are still uncertain.

Structural and functional aging of the brain have functional implications. Depending on the areas of the brain affected by the passing of time in a certain person, behavior, cognition, and emotions are affected. However, this is not the purpose of this work but rather the subject of following chapters.

REFERENCES

1. Vogt, C. and Vogt, O., Importance of neuroanatomy in the field of neuropathology, *Neurology*, 1, 205–218, 1951.
2. Shimada, A., Age-dependent cerebral atrophy and cognitive dysfunction in SAMP10 mice, *Neurobiol. Aging*, 20, 125–136, 1999.
3. Oguro, H. et al., Sex differences in morphology of the brain stem and cerebellum with normal aging, *Neuroradiology*, 40, 788–792, 1998.
4. Woo, J. I., Kim, J. H., and Lee, J. H., Age of onset and brain atrophy in Alzheimer's disease, *Int. Psychogeriatr.*, 9, 183–196, 1997.
5. Murphy, D. et al., Age-related differences in volumes of subcortical nuclei, brain matter, and cerebro-spinal fluid in healthy men as measured with magnetic resonance imaging (MRI), *Arch. Neurol.*, 49, 839–845, 1996.
6. Salonen, O. et al., MRI of the brain in neurologically healthy middle-aged and elderly individuals, *Neuroradiology*, 39, 537–545, 1997.
7. Raz, N., Neuroanatomy of the aging brain observed *in vivo*: a review of structural MRI findings, in *Neuroimaging II: Clinical Applications*, Bigler, E. D., Ed., Plenum Press, New York, 1996, chap. 6.
8. Kozachuck, W. E. et al., White matter hyperintensities in dementia of Alzheimer's type and in healthy subjects without cerebrovascular risk factors, *Arch. Neurol.*, 42, 1306–1310, 1990.

9. Leys, D. et al., Periventricular and white matter magnetic resonance imaging hyper-
    intensities do not differ between Alzheimer's disease and normal aging, *Arch. Neurol.*,
    47, 524–527, 1990.
10. Yamashita, K. et al., The relationship between cerebral white matter changes, mental
    function and blood pressure in normal elderly, *Jpn. J. Geriatr.*, 28, 546–550, 1991.
11. Araki, Y. et al., MRI of the brain in diabetes mellitus, *Neuroradiology*, 36,
    101–103, 1994.
12. Schmidt, R. et al., Magnetic resonance imaging signal hyperintensities in the deep
    and subcortical white matter, *Arch. Neurol.*, 49, 825–827, 1992.
13. Bronge, L. et al., White matter lesions in Alzheimer patients are influenced by
    apolipoprotein E genotype, *Dement. Geriatr. Cogn. Disord.*, 10, 89–96, 1999.
14. Wen, G. Y., Wisniewski, H. M., and Kassack, R. J., Biondi ring tangles in the choroid
    plexus of Alzheimer's disease and normal aging brains: a quantitative study, *Brain
    Res.*, 832, 40–46, 1999.
15. Kitagaki, H. et al., CSF spaces in idiopathic normal pressure hydrocephalus: mor-
    phology and volumetry, *Am. J. Neuroradiol.*, 19, 1277–1284, 1998.
16. Foundas, A. L., Zipin, D., and Browning, C. A., Age-related changes of the insular
    cortex and lateral ventricles: conventional MRI volumetric measures, *J. Neuroimag-
    ing*, 8, 216–221, 1998.
17. Bakshi, R. et al., Intraventricular CSF pulsation artifact on fast fluid-attenuated
    inversion-recovery MR images: analysis of 100 consecutive normal studies, *Am. J.
    Neuroradiol.*, 21, 503–508, 2000.
18. Berardi, A. et al., Face and word memory differences are related to patterns of right
    and left lateral ventricle size in healthy aging, *J. Gerontol. B Psychol. Sci. Soc. Sci.*,
    52, 54–61, 1997.
19. Seno, H. et al., Computed tomographic study of aged schizophrenic patients, *Psy-
    chiatr. Clin. Neurosci.*, 51, 373–377, 1997.
20. Garver, D. L. et al., Atrophic and static (neurodevelopmental) schizophrenic psycho-
    ses: premorbid functioning, symptoms and neuroleptic response, *Neuropsychophar-
    macology*, 21, 82–92, 1999.
21. Hanyu, H. et al., Age-related changes of diffusional anisotropy in the cerebral white
    matter in normal subjects, *No To Shinkei*, 49, 331–336, 1997.
22. Silver, N. C. et al., Magnetisation transfer ratio of normal brain white matter: a
    normative database spanning four decades of life, *J. Neurol. Neurosurg. Psychiatr.*,
    63, 223–228, 1997.
23. Salat, D. et al., Sex differences in the corpus callosum with aging, *Neurobiol. Aging*,
    18, 191–197, 1997.
24. Davatzikos, C. and Resnick, S. M., Sex differences in anatomic measures of inter-
    hemispheric connectivity: correlations with cognition in women but not men, *Cereb.
    Cortex*, 8, 635–640, 1998.
25. Teipel, S. J. et al., Region-specific corpus callosum atrophy correlates with the
    regional pattern of cortical glucose metabolism in Alzheimer disease, *Arch. Neurol.*,
    56, 467–473, 1999.
26. Hampel, H. et al., Corpus callosum atrophy is a possible indicator of region- and cell
    type-specific neuronal degeneration in Alzheimer disease: a magnetic resonance imag-
    ing analysis, *Arch. Neurol.*, 55, 193–198, 1998.
27. Thompson, P. M. et al., Cortical variability and asymmetry in normal aging and
    Alzheimer's disease, *Cereb. Cortex*, 8, 492–509, 1998.

28. Raz, N., Millman, D., and Sarpel, G., Cerebral correlates of cognitive aging: gray–white matter differentiation in the medial temporal lobes, and fluid vs. crystallized abilities, *Psychobiology*, 18, 475–481, 1990.

29. Santi, S. et al., Frequency of hippocampal formation atrophy in normal aging and Alzheimer's disease, *Neurobiol Aging*, 18, 1–11, 1997.

30. Mu, Q. et al., A quantitative MR study of the hippocampal formation, the amygdala, and the temporal horn of the lateral ventricle in healthy subjects 40 to 90 years of age, *Am. J. Neuroradiol.*, 20, 207–211, 1999.

31. Raz, N. et al., Neuroanatomical correlates of cognitive aging: evidence from structural magnetic resonance imaging, *Neuropsychology*, 12, 95–114, 1998.

32. Levine, B., Stuss, D. T., and Milberg, W. P., Effects of aging on conditional associative learning: process analyses and comparison with focal frontal lesions, *Neuropsychology*, 11, 367–381, 1997.

33. Esposito, G. et al., Context-dependent, neural system-specific neuropsychological concomitants of aging: mapping PET correlates during cognitive activation, *Brain*, 122, 963–979, 1999.

34. Pfefferbaum, A. et al., A controlled study of cortical gray matter and ventricular changes in alcoholic men over a 5-year interval, *Arch. Gen. Psychiatr.*, 55, 905–912, 1998.

35. Brennan, M., Welsh, M. C., and Fisher, C. B., Aging and executive function skills: an examination of a community-dwelling older adult population, *Percept. Mot. Skills*, 84, 1187–1197, 1997.

36. Kramer, A. F., Hahn, S., and Gopher, D., Task coordination and aging: explorations of executive control processes in the task switching paradigm, *Acta Psychol.* (Amsterdam), 101, 339–378, 1999.

37. Johnson, J. K. et al., Clinical and pathological evidence for a frontal variant of Alzheimer disease, *Arch. Neurol.*, 56, 1233–1239, 1999.

38. West, R. L., An application of prefrontal cortex function theory to cognitive aging, *Psychol. Bull.*, 120, 272–292, 1996.

39. Alheid, G. E., Switzer III, R. C., and Heimer, L., Basal ganglia, in *The Human Nervous System*, Paxinos, G., Ed., Academic Press, San Diego, 1990, 483–583.

40. Raz, N., Torres, I., and Acker, J. D., Age, gender, and hemispheric differences in human striatum: a quantitative review and new data from *in vivo* MRI morphometry, *Neurobiol. Learning Memory*, 63, 133–142, 1995.

41. Milton, W. J. et al., Deep gray matter hypointensity patterns with aging in healthy adults: MR imaging at 1.5 T, *Radiology*, 181, 715–719, 1991.

42. Ellis, R. S., Norms for some structural changes in human cerebellum from birth to old age, *J. Comp. Neurol.*, 32, 1–33, 1920.

43. Torvik, A., Torp, S., and Lindboe, C. F., Atrophy of the cerebellar vermis in aging: a morphometric and histological study, *J. Neurol. Sci.*, 76, 283–294, 1986.

44. Blinkov, S. M. and Glezer, I. I., *The Human Brain in Figures and Tables*, Basic Books, New York, 1968.

45. Raz, N. and Acker, J. D., Differential aging of subcortical structures observed *in vivo*: a prospective study, paper presented at the Annual Meeting of the European Neuroscience Association, Vienna, Austria, September, 1994.

46. Shah, S. A. et al., Posterior fossa abnormalities in major depression: a controlled magnetic resonance imaging study, *Acta Psychiatr. Scand.*, 85, 474–479, 1992.

47. Carper, R. A., Kaye, J. A., and Janowsky, J. S., Quantitative MRI analysis of normal and abnormal brain aging, *Soc. Neurosci. Abstr.*, 19, 179, 1993.

Part II

Cognition and Behavior
in Elderly People

Part II

Cognition and Behavior in Elderly People

5 General Cognitive Changes with Aging

Linas A. Bieliauskas

CONTENTS

5.1   Introduction 85
5.2   General Sensory Changes 86
5.3   Some General Cognitive Changes 89
5.4   General Processing Resources 92
5.5   Age-Related Decline in Specific Cognitive Abilities................................96
    5.5.1   Memory 96
    5.5.2   Visuospatial Processing...99
    5.5.3   Reasoning and the Frontal Aging Hypothesis...............................100
    5.5.4   Attention..102
5.6   Summary and Conclusions 102
References..104

5.1 INTRODUCTION

Why, at the grocery store or bank, do younger people avoid standing in a line that contains one or more elderly persons or where the individual collecting payment is quite elderly? After all, these are normal older citizens, going about their daily business, and these are people who generally attend to their daily affairs in a competent fashion, performing tasks without serious errors. Nevertheless, their younger peers often perceive them as less efficient and slower in many of their activities, requiring patience and understanding. Unfortunately, in population studies, even brief measures of cognitive efficiency of those 75 years of age and older reveal that there is indeed substantial cognitive decline present and that it is under-estimated.[86] This chapter reviews the general cognitive changes that occur with normal aging and lead to the perceptions such as those described. Because of the voluminous literature, the review will be selective, although an attempt is made to cover the most recent studies in the domains surveyed. It is not the purpose here to address cognitive declines or impairments associated with dementing conditions. To put these changes in context, the chapter first briefly examines some general sensory changes related to aging.

0-8493-2066-/01/$0.00+$1.50
© 2001 by CRC Press LLC

5.2 GENERAL SENSORY CHANGES

Storandt[1] provides a concise general review of the kind of changes all people undergo as they age, important information for those making psychological or health-related recommendations. Vision certainly begins to decline after the halcyon years of the 30s. More and more people have trouble reading small print as they become older; with increased age, the lens of the eye becomes more rigid and is less able to change shape to achieve focus on close objects (Figure 5.1). Along with this, the yellowing of the lens of the eye makes it more difficult for older people to distinguish shades of blue and green, thus diminishing appreciation for color. Difficulty seeing in dim light becomes a major difficulty by the time most reach 80. In fact, the overall transmission of different wavelengths of light drops quite dramatically with aging (Figure 5.2). In addition, visual processing speed tends to slow, affecting both reading and response time on visual tasks. The ability to hear sound at different frequencies drops significantly (Figure 5.3).

As one might guess, there are practical implications of these changes — which are obvious. In an activity such as driving, the changes mentioned above would lead to differences in the way information and direction signs on expressways are interpreted by older and younger drivers. Older drivers cannot instantly comprehend

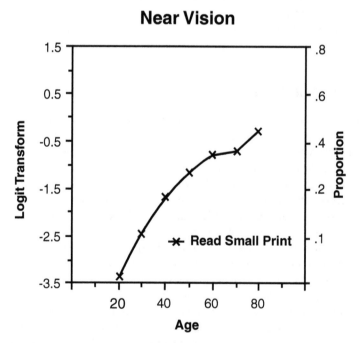

Near Vision

FIGURE 5.1 Proportion of survey respondents reporting difficulty with reading small print. (From Kosnik, W. et al., *J. Gerontol. Psychol. Sci.*, 43, P68, 1988. ©1988 by The Gerontological Society of America. Reprinted with permission.)

signs on the expressway as they hurtle down the highway at 60 mph; maps become difficult to read, especially while driving; and road markers, warning signals, and geographic features become more difficult to distinguish as evening approaches. Is it any surprise that one's grandfather might tend to study maps to some extent before leaving on a trip, drive slowly, stare at road signs for long periods, not pay much attention to honking horns, and dislike driving at night?

Or, to extend the initial example in this context, the older individual in line to pay at a grocery store might have some trouble hearing the verbalizations of the seller, might have difficulty seeing inside her purse to separate change, and might have difficulty making out the different denominations of the currency in his wallet.

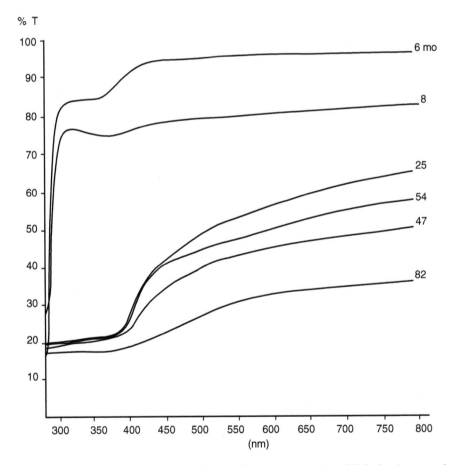

FIGURE 5.2 Percentage transmission (T) of different wavelengths of light by the normal human lens at different ages ranging from 6 months to 82 years. (From Lerman, S., *J. Gerontol.*, 38, 295, 1983. © 1983 by The Gerontological Society of America. Reprinted with permission.)

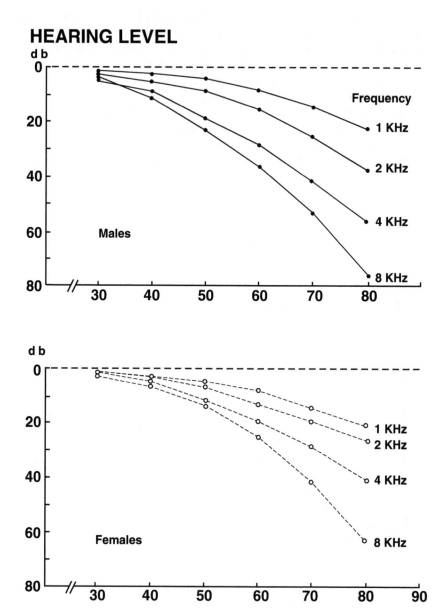

FIGURE 5.3 Age differences in hearing loss at higher frequencies from 1 to 8 kHz. The data from eight published surveys compiled by Spoor[95] and converted to ANSI-1969 standards by Lebo and Reddell.[96] (From Ordy, J. M. and Brizzee, K. R., Eds., *Aging, Vol. 10, Sensory Systems and Communications in the Elderly*, Raven Press, New York, 1979, 156. © Raven Press. Reprinted with permission.)

5.3 SOME GENERAL COGNITIVE CHANGES

As with other physically related functions, cognitive efficiency unfortunately declines with normal aging, and may well account for more functional difficulties than the sensory changes described above.

Declines in cognitive efficiency should not be surprising since changes in the physiological substrates for cognition are apparent. Increasing age has been associated with (1) decreasing volumes of the cerebral hemispheres (up to 0.55% per year); (2) increasing volumes of the third ventricle and the lateral ventricles (up to 3% per year); and (3) increasing odds of cortical atrophy and lateral ventricular enlargement (up to 9% per year).[2] More specific functionally related changes in brain substrate have been reported. Raz et al.[3] reported shrinkage on volumetric measures of the cortex correlated with functions as follows: prefrontal cortex with age-related increases in perseveration; visual processing areas with performance on nonverbal working memory tasks; limbic structures with decline in explicit memory. Brain weight is also reported to decline with age, although this may be due to a reduction in neuronal size rather than to a loss of neurons.[4]

Although most cognitive abilities seem to decline with age, they do not all do so at the same rate, and decline as measured by cognitive tests may not reflect the real-world impact of abilities measured by those tests.[5] Some of the nicest work in documenting changes in cognition has been done by Powell,[6] the head of the team that originated the current state-of-the-art neuropsychological testing software MicroCog™, which is currently marketed by The Psychological Corporation. The next few sections borrow from Powell's book, *Profiles in Cognitive Aging*, which describe these changes.

A good place to begin is the WAIS Full Scale IQ (Figure 5.4). IQ might best be conceptualized as representing a person's general level of information-processing

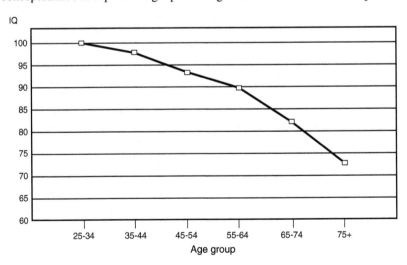

FIGURE 5.4 Average WAIS Full Scale IQ scores for age groups 25 to 34 and 75+. (From Kaufman, A. S., *Assessing Adolescent and Adult Intelligence*, Allyn & Bacon, Boston, 1990, 185. With permission.)

efficiency.[8] The values obtained for IQ result from entering the mean score from the scale scores of these age groups into the WAIS IQ table for 25- to 34-year-olds. It is easy to forget that the WAIS-related IQ scores that result are *age-corrected.*[9] If age is not corrected for, a fairly dramatic decline occurs in the general level of information-processing efficiency. Nevertheless, if one looks at the raw score values determining IQs with aging, it is clear that verbal and performance abilities decline differentially, with verbally related tasks being much more resistant to the effects of aging than spatially, timed, and motor-related tasks. This is immediately clear from simply plotting out declines in Verbal IQ vs. Performance IQ based on the WAIS tables (Figure 5.5). This has also been recently confirmed in studies that looked at verbal and visuospatial processing speed tasks[10] and verbal and visuospatial speed tasks, working memory tasks, and paired-associate learning tasks by Jenkins et al.[11] These authors conclude that "visuospatial cognition is generally more affected by aging than verbal cognition" (p. 157).

The three general areas of ability that seem to be most susceptible to the effects are general visuospatial ability, inductive reasoning, and verbal memory (Figure 5.6). The data in this figure are adapted from a reanalysis by Salthouse[12] of 5000 subjects from the Seattle Longitudinal Study,[13] under untimed or slightly timed conditions with relatively highly educated subjects. Thus, these declines occur independently of the effects of perhaps general cognitive slowing and show that even highly educated individuals are susceptible to the cognitive declines described above. Salthouse[12] went on to look at two different groups of subjects, one healthy and the other less healthy, and found similar declines in memory, spatial, and reasoning abilities, thus suggesting that health status had little effect on these cognitive domains.

Similarly, Powell,[6] in reporting data for the MicroCog, also demonstrated a high correlation for age between the total MicroCog score and specific subtest scores measuring reasoning skills (Analogies), visuospatial facility (Tictac), and verbal memory (Stories: Delayed Recall) (Figure 5.7). He notes, however, that the total MicroCog score correlates more strongly with age than any subtest score, suggesting "that the decline of specific skills is nested in a global trend downward" (p. 74). The idea of a generalized factor of cognitive decline in aging is discussed further in the next few sections.

Interestingly, Powell[6] also looked at MicroCog test scores in terms of levels of education. He compared performance of physicians ($n = 1002$) with less-educated individuals (average of 14.13 years of education; $n = 581$) and found that while there appeared to be less of an absolute decline in more highly educated groups, the slope of change is nevertheless the same (Figure 5.8). This slope, however, increases with older ages. For example, at age 70, the overall scores for the physicians in the sample were about 14% lower than for the youngest physicians; at age 75+, they were about 26% lower. Again, for the less educated individuals, the absolute scores were lower, with this cohort scoring at about the same level as physicians 10 years older in the two decades after age 60.

Others maintain, however, that there are some declines associated with aging in most cognitive domains, including "attentional processing, memory (both verbal and

Verbal IQ

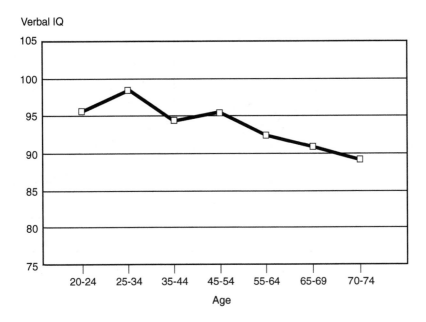

Performance IQ

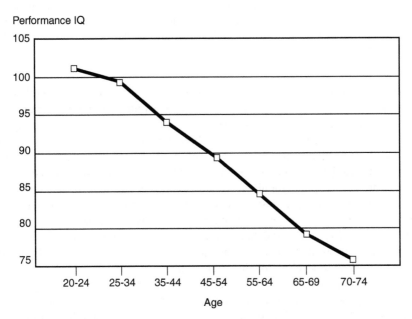

FIGURE 5.5 Change in WAIS-R Verbal and Performance IQs from 20 to 74 years (IQs based on norms for ages 25 to 34). (From Kaufman, A. S., *Assessing Adolescent and Adult Intelligence*, Allyn & Bacon, Boston, 1990, 935. With permission.)

Young standard deviation units

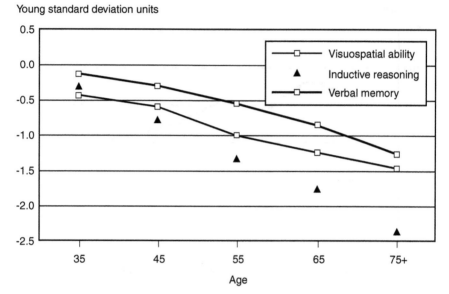

FIGURE 5.6 Age-related differences in memory, reasoning, and visuospatial ability of subjects aged 35 to 75; decline expressed in young adult (22 to 28) standard deviations. (From Powell, D. H., *Profiles in Cognitive Aging*, Harvard University Press, Cambridge, MA, 1997, 87. With permission.)

spatial), and the sensorimotor domain, particularly motor speed."[5] A recently completed longitudinal study of effects of aging within four different age cohorts also reflects general tendencies for decreased performance in "non-verbal learning and memory, retention of verbal material, psychomotor speed and speed of visuospatial processing, and concentration" (Reference 94, p. 68). Nevertheless, it has long been pointed out that these declines represent averages of group performance and that the declines are not inevitable for all individuals. Benton et al.[15] in reviewing test scores on nine neuropsychological instruments, in 162 older individuals, found that if one looks at percentages of age groups that render defective performance, 70% of those over 80 years of age showed deficient performance in no more than one test. They interpreted their results to indicate "that normal aging does not necessarily involve a general decline in level of cognitive functioning" (p. 33).

It is thus important to consider whether cognitive changes seen with aging may represent a general factor affecting most cognitive domains or whether there are differential effects, depending on which area of cognitive functioning is examined.

5.4 GENERAL PROCESSING RESOURCES

Salthouse[12] hypothesized that differentiating between age-related cognitive changes on different categorizations (and related tasks) such as speed of processing, divided

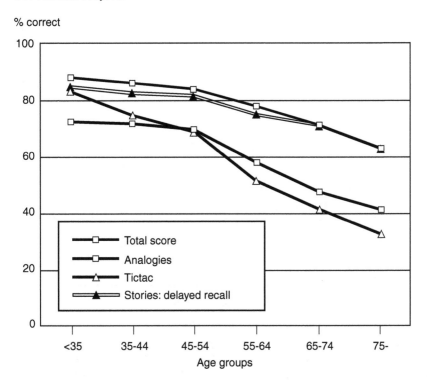

FIGURE 5.7 MicroCog aptitude scores that decline significantly by decade compared with total. (From Powell, D. H., *Profiles in Cognitive Aging*, Harvard University Press, Cambridge, MA, 1994, 75. With permission.)

attention, and working memory capacity may be somewhat arbitrary if they are relatively equivalent. As he indicates, "The processing resources perspective is based on the simple but appealing idea that a small number of factors may be responsible for many of the age differences observed in measures of cognitive functioning" (p. 348). Salthouse[14] proposes that decreased speed of information processing may be the underlying change primarily responsible for the changes seen in multiple cognitive domains. Salthouse and Coon[16] have suggested that there appears to be a decrease in the speed of executing many cognitive processes, even in memory tasks, and not decreased speed of one or two processes. This general processing speed is viewed as a "fundamental component of the architecture of human cognition" and relates to basic cognition components in which elements of working memory are compared with data stored in long-term memory (Reference 18, p. 222). This comparison, or recognition cycle, has been viewed as underlying cognition as a fundamental.[19] Thus, the speed at which such recognition cycles occur would itself slow with aging, thus essentially affecting all cognition. Salthouse summarizes:

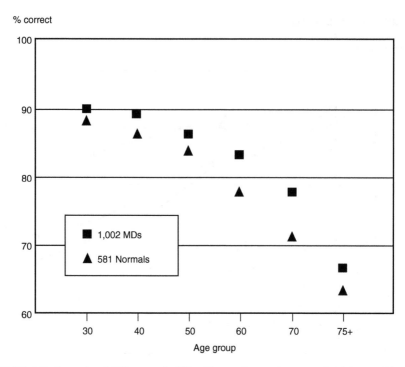

FIGURE 5.8 Age-related differences in MicroCog total score between physicians and lesser-educated individuals (average 14.13 years of education). (From Powell, D. H., *Profiles in Cognitive Aging*, Harvard University Press, Cambridge, MA, 1994, 71. With permission.)

> Increased age in adulthood is associated with a decrease in the speed with which many processing operations can be executed and that this reduction in speed leads to impairments in cognitive functioning because of what are termed the limited time mechanism and the simultaneity mechanism. That is, cognitive performance is degraded when processing is slow because relevant operations cannot be successfully executed (limited time) and because the products of early processing may no longer be available when later processing is complete (simultaneity). (Reference 14, p. 403)

In supporting research, Kray and Lindenberger[98] suggest "that the ability to efficiently maintain and coordinate 2 alternating task sets in working memory instead of 1 is more negatively affected by advancing age than the ability to execute the task switch itself" (p. 126).

Nevertheless, on the less pessimistic side, Salthouse and Somberg[17] had earlier pointed out that while older individuals require more time to perform a number of cognitive tasks, they can learn and produce accurate responses at a level comparable to younger adults. More recently, Salthouse[20] analyzed data sets of tests of reasoning and found that relations between age and accuracy of solutions in these tests did not vary by item difficulty although he felt there was evidence for some independent age-related influences on more difficult test items. Nevertheless, again using statistical inference, Salthouse and Czaja[29] observe that many cognitive abilities seem to share age-related variance with each other, with rather small unique, ability-specific age effects. They argue that it is important to consider the structure in which a variable operates.

Undoubtedly, the conclusions of Salthouse and colleagues would be consistent with the introduction to this chapter, i.e., the observation of slowed everyday task performance among elderly people. There is little doubt that speed of processing, as measured by tasks such as reaction time, slows with age. Birren et al.,[21] in a review of the literature, suggest that there is about a 20% slowing of reaction time from the 20s to the 60s, and indicate that this is a much-replicated finding. Studies seem consistently to demonstrate slowing of simple and choice reaction times between young and middle age, and middle and old age.[23] Gottsdanker[22] also reports that simple reaction time shows significant increases between age 18 and 93, although with optimal conditions, he found only a slowing of about 2 ms/decade.

It should be noted, however, that arguments made by those who favor slowed information processing as a fundamental overall effect of aging on cognition are making the argument on a statistical basis. Path analysis, structured equations, and regression models are employed to examine the degree of variance in performance on one task that can be accounted for by performance on another.[14,24,25] While the analyses are elegant in and of themselves and undoubtedly demonstrate significant relationships between performance on multiple cognitive tasks, if one covaries a highly age-related variable, such as reaction time, with performance on other tasks, the variance in the second task that is accounted for by the age-related task will inherently be high. For example, if one covaries reaction time with age-related changes on memory tasks, it becomes quite likely that the amount of variance in a memory task that is accounted for by age, after removing the variance accounted for by reaction time, will be small. For example, Earles and Kersten[26] found that age-related variance on delayed recall of activities was reduced 52% by the statistical control of perceptual speed and, in immediate activity recall, this variance was reduced by 91%.

Obviously, one can make the inference that if speed-of-processing variables account for most of the variance related to age on multiple tasks, then speed of processing is a fundamental factor in cognitive architecture. One can, however, imagine another scenario. Suppose that another factor that is highly related to aging, such as graying of the hair, is chosen. If one then covaries the variance related to grayness of hair with performance on cognitive tasks such as a memory task, the amount of variance on the task accounted for by age is small when the variance attributed to grayness of hair is removed. Can it then be concluded that grayness of hair is a fundamental part of cognitive architecture? The argument made here is that the inference of a general factor of speed of processing that affects multiple cognitive domains is based on correlational relationships; thus it is suggestive but not conclusive. Therefore, although there clearly is slowing in measures of reaction time and in processing certain kinds of information such as lexical stimuli,[27] others point out limits to the notion that underlying processing speed affects all cognitive domains. Swearer and Kane[28] demonstrate that although older adults were slower than younger ones in simultaneous matching-to-sample tasks, this was not true for delayed matching-to-sample tasks. Thus, in overview, it is possible that slowed speed of processing by itself may be responsible for performance on simultaneous processing tasks, but may not independently affect the specific cognitive domain under study. In a memory task, for example, if an individual is slow to absorb a paragraph that is read, and the reader speaks quickly, it is likely that not all the verbal information is made accessible to storage. What looks like a memory deficit can result. When the paragraph is read more slowly, the paragraph may well be accessible to storage and no memory deficit is observable. Does this mean that speed of processing itself underpins memory or does it mean that speed of processing independently affects incoming information without affecting memory itself?

5.5   AGE-RELATED DECLINE
IN SPECIFIC COGNITIVE ABILITIES

5.5.1   MEMORY

Studies have generally demonstrated that speed of retrieval from memory stores is negatively affected by age, as is working memory and encoding and retrieval of newly acquired information.[30–32] Fisk and Warr[74] support the notion that older persons have more difficulty in forming associations as rapidly as younger persons and that this primarily accounts for the age effects seen in short-term forgetting. When looking at younger (ages 20 to 35) vs. older (ages 60 to 80) subjects, it is clear that memory loss for the recency effect on word-list learning is greater among elderly people after a delay,[33] thus confirming the long-standing finding of the sensitivity of delayed memory to decline with aging.[34] It is also evident that recall is far more affected than registration per se. Schugens et al.[35] examined explicit and implicit memory in younger (20s) vs. older (60s) subjects, and found that ability to recall verbal or visual materials declined steadily with age at both immediate and delayed testing, while there did not appear to be consistent age differences when recognition tasks are employed. The difference between the larger decline in recall vs. recognition test scores by age for a figure memory task can be seen in Figure 5.9.[97] Thus, in terms of memory, there appears to be evidence of age-related decline in retrieval and in encoding of recent memory into long-term memory, and specific decline is seen on delayed memory tasks. Recognition of previously presented stimuli, once encoded, does not appear to be differentially sensitive to the effects of aging. Whiting and Smith[36] have more recently confirmed, using primary and secondary memory tasks, that recall requires greater processing capacity than recognition, and that older subjects seem to have more limitations in this processing capacity. Recall tasks also provide little or no contextual information to the individual and it appears that age differences are magnified when little contextual information is provided.[88] Thus, recall tasks are seen to place a greater burden on processing resources.[89] Nevertheless, the inference of memory deficit in aging appears to depend, at least in part, on the nature of the task employed to study it. The studies noted in the paragraph above generally utilized fairly traditional tasks such as word lists or paired stimuli. A widely

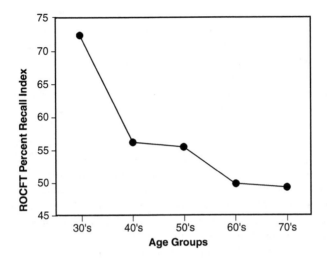

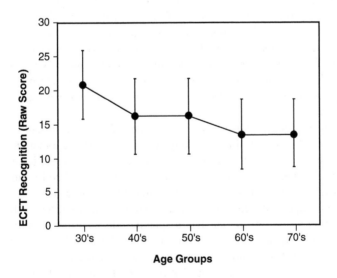

FIGURE 5.9 Extended Complex Figure Test percent recall index (recall/copy × 100) and recognition scores, by age group. (From Fastenau, P. et al., in *The Rey-Osterrieth Complex Figure Test: Clinical and Research Applications*, Knight, J. A. and Kaplan, E., Eds., Psychological Assessment Resources, Odessa, FL, in press. With permission.)

acknowledged model of decline in memory abilities postulates that retrieval is less efficient in elderly people as a result of an inability to screen irrelevant information from working memory.[37] This is called the "fan effect" and in the paradigm used to study it participants are required to distinguish between pairs of stimuli that had been presented to them before and foils representing irrelevant pairings of these stimuli.[38] When target facts that an individual has to remember are arbitrary, such as "the butcher drove home" and "the policeman bought groceries," the foil can be an item such as "the policeman drove home." Basically, the fan effect refers to deterioration in accurate memories the more facts are included; this is true for anyone, although it is differentially affected by age. Gerard et al.[39] demonstrated that with speeded recognition, the detrimental effect of fan size is larger on older adults, leading to the inference that, with age, there is a decline in the ability to screen irrelevant information from working memory. In other words, as one ages, separating stimuli targeted for learning from distracting or irrelevant stimuli becomes more difficult. It is not clear whether this reflects a speed-of-processing matching function or a specific difficulty with screening irrelevant information from memory; in either case, it does appear that working memory is involved in these findings.

It has also been posited that differences may exist between younger and older individuals in automatic vs. effortful memory processing. Automatic processing would refer to encoding of information that requires little or no effort, while effortful processing would require designation of attentional capacity for encoding to occur.[40] It has been suggested that restriction of this attentional capacity may affect the ability of older persons to encode information effortfully, but not the ability for automatic encoding.[41] Rohling et al.[42] reported that on a picturebook memory task requiring effort, there did not appear to be differences between younger and older subjects, although there was a difference between older subjects and patients with organic brain conditions. Again, there appears to be some difference in interpretation of data depending on the nature of tasks used, and it is not certain that there is a unitary memory deficit.

The same can be true for popular conceptions of memory difficulties in old age having to do with retrieval of names. Maylor[43] studied this phenomenon, taking into account the effect of age on other tasks such as more semantic retrieval. She found that there was no independent effect; i.e., the effect of age on face-to-name matching was predictable from general effects of aging on semantic name retrieval. This finding would support the earlier-discussed notion of a more general effect of aging on information processing rather than a specific effect on the particular ability to recall names of acquaintances. In a related study, Au et al.[44] document a general decline in confrontation naming with age and that this may reflect "more than simply a breakdown in lexical retrieval and that perceptual and semantic processing may be implicated" (p. 300). In addition, older individuals (over 60) report more "tip of the tongue" phenomena,[90] and individuals over 80 make more errors on naming-to-confrontation tasks.[91] Altogether, there appears little doubt that older individuals often experience increased word-finding problems.[92]

Finally, Zelinski and Stewart[45] have looked at whether reasoning and vocabulary would predict changes in recall and recognition of text over a 16-year period in adults who were 55 to 81 years old at baseline. They found that male gender and decline in vocabulary were related to declines in word list recall, while there did not seem to be reliable predictors of recognition memory. The authors suggest that declines in other cognitive abilities may be predictive of declines in various memory tasks, but that these predictions are task specific and reflect individual differences between subjects. Nevertheless, using structural equation modeling in studying individual differences on a lengthy cognitive battery in subjects ranging from 20 to 90 years of age, Park et al.[46] again report that both speed of processing and working memory account for large amounts of age-related variance in long-term episodic memory.

5.5.2 Visuospatial Processing

As discussed earlier, visuospatial processing ability also seems particularly influenced by aging, far more so than verbal cognition.[11] Dobson et al.[47] examined the interaction among age, complexity of a figure comparison task, and perceptual speed. Their findings supported the commonly reported observation that older individuals had more difficulty with more complex tasks. Perceptual speed, however, was a predictor of age-related task performance only for the men in the study, not for the women. As with the study of Zelinski and Stewart,[45] it appeared that more general cognitive predictors were related to performance on the specific task of study for males only, with Dobson et al. suggesting that gender differences in performance were far more pervasive for older than for younger subjects.

Erber et al.[48] showed that there appears to be a particular weakness for performance on a digit–number matching test for elderly people that cannot be explained by memory or specific perceptual factors. Newman and Kaszniak[49] attempted to document further visuospatial memory changes in a maze-learning task in young (18 to 30) vs. older (61 to 82) subjects. Differences between the groups were not significant for a practice trial that could be solved verbally, whereas differences emerged for subsequent trials depending on spatial memory, with the older adults performing significantly worse. This suggested a more specific decline in the visuospatial component of memory per se. Fastenau and colleagues,[50,51] however, when statistically controlling for processing speed and isolating retrieval efficiency, report that, while there is a reduction in age-related retrieval with such statistical control, the age effect is less changed for visuospatial material than for verbal, thus suggesting that retrieval of verbal material may be more susceptible to general declines related to speed of processing.

These somewhat inconsistent findings do not mitigate the well-known decrements in performance on visuospatial tasks as mentioned at the start of this chapter. In addition to the very clear declines in performance IQ seen on the Wechsler Scales with age, Roper et al.[52] showed similarly poor performance in older vs. younger individuals on a figure-ground perception task and Koss et al.[53] showed evidence of impaired visuospatial functioning with preserved language-related functioning with older age.

There are other factors, however, that are potentially related to visuospatial task performance. First, there does indeed seem to be somewhat of a novelty effect, which particularly affects elderly people. Wadsworth Denney and Pearce[54] compared young, middle-aged, and older adults on a figure-matching test and showed that whereas older adults made more errors at the start of the test, with practice, their error rate decreased to the level of those younger. Thus, practice (familiarity) with the test was of significant benefit to older individuals while it did not affect performance for younger subjects. A much earlier but related finding was reported of older individuals having significantly more perceptual difficulty than younger subjects, seen primarily as a significantly slower response time with visual stimuli of increasing complexity.[55]

As mentioned at the start of this chapter, it is also important to take into consideration the changes in vision that occur with increasing age. As the example shown in Figure 5.1 suggests, there are declines in ability to read small print, in visual processing speed, and in ability to see with dim illumination.[56] It is pointed out, however, that functional abilities beyond those related to visual acuity are affected and that all spatial vision functions show a similar rate of decline with age, including tests of stereoacuity, recovery from glare, color vision, contrast sensitivity, etc.[57] Steinman et al.[58] report that activation of transient visual attention is slower and weaker in elderly people, suggesting visual attention deficits even in "visually normal" older individuals. Finally, it has also been demonstrated that elderly individuals have difficulty in searching for peripheral visual targets, and this measure, called "the useful field of view" appears to be predictive of risk of accidents when driving.[59–61]

5.5.3 REASONING AND THE FRONTAL AGING HYPOTHESIS

As described by Powell's[6] work, reasoning, as measured by analogy-like tasks, also seems to decline with older age. Mittenberg et al.[62] reported that when performance on a number of neuropsychological tests was analyzed in younger and older subjects, declines in performance were reflected not in any lateralizing pattern, but on tests particularly sensitive to frontal lobe functions; they suggested that age-related neuropsychological changes are primarily reflected in frontal lobe-related abilities. Similarly, in examining age-related changes in semantic episodic memory, Mayr and Kliegl[63] report that nonsemantic components of a memory task involving the function of retrieval position were the primary aspects affected by age, not the semantic retrieval itself. They also raise the issue that executive control of retrieval is the primary area affected by age.

These observations of age-related declines in executive functioning tasks have led to the postulation of a frontal aging hypothesis. Dempster[64] has suggested "the prefrontal cortex leads most, if not all, other areas in the aging process" (p. 51), and Moscovitch and Winocur[65] indicate that changes in frontal systems, as well as hippocampal, lead to decline in memory with age. Greenwood,[66] in a critical review of studies related to this hypothesis, finds that, although frontal areas and functions are subject to age-related decline, "there is only weak and conflicting evidence that frontal regions are selectively and differentially affected by age" (p. 705). Rather, Greenwood argues for a network-based theory of cognitive aging, where the frontal lobes are recruited under conditions of high task demand such as with executive functions. Thus, although weakness on such tasks might appear to reflect weakness in the frontal lobes, it is argued that it more likely affects changes in functional networks that are more widely distributed. Similarly, Parkin and Java[67] specifically report age-related declines on a number of frontal lobe–related measures leading to the conclusion that the noted age-related variance is more likely attributed to a more general factor in cognitive aging. Daigneault and Braun[82] suggest that an active attentional processing deficit, associated with prefrontal functional decline, is responsible for age-related impairment in working memory. West,[68] however, argues that evidence for age-related volumetric decline (e.g., Raz et al.[69]) as well as age-related changes on frontally related tasks support the concept of a decline in processes supported by the frontal lobes rather than a generalized decline in functions that this area happens to support. Keys and White[85] examined performance of older and younger adults on two tasks that were generally equated for task demands, one measuring primarily executive functioning and another speed of processing. They reported that even though psychomotor speed somewhat reduced the amount of variance in executive functioning attributed to age, there was still a substantial and unique portion of variance in executive functioning that was age related. From a different perspective, Stuss et al.[83] have found that older normal subjects perform similarly to younger patients with frontal damage on a list-learning task, thus also supporting that frontal system dysfunction is related to aging.

Some additional clues to the nature of how the aging brain reorganizes function is emerging from work with functional neuroimaging. Smith and Jonides[70] have elegantly demonstrated that short-term storage (working memory) and executive processing (operating on the contents of this storage) are major functions of the frontal lobes. And, as can be deduced from earlier discussion in this chapter, these functions appear to be particularly susceptible to aging. A recent study by Reuter-Lorenz et al.[71] suggests that larger areas of the frontal cortex are recruited as compensation for age-related neural decline in older vs. younger people on letter-matching tasks. These findings were further extended by a demonstration that a verbal working memory task tended to activate the left frontal cortex in younger adults and a visuospatial working memory task tended to activate the right frontal cortex, whereas both kinds of task tended to activate the frontal cortex bilaterally in older adults.[72] However, the picture may be more complicated. Grachev and Apkarian[73] have very recently studied chemical intercorrelations among neurotransmitters in younger and middle-aged adults and suggest that, although there is an increase of overall chemical correlation between brain regions with advancing age, there is a pattern of negative chemical connectivity across (within) brain regions that becomes weaker in middle-aged subjects. They suggest that the "decreased level of overall negative connectivity across brain regions may be a reflection of reduced inhibitory control mechanisms of aging" (p. S83). In functional imaging, increased blood flow may thus represent increased activity in areas that are normally inhibited in the efficient performance of a task. Thus, it is possible that what appears to be increased areas of activation associated with task performance, in a region such as the frontal lobes in elderly people, when compared with younger individuals performing the same task, may instead reflect *decreased* inhibition. In either case, there does appear to be decreased efficiency of functioning in the frontal lobes with aging, although it is unclear whether this reflects frontal-specific decline or decreased efficiency of more general function that the frontal lobes support.

5.5.4 ATTENTION

Different aspects of attention seem to decline with age.[32] Specifically, divided attention (the ability to attend to two different tasks at the same time) has been shown to decline in elderly people over multiple studies.[75] This would also be consistent with the fan effect model of memory interference supported by Hasher and Zacks.[37] Selective attention, the ability to disregard unnecessary, irrelevant, or distracting stimuli, is also more susceptible to disruption in older adults.[76–78] There appears to be a greater age-related deficit in selective attention than can be explained by generalized cognitive slowing alone, especially for more demanding tasks.[84] Sustained attention, or the ability to attend to a stimulus over time, does not generally seem to demonstrate the same kind of age-related decline,[76] although there have been some observations to the contrary.[79]

There has been some controversy about the ability of elderly people to switch attention between tasks, with older individuals showing decline of this ability in the auditory modality but not the visual modality.[32] Recent evidence, however, suggests that there does appear to be a specific decline in this kind of task both in the very old[80] and in individuals with early dementia of the Alzheimer type.[81] Specifically, the attentional deficit noted by Parasuraman and colleagues in these studies is one of inability to *disengage* attention efficiently from one stimulus to focus upon another. In other words, with increased age, individuals seem to have difficulty with stopping the fixation of attention on one object and shifting that attention to another. Parenthetically, with the earlier discussion on changes in vision and how this could affect driving ability in elderly people, a deficit in the ability to disengage attention may potentially underlie many difficulties the older people have when making left turns or judging the flow of traffic in busy driving situations.

Finally, note is again made of Hasher and Zacks'[40] distinction between automatic vs. effortful processing in attentional capacity, wherein they postulate that familiar, commonly used skills necessitate little attentional capacity while tasks requiring an individual to deal with more complex or unusual stimuli would be more taxing and demand more attentional capacity. Effortful tasks seem much more affected in elderly people.[42,87]

5.6 SUMMARY AND CONCLUSIONS

It seems a fact that cognitive efficiency decreases with old age, especially past the age of 75. Nevertheless, it is clear that there are significant individual differences in both the magnitude and rate of cognitive decline. While some eventual decline may be inevitable with aging, the degree of impairment and when it occurs is variable in individuals.

There is both evidence for a generalized factor of cognitive aging, which affects multiple functions, and evidence of more specific decline in various functions themselves. The evidence for a generalized factor of declining processing speed is largely statistically based and may overstate its influence or component value on other cognitive processes. Nevertheless, there is no question that processing speed is very much related to age and that it has a significant relationship to other cognitive capabilities. In this same vein, the frontal aging hypothesis suggests that deterioration in the functioning of the frontal cortex is selectively related to age and that it either influences or supports age-related cognitive decline. That the frontal cortex undergoes significant change appears assured, although it remains controversial whether this part of the brain and associated functions are preferentially susceptible to the effects of aging. There does not seem to be a question that executive functions are significantly affected with aging.

In terms of more specific conclusions:

1. People clearly undergo significant adverse sensory changes in vision, visual processing speed, and hearing.
2. Memory is affected, with recall being far more affected than recognition memory. This is postulated, in part, to be due to difficulty with original encoding of information and with the speed of encoding in working memory. In addition, the older people are, the more difficulty they have remembering relevant vs. irrelevant stimuli or remembering more complex arrays of stimulus relationships.
3. Visuospatial information processing appears to be more affected than verbal information processing, although this may well depend on the type of task on which such ability is measured.[93] It is not clear whether this is due to the visuospatial nature of the information or whether visuospatial information itself is more complex than verbal information. It is not clear whether visuospatial memory is more affected than verbal memory. In addition, there is a very clear change in characteristics with age, and this may affect information processing from a peripheral standpoint.
4. Analogy-like reasoning and executive function, i.e., planning, arranging, and initiating, also appear to undergo age-related decline. A decline in working memory capacity appears to be related to this change. Evidence from functional neuroimaging studies appears to implicate a perhaps greater recruitment of frontal cortical areas among elderly individuals in performing the same task as younger individuals. However, the specter is raised that what appears to be greater activation on neuroimaging may reflect decreased inhibition, and thus lowered efficiency.
5. Divided attention and selective attention appear to undergo more decline than the ability to sustain attention. There appears to be some difficulty experienced with age with switching between tasks and there is specific evidence that a particular attentional deficit seen in elderly people is the inability to disengage attention from one stimulus to engage another. Finally, there appears to be more of an age-related decline in efficiency in attention-related tasks that require greater effort as opposed to those that require little effort.

The body of knowledge in cognition and aging is growing exponentially, and it appears that some general principles underlying the characteristics of cognitive change are emerging. The areas of controversy about change that reflects general vs. specific cognitive change or localized vs. generalized brain involvement will likely continue for some time and may not reflect mutually independent processes. The hope is that there will be continued progress in understanding the neural and neurophysiological underpinnings of the cognitive changes that take place, leading to potential interventions to assuage or temper them.

REFERENCES

1. Storandt, M., General principles of assessment of older adults, in *Neuropsychological Assessment of Depression and Dementia*, Storandt, M. and Vandenbos, G. R., Eds., American Psychological Association, Washington, D.C., 1994, chap. 2.
2. Coffey, C. E. et al., Quantitative cerebral anatomy of the aging human brain: a cross-sectional study using magnetic resonance imaging, *Neurology*, 42, 527–536, 1992.
3. Raz, N., Gunning-Dixon, F. M., Head, D., Dupuis, J. H., and Acker, J. D., Neuroanatomical correlates of cognitive aging: evidence from structural magnetic resonance imaging, *Neuropsychology*, 12, 95–114, 1998.
4. Morris, J. C. and McManus, D. Q., The neurology of aging: normal versus pathological change, *Geriatrics*, 46, 47–64, 1991.
5. Gur, R. C., Mobert, P. J., and Gur, R. E., Aging and cognitive functioning, in *Geriatric Secrets*, Forciea, M. A. and Lavizzo-Mourey, R. J., Eds., Hanley & Belfus, Philadelphia, 1996, 126–129.
6. Powell, D. H., *Profiles in Cognitive Aging*, Harvard University Press, Cambridge, MA, 1994.
7. Powell, D. H. et al., *MicroCog: Assessment of Cognitive Functioning*, The Psychological Corporation, San Antonio, TX, 1993.
8. Lezak, M. D., *Neuropsychological Assessment*, Oxford, New York, 1976.
9. Kaufman, A. S., *Assessing Adolescent and Adult Intelligence*, Allyn & Bacon, Boston, 1990.
10. Lawrence, B., Myerson, J., and Hale, S., Differential decline of verbal and visuospatial processing speed across the adult life span, *Aging Neuropsychol. Cogn.*, 5, 129–146, 1998.
11. Jenkins, L., Myerson, J. U., Joerding, J. A., and Hale, S., Converging evidence that visuospatial cognition is more age sensitive than verbal cognition, *Psychol. Aging*, 15, 157–175, 2000.
12. Salthouse, T. A., *Theoretical Perspectives on Cognitive Aging*, Lawrence Erlbaum Associates, Hillsdale, NJ, 1991.
13. Schaie, K. W., The course of adult intellectual development, *Am. Psychol.*, 49, 304–313, 1994.
14. Salthouse, T. A., The processing-speed theory of adult age-differences in cognition, *Psychol. Rev.*, 103, 403–428, 1996.
15. Benton, A. L., Eslinger, P. J., and Damasio, A. R., Normative observations on neuropsychological test performances in old age, *J. Clin. Neuropsychol.*, 3, 33–42, 1981.
16. Salthouse, T. A. and Coon, V. E., Influence of task-specific processing speed on age differences in memory, *J. Gerontol. Psychol. Sci.*, 48, P245–P255, 1993.

17. Salthouse, T. A. and Somberg, B. L., Time-accuracy relationships in young and old adults, *J. Gerontol.*, 37, 349–353, 1982.
18. Kail, R. and Salthouse, T. A., Processing speed as a mental capacity, *Acta Psychol.*, 86, 199–225, 1994.
19. Klahr, D., Information-processing approaches, *Ann. Child Dev.*, 6, 133–185, 1989.
20. Salthouse, T. A., Item analyses of age relations on reasoning tests, *Psychol. Aging*, 14, 3–8.
21. Birren, J. E., Woods, A. M., and Williams, M. V., Behavioral slowing with age: causes, organization, and consequences, in *Aging in the 1980's: Psychological Issues*, Poon, L. W., Ed., American Psychological Association, Washington, D.C., 1980.
22. Gottsdanker, R., Age and simple reaction time, *J. Gerontol.*, 37, 342–348, 1982.
23. Era, P., Jokela, J., and Heikkinen, E., Reaction and movement times in men of different ages: a population study, *Percept. Mot. Skills*, 63, 111–130, 1986.
24. Salthouse, T. A. and Meinz, E. J., Aging, inhibition, working memory, and speed, *J. Gerontol. Psychol. Sci.*, 50B, P207–P306, 1995.
25. Salthouse, T. A., Where in an ordered sequence of variables do independent age-related effects occur? *J. Gerontol.: Psychol. Sci.*, 51B, P166–P178, 1996.
26. Earles, J. L. and Kersten, A. W., Processing speed and adult age differences in activity memory, *Exp. Aging Res.*, 25, 243–253.
27. Hale, S. and Myerson, J., Fifty years older, fifty percent slower? Meta-analytic regression models and semantic context effects, *Aging Cogn.*, 2, 132–145, 1999.
28. Swearer, J. M. and Kane, K. J., Behavioral slowing with age: boundary conditions of the generalized slowing model, *J. Gerontol.*, 51B, P189–P200, 1996.
29. Salthouse, T. A. and Czaja, S. J., Structural constraints on process explanations in cognitive aging, *Psychol. Aging*, 15, 44–55, 2000.
30. Kas:zniak, A. W., The neuropsychology of dementia, in *Neuropsychological Assessment of Neuropsychiatric Disorders*, Grant, I. and Adams, K. M., Eds., Oxford University Press, New York, 1986, 172–220.
31. Hultsch, D. F. and Dixon, R. A., Learning and memory in aging, in *Handbook of the Psychology of Aging*, Birren, J. E. and Schaie, K. W., Eds., Academic Press, New York, 1990, 258–274.
32. Zec, R. F., The neuropsychology of aging, *Exp. Gerontol.*, 30, 431–442, 1995.
33. Carlesimo, G. A., Sabbadini, M., Fadda, L., and Caltagirone, C., Word-list forgetting in young and elderly subjects: evidence from age-related decline in transferring information from transitory to permanent memory conditions, *Cortex*, 33, 155–166, 1997.
34. Poon, L. W., Differences in human memory with aging: nature, causes, and clinical implications, in *Handbook of the Psychology of Aging*, Birren, J. E. and Schaie, K. W., Eds., Van Nostrand Reinhold, New York, 1985, 427–462.
35. Schugens, M. M., Daum, I., Spindler, M., and Birbaumer, N., Differential effects of aging on explicit and implicit memory, *Aging, Neuropsychol. Cogn.*, 4, 33–44, 1997.
36. Whiting, W. L. and Smith, A. D., Differential age-related processing limitations in recall and recognition tasks, *Psychol. Aging*, 12, 216–224, 1997.
37. Hasher, L. and Zacks, R. T., Working memory, comprehension, and aging: a review and new view, in *The Psychology of Learning and Motivation*, Bower, G. H., Ed., Academic Press, New York, 1988, 193–225.
38. Anderson, J. R., *The Architecture of Cognition*, Harvard University Press, Cambridge, MA, 1983.
39. Gerard, L., Zacks, R. T., Hasher, L., and Radvansky, G., Age deficits in retrieval: the fan effect, *J. Gerontol. Psychol. Sci.*, 46, P131–P136, 1991.

40. Hasher, L. and Zacks, R. T., Automatic and effortful processes in memory, *J. Exp. Psychol.*, 108, 356–388, 1979.
41. Hasher, L. and Zacks, R. T., Automatic processing of fundamental information, *Am. Psychol.*, 39, 1372–1388, 1984.
42. Rohling, M. L., Ellis, N. R., and Scogin, F., Automatic and effortful memory processes in elderly persons with organic brain pathology, *J. Gerontol. Psychol. Sci.*, 46, P137–P143, 1991.
43. Maylor, E. A., Proper name retrieval in old age: converging evidence against disproportionate impairment, *Aging Neuropsychol. Cogn.*, 4, 221–226, 1997.
44. Au, R., Joung, P., Nicholas, M., Obler, L. K., Kass, R., and Albert, M. L., Naming ability across the adult life span, *Aging Cogn.*, 2, 300–311, 1995.
45. Zelinski, E. M. and Stewart, S. T., Individual differences in 16-year memory changes, *Psychol. Aging*, 13, 622–630, 1998.
46. Park, D. C. et al., Mediators of long-term memory performance across the life span, *Psychol. Aging*, 11, 621–637, 1996.
47. Dobson, S. H., Kirasic, K., and Allen, G. L., Age-related differences in adults' spatial task performance: influences of task complexity and perceptual speed, *Aging Cogn.*, 2, 19–38, 1995.
48. Erber, J. T., Botwinick, J., and Storandt, M., The impact of memory on age differences in Digit Symbol performance, *J. Gerontol.*, 36, 586–590, 1981.
49. Newman, M. C. and Kaszniak, A. W., Spatial memory and aging: performance on a human analog of the Morris water maze, *Aging Neuropsychol. Cogn.*, 7, 86–93, 2000.
50. Fastenau, P. S., Denburg, N. L., and Abeles, N., Age differences in retrieval: further support for the resource-reduction hypothesis, *Psychol. Aging*, 11, 140–146, 1996.
51. Fastenau, P. S., Denburg, N. L., and Abeles, N., The role of attention in aging retrieval: relative sparing with greater visual involvement, *Brain Cogn.*, 30, 393–396, 1996.
52. Roper, B. L., Bieliauskas, L. A., Basso, M., and Colman, S., The influence of age and impairment status on the Southern California Figure-Ground Visual Perception Test (FG), *J. Int. Neuropsychol. Soc.*, 1, 169, 1995.
53. Koss, E. et al., Patterns of performance preservation and loss in healthy aging, *Dev. Neuropsychol.*, 7, 99–113, 1991.
54. Wadsworth Denney, N. and Pearce, K. A., Effects of practice on the matching familiar figures test: a comparison of young, middle-aged and elderly adults, *Aging Cogn.*, 1, 177–187, 1994.
55. Birren, J. E. and Botwinick, J., Speed of response as a function of perceptual difficulty and age, *J. Gerontol.*, 10, 433–436, 1955.
56. Kosnik, W. et al., Visual changes in daily life throughout adulthood, *J. Gerontol. Psychol. Sci.*, 43, P63–P70, 1988.
57. Haegerstrom-Portnoy, G., Schneck, M. E., and Brabyn, J. A., Seeing into old age: vision function beyond acuity, *Optometr. Vision Sci.*, 76, 141–158, 1999.
58. Steinman, S. B., Steinman, B. A., Trick, G. L., and Lehmkuhle, S., A sensory explanation for visual attention deficits in the elderly, *Optometr. Vision Sci.*, 71, 743–749, 1994.
59. Scialfa, C. T., Thomas, D. M., and Joffe, K. M., Age differences in the useful field of view: an eye movement analysis, *Optometr. Vision Sci.*, 71, 736–742, 1994.
60. Owsley, C., Vision and driving in the elderly, *Optometr. Vision Sci.*, 71, 727–735, 1994.
61. Owsley, C., Visual processing impairment and risk of motor vehicle crash among older adults, *JAMA*, 279, 1083–1088, 1998.

62. Mittenberg, W., Seidenberg, M., O'Leary, D. S., and DiGiulio, D. V., Changes in cerebral functioning associated with normal aging, *J. Clin. Exp. Neuropsychol.*, 11, 918–932, 1989.

63. Mayr, U. and Kliegl, R., Complex semantic processing in old age: does it stay or does it go? *Psychol. Aging*, 15, 29–43, 2000.

64. Dempster, F. N., The rise and fall of the inhibitory mechanism: toward a unified theory of cognitive development and aging, *Dev. Rev.*, 12, 45–75, 1992.

65. Moskovitch, M. and Winocur, G., The neuropsychology of memory and aging, in *The Handbook of Aging and Cognition*, Craik, F. I. M. and Salthouse, T. A., Eds., Lawrence Erlbaum Associates, Hillsdale, NJ, 1992, 315–372.

66. Greenwood, P. M., The frontal aging hypothesis evaluated, *J. Int. Neuropsychol. Soc.*, 6, 705–726, 2000.

67. Parkin, A. J. and Java, R. I., Deterioration of frontal lobe function in normal aging: influences of fluid intelligence versus perceptual speed, *Neuropsychology*, 13, 539–545, 1999.

68. West, R., In defense of the frontal lobe hypothesis of cognitive aging, *J. Int. Neuropsychol. Soc.*, 6, 727–729, 2000.

69. Raz, N., Gunning-Dixon, F. M., Head, D., Dupuis, J. H., McQuain, J., Briggs, S. D., Loken, W. J., Thornton, A. E., and Acker, J. D., Selective aging of the human cerebral cortex observed *in vivo*: differential vulnerability of the prefrontal gray matter, *Cerebral Cortex*, 7, 268–282, 1997.

70. Smith, E. E. and Jonides, J., Storage and executive processes in the frontal lobes, *Science*, 283, 1657–1661, 1999.

71. Reuter-Lorenz, P. A., Stanczak, L., and Miller, A. C., Neural recruitment and cognitive aging: two hemispheres are better than one, especially as you age, *Psychol. Sci.*, 10, 494–500, 1999.

72. Reuter-Lorenz, P. A. et al., Age differences in the frontal lateralization of verbal and spatial working memory revealed by PET, *J. Cogn. Neurosci.*, 12, 174–187, 2000.

73. Grachev, I. D. and Apkarian, A. V., Chemical network of the human brain: evidence of reorganization with aging, *Neuroimage*, 11, S83, 2000.

74. Fisk, J. E. and Warr, P. B., Associative learning and short-term forgetting as a function of age, perceptual speed, and central executive functioning, *J. Gerontol. Psychol. Sci.*, 53B, P112–P121, 1998.

75. Somberg, B. L. and Salthouse, T. Z., Divided attention abilities in young and old adults, *J. Exp. Psychol. Hum. Perception Performance*, 8, 651–663, 1982.

76. McDowd, J. M. and Birren, J. E., Aging and attentional processes, in *Handbook of the Psychology of Aging*, Birren, J. E. and Schaie, K. W., Eds., Academic Press, New York, 1990, 222–233.

77. Hartman, M. and Dusek, J., Direct and indirect memory tests: what they reveal about age differences in interference, *Aging Cogn.*, 1, 292–309, 1994.

78. McDowd, J. M. and Filion, D. L., Aging, selective attention, and inhibitory processes: a psychophysiological approach, *Psychol. Aging*, 7, 65–71, 1992.

79. Mazaux, J. M. et al., Visuo-spatial attention and psychomotor performance in elderly community residents: effects of age, gender, and education, *J. Clin. Exp. Neuropsychol.*, 17, 71–81, 1995.

80. Greenwood, P. M. and Parasuraman, R., Attentional disengagement deficit in nondemented elderly over 75 years of age, *Aging Cogn.*, 1, 188–202, 1994.

81. Parasuraman, R. et al., Visuospatial attention in dementia of the Alzheimer type, *Brain*, 115, 711–733, 1992.

82. Daigneault, S. and Braun, C. M. J., Working memory and the self-ordered pointing task: further evidence of early prefrontal decline in normal aging, *J. Clin. Exp. Neuropsychol.*, 15, 881–895, 1993.

83. Stuss, D. T. et al., Comparison of older people and patients with frontal lesions: evidence from word list learning, *Psychol. Aging*, 11, 387–395, 1996.

84. Foster, J. K., Behrmann, M., and Stuss, D. T., Aging and visual search: generalized cognitive slowing or selective deficit in attention? *Aging Cogn.*, 2, 279–299, 1995.

85. Keys, B. A. and White, D. A., Exploring the relationship between age, executive abilities, and psychomotor speed, *J. Int. Neuropsychol. Soc.*, 6, 76–82, 2000.

86. Brayne, C. et al., Estimating the true extent of cognitive decline in the old old, *J. Am. Geriatr. Soc.*, 47, 1283–1288, 1999.

87. Tun, P. A. and Wingfield, A., Does dividing attention become harder with age? Findings from the divided attention questionnaire, *Aging Cogn.*, 2, 39–66, 1995.

88. Craik, F. I. M., A functional account of age differences in memory, in *Human Memory and Cognitive Capabilities*, Kilx, F. and Hagendorf, H., Eds., North-Holland, Amsterdam, 1986, 409–422.

89. Huppert, F. A., Memory function in dementia and normal aging — dimension or dichotomy? in *Dementia and Normal Aging*, Huppert, F. A., Brayne, C., and O'Connor, D. W., Eds., Cambridge University Press, New York, 1994, 291–330.

90. Burke, D. M. et al., On the tip of the tongue: what causes word finding failures in young and older adults? *J. Mem. Language*, 30, 542–579, 1991.

91. Albert, M. S., Heller, H. S., and Milberg, W., Changes in naming ability with age, *Psychol. Aging*, 3, 173–178, 1988.

92. Kempler, D. and Zelinski, E. M., Language in dementia and normal aging, in *Dementia and Normal Aging*, Huppert, F. A., Brayne, C., and O'Connor, D. W., Eds., Cambridge University Press, New York, 1994, 291–330.

93. Filoteo, J. V. et al., Visuospatial dysfunction in dementia and normal aging, in *Dementia and Normal Aging*, Huppert, F. A., Brayne, C., and O'Connor, D. W., Eds., Cambridge University Press, New York, 1994, 291–330.

94. Laursen, P., The impact of aging on cognitive functions. An 11 year follow-up study of four age cohorts, *Acta Neurol. Scand. Suppl.*, 96, 1–75, 1997.

95. Spoor, A., Presbycusis values in relation to noise-induced hearing loss, *Int. Audiol.*, 6, 48–57, 1967.

96. Lebo, C. P. and Reddell, R. C., The presbycusis component in occupational hearing loss, *Laryngoscope*, 82, 1399–1409, 1972.

97. Fastenau, P. S., Denburg, N. L., and Abeles, N., The ROCFT and the Extended Complex Figure Test: a lifespan perspective, in *The Rey-Osterrieth Complex Figure Test: Clinical and Research Applications*, Knight, J. A. and Kaplan, E., Eds., Psychological Assessment Resources, Odessa, FL, in press.

98. Kray, J. and Lindenberger, U., adult age differences in task switching, *Psychol. Aging*, 15, 126–147, 2000.

6 Memory and Executive Dysfunction in Elderly People: The Role of the Frontal Lobes

Ingrid C. Friesen and Catherine A. Mateer

CONTENTS

6.1   Introduction 109
6.2   Neuropathology and Neuroimaging.. 110
6.3   Neuropsychology 111
      6.3.1   Disorders Involving Primarily Memory Functioning...................... 111
              6.3.1.1   Normal Aging 111
              6.3.1.2   Alzheimer's Disease 112
      6.3.2   Disorders Involving Primarily Executive Functions 113
              6.3.2.1   Normal Aging 113
              6.3.2.2   Frontal Lobe Dementias and Pick's Disease 114
              6.3.2.3   Parkinson's Disease 114
              6.3.2.4   Traumatic Brain Injury 115
6.4   Interventions for Declines in Memory Functioning.................................... 116
6.5   Interventions for Executive Dysfunctions 118
6.6   Interventions for Neuropsychiatric Symptoms.. 119
6.7   Summary 119
References... 120

6.1   INTRODUCTION

In recent years there has been an increasing number of studies that have examined the role of the frontal lobes in the cognitive abilities of older adults. Essentially, the data from these studies have led to the theory that the cognitive changes that are observed in older adults are similar to those observed in patients with damage to the frontal lobes.[1] The data suggest tasks that are believed to reflect frontal lobe functioning are the first to decline with advancing age.[2] Moreover, there is considerable evidence that demonstrates neuropathological and pathophysiological changes occur in the frontal lobes in older adults in advance of changes elsewhere in the brain.

This chapter addresses the neuropathological changes that occur in normal and pathological aging. Specific attention is paid to the changes that occur in the frontal lobes and the concomitant cognitive and psychiatric changes that occur. In addition, interventions that address executive and memory dysfunctions as well as psychiatric disturbances are discussed.

6.2 NEUROPATHOLOGY AND NEUROIMAGING

From early adulthood through the mid-50s, there is usually little evidence for major structural or functional changes in the brain. Brain volume peaks in the early 20s and declines very gradually until about age 55, when a much more rapid rate of shrinkage begins. Signs of cortical shrinkage include sulcal seining, narrowing of gyri, and thinning of the cortical mantle. Volumes are also reduced in subcortical structures including anterior diencephalic structures and portions of the basal ganglia. Over the entire brain, volume reduction has been estimated at about 5%.[3] Volume reduction is highly variable, however, across brain regions. The frontal cortex is by far most affected, with an estimated 17% loss, as compared with losses in the basal ganglia of 8% and even smaller losses in the temporal, parietal, and occipital cortices in the range of only 1%.[4]

Neuronal counts actually remain relatively stable over the life span, suggesting that reductions in brain volume result more from shrinkage than from actual loss of neurons.[4] The decreasing cell volumes are thought to result from both a loss of dendritic extension and a reduction in the number of synapses. Before age 40, there is little change in cell size, but, thereafter, shrinkage of cortical neurons, especially in the prefrontal cortex, begins. This process becomes most pronounced after age 65, and is particularly evident in the prefrontal region.

White matter loss also accounts for a significant amount of brain shrinkage. White matter lesions, termed leukoaraiosis, are seen in anterior frontal horns of the lateral ventricles in as many as 10% of healthy individuals over 65 years of age.[5] A relationship has been shown between the extent of white matter lesions and disturbances in attention and executive function.[6]

In addition to the neuropathological changes, there is evidence for changes in functional brain activity in elderly people. In young and middle-aged adults, greater blood flow is typically seen in anterior or posterior brain regions, a pattern sometimes termed *hyperfrontality*.[7] In older individuals, this pattern is often reversed, and called *hypofrontality*.[8] Shaw et al.[9] conducted a 4-year longitudinal study in which cerebral blood flow was measured in healthy elderly adults. Blood flow reductions were prominent in the prefrontal cortex, but only minimal in motor, frontotemporal, temporal, or occipital regions. In functional imaging studies, tasks that reliably result in blood flow activations in young adults result in diminished activation in older adults.

In summary, normal aging appears to be associated with both structural and functional changes in the brain, with greater volume reductions, neuronal loss, and blood flow reductions evident in the prefrontal cortex than in other cortical regions. These findings have led to the frontal lobe hypothesis of aging, which proposes that structural and functional changes in the frontal lobes result in an earlier and more severe decline in frontally based cognitive and behavioral functions than those supported by other brain regions.[2,10]

6.3 NEUROPSYCHOLOGY

Changes in cognition that have been reported in normal aging and in various neurological disorders, and which are thought to be associated with frontal lobe functioning, are discussed in the following sections. The neuropsychological findings are divided into disorders of memory and those of executive functioning.

6.3.1 DISORDERS INVOLVING PRIMARILY MEMORY FUNCTIONING

The processes involved in memory functioning have been mapped to the medial temporal and prefrontal regions.[11,12] As indicated above, these structures show atrophy or shrinkage in normal aging[13] and even more so in Alzheimer's disease.[14] These regions also show reductions in blood flow and glucose metabolism with advancing age.[15]

Disruptions to the frontal lobes affect some aspects of memory functioning. Patients with frontal lobe damage typically have difficulty with free recall tasks but less so with recognition tasks.[16] The difficulty with free recall tasks may be due to the inability to access or retrieve the information without cueing.[17] The frontal lobes are also involved in the use of elaborate encoding strategies that enhance memory.

6.3.1.1 Normal Aging

The most common complaint regarding cognitive functioning in later life is diminished memory abilities. Empirical findings suggest that there is validity to these complaints as there appear to be some robust cognitive changes with advancing age. This is particularly true for the old-old group, those over the age of 75 years. The decline in memory ability, however, is not pervasive as different aspects of memory decline at varying rates. The ability to recall information immediately after it has been presented, often referred to as short-term memory, has been shown to decline with age. Studies have demonstrated this age-related difference using a variety of tasks, including story recall,[18] word recall,[19] sentence recall,[20] and verbal paired associates.[21] Long-term or delayed memory also shows age-related decline. Studies have demonstrated that older adults perform more poorly than younger adults when a delay has occurred between the presentation and the recall of stories[22] and word lists.[23]

Age differences are attenuated, however, when there are high degrees of environmental or contextual support.[24] That is, fewer age differences are observed for tasks that involve recognition or, to a lesser extent, cued recall. Larger age differences are observed when there is little or no environmental support, such as for free recall tasks. Craik[24] asserts that this is the case because tasks with lower levels of environmental support require greater self-initiation and therefore utilize more cognitive resources. The magnitude of age differences on memory tasks, however, is mediated by verbal skills as those older adults with high verbal skills tend to perform similar to younger adults.[21,25]

The age differences in memory performance appear to be due to changes in encoding processes rather than in retrieval. When younger and older adults are equated in terms of initial learning (i.e., encoding) recall of information or the rate of forgetting is about the same across age groups.[21] Active encoding strategies are believed to be mediated by the prefrontal cortex, and recent research suggests that this area of the brain shows age-related decline before other areas.[26,27] Some assert that the changes that occur in normal aging are analogous to those found in patients with frontal lobe damage.[1,2,28]

6.3.1.2 Alzheimer's Disease

The neuropathology of Alzheimer's disease includes grossly atrophic regions of the brain, particularly in the temporoparietal and anterior frontal regions.[14] Other neuropathological findings include amyloid plaques, neurofibrillary tangles, and granulovacuolar degeneration.[29]

Disturbances in memory functioning and the inability to encode new information typically are the first symptoms of Alzheimer's disease. In particular, the memory for newly learned information is significantly worse than the memory for information or events that occurred in the distant past. For example, patients with Alzheimer's disease may be able to recall events from childhood but have difficulty in remembering the events that occurred yesterday. In contrast, overlearned skills, such as eating and dressing, typically remain intact until the late stages of the disease.

Changes in linguistic functions and visual spatial skills also become evident as Alzheimer's disease progresses. Verbal fluency becomes progressively impaired with greater deficits observed in letter fluency than in category fluency. Anomia or word-finding difficulties also become apparent in the early stages of the disease.

Changes in personality and the emergence of psychiatric symptoms may occur in Alzheimer's disease, particularly in the mid to late stages. In addition to an uncomplicated progression of the disease, the DSM-IV identifies three subgroups of patients with Alzheimer's disease: those with delirium, delusions, or depression. Delirium, or an acute confusional state, commonly occurs in Alzheimer's disease. In patients with dementia, the delirium typically is due to infections, fluid and electrolyte imbalances, or medication toxicity.[30] About half of patients develop psychosis or delusions during the course of the disease.[31] The delusions are usually persecutory in nature and involve fears of personal harm, theft of property, or infidelity. The presence of depression in Alzheimer's disease is controversial as many of the symptoms, such as weight loss, difficulty sleeping, loss of interest, and agitation, are common to both depression and Alzheimer's disease.[14] Patients, however, may exhibit mild to moderate depression, particularly early in the disease as they begin to become aware of the cognitive changes that are taking place. In addition, patients may develop agitation that includes physical or verbal aggression, restlessness, pacing, and screaming.

6.3.2 DISORDERS INVOLVING PRIMARILY EXECUTIVE FUNCTIONS

Executive functions comprise a superordinate system that mediates self-initiated behavior, and governs the planning, regulation, efficiency, and appropriateness of task performance. Important component processes supporting executive function include working memory, interference control, inhibition of prepotent responses, and prospective memory. Working memory refers to the ability to hold on to information while manipulating or reorganizing it. Impairments in working memory result in behaviors that are not guided by internal representations and instead become stimulus bound. Individuals with impaired working memory, therefore, appear to be distractable and impulsive. Interference control refers to the ability to ignore or clear information that is no longer relevant and to suppress interfering information from the internal or external environments.[2] Patients may continue to respond with a behavior that was once successful but is no longer appropriate. Inhibition of prepotent responses refers to the ability to allow for the inhibition of inappropriate responses that may be cued by the external or internal environment. Problems with inhibition may lead to impulsive behaviors. Prospective memory, which can be separated from retrospective memory, is the ability to carry out a prior intention. It can be initiated by either internal or external cues. Neuroanatomical correlates of executive functions involve primarily the frontal lobes,[32] which have an elaborate network of synaptic connections with the brain stem, thalamus, and cortex. Executive functions often are disrupted in dementias involving the frontal lobes, such as Pick's disease, Parkinson's disease, and traumatic brain injury.

6.3.2.1 Normal Aging

Many of the component processes that support executive functions show age-related declines. This observation has led to the model that the cognitive changes that are observed with advancing age are analogous to those observed in patients with frontal lobe damage.[1,2] In the extreme form of the model, the two are the same. In weaker forms of the model, however, older adults show greater deficits on tests designed to measure frontal lobe functioning compared with other cognitive tests.

Working memory involves the online processing of information. There are numerous studies that have shown age-related declines in this ability.[33] The amount of information that older adults can hold in short-term storage is not decreased. Rather, it is the act of manipulating the information that shows age-related declines.

Tasks that measure the ability to inhibit prepotent responses show declines with age. Difficulty in inhibiting prepotent responses are first observed in the sixth and seventh decades and increase steadily in the later decades.[34] Older adults also perform more poorly on tasks that require mental flexibility or a set shift according to changing environmental demands.[35]

Prospective memory, or the memory for an intended action, has been shown to be inferior in older adults compared with younger adults.[36-38] Older adults seem to do most poorly on the prospective memory tasks that require the greatest self-initiation, namely, time-based tasks. Time-based prospective memory tasks require that the individual monitor the passage of time prior to executing the appropriate response. This is in contrast to event-based prospective memory tasks in which a cue in the external environment prompts the individual to carry out the task at the appropriate time.

6.3.2.2 Frontal Lobe Dementias and Pick's Disease

Frontal lobe dementias (FLD) comprise a group of cortical degenerative diseases, all with similar clinical, pathological, and imaging presentations.[39] Pick's disease is classified as distinct from the other FLD because of pathological differences. At autopsy, Pick's bodies are only found in the brains of patients with Pick's disease.[39] Clinically, however, it is difficult, if not impossible, to separate Pick's disease from FLD.

Changes in personality and social behavior are the first signs of FLD and Pick's disease. Initially, the patient may become withdrawn and show little interest in social interactions. The individual may become socially disinhibited resulting in uncharacteristic behaviors, such as sexual promiscuity. Lack of insight also is common. As the disease progresses, a reduction in drive occurs. The personality changes typically occur years in advance of obvious cognitive changes.[40]

Initially, cognitive changes in FLD and Pick's disease are mild. Language problems are first observed with common changes including anomia and circumlocutions. These changes result in empty speech in which the individual is verbose because she or he cannot find the words needed. As FLD or Pick's disease progresses, comprehension becomes impaired and the quality of speech diminished, characterized by echolalia and perseverations. Memory disturbances occur after the initial language deficits and are similar to those found in Alzheimer's disease. Specifically, learning for new information and memory for recent events are most impaired.

6.3.2.3 Parkinson's Disease

In Parkinson's disease, the substantia nigra shows the greatest neuropathological and pathophysiological changes and there are Lewy bodies present throughout much of the brain.[14,39] At autopsy, atrophy is typically found in frontal regions of the brain.[41] The cognitive sequelae of Parkinson's disease are varied, with some individuals showing no deficits, others showing specific deficits in memory, executive functions, and visuospatial abilities, while a third group has global impairment.

Specific executive function deficits in patients with Parkinson's disease include planning and then executing the intended behavior. Difficulties in forming concepts and then shifting from one concept to another are common. Deficits also are observed in divided attention tasks and patients have difficulty in tasks requiring inhibition.

With regard to memory functioning, patients with Parkinson's disease appear to have preserved encoding processes but impaired retrieval processes. Evidence for this comes from normal performance on recognition tasks but impaired performance on tasks of free recall. That is, with cueing, patients are often able to recall the information, which is not the case in Alzheimer's disease. This pattern of memory impairment is consistent with frontal lobe dysfunction.

There is evidence to suggest that patients with Parkinson's disease have deficits in visuomotor tasks that require drawing complex figures. Other visuospatial deficits include difficulty with tasks of line orientation, pattern tracing and construction, and mental imagery. The impairments in visuomotor tasks are evident even when the contribution of the motor disability is taken into account and reflect the involvement of the frontal lobes.[42]

In addition to the cognitive changes that occur in Parkinson's disease, depression is common and affects about 40% of patients. The level of depression does not appear to be correlated with the severity of Parkinson's disease and therefore is believed to be an integral part of the disease rather than simply a reaction to it.[14]

6.3.2.4 Traumatic Brain Injury

Depending on the location or extent of injury, a variety of cognitive, emotional, and behavioral sequelae may be observed. It is well known that the frontal lobes are particularly vulnerable in situations involving falls or acceleration/deceleration injuries that are typical in motor vehicle accidents. Because relatively few studies have examined the effects of traumatic brain injury (TBI) in elderly people, the degree to which older adults may be more vulnerable to the primary or secondary effects of TBI compared with younger adults is not yet well established. However, one study found that adults over the age of 65 who experienced a mild or moderate TBI were three times more likely to develop intracranial hematomas compared with those under the age of 65 years.[43] Hemorrhages also have been found to be more common in older adults following TBI.[44] As discussed in Fields and Coffey,[45] Fields[46] found that older adults, particularly those over 75 years of age, had a considerably higher mortality rate following mild or severe TBI than younger adults. In this latter study, 12% of older adults with mild TBI died, whereas death occurred in less than 2% of the young group.

TBI is often associated with a wide range of cognitive, behavioral, and emotional sequelae. In the cognitive domain, deficits in attention are very common.[45,47] This is particularly true for complex tasks of attention, such as sustained vigilance,[48] shifting from one task to another or dividing attention between tasks.[49] There is reliable evidence that several aspects of attention decline with normal aging. Both completion times and error rates increase on cancellation tasks beginning after age 40,[50] indicating age-related declines in ignoring irrelevant information. Older individuals are also less able to inhibit processing of redundant information on choice reaction time tasks; while simple reaction time changes little with age, choice reaction time increases with age.[49] As a consequence of these anticipated changes in attentional processing, it is often difficult to sort out the effects of normal aging vs. TBI on attention. Unfortunately, there have been relatively few studies that have examined cognitive effects of TBI in elderly people. In a recent study, Richards[51] found an affect of even mild TBI on omission and commission errors on the Digit Symbol Test, over and above any effects attributable to age.

Deficits in memory are also very common following TBI, although memory and learning following TBI in older adults have not been well studied. Raskin and colleagues[52] reported that subjects with mild TBI who were over 40 years of age did less well than those under 40 on the California Verbal Learning Test (CVLT). In another study using the CVLT, Goldstein et al.[53] found that elderly TBI subjects and controls exhibited similar learning curves, but that the TBI patients with TBI demonstrated significantly less categorical clustering than controls. This suggests a selective vulnerability of the executive aspects of verbal learning that are already in decline as a result of normal aging.

Another area of functioning, which has been perhaps most strongly implicated in TBI, is executive functioning. Although the vulnerability of executive functions is well known with respect to normal aging, the limited data available suggest further and potentially independent declines in some executive functions in elderly persons who sustain TBI. Richards[51] compared young and elderly controls and young and elderly subjects with mild TBI. He reported deficits in switching aspects of verbal fluency and on the Trail Making Test Part B in elderly subjects with mild TBI, and both age and TBI effects on the ability to hold information in mind over distraction. He argued that deficits in attention, memory, and executive function were additive rather than interactive in nature in elderly subjects, such that age and TBI generally produced independent cognitive decrements.

Depression is another common outcome of TBI with prevalence rates varying between 6 and 39%.[54] Personality changes, including irritability, agitation, aggression, and impaired social judgment, occur in about two thirds of patients who have sustained a severe TBI.[55] Many of these changes in mood, personality, and social behavior are thought to reflect alterations in frontal lobe dysfunction. Although some of these types of changes can be seen in normal aging, it may well be that there are separable effects of aging and TBI in these domains as well as in cognitive domains.

6.4 INTERVENTIONS FOR DECLINES IN MEMORY FUNCTIONING

Neuropsychological interventions have been aimed at either improving underlying memory functioning or alleviating some of the practical problems that result from deficits in memory. Interventions aimed at improving memory function have sometimes utilized repetitive practice or training in memory and learning strategies. Compensatory memory strategies have focused on using external aids to assist in reminding the individual of information or intentions to be remembered, or in organizing and displaying information that might not otherwise be retrieved.[56,57] Most of these techniques and studies of their efficacy have been carried out in younger adults with acquired brain injury. Glisky and Glisky[58] point out that relatively few rehabilitation efforts have been directed at older adults.

With respect to memory-enhancing techniques, the idea that repetition of to-be-remembered information results in an improvement in memory functioning is not new. Such techniques involve reviewing and organizing specific information, such as short stories, presumably to foster deeper encoding and later retrieval of information.[59] Typically, patients engage in numerous drills each day over an extended period of time. Although these types of repetitive exercises still find favor with some clinicians, empirical data supporting their usefulness in improving general memory functioning are lacking.[56]

Another approach to memory improvement is the use of specific internally generated mnemonic techniques, such as visual imagery. Unfortunately, such techniques have not shown empirical support either. In part, this reflects the fact that such techniques often require a high level of abstraction or executive control for initiation and monitoring. Such techniques are also difficult to adapt to the practical memory requirements of everyday life.

The method of loci, for example, is an internal compensatory strategy that involves making a visual image of the to-be-remembered information with a geographic site that is well known to the individual. A series of studies have examined the efficacy of the method of loci.[60–62] These studies demonstrate that the method of loci can improve the amount of information older adults recall, and follow-up studies show that the older adults may spontaneously continue to use the technique up to 3 years later. Generally, however, the benefits are observed only on the experimental tasks with little or no generalization to other tasks, including everyday ones.[58]

Compensatory strategies using external memory aids are usually more effective. External memory aids include diaries, calendars and appointment books, notebooks and lists, alarm watches and timers, and pill-management devices. External memory aids generally are more efficacious than those that rely solely on internal resources.

External memory aids have been shown to be very effective in increasing the medication compliance of old-old adults. For example, older adults who were instructed to use a medication organizer and an organizational chart that described how the medications were to be taken increased their medication compliance significantly.[63]

In a study of prospective memory, Maylor[64] found that the most effective compensatory strategies for healthy adults were ones in which the target task was routinely completed in conjunction with another regularly performed activity. For example, medications might be most reliably taken when paired with the morning meal. External cues, such as writing notes, also were effective in helping older adults remember the target task, although to a lesser extent than the conjunctive cues. The least effective strategies were those that involved internal cues. The bulk of the data suggests that explicit, externally generated cues, embedded in functional everyday activities are the most effective at cueing memory and behavioral follow-through.

Reality orientation has been used, especially in long-term-care facilities, with individuals suffering from severe memory loss. This technique consists of explicit and repeated orientation to the physical and social environment through continual verbal communication.[65] Essentially, the caregiver provides constant repetition of information about the individual's name, where he or she is, and what is about to happen. There is no evidence that reality orientation improves underlying memory functioning, but Blazer[65] asserts that less medication may be necessary for controlling agitated behaviors when the individual is given specific information about what the caregiver is about to do.

6.5 INTERVENTIONS FOR EXECUTIVE DYSFUNCTIONS

The rehabilitation of individuals with executive function deficits is often extremely challenging. Individuals with frontal lobe dysfunction and executive disorders can appear very different depending on the nature and degree of impairment. Individuals with initiation problems may sit quietly and remain unengaged in their surroundings, whereas individuals with impulsivity or agitation may pace, wander, or respond unpredictably, putting themselves or others at risk. In addition, since executive functions include a wide variety of different areas of ability including attention, working memory, organization, planning, self-monitoring, and self-awareness, each of these areas may need to be addressed specifically in an intervention program.

One of the most important avenues of intervention involves education for the individuals and/or for family and caregivers to help them understand and cope with changes in the individual's function. A major problem that encumbers rehabilitation of difficulties related to frontal lobe dysfunction is the fact that such individuals frequently demonstrate altered self-awareness. In fact, the more severe the dysfunction, often the less aware the individuals are of ways in which their abilities and behavior have changed. This lack of insight makes rehabilitation extremely challenging, as patients may not appreciate the extent of their difficulties. This unawareness may keep individuals from feeling anxiety regarding their altered level of functioning, but it certainly does not decrease the stress on the patients' caregivers, spouses, and/or rehabilitation workers. Unfortunately, frontal lobe injuries or impairment can lead to personality changes and social deficits that are often confusing and frustrating for family members and caregivers. It may seem to family members that the patients are being manipulative, uncaring, or stubborn, when the patients are actually experiencing an organic unawareness, and an inability to regulate their own behavior.

When patients are minimally aware of their difficulties or have little self-regulation or direction, techniques that work best focus on changing the individuals' environment. Cues or prompting from caregivers can be effective for patients who have problems with initiation or volition.[32] External cues can be used to help initiate, guide, and sequence behavior. For example, a list of tasks to be done during a morning dressing and bathing routine can be used to prompt and keep on track an effective behavioral sequence. Problems may also arise if the person is overstimulated, and it is often helpful to reduce distractions. Frustration, behavioral outbursts, and disorganized behavior can result when the patients are not given enough information or support to perform tasks or when too much is asked of them. It is helpful to pay attention to signs the patients are getting overloaded or are uncertain what to do. Providing a lot of structure and routine is often useful in reducing the potential negative impact of executive function impairment. Behavioral strategies are often useful in shaping and reinforcing adaptive behaviors and routines.

When individuals with frontal injury are more aware of their difficulties and have some capacity for self-regulation, it is often useful to increase the individuals' ability to better self-manage their cognitive functioning, behavior, and mood. In the cognitive domain, individuals can be taught to avoid distractions, concentrate for longer and longer periods of time, and think more flexibly.[47,57] In the behavioral domain, they can be taught skills for dealing more effectively with depression, irritability, frustration, and anger. For such patients, cognitive–behavioral interventions have often been found to be quite effective.

6.6 INTERVENTIONS FOR NEUROPSYCHIATRIC SYMPTOMS

The neuropsychiatric symptoms that occur with dementia of the Pick's or Alzheimer's type, Parkinson's disease, and TBI are difficult to manage and often require more attention from caregivers than the cognitive symptoms.[66] Interventions generally fall into two categories: pharmacological and changes to the external environment.

Prior to introducing a pharmacological treatment, it is important to consider the changes in absorption, body mass, and metabolism that occur in older adults.[14] These changes can lead to toxicity if inappropriate dosages are administered.[66] For this reason, it is recommended that nonpharmacological interventions should be used whenever possible and the use of pharmacological ones minimized.[66,67]

Eliminating excessive visual and auditory stimulation in the environment can reduce agitation.[66] Specifically, visual stimulation can be reduced through the use of soft lighting and calm colors, such as peach and tan, restricting mirrors to bathrooms, and avoiding abstract or complex designs.[68] Swanwick[68] recommends using carpeting to absorb sound and avoiding the use of loud telephone bells to reduce auditory stimulation. According to Leiter and Cummings,[66] low doses of neuroleptics can be effective in treating agitated behaviors such as excitement, hostility, belligerence, and emotional lability.

Sensory deficits, particularly impaired vision and hearing, can cause hallucinations or delusions in the older adult with dementia. Prior to treating hallucinations or delusions, therefore, the individual's vision and hearing should be tested.[66] Wright and Cummings[69] recommend the use of neuroleptics or physostigmine as a pharmacological intervention for hallucinations and delusions in Alzheimer's disease.

6.7 SUMMARY

Structural and functional changes in the brain become more rapid starting in about the sixth decade of life. Although these changes occur throughout the brain, the frontal lobes show disproportionate cell loss and reduced blood flow. In pathological aging, such as in Alzheimer's or Parkinson's disease, these changes may become accelerated. Concomitant with the neuropathological alterations, myriad cognitive changes are observed in both healthy and pathological aging. Memory declines observed in healthy aging appear to be due largely to retrieval problems or inefficient encoding strategies. This pattern is similar to that observed in patients with frontal lobe damage. Moreover, older adults perform more poorly on tasks that are believed to measure frontal lobe function relative to other cognitive tasks. Memory deficits are the first to emerge in Alzheimer's disease but, unlike healthy aging, encoding rather than retrieval appears to be the primary problem. In contrast, executive functions are the first cognitive deficits observed in Pick's disease, Parkinson's disease, and TBI. To date, few interventions have been designed and empirically validated for older adults suffering from the behavioral sequelae of memory and executive dysfunction. Although the interventions may lead to improvements in the specific skill taught, they typically do not improve general memory or executive functions.

REFERENCES

1. Perfect, T., Memory aging as frontal lobe dysfunction, in *Cognitive Models of Memory*, Conway, M. A., Ed., MIT Press, Cambridge, MA, 1997.
2. West, R. L., An application of prefrontal cortex function theory to cognitive aging, *Psychol. Bull.*, 120, 272–292, 1996.
3. Freedman, M., Knoefel, J., Naser, M., and Levin, H., Computerized axial tomography in aging, in *Clinical Neurology of Aging*, Albert, M. L., Ed., Oxford University Press, New York, 1984, 139–148.
4. Haug, H. and Eggers, R., Morphometry of the human cortex cerebri and corpus striatum during aging [comment], *Neurobiol. Aging*, 12, 336–338, 1991.
5. Hachinski, V. C., Potter, P., and Merskey, H., Leudo-ariosis, *Arch. Neurol.*, 44, 21–23, 1987.
6. Boone, K. B., Miller, B. L., Lesser, I., Mehringer, M., Hill-Gutierrez, E., Goldberg, M. A., and Berman, N. G., Neuropsychological correlates of white-matter lesions in healthy elderly subjects: a threshold effect, *Arch. Neurol.*, 49, 549–554, 1992.
7. Hagstadius, S. and Risberg, J., Regional cerebral blood flow characteristics and variations with age in resting normal subjects, *Brain Cogn.*, 10, 28–43, 1989.
8. Dupui, P., Guell, A., and Bessoles, G., Cerebral blood flow in aging: decrease of hyperfrontal distribution, in *Monographs in Neural Sciences*, Cohen, M. M., Ed., Karger, Basel, Switzerland, 1984, 131–138.
9. Shaw, T. G., Mortel, K. F., Meyer, J. S., Rogers, R. L., Hardenberg, J., and Cutaia, M. M., Cerebral blood flow changes in benign aging and cerebrovascular disease, *Neurology*, 34, 855–862, 1984.
10. Albert, M. and Kaplan, E., Organic implications of neuropsychological deficits in the elderly, in *New Directions in Memory and Aging: Proceedings of the George A. Talland Memorial Conference*, Poon, L. W., Ed., Lawrence Erlbaum Associates, Hillsdale, NJ, 1980, 403–432.
11. Schacter, D. L., Savage, C. R., Alpert, N. M, Rauch, S. L., and Albert, M. S., The role of the hippocampus and frontal cortex in age-related memory changes: a PET study, *Neuroreport*, 7, 1165–1169, 1996.
12. Shallice, T., Fletcher, P., Frith, C. D., Grasby, P., Frackowiak, R. S. J., and Dolan, R. J., Brain regions associated with acquisition and retrieval of verbal episodic memory, *Nature*, 368, 633–635, 1994.
13. Coffey, C. E., Wilkinson, W. E., Parashos, I. A., Soady, S. A. R., Sullivan, R. J., Patterson, L. J., Figiel, G. S., Webb, M. C., Spritzer, C. E., and Djang, W. T., Quantitative cerebral anatomy of the aging human brain: a cross-sectional study using magnetic resonance imaging, *Neuropsychology*, 42, 527–536, 1992.
14. Cummings, J. L. and Benson, D. F., *Dementia: A Clinical Approach*, 2nd ed., Butterworth-Heinemann, Boston, 1992.

15. Martin, A. J., Friston, K. J., Colebatch, J. G., and Frackowiak, R. S. J., Decreases in regional cerebral blood flow with normal ageing, *J. Cerebral Blood Flow Metab.*, 11, 684–689, 1991.

16. Stuss, D. T., Eskes, G. A., and Foster, J. K., Experimental neuropsychological studies of frontal lobe functions, in *Handbook of Neuropsychology*, Vol. 9, Boller, F. and Grafman, J., Eds., Elsevier Press, Amsterdam, 1994.

17. Dawson, D., Winocur, G., and Moscovitch, M., Psychosocial factors influence cognitive enhancement in normal old people, in *Cognitive Neurorehabilitation*, Stuss, D. T., Winocur, G., and Robertson, I., Eds., Oxford University Press, New York, 1999.

18. Dixon, R. A., Hultsch, D. F., Simon, E. W., and von Eye, A., Verbal ability and text structure effects on adult age differences in text recall, *J. Verbal Learning Verbal Behav.*, 23, 569–578, 1984.

19. Craik, F. I. M., Age differences in human memory, in *Handbook of the Psychology of Aging*, Birren, J. E. and Schaie, K. W., Eds., Van Nostrand Reinhold, New York, 1977.

20. Bäckman, L. and Nilsson, L. G., Aging effects in recall: an exception to the rule, *Hum. Learning*, 3, 53–69, 1984 .

21. Craik, F. I. M., Byrd, M., and Swanson, J. M., Patterns of memory loss in three elderly samples, *Psychol. Aging*, 2, 79–86, 1987.

22. McCarty, S. M., Siegler, I. C., and Logue, P. E., Cross-sectional and longitudinal patterns of three Wechsler Memory Scale subtests, *J. Gerontol.*, 37, 169–175, 1982.

23. Wiederholt, W. C., Cahn, D., Butters, N. M., Salmon, D. P., Kritz-Silverstein, D., and Barrett-Conner, E., Effects of age, gender, and education on selected neuropsychological tests in an elderly community cohort, *J. Am. Geriatr. Soc.*, 41, 639–647, 1993.

24. Craik, F. I. M., A functional account of age differences in memory, in *Human Memory and Cognitive Capabilities, Mechanisms, and Performances*, Klix, F. and Hagendorf, H., Eds., Elsevier, Amsterdam, 1986.

25. Hultsch, D. F. and Dixon, R. A., Text processing in adulthood, in *Life Span Development and Behavior*, Vol. 6, Baltes, P. B. and Brim, O. G., Jr., Eds., Academic Press, New York, 1984.

26. Schacter, D. L., Kaszniak, A. W., Kihlstrom, J. F., and Valdiserri, M., The relation between source memory and aging, *Psychol. Aging*, 6, 559–568, 1991.

27. Shimamura, A. P. and Jurica, P. J., Memory interference effects and aging: findings from a test of frontal lobe function, *Neuropsychology*, 8, 408–412, 1994.

28. Baddeley, A. D. and Wilson, B., Frontal amnesia and the dysexecutive syndrome, *Brain Cogn.*, 7, 212–230, 1988.

29. Terry, R. D. and Katzman, R., Senile dementia of the Alzheimer type, *Ann. Neurol.*, 14, 497–506, 1983.

30. Purdie, F. R., Honigman, B., and Rosen, P., Acute organic brain syndrome: a review of 100 cases, *Ann. Emerg. Med.*, 10, 455–461, 1981.

31. Wragg, R. E. and Jeste, D. V., Overview of depression and psychosis in Alzheimer's disease, *Am. J. Psychiatr.*, 146, 577–587, 1989.

32. Mateer, C. A., The rehabilitation of executive disorders, in *Cognitive Neurorehabilitation*, Stuss, D. T., Winocur, G., and Robertson, I. H., Eds., Cambridge University Press, Cambridge, U.K., 1999.

33. Tuokko, H. and Hadjistavropoulos, T., *An Assessment Guide to Geriatric Neuropsychology*, Lawrence Erlbaum Associates, Mahwah, NJ, 1998.

34. Houx, P. J., Jolles, J., and Vreeling, F. W., Stroop interference: aging effects assessed with the Stroop Color-Word Test, *Exp. Aging Res.*, 19, 209–224, 1993.

35. Axelrod, B. N. and Henry, R. R., Age-related performance on the Wisconsin Card Sorting, Similarities, and Controlled Oral Word Association Tests, *Clin. Neuropsychol.*, 6, 16–26, 1992.
36. Einstein, G. O. and McDaniel, M. A., Retrieval processes in prospective memory. Theoretical approaches and some new empirical findings, in *Prospective Memory: Theory and Applications*, Brandimonte, M., Einstein, G. O., and McDaniel, M. A., Eds., Lawrence Erlbaum Associates, Mahwah, NJ, 1992.
37. Einstein, G. O., McDaniel, M. A., Richardson, S. L., and Guynn, M. J., Aging and prospective memory: examining the influences of self-initiated retrieval processes, *J. Exp. Psychol. Learning Mem. Cogn.*, 21, 996–1007, 1995.
38. Park, D. C., Hertzog, C., Kidder, D. P., Morrell, R. W., and Mayhorn, C. B., Effects of age on event-based and time-based prospective memory, *Psychol. Aging*, 12, 314–327, 1997.
39. Miller, B. L., Chang, L., Oropilla, G., and Mena, I., Alzheimer's disease and frontal lobe dementias, in Coffey, C. E. and Cummings, J. L., Eds., *Textbook of Geriatric Neuropsychiatry*, American Psychiatric Press, Washington, D.C., 1994.
40. Miller, B. L., Cummings, J. L., and Villanueva-Meyer, J., Frontal lobe degeneration: clinical, neuropsychological and SPECT characteristics, *Neurology*, 41, 1374–1382, 1991.
41. Alvord, E. C., The pathology of Parkinsonism. Part II. An interpretation with special reference to other changes in the aging brain, in *Recent Advances in Parkinson's Disease*, McDowell, F. H. and Markham, C. H., Eds., F. A. Davis, Philadelphia, 1971.
42. Koller, W. C. and Megaffin, B. B., in *Textbook of Geriatric Neuropsychiatry*, Coffey, C. E. and Cummings, J. L., Eds., American Psychiatric Press, Washington, D.C., 1994.
43. Pentland, B., Jones, P. A., Roy, C. W., and Miller, J. D., Head injury in the elderly, *Age Ageing*, 15, 193–202, 1986.
44. Vollmer, D. G. et al., Age and outcome following traumatic coma: why do older patients fare worse? *J. Neurosurg.*, 75 (Suppl.), S37–S49, 1991.
45. Fields, R. B. and Coffey, C. E., Traumatic brain injury, in *Textbook of Geriatric Neuropsychiatry*, Coffey, C. E. and Cummings, J. L., Eds., American Psychiatric Press, Washington, D.C., 1994.
46. Fields, R. B., The effects of head injuries on older adults, *Clin. Neuropsychol.*, 5, 252, 1991.
47. Mateer, C. A., Rehabilitation of individuals with frontal lobe impairment, in *Neuropsychological Rehabilitation: Fundamentals, Innovations, and Directions*, León-Carrión, J., Ed., St. Lucie Press, Delray Beach, FL, 1997.
48. Van Zomeren, A. H. and Brauwer, W. H., *Clinical Neuropsychology of Attention*, Oxford University Press, New York, 1994.
49. Stuss, D. T., Stethem, L. L., Hugenholtz, H., Picton, T., Pivik, J., and Richard, M. T., Reaction time after head injury: fatigue, divided and focused attention, and consistency of performance, *J. Neurol. Neurosurg. Psychiatr.*, 52, 742–748, 1989.
50. Lezak, M. D., *Neuropsychological Assessment*, 3rd ed., Oxford University Press, New York, 1995.
51. Richards, B., The Effects of Aging and Mild Traumatic Brain Injury on Neuropsychological Performance, Doctoral dissertation, York University, Toronto, Ontario, 2000.
52. Raskin, S. A., Mateer, C. A., and Tweeten, R., Neuropsychological assessment of individuals with mild traumatic brain injury, *Clin. Neuropsychol.*, 12, 21–30, 1998.
53. Goldstein, F. C., Levin, H. S., Presley, R. M., Searcy, J., Colohan, A. R. T., Eisenberg, H. M., Jan, B., and Bertolino-Kusnerik, L., Neurobehavioral consequences of closed head injury in older adults, *J. Neurol. Neurosurg. Psychiatr.*, 7, 961–966, 1994.

54. Jennett, B. and Teasdale, G., *Management of Head Injuries*, F. A. Davis, Philadelphia, 1981.

55. Silver, J. M., Hales, R. E., and Yudofsky, S. C., Neuropsychiatric aspects of traumatic brain injury, in *Textbook of Neuropsychiatry*, 2nd ed., Yudofsky, S. C. and Hales, R. E., Eds., American Psychiatric Press, Washington, D.C., 1992.

56. Schacter, D. L. and Glisky, E. L., Memory remediation: restoration, alleviation, and the acquisition of domain-specific knowledge, in *Clinical Neuropsychology of Intervention*, Uzzell, B. P. and Gross, Y., Eds., Martinus Nijhoff Publishing, Boston, MA, 1986.

57. Sohlberg, M. M. and Mateer, C. A., Effectiveness of an attention training program, *J. Clin. Exp. Neuropsychol.*, 19, 117–130, 1987.

58. Glisky, E. L. and Glisky, M. L., Memory rehabilitation in the elderly, in *Cognitive Neurorehabilitation*, Stuss, D. T., Winocur, G., and Robertson, I. H., Eds., Cambridge University Press, Cambridge, U.K., 1999.

59. Prigatano, G. P., Fordyce, D. J., Ziener, H. K., Roueche, J. R., Pepping, M., and Wood, B. C., Neuropsychological rehabilitation after closed head injury in young adults, *J. Neurol. Neurosurg. Psychiatr.*, 47, 505–513, 1984.

60. Anschutz, L., Camp, C. J., Markley, R. P., and Kramer, J. J., Maintenance and generalization of mnemonics for grocery shopping by older adults, *Exp. Aging Res.*, 11, 157–160, 1985.

61. Neely, A. S. and Bäckman, L., Long-term maintenance of gains from memory training in older adults: two $3^1/_2$-year follow-up studies, *J. Gerontol. Psychol. Sci.*, 48, P233–237, 1993.

62. West, R. L. and Crook, T. H., Video training of imagery for mature adults, *Appl. Cogn. Psychol.*, 6, 307–320, 1992.

63. Park, D. C., Morrell, R. W., Frieske, D., and Kincaid, D., Medication adherence behaviors in older adults: effects of external cognitive supports, *Psychol. Aging*, 7, 252–256, 1992.

64. Maylor, E. A., Age and prospective memory, *Q. J. Exp. Psychol.*, 42A, 471–493, 1990.

65. Blazer, D., *Emotional Problems in Later Life: Intervention Strategies for Professional Caregivers*, Springer-Verlag, New York, 1990.

66. Leiter, F. L. and Cummings, J. L., Pharmacological interventions in Alzheimer's disease, in *Cognitive Neurorehabilitation*, Stuss, D. T., Winocur, G., and Robertson, I. H., Eds., Cambridge University Press, Cambridge, U.K., 1999.

67. Fishman, L., Rehabilitation of elderly patients after traumatic brain injury, in *Rehabilitation of the Aging and Elderly Patient*, Felsenthal, G., Garrison, S. J., and Steinberg, F. U., Eds., Williams & Wilkins, Baltimore, MD, 1994.

68. Swanwick, G. R. J., Nonpharmacological treatment of behavioral symptoms, in *Behavioral Complications in Alzheimer's Disease*, Lawlor, B. A., Ed., American Psychiatric Press, Washington, D.C., 1995.

69. Wright, M. T. and Cummings, J. L., Neuropsychiatric disturbances in Alzheimer's disease and other dementias: recognition and management, *Neurologist*, 2, 207–218, 1996.

7 Motor Functions and Praxis in the Elderly

María J. Mozaz and Inés Monguió

CONTENTS

7.1 Introduction 125
7.2 Anatomy of Motor Functions 127
    7.2.1 Cortical Areas... 127
        7.2.1.1 Primary Motor Area... 127
        7.2.1.2 Supplementary Motor Area 127
        7.2.1.3 The Premotor Cortex 128
    7.2.2 Noncortical Structures.. 129
7.3 Theories on Motor Programs... 130
    7.3.1 The Functional System Theory... 131
        7.3.1.1 Perceptual and Motor Integration... 131
        7.3.1.2 Variability.. 131
        7.3.1.3 Sequencing 132
    7.3.2 The Neural Network Model.. 133
7.4 Age-Related Changes in Motor Skills: Functional Changes 133
    7.4.1 Upper and Lower Limbs... 135
    7.4.2 Gait... 136
    7.4.3 Oral Motor Skills 137
    7.4.4 Manual Skills 137
    7.4.5 Motor Learning 139
7.5 Limb Praxis Characteristics of Healthy Elderly People 140
    7.5.1 Quantitative Analysis 141
    7.5.2 Qualitative Analysis 143
7.6 Summary and Conclusions 145
References.. 146

7.1 INTRODUCTION

Purposeful and automatic body movements comprise a large variety of behaviors crucial for daily living that are produced to accomplish different behavioral goals (e.g., locomotion, speech, reaching and manipulating objects, and nonverbal communication, among others). Perhaps because of the mundane quality of the behaviors,

0-8493-2066-/01/$0.00+$1.50
© 2001 by CRC Press LLC

motor functions and praxis are subjects often neglected in edited volumes. Yet, movement, as one of the most explicit components of behavior, is one of the most objectively measurable manifestations of physiological, psychological, and cognitive processes. Movement in the external space is presumably one of the most crucial variables in evolution, and probably the most common behavioral outcome in animals, that implies a functional goal.

Movement can be broadly classified as voluntary and involuntary, conscious and unconscious. Unlike other cognitive functions that seem to require a certain level of central nervous system maturation, such as object permanence, speech, and concepts, movement probably produces the most striking synergy in the phylogenetic and ontogenetic evolution of the nervous systems at the phylogenetic and ontogenic levels.

Neuropsychology has generally used brain lesion paradigms when studying cognitive functions. This static, localization approach may work for circumscribed functions. However, all behavior, observable or not, is influenced in the ontogenic evolution within individuals by mental and physical experience. Therefore, developmental studies can contribute to understanding of neuropsychological functions. It is not possible to state that elderly people are apraxic unless there is an underlying neurological process responsible for the changes in the execution of voluntary movements. Aging, as a physiological process, is not just a decline process, but also a developing process, which affects brain functions and thus movement. Attending to how elderly people accomplish the execution of motor movements can offer rich information not only about its characteristics, but also about development in general. The neuropsychology of aging is interested in evaluating the brain–praxis relationship as a function of age, not necessarily of lesions or deterioration. However, to the authors' knowledge there are no studies addressing specifically normal age-related changes in praxis.

Movement in space does not belong to just one class of behaviors. The most common classification of movements distinguishes between movements that are initiated or stopped without conscious volition (involuntary) and those that can be suppressed or not initiated at will (voluntary).[1] Voluntary movements have been further separated into learned and unlearned movements.[2] The performance of voluntary movements depends on the participation of several anatomical structures in the nervous system and periphery. In addition to the motor neurons, the striated muscles, the specific body parts involved in the motion, and the central nervous system (CNS) are involved in the organization of the behavior and participate in the execution of voluntary movement. This complex process requires the coactivation of motor, planning, and organizational structures together with sensory structures in the CNS. Because of the multiple components involved in the execution of voluntary movement, it is difficult to identify the cerebral structures that are exclusively responsible for motor behavior. This chapter describes the cortical and subcortical structures involved in the execution of voluntary movement, and reviews some of the current theories on motor systems.

A complete review of the evolution of all motor activities is beyond the scope of this chapter. The review here is limited to human motor functions that affect activities of daily living when the quality of the movement changes. Reviewed are gait, crucial in independent functioning; swallowing and oral-motor skills because of their importance in feeding and verbal communication; studies of normal elderly subjects in the execution of upper limb movements, including manual motor skills; and the effects of aging on learning new motor skills. Finally, this chapter reviews some of the most relevant studies in apraxia, defined as a neurological disorder of learned purposive behavior movement skill that is not explained by deficits in elemental motor or sensory systems[3] and describes praxis in normal elderly subjects that were used as control groups in research.

7.2 ANATOMY OF MOTOR FUNCTIONS

Among the cortical structures involved in voluntary movements, the frontal cortex contains the primary motor cortex (MI), which corresponds to area 4 of Brodman, the supplementary motor area (SMA), which conforms to the lateral and medial premotor cortex in the medial part of area 6, and the premotor cortex (PM), also called the dorsal prefrontal cortex, above the frontal eye field (areas 9 and 46). The basal ganglia and the cerebellum are the two major noncortical components of the motor system.

7.2.1 CORTICAL AREAS

7.2.1.1 Primary Motor Area

The neurons of the MI connect to spinal and bulbar motor neurons and receive afferent impulses from the premotor area (PM), SMA, and cerebellum. Studies in cerebral blood flow (CBF) and cerebral metabolism (CMR) show that, except for voluntary eye movements, all other types of voluntary activity of the limbs, head, and face increase regional cerebral blood flow (rCBF), regional cerebral metabolism (rCMR), or open regional calcium channels (Ca^{2+}) in the somatotopical field of the MI.[4] These signs of increased energy utilization of areas in MI during voluntary motor activities of the limbs is mostly contralateral, although in the early phases of motor learning small activation can appear in the ipsilateral MI areas.[4]

MI provides a mechanism for the execution of fine variants selected in voluntary action, so that although active while reaching and walking, MI does not seem to be essential for the execution of these movements. It appears that subcortical structures are sufficient to perform such nonlearned movements, even in the absence of the motor cortex.[2] Joint activation of the SMA and the PM usually accompanies the activation of MI.[4] Thus, it is unlikely MI alone is able to control and produce voluntary motor activity, although without it, subtle variations in the quality of learned behaviors may be absent (Figure 7.1).

7.2.1.2 Supplementary Motor Area

In humans, the SMA, also known as the lateral and medial premotor cortex, seems to have close connections with the contralateral SMA, the cingulate, and the superior prefrontal cortices. Roland[4] stated that anatomically and functionally SMA is a higher-order motor structure than MI, and proposed that the role of the SMA is that

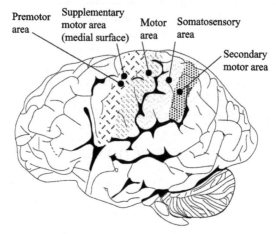

Premotor area — Supplementary motor area (medial surface) — Motor area — Somatosensory area — Secondary motor area

FIGURE 7.1   The sensory-motor cortex. (Courtesy of Jésus Pérez Lerga.)

of programmer of motor subroutines in intrapersonal space. Many learned skills consist of motor subroutines, which can be executed without any significant sensory feedback, once the synaptic changes in the SMA have established a memory. Data from lesion studies suggest that the SMA is specialized for the direction of self-generated movements that do not depend on external cues.[4] Functional brain imaging data offer additional tentative evidence that the SMA is particularly activated during the performance of overlearned motor sequences that do not require visual cues for execution. Furthermore, during prelearned performance, the SMA is more involved in the experimental motor sequence task than in the experimental visual conditional task.[2] These observations suggest that activation of SMA seems to be associated more with the sequential aspect of the motor task than with motor-visual integration.

However, since the initial attempts while learning motor skills are carried out totally under the guidance of sensory information, in order for the SMA to be a programmer of subroutines, it must also work together with somatosensory areas that become involved in the initial generation of patterns in the acquisition of new learning. Positron emission tomography (PET) studies have shown that during the early phases of learning there is more activity in the lateral premotor cortex than in the SMA itself.[2]

7.2.1.3 The Premotor Cortex

PM seems to be specifically activated only when sensory information is needed to build the motor program mainly in extrapersonal space, or when the motor program is modulated through incoming sensory information.[4] Lesion studies suggest that visual cues influence the motor system via the PM, and functional brain imaging data also offer tentative evidence that the dorsal PM is activated when a task is first learned and when the subject must pay attention to the visual cues relevant to the motor routine.[5] Single-cell recording studies have shown learning-related changes in over half of the PM neurons in monkeys,[6] suggesting that the PM participates in the learning process. Finally, the role of the PM in visuomotor associations has been underlined both in monkeys and in humans.[7] Thus, it seems to be clear that the dorsal PM integrates external sensory information during the formation of motor routines.

7.2.2 NONCORTICAL STRUCTURES

The basal ganglia are among the most complex structures in the brain and the study of the contribution of the basal ganglia to the planning and execution of voluntary movements is a real challenge. Studies of activation in the human brain of rCBF and rCMR have concentrated mainly on the caudate nucleus, the input striatum nucleus of the basal ganglia (putamen), and the output nucleus of the basal ganglia (globus pallidus). No information is available on the basal ganglia and the subthalamic nucleus as relates to voluntary action. But it is known that decreases in or near the substantia nigra occur during motor learning.[8] Some authors consider that the increased activity in the basal ganglia during a motor task depends upon the amount of learning already involved in the performance of the task and note that the globus pallidus flow increases moderately after learning has taken place.[4] The red nucleus in the mesencephalum seems to play a role in the control of movement.[4]

The internal segment of the globus pallidus transmits information from the motor cortices to the ventrolateral (VL) nucleus of the thalamus.[9] However, it seems that the only indicator that the thalamus is engaged in the preparation of voluntary movements has been provided by Decety et al.,[10] who found an increase in the left ventrolateral thalamus when subjects were preparing for a reaching movement with their right arm. One additional structure involved in voluntary movement is the cerebellum, which receives information from the motor cortex, the somatosensory cortices, the posterior prefrontal cortex, and in a smaller part from the visual association cortex via the pontine nuclei. The somatotopical field laterally in the anterior lobe of the cerebellum is activated when performing motor and sensoriomotor tasks, whereas the deep nucleus, the dentate, is only activated by sensorimotor tasks (Figure 7.2).

The manner and degree of participation among the different cortical and subcortical structures described above when executing movements are not yet fully understood. For example, changes in rCBF or rCMR during unilateral limb movements have been found both in ipsilateral and contralateral cortical and subcortical structures. Nevertheless, it has been suggested that of all the structures mentioned above, only the motor cortices PM, ipsilateral and contralateral SMA, and the contralateral MI are specialized for motor functions.[4] In contrast, the basal ganglia, cerebellum, and thalamus, as well as functionally heterogeneous structures like the putamen, the contra- and ipsilateral globus pallidus, and the contralateral substantia nigra, contain sections involved in motor functions, possibly through the contribution of sensory and proprioceptive information, but are not motor structures per se. Furthermore, when learning a movement, the participation of other structures involved in the analysis of somatosensory information is also needed. The posterior VL thalamus, the left somatosensory hand area in the postcentral gyrus, the somatosensory association areas in the anterior part of the parietal lobe, the supplementary

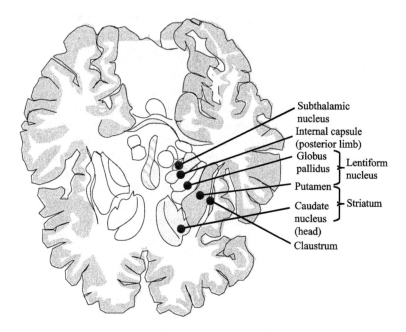

Subthalamic
nucleus
Internal capsule
(posterior limb)
Globus
pallidus   } Lentiform
                    nucleus
Putamen
Caudate   } Striatum
nucleus
(head)
Claustrum

FIGURE 7.2   The basal ganglia. (Courtesy of Jésus Pérez Lerga.)

sensory area, and the cortex in the anterior part of the intraparietal sulcus, likely participate in such analysis.[4]

As described in the sections above, much is known about the different areas of the brain that are activated during the learning and subsequent performance of voluntary movements. However, it is not known how the contribution from all of these motor and nonmotor structures is organized to produce voluntary movements. Neither is it known where in the brain motor programs are stored. The following reviews current theories on these topics.

7.3   THEORIES ON MOTOR PROGRAMS

Because of the complexity and heterogeneous nature of the behavior, describing and understanding voluntary movement is a challenging topic in behavioral, neural, and theoretical model research. One of the most difficult questions to be answered is how such diverse brain structures as the cerebral cortex, basal ganglia, and cerebellum cooperate to produce graceful, accurate, and seemingly effortless purposeful reaching movements.[7] Disruption of praxis has been traditionally associated with left hemisphere lesions.[11] The likelihood that cortical and/or subcortical left hemisphere structures are involved in praxis has been supported by several authors (for example, References 12 and 13) who have reported patients who suffered left subcortical lesions and who showed apraxia. However, the participation of both hemispheres in the organization of movements[14] and the role of the right hemisphere in controlling the limbs[15,16] has also been demonstrated. In addition, Mozaz et al.[17] have reported on a patient with a right subcortical lesion, and more recently, several hypotheses has been offered regarding the role of the subcortical structures in the organization of praxis.[18]

Different attempts have been made to explain how those different structures participate in the different components of a movement, and how the structures involved in movement are organized when performing voluntary movements.

7.3.1 THE FUNCTIONAL SYSTEM THEORY

One approach to explain the relationship among the multiple structures involved in purposeful movement considers the unit-system as a functional one composed of multiple components that may have independent neuroanatomical and functional natures. The components in the larger system may have functional independence but can come together as a functional unit to perform tasks of certain complexity, yet remain independent to afford collaboration when their input is needed for other classes of behaviors. One theory takes a page from memory systems paradigms and proposes that, when systems are defined functionally, then considering multiple systems as involved in the performance of movements is useful. Thus, evidence of functional and neuroanatomical independence for the different systems does not negate functional collaboration in certain behaviors.[7] Willingham,[7] using parallels between the motor skill and motor control systems, outlined three main functional processes in motor movement that involve cooperation of varied brain structures: perceptual and motor integration, excess degrees of freedom or variability, and serial ordering or sequencing. The following elaborates on each of the main functional processes posited by Willingham.[7]

7.3.1.1 Perceptual and Motor Integration

The first task to be accomplished in the successful execution of voluntary movement is that of perceptual and motor integration. This can be accomplished in at least two ways: (1) visuomotor association, by which perceptual information prescribes the movement to be done, and/or (2) visual guidance, which provides feedback about an ongoing movement. As mentioned previously, the parietal cortex participates in the analysis of somatosensory information. Various studies have found support for this, reporting that the PM receives projections directly from area 7a in the posterior parietal cortex. Area 7a also projects to cells in the pons that respond to visual information. These pontine cells project to the contralateral cerebellar hemisphere and the PM receives cerebellar input via nucleus X of the VL thalamus.[7] Thus, PM, area 7a of the posterior parietal cortex, and the cerebellum are relevant in the integration of perceptual and motor information. This collaboration occurs regardless of whether the integration is of visuomotor association areas or of visual guidance during an ongoing motor act.

7.3.1.2 Variability

The challenge of some motor skills, dancing, for example, is to gain expertise by reducing the spatial and temporal variability of a movement. It seems that the various systems involved in motor behavior reduce variability by organizing action in terms of muscle groups rather than individual muscles. Data suggest that synergy may operate at several levels, from simple conjunction of muscle flexion (such as at the wrist in preparation for a finger movement), to the more complex synergy involving timing, direction, and amplitude to maintain posture or to displace oneself in space (see Reference 7). The cerebellum is likely involved in these synergies, and the clinical interpretation of cerebellar ataxia as a degeneration of motor synergies[19] supports this view. Willingham[7] concluded, however, that there is no clear evidence for a motor skill system responsible for developing synergies, or how synergies are acquired.

7.3.1.3 Sequencing

Movements must be executed in the correct order to be operative. Patients with Parkinson's and Huntington disease, who suffer dopamine depletion to the striatum and striatal atrophy, respectively, seem to have difficulties with sequencing (see Reference 7 for a review), and, although for different causes, patients with ideomotor apraxia[20] have difficulty with sequencing as well. It has been suggested[20] that neurologically intact individuals parse serial events into subgroups to organize the sequence. Willingham[7] offered evidence that the SMA is involved in the sequencing of motor acts, and based on clinical evidence, suggested that the basal ganglia–SMA circuit participates in the sequencing of movements when visual feedback or cues are not needed. From his point of view, the basal ganglia–SMA circuit may be better described as a high-level planner than as a simple sequencer of motor actions. Further evidence that this last circuit may be involved in the management of the activity of various circuit activation can be found in the research of Harrington and Haaland.[20] These authors suggest that the basal ganglia and the thalamocortical connections may regulate mechanisms that are responsible for switching between different motor programs (Figure 7.3).

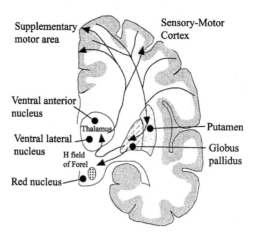

FIGURE 7.3 Circuit motor. (Courtesy of Jésus Pérez Lerga.)

7.3.2 The Neural Network Model

Another approach based on a neural network modeling proposes the existence of a general-purpose network involved in all types of movements,[21] regardless of whether or not they are memorized. The proposed motor system need not carry information about memorized trajectories or specific characteristics. If activated on its own, the system would produce straight-line trajectories. More recently, the existence of networks highly specific for a particular trajectory has been offered for consideration. These highly specialized subnetworks would interconnect to the general-purpose network, fusing in a new network able to produce the desired trajectory.[1] But, how such networks may be generated has not been explained. This theory assumes that the general-purpose network is present at birth, and that exposure to specific motor learning would result in selection of specific subnetworks from the vast number of choices available.[1] Georgopoulos[1] offered an alternative to his own hypothesis to explain voluntary movement. In this alternative, the organism starts out with motor shape primitives, which combine with the general network. The most complex trajectories resulting from this primitive combination become themselves very specialized and behave as such in other associations giving place to new trajectories. The new trajectories would give rise to neural subsystems for motor programs, defined as abstract representation of intended movements that describe the relationship among the goal of an action, the external event or objects it is directed toward, and the organism's interactions with the external event.[20]

In summary, although there appears to be evidence for independent anatomical systems in motor skills, explanatory theories are not conclusive and further research is needed regarding processes as well as in neuroanatomy, neurophysiology, and imaging techniques, to understand the real-time, dynamic cooperation of brain areas in planning, initiating, and controlling voluntary movements.[1]

7.4 AGE-RELATED CHANGES IN MOTOR SKILLS: FUNCTIONAL CHANGES

There are various reasons to investigate the functional changes that emerge during the aging process. Developmental neuropsychology is interested in establishing the normal pattern of behavior in healthy subjects all along their life process, with the goal of describing normal variations within determined age ranges, and to offer clues useful in diagnosing pathology. Developmental studies in neuropsychology are also interested in evaluating the effect of rehabilitation programs, to establish realistic expectations for rehabilitation efforts.

In addition to the useful information to be gathered from developmental studies regarding normal and pathological parameters, studying the elderly population is of interest for psychosocial reasons. The aging of the population represents a significant demographic shift that has an impact on economic and social systems in many industrialized countries all around the world. The low fertility rate with the subsequent potential reduction of labor force, and the potential reduction in the economy in those countries, create an area of concern that is not always properly considered. The reintroduction of previously retired employees into the workforce and the retraining of existing employees have been contemplated as possible solutions. However, current widely held beliefs that aging represents a decrement in functions could prevent social engineers from pursuing these alternatives.[22]

Many body systems change with age and it has been stated that most physiological functions decline at a rate of 1% per year beginning at age 30. Nerve conduction speed decrease, gross muscular atrophy, loss of balance related to postural sway, and changes in neurotransmitter systems of unknown significance are considered "normal." These changes only partly account for the observed decline in motor functions.[23] Depletion in dopamine in subcortical structures is related, as mentioned before, to motor deficits in Parkinson's disease. In normal aging no consistent age-related alteration in the dopamine D_1 receptor subtype has been reported,[24] but PET studies have measured a decrease of dopamine D_2 receptor subtype in the caudate and the putamen. These changes in D_2 receptors are related to deterioration of motor performance in older human subjects.[25]

Separately from changes in neurotransmitter availability or utilization, the activity of different regions of the normal brain changes moment to moment on a short-term basis, and upon learning and aging on a more long-term basis. Brain changes promote body changes and the evolution that comes with age involves changes in the characteristics of performance of very different behaviors. It is understood that changes in performance are not necessarily abnormal.

A common social belief has been formalized in the decremental theory of aging.[26] This theory predicts that as ability declines with age, so too will performance. However, there is still no clear data to support that normal declines in body functions affect the performance of functional activities. According to the 1991 U.S. Bureau of Labor Statistics older workers receive less training than all other age groups[22] and, although work needs and preference may change with age, older workers have been found to have work attitudes and to demonstrate work behaviors consistent with effective organizational functioning.[22] Instead of deterioration due to aging, fatigue, inactivity, and disuse, depression due to isolation and other factors not yet identified could be the largest contributors to losses in motor functions.[23] Therefore, sensible research is needed to better understand the real pattern of changes, and to reduce the dominate influence of the decremental theory of aging.[22]

It is possible that data from studies lacking control of extraneous factors, as proposed above, have been integrated into theories similar to the decremental theory of aging. But in the absence of controlling for fatigue, depression, medication use, musculoskeletal problems, and depression, conclusions regarding the presence or absence of abnormality are unwarranted. In the authors' opinion, when evaluating the functional ability of elderly people it is necessary to determine their sensory, physical conditions and their capacity for normal movement. It is also necessary to have in mind possible side effects due to medication and fatigue. It is generally accepted that response times are increasingly slowed with advancing age;[27] thus, interpretation of timed tests requires age norms, and if such norms are not available, only qualitative interpretation is advisable for cognitive and motor functions.

7.4.1 UPPER AND LOWER LIMBS

Lower (LE) and upper extremities (UE) are essential for physical independence. Decline of speed occurs at different rates in upper and lower limbs and a significant effect of age has been reported.[28] The elderly people showing poorest overall performance also had relatively slower response in their LE than in their UE. Regardless of gender, the rate of decline in leg and trunk muscles among elderly people was greater than in arm and handgrip muscles.[29] Several explanations can account for this finding.

The relative difference in decline of lower vs. upper limbs may be due to the difference in brain structures involved in the execution of movements using UE and LE. Some neurological studies reported that, whereas movement-related potentials are primarily in the cortex contralateral to the moving hand, they are ipsilateral to the moving foot.[30] More recently, a combination of functional magnetic resonance imaging (fMRI) and transcranial magnetic stimulation (TMS) techniques have been used as fMRI alone cannot differentiate between activation of corticospinal tract cells and other neural networks involved in motor planning.[31] fMRI activation of the motor cortex ipsilateral to the moving hand in normal subjects has been found, while during TMS of that same cortical motor area, no response in the ipsilateral hand occurred. Bilateral activation in cortical motor networks has been shown to be present during the execution of complex, rather than simple motor tasks.[31] Thus, it may be that a different level complexity of the task performed with the hands and those performed with the foot could account for the differences between reports of studies that have found decreases in motor functions of upper and lower limbs in elderly people. It may also explain the difference in the cortex between response to motor activities performed with the upper limbs and those performed with the lower limbs.

From the perspective of neural mechanism, fewer neural resources are involved in leg and foot control than in arm and hand control.[32] It is well known that the cortical area of projection of the hands and arms is more extensive than the cortical area of projection of the feet and legs. It might be that the function of lower limbs is more sensitive to the losses in efficiency in the CNS than is the function of the upper limbs. The decline in LE functioning may also be due to causes not immediately related to motor activity. For example, 40% reduction in sensory cells within the vestibular systems in people age 70 or older has been found,[33] which could affect postural control and balance. Visual and somatosensory deterioration are common in elderly people, and any or a combination of these sensory losses could account for motor decline. Control of hand movement is basically free of the requirements of postural control, whereas control of foot movement involves postural control mechanism, thus accounting again for the differences between upper and lower limb performance in aging. Postural response progressively deteriorates from the 50s onward,[23] and older adults had longer movement times, longer path lengths, and shorter distances of functional reach when compared with younger adults.[34] These findings suggest that, since all measures studied to identify age-related changes on postural control are sensitive to age, measures must be designed that are independent of age to clarify what changes and what stays the same as individuals age.

7.4.2 GAIT

The movements of the upper and the lower limbs are coordinated when walking. When the left leg is advanced, the right arm swings forward and the left arm swings backward with the purpose of decelerating rotation of the body and counterbalancing the forward swinging of the leg.[35] The total range of shoulder and elbow motion ranges from 28 to 34° and from 27 to 35°, respectively, in both young and older adults at free speed.[36] At faster speed, older subjects show a decreasing amplitude of shoulder and elbow movements.[35]

Studies comparing free-speed gait patterns of healthy younger women vs. elderly women reported significant smaller values of step length, stride length, ankle range of motion, pelvic obliquity, and velocity in older women. The same variables as well as vertical and horizontal excursions of the center of gravity were compared between young and elderly men.[37] The younger men demonstrated a significantly larger stride width than the elderly men, but there were no significant differences for the rest of the measures, suggesting that both young and older men have similar gait characteristics. When considering the variable of gender, the free-speed cadence for women is faster than that of men for both the younger and older populations, so that the faster cadence in women nearly compensates for their stride length.[35]

With reference to other gait factors, it has been reported that walking velocity decreases with age, while free-speed gait and fast velocities appear relatively stable until the seventh decade, after which they decline at a rate of 12 to 16% and 20% per decade, respectively (see Reference 35 for a review). There are other changes in factors relevant to the gait characteristics in elderly people. For example, older adults set a lower average fast walking speed (90 m/min) compared with younger adults (106m/min), probably as a way to economize their energy expenditure.[38] Healthy elderly people demonstrate a less vigorous push-off and a more flat-footed landing; this characteristic is thought to be caused by reductions in ankle motion resulting from a change in kinematics.[35] As an example of gravity control, it has been reported that healthy older adults use a more conservative strategy such as using slower crossing speed, shorter step lengths, and shorter obstacle–heel strike distances, when crossing obstacles.[39] Keeping in mind the kinematics of the trunk and extremities, it has been noted that in older subjects the movement of the trunk during gait tends to be slighter and the position of their head slightly backward when compared with younger people.[40] Considering all the above information, the authors agree with Hageman[35] in concluding that the gait characteristics of older healthy adults may be an adaptation toward a safer, less-energy-consuming gait pattern, not necessarily indicative of pathology, deficit, disability, or abnormality. Rather, changes in gait may represent successful adaptation that should be reinforced, rather than stigmatized. Physicians and physical therapists should not establish similar expectations for younger women and for elderly women during gait rehabilitation.[41] From the authors' point of view, the differences in gait characteristics between men and women as well as between healthy younger and older men must be taken into account when considering diagnosis and rehabilitation goals.

7.4.3 ORAL MOTOR SKILLS

Swallowing dysfunction, also known as dysphagia, which involves difficulties in eating or drinking, appears to increase with age as well as changes in mastication, tongue mobility, and lip movements.[42] There is no agreement, however, on the number of elderly people who experience difficulties in oral motor skills. Some authors report that only the 8% of people 60 to 95 years old have dysphagia,[43] while others have found that in long-term chronic-care facilities dysphagia may be as high as 79%.[44]

A group of 79 healthy people between 60 and 97 years old participated in a 3-year study conducted to identify changes in functional feeding and oral praxis abilities.[42] Of the subjects, 60 were living in their own homes and 19 in group homes. Information on denture wear, use of hearing aids and glasses, as well as about types of foods avoided, was registered. Results showed that there was no correlation between functional feeding ability and oral praxis skills. The author concluded that these two skills represent different domains of oral motor behavior. Healthy older people as a group maintained functional feeding skills over the four decades of life studied, and these skills were more dependent on the condition of dentures than on age. Results in oral praxis skills correlated significantly with age, but not with hearing aid use, suggesting that healthy elderly people maintain their oral praxis skills as well as feeding skills.

Oral praxis skills are involved in the production of speech, and some researchers reported fluency to be stable with aging (see Reference 27). More recently, an increase in vocal reaction time observed in aged subjects has been considered likely to be related to altered biomechanics and reduced efficiency of CNS motor processing.[45] Other authors have reported that only in stressful conditions elderly speakers become much more disfluent than younger speakers.[46]

A possible conclusion is that swallowing and oral praxis difficulties are not necessarily common signs of healthy aging and that they may be secondary to medical conditions, decreased sensitivity in both the oral and pharyngeal cavities,[46] use of medication, bad condition of dentures,[42] and hearing aid use. Regarding speech, and taking into account the studies mentioned above, it is likely that aging has no direct negative influence on speech fluency.

7.4.4 MANUAL SKILLS

Activities of daily living require a remarkable involvement of UE and manual ability considered to be essential for independence. UE motor coordination, manual dexterity, muscle strength, and sensibility are prerequisites for competent manual skill performance.[47,48] This section addresses the results of two recent unusual studies that measured gross, fine, and complex manual motor skills in healthy older people. The purpose of this section is to encourage a realistic understanding of normal results in healthy older people, rather than to consider normal variations in elderly people as deficient. If this is successful, the clinician may be helped to question the influence of the decremental theory of aging when assessing elderly people.

Using a longitudinal design, Desrosiers et al.[48] examined age-related changes in the UE sensoriomotor performance of 264 elderly people over a 3-year period. The study is a comprehensive UE evaluation that offers normative data for elderly people for each test. Tests administered were designed to measure gross and fine manual dexterity, global performance, motor coordination, grip strength, tactile recognition, static and moving two-point discrimination, and touch-pressure threshold. Statistically significant declines for most of the tests administered were found, but some test results were considered more clinically useful than others. For example, the tests showing lower rates of decline, such as some of the global performance tasks, were more consistently associated with the presence of deficits than those showing higher declines. Results revealed that gender is related to performance decline with age in some, but not all, tests or subtests. In addition, the better the score at first testing, the greater the decline at second testing, regardless of gender. The decline was considered to be related to initial score but not to age, suggesting that factors other than age may best account for the decline in functions measured. It might be that decrease of functions is biologically set within each individual and that, although the onset of deterioration may vary within individuals, once the decline begins, the changes in function follow a certain rapid slope that stabilizes to a slower decline later in the process. However, it may also be that elderly people with good upper limb functions become disheartened, depressed, or anxious when first experiencing decline in functions. While emotional responses are present during the effort to adapt to changes in functioning, the elderly individual may show a decline in physical functions over and beyond what may be strictly due to the physical deterioration itself (see Chapter 9 by Monguió). For example, patients first experiencing problems in daily function may be more vulnerable to developing depressed or anxious affect that may influence praxis, perhaps because of volitional or attention factors. Obviously, more research is needed in this area, including psychological status and other variables when studying physical functioning.

Kluger and colleagues[49] set out to assess, among other research hypotheses, the extent to which motor/psychomotor performance can distinguish normal elderly from mildly impaired subjects, and both groups from patients with a clinical diagnosis of mild or probable Alzheimer's disease. Complex motor functions were measured by the Head Tracking Assembly Test of Purdue Pegboard Test, Digit Symbol subtest from the WAIS, and Alternating Hand Movements or diadiokinesis. Gross motor functions were measured by Gross Motor Speed, Hand and Head Steadiness, and Hand Dynamometer. Fine motor functions were measured by the Purdue Pegboard and Grooved Pegboard Tests. Results showed that fine motor functions but not gross motor functions differentiate among the nondemented groups. Complex motor functions constituted the best measure that correctly classified subjects into the three different groups. The study also showed that control of complex motor functions is relatively independent of the influence of the more rudimentary aspects of motor control, thus suggesting that factors other than simply deterioration of motor functions could account for the differences in the performance of the three types of motor tasks among the three groups of subjects.

Given the results of the two studies reviewed here, it seems important to keep in mind that elderly people may demonstrate normal changes in motor functions that do not need to be considered pathological. Considering that normal changes related to age can lead to better prediction of expectations of future functions in nondemented elderly people,[49] attending to normal variations in motor performance among elderly people will result in more realistic expectations of their functioning, and this in turn can lead the clinician to identify factors in each individual that may be amenable to therapeutic interventions to help the individual maintain good upper limb mobility.[48]

7.4.5 MOTOR LEARNING

This chapter previously described how different areas of the brain participate in the generation and management of motor functions, some more active when the movement sequence is being learned, or is already learned. To keep the scope of this chapter to a manageable size, this section is limited to reviewing some recent studies that have addressed age-related factors affecting motor learning. Healthy older subjects (average age 66.2 years) can learn tasks as well as younger subjects (average age 19.8 years). The differences found were related to the effects of speed requirements in the learning of the task, but not in the learning of the task itself.[50] Perhaps anxiety or expectations of failure when speed is a factor in a task affects elderly more than younger subjects.

Wishart et al.[50] reported age-related differences for movement accuracy and consistency of acquisition measures, as well as on retention of material. However, transfer of learned skills was not related to age. These results are explained by Wishart et al.[50] as due to decrements in a central time-keeping mechanism responsible for motor outflow, or to a decrease in proprioceptive information feedback necessary for accurate timing. Wishart and colleagues concluded that older adults can learn a movement task with timing constraint as well as younger individuals whether feedback on results was infrequent or frequent. Results suggest that external feedback on performance accuracy had neither a positive nor a negative influence in younger or older adults.

Using different models of feedback, Swinnen et al.[51] found that relative phase accuracy was highest for adolescents (mean age 18.8) and elderly (mean age 72.70) subjects during augmented visual feedback in a motor learning task, in contrast to normal vision and blindfolded feedback conditions. The decrease in performance during the nonaugmented conditions was larger for elderly subjects, which could be explained by their reduced quality of sensory information. Results also showed that both the performance levels and the rate of improvement in elderly people were lower than in adolescent subjects. The authors hypothesize that the difference between older and younger subjects could be due to the increased difficulty of elderly people in overcoming previous patterns, as required for effective development or acquisition of new patterns. This reduced capability in elderly people may reflect an age-related decrease in efficiency associated with changes in frontal lobe functioning.[51]

Adolescent subjects in the study by Swinnen et al.[51] had a mean average age of 18.8 years. In a very recent study, a significant age effect was found in frontalization of functions, a CNS maturation task that may not be completed until the mid-20s.[52] According to the results of Rubia and colleagues,[52] the process of frontalization of the subjects in the Swinnen study was likely not yet completed. Yet, in the Swinnen study the adolescent subjects performed better than the healthy elderly subjects. It is possible that frontalization of functions that are most related to phylogenetic survival occur faster than those more typical of the "luxury" of being human. Therefore, individuals of 18 could have accomplished frontalization of other functions instead of the task. Speed of processing, lack of concerns regarding ability to succeed at physical tasks, and general level of energy could have resulted in the difference in scores between elderly and adolescent subjects in the Swinnen study. It is difficult to integrate the current information in this field with the knowledge of the development of motor functions that neuropsychology has clarified. The data from the Swinnen and the Rubia studies could be explained by the use of different methodology, or differences in functions measured. More research is needed to understand the age-related frontalization process, and how the changes in those processes affect functional motor activity in healthy subjects at various ages.

7.5 LIMB PRAXIS CHARACTERISTICS OF HEALTHY ELDERLY PEOPLE

The entire upper limbs are essential for the performance of limb praxis, those voluntary movements that include meaningless postures (e.g., hand under chin) and meaningful movements or gestures (e.g., pantomime of functional activity or non-verbal communication). Gestures are learned patterns of behavior, and may be defined as the result of a complex integration of an idea of the movement and of its execution in time and space. A gesture can be classified as transitive, involving object manipulation (e.g., comb hair), or intransitive, which relates to symbolic communication (e.g., wave goodbye).

The apraxias, agnosias, and aphasias have been the cornerstones upon which neuropsychology has developed as a specific discipline. Neuropsychology has been interested mostly in those changes resulting from CNS injuries when researching voluntary movements, that is, the apraxias. In 1870, Steinthal (see Reference 53) was probably the first to use the term *apraxia* to name the disorders not of primary motor skills, but of the ability to perform motor activity correctly on command. At the beginning of the 20th century, Liepman (see Reference 54) elaborated the first anatomoclinical and psychophatological theory of apraxia. From Liepman's point of view, apraxia was a unitary phenomenon, with the different varieties being different levels of dysfunction of the same mechanism. He distinguished three distinct types:

1. Melokinetic apraxia, which describes the loss of kinetic engrams for certain sections of the body. This type of apraxia is difficult to distinguish from a mild form of paresis.[55]

2. Ideomotor apraxia, which involves a dissociation of optic, tactile, and kinetic components for different parts of the body that must work in cooperation to produce a required movement.
3. Ideational apraxia, which refers to disorders to the ideational plan of the movement.

In addition to this classification, other varieties of apraxia, such as constructional apraxia, dressing apraxia, limb apraxia, and gait apraxia, among others, have been proposed, and not all of them follow Liepman's original definition of the disorder. Gait apraxia, for example, is not considered a disorder of learned skilled movements; dressing and constructional apraxia, although both have limb involvement, may be induced by visuospatial disorder or neglect,[56] thus seemingly involving more than the motor control systems in planning and execution of the movements.

One of the most controversial areas in the history of apraxia research is that of differentiating between ideomotor and purely ideational apraxia. A critical review of the different criteria, as well as an evaluation of the different methods of testing (verbal command, imitation, and real use of objects) and how those affect patients' responses, have been offered.[57] The author emphasized the importance of a qualitative analysis of the responses to the different methods of testing the patient with limb apraxia to clarify the mechanism underlying the deficit in voluntary movement. Recently, it has been concluded that patients with ideomotor apraxia make spatial and temporal errors, and that the term *ideational apraxia* should be used to denote the inability of patients to perform a series of acts leading to a goal (e.g., making a sandwich). In contrast, the term *conceptual apraxia* should be used when the disorder is characterized by content errors (a loss of tool–action associative knowledge).[56]

Although the study of disorders of voluntary movement helps to understand the nature of the problems, it is not sufficient to elucidate the mechanism underlying voluntary movement control in normal subjects. Cognitive neuropsychology has offered a model that explains the systems that mediate performance of learned, skilled movements.[54] The authors of this chapter concur with Gonzalez-Rothi and colleagues[54] who encouraged more collaboration between studies on disorders of voluntary movement and those investigating normal voluntary motor control. The following sections review some of the most relevant studies on limb apraxia with the goal of presenting data from normal subjects when performing limb praxis as control subjects. The intent is to raise awareness of what constitutes normal praxis in the elderly population,

7.5.1 QUANTITATIVE ANALYSIS

There are a series of tests used by different researchers to explore gestural praxis, but only the Test of Imitation of Gestures[58] is standardized, although the norms are those for children aged 3 to 6. The majority of studies have used the average scores obtained by normal control subjects minus two or three standard deviations to arrive at a cutoff score that classifies praxis as impaired. A list of tests used in the literature has been reviewed by Mozaz[59] (mentioned here as most relevant are those included in the Luria neuropsychological diagnostic,[60] the Test of Imitation of Gestures,[61] and the Test of Praxis[62]). There is available an interesting revision of the original methods by De Renzi[63] and a more recent version of the multiple object test[64] to assess the nature of the apraxias.

Mozaz et al.,[17,65,66] aware that a variety of instruments measuring praxis assess performance of movements considered to be of varied nature (for example, meaningful gestures and meaningless postures; transitive and intransitive movements) in one measure, proposed a method for exploring this area that separates into specific subtests measures for different types of movements, and proposed that results are comparable only when they are obtained under the same research conditions (verbal command, imitation, and real use of objects for transitive gestures). Recently, the Florida Battery, which is continuously revised and expanded,[67] although not yet standardized, offers an exhaustive assessment approach that includes the Florida Apraxia Screening Test and tests of Gesture Reception, Gesture Production, Praxis Imitation, and different tasks to measure Action Semantics. A new task measuring Postural Knowledge[68] has been developed recently for inclusion in the Florida Battery.

As mentioned above, the lack of standardized test for limb praxis makes it difficult to offer a thorough analysis of praxis characteristics in normal elderly people. The vast majority of studies on apraxia have been carried out on patients with focal lesions as subjects with an average age for control and impaired subjects under 65 years. Taking this age of 65 as the operational definition of "elderly," this chapter next reviews the research on praxis disorders, mainly, but not exclusively, those of patients diagnosed with Alzheimer's dementia. The goal of this review is to extract from those studies the results of the measures of praxis in the control groups, healthy subjects age 65 or older (Table 7.1). It is necessary to note that these studies use a variety of assessment and scoring methods. To render results more comparable among studies the average scores for transitive and intransitive gestures will be transformed to percentages of correct responses whenever possible. The results obtained under verbal command are differentiated from those in response to imitation. The reader is referred to the original articles for more detailed information.

In general, the results are those of subjects using the right dominant limb for the performance of the praxis. Control subjects scored within normal limits in the Mini Mental State Examination (MMSE),[69,70] or in the Spanish version of the same.[71] In the studies of patients with Alzheimer's disease, as in the patients with focal lesions, control subjects had a negative history of neurological or psychiatric illness.[72–74]

It is important to note that there is evidence of significant differences in the results of measuring the performance of transitive or intransitive gestures in patients[75] and in healthy elderly subjects.[76,77] As a possible explanation for this difference, some authors have suggested that transitive gestures require a larger participation of the limb joints, and therefore imply a greater motor complexity than intransitive gestures.[76] However Mozaz et al.[77] have found that when their normal elderly subjects were asked to discriminate between correct and incorrect postures, even though this task does not require movement, subjects had more difficulties selecting the correct

TABLE 7.1
**Percentage of Correct Responses by Control Subjects
in Various Studies**

Author	N	Mean Age	Mean MMSE	VC	IMI
Rapcsak et al. (1989)[72]	23	74			94
Ochipa et al. (1992)[73]	32	72.97		89	
Heilman et al. (1997)[74]	10	69.4	87		
Mozaz et al. (1999)[66]	20	72.10	28.40		98

Note: MMSE = Mini Mental State Examination; VC = verbal command; IMI = imitation.

posture for the transitive gestures than they did for the intransitive gestures. It appears that transitive and intransitive gesture representation systems could be separate from each other, at least in part. These researchers also found that there were no significant differences in the production of transitive and intransitive gestures between younger-elderly (66- to 76-year-old) and older-elderly (78- to 87-year-old) groups of normal subjects. These findings suggest that the production systems for transitive and intransitive gestures do not seem to be sensitive to age. The representational system for intransitive gestures was found to change with age; the one for transitive gesture does not.[77] The results of this research support the hypothesis that at some level there are different systems for representational and production programs for transitive and intransitive gestures.

7.5.2 QUALITATIVE ANALYSIS

Another important factor in the analysis of praxis is qualitative analysis, that is, the examination of the kind of response produced by the subjects when performing praxis. Some authors have looked at the different types of responses shown by patients with cortical lesions[11,64,78–81] and subcortical lesions.[12,17,75,82] However, to the authors' knowledge there is no available research analyzing the qualitative pattern of responses in normal elderly people. Thus, Table 7.2 offers an example of the type of responses displayed by control subjects 65 or older under verbal command when asked to pantomime to use a tool in the absence of the tool or object. The table summarizes the results of the studies that lent themselves to this type of analysis. Because subjects could make more than one error per item, the numbers of errors in each category do not add up to the total number of items. Not all articles used the same level of specificity when classifying the various types of responses, so an "Other" category is supplied to include unrecognizable responses[75] and "inaccuracy" responses.[83]

The body-part-as-object (BPO) response (i.e., subjects use a part of their bodies as an object, for example, index finger as a toothbrush) was the most frequent response by the control subjects in the different studies summarized above (Total 31). The next most common types of response, in order, were unrecognizable response or inaccuracy: "Other" (Total 18), followed by internal configuration (IC) response,

TABLE 7.2

Error Patterns by Control Subjects on the Verbal Command Modality in Different Studies: Transitive Gestures

Author Modality	No. of Subjects Older Than 65	Mean Age	Total Errors	Error Type
Gonzalez et al. (1988)[75]	4	74	16	BPO(7) ECO(2) C(2)[a] M(2) A(1) O(1) Other (1)
McDonald et al. (1994)[83]	24	71.2	34	BPO(17) Other (17)
Poole et al. (1997)[84]	10	68.6	30	BPO(7) ECO(7) IC(11)

[a] BPO = body-part-as-object; ECO = external configuration orientation; C = content; M = movement; A = amplitude; O = occurrence; Other = unrecognizable response and inaccuracy; IC = internal configuration.

or inexact relationship of the finger/hand to the object (i.e., no space allowed to handle the imagined toothbrush; Total 11); external configuration (ECO) (i.e., imprecision in considering the length of the object, as when asked to pretend to brush the teeth the subject holds the hand next to the mouth with no space between the hand and the teeth to accommodate the imagined toothbrush; Total 9); Content (C) (i.e., perseveration, when including all or part of a previously produced pantomime when a new gesture is required; Total 2); Movement (M) (i.e., disturbance of the characteristic movement; Total 2); and least common errors Amplitude (A) (i.e., any modification of the standard amplitude of the gesture; Total 1) and Occurrence (O) (i e., any multiplication of single cycles or any reduction of a repetitive cycle to a single event; Total 1).

BPO responses were first reported by Goodglass and Kaplan[11] in patients with brain damage and it was considered to be a primary sign of neuropathology. In addition to the data included in Table 7.2, BPO errors have also been reported in normal adults with a mean age of 63.3 years,[85] mean age of 56.7,[65] and mean age of 21.65[84] when performing transitive gestures under verbal command. On imitation Ska and Nespoulous[86] reported that BPO appears often in old normal control subjects (mean age 70) and seldom in middle-aged (mean age 44.1) and younger (mean age 26.3) normal control subjects, while Mozaz et al.[65] did not report BPO on imitation in the same population. Other researchers have found results consistent with the research findings of Mozaz. Poole and colleagues[84] found that only one of ten normal control subjects (mean age of group 68.6) showed BPO when imitating gesture movements. Thus far, the most severe praxis errors have been described only in patients with documented brain injury of varied etiology. This population showed a type of BPO response that demonstrated errors in the functional use of real objects (DBO), for example, using a saw on their thigh when asked to demonstrate its use.[87] Thus, it appears that when assessing disorders of praxis a distinction must be made between transitive and intransitive gestures, imitation vs. production on verbal command, and gestures in the presence or absence of the tool whose use is to be demonstrated by the patient.

It was suggested that EC, IC, DOB responses, and the use of irrelevant objects to demonstrate the use of an object (IO)[66,86,87] (e.g., using a pencil as a hammer when asked to pantomime a hammer) could be related to CNS conditions that underlie BPO responses.[57] They were considered to indicate different manifestations of impairment of the propositional use of objects.[88] BPO responses are common in the 4-year-old child, while external configuration (EC) errors, a less-primitive response, are more commonly made by 8-year-olds.[81] EC and IC errors in praxis have also been considered to have spatial components.[75,89] which would indicate dysfunction in the system involved in the production of voluntary movements. Further, level of education could affect the occurrence of BPO responses. But studies have failed to find differences between normal subjects without schooling and those with at least 4 years of schooling,[65,85] suggesting that developmental processes (e.g., sensorimotor stage[90]), more than education or cultural milieu,[91] contribute to the organization of the internal representation of objects and their utilization.

In summary, BPO, EC, and IC responses have been reported in normal adult and older subjects, as well as IO responses.[66,86] Thus, the incidence of these types of responses suggest that their presence per se can no longer be considered specific enough to be considered pathognomic for apraxia.[65] More research is needed to clarify the issues outlined above. It is necessary to better understand the variables that affect the mechanisms underlying BPO and related errors in healthy individuals at various ages. Once this information is available we could then begin to understand the responses of elderly subjects and of patients with brain lesions.

7.6 SUMMARY AND CONCLUSIONS

Aging brings physiological changes that can impact the functional characteristics of individuals in this phase of life. But aging is not a homogeneous process whether seen from the neurological or functional point of view. The preponderance of lost neurons due to age or of new neuronal connections within the capacity of the CNS would determine whether individuals age healthily or not. In addition, there are factors concomitant with aging that can influence negatively how elderly people function. In terms of motor function factors, the focus of this chapter, variables such as medication, fatigue, depression must be considered. In the elderly female, hormonal factors can contribute to the deterioration of motor functions because of osteoporosis.

Barring the conditions mentioned above that may affect motor functions, it is the position of the authors that the characteristics of the motor responses in elderly people may not represent deterioration. To diagnose accurately, to design realistic rehabilitation programs, and to assess progress, it is necessary to have reliable criteria of what is normal at different ages. This chapter has reviewed some of the most relevant investigations of various motor functions. On the basis of the review, the following conclusions are proposed:

- Postural control is sensitive to age.
- There are differences in gait characteristics between young women and elderly women, between men and women, and between healthy younger

and older men. Older healthy people develop compensating strategies for changes in speed and straight-line, which are not necessarily abnormal.

- Aging per se seems not to have a negative influence in swallowing, oral praxis, or speech.
- Decline with age in manual skills differs for men and women. The findings of faster decline in individuals with better initial functions are difficult to understand, given the available information. Decline in complex manual motor control tasks seems a more accurate measure of pathology than other measures.
- Sensory deterioration and timed tasks can negatively affect motor learning in elderly people. When these factors are not present, there seems to be no notable difference in the capacity to learn between the older and younger people.

This chapter has reviewed data and provided observations regarding gesture praxis. The goal is to encourage readers to consider and perhaps include in their investigation variables important to clarify this complex and relevant aspect in developmental neuropsychology. Future research should analyze changes that occur in the praxis of healthy elderly people so that norms can be developed to use for adequate diagnosis and rehabilitation. In addition, the availability of norms would help the clinician identify deteriorating praxis that may signal grave risk to the patient in the use of tools of daily living.

In conclusion, aging implies inevitable changes. The authors agree with the postmodern approach[92] that society needs to enable elderly people to cope effectively with personal and social changes. Successful aging is not a fantasy, but a real experience for many people. From this point of view successful aging, as successful living, means the ability of people to adjust to the continuous changes inside and all around them. People learn to cope with specific limitations, and to enhance the learning and skills that are specific to each age. Neuropsychological research holds in its hands the opportunity to change stereotypes that negatively influence expectations about old age and can offer a realistic view of the process of aging.

REFERENCES

1. Georgopoulos, A. P., Voluntary movement: computational principles and neural mechanisms, in *Cognitive Neuroscience*, Rugg, M. D., Ed., Psychology Press, Hove, East Sussex, U.K., 1997, chap. 5.
2. Passighan, R., *The Frontal Lobe and Voluntary Action*, Oxford Psychology Series, New York, 1993, chap. 2.
3. Gonzalez Rothi, L. J. and Heilman, K. M., A introduction to limb apraxia, in *Apraxia, the Neuropsychology of Action*, Rothi, L. J. G. and Heilman, K. M., Eds., Psychology Press, Hove, East Sussex, U.K., 1997, chap. 1.
4. Roland, P. E., *Brain Activation*, Wiley-Liss, New York, 1993, chap. 8.
5. Passighan, R., Functional organization of the motor system, in *Human Brain Function*, Frackowiak, R. S. J., Friston, K. J., Frith, C. D., Dolan, R. J., and Mazziotta, J. C., Eds., Academic Press, New York, 1997, chap. 11.

6. Mitz, A. R., Godschalk, M., and Wise, S. P., Learning-dependent neural activity in the premotor cortex: activity during the acquisition of conditional motor association, *J. Neurosci.*, 11(6), 1991.

7. Willingham, D. B., Systems of motor skills, in *Neuropsychology of Memory*, Squire, L. R. and Butters, N., Eds., Guilford Press, New York, 1992, chap. 14.

8. Seitz, R. J. et al., Motor learning in man: a positron emission tomographic study, *NeuroReport*, 1(1), 1990.

9. Alexander, G. E., DeLong, M. R., and Strick, P. L., Parallel organization of functionally segregated circuits linking basal ganglia and cortex, *Annu. Rev. Neurosci.*, 9, 357–381, 1986.

10. Decety, J. et al., Preparation for reaching: a PET study of the participating structures in the human brain, *NeuroReport*, 3(9), 761–764, 1992.

11. Goodglass, H. and Kaplan, E., Disturbance of gestures and pantomime in aphasia, *Brain*, 86, 703–720, 1963.

12. De Renzi, E. et al., Limb apraxia in patients with damage confined to the left basal ganglia and thalamus, *J. Neurol. Neurosurg. Psychiatry*, 49, 1030–1038, 1986.

13. Gonzalez Rothi, L. et al., Subcortical ideomotor apraxia. Abstract poster, *J. Clin. Exp. Neuropsychol.*, 10, 1988.

14. Kimura, D. and Humphrys, C. A., A comparison of left and right arm movements during speaking, *Neuropsychologia*, 19, 1981.

15. Wyke, M., The effects of brain lesions on the performance of bilateral arm movements, *Neuropsychologia*, 9, 33-42, 1971.

16. Zaidel, D., Zaidel, E., and Sperry, R. W., Ipsilateral hand finger control in commissurotomy patients, *Biol. Annu. Rep.*, 84, 1975.

17. Mozaz, M. et al., Apraxia in a patient with lesion located in right sub-cortical area. Analysis of errors, *Cortex*, 26, 651–655, 1990.

18. Crosson, B., Subcortical limb apraxia, in *Apraxia, the Neuropsychology of Action*, Rothi, L. J. G. and Heilman, K. M., Eds., Psychology Press, Hove, East Sussex, U.K., 1997, chap. 12.

19. Brooks, V. B. and Trach, W. T., Cerebellar control of posture and movement, in *Handbook of Physiology: Section 1. The Nervous System*, vol. 2, *Motor Control*, Brooks, V. B., Ed., American Physiological Society, Bethesda, MD, 1981, Part 2.

20. Harrington, D. L. and Haaland, K.Y., Representations of action in ideomotor limb apraxia: clues for motor programming and control, in *Apraxia, the Neuropsychology of Action*, Rothi, L. J. G. and Heilman, K. M., Eds., Psychology Press, Hove, East Sussex, U.K., 1997, chap. 9.

21. Lukhasing, A. V., Wilcox, G. L., and Georgopoulos, A. P., Overlapping neural networks for multiple motor programs, *Proc. Natl. Acad. Sci. U.S.A.*, 91(18), 8651–8654, 1994.

22. Seifert, C. F. and Kavanagh, M. J., Age and performance: implications in an organizational setting, available at http://www.siena.edu/seifert/research__age_and _performance.htm.

23. Schut, L. J., Motor system changes in aging brain: what is normal and what is not, *Geriatrics*, 53(Suppl. 1), 516–519, 1998.

24. Strong, R., Neurochemical changes in the aging human brain: implications for behavioral impairment and neurodegenerative disease, *Geriatrics*, Suppl. 1, 1998.

25. Volkow, N. D. et al., Association between decline in brain dopamine activity with age and cognitive and motor impairment in healthy individuals, *Am. J. Psychiatr.*, 155, 3, 1998.

26. Ginger, S., Dispenzieri, A., and Eisenberg, J., Age, experience and performance on speed and skill jobs in an applied setting, *J. Appl. Psychol.*, 68, 1983.
27. Lezak, M. D., *Neuropsychological Assessment*, 3rd ed., Oxford University Press, New York, 1995, chaps. 8, 16.
28. Li, Y., McGolgin, C., and Van Oteghen, S. L., Comparison of psychomotor performance between the upper and the lower extremities in three age groups, *Percept. Mot. Skills*, 87(3), 1, 1998.
29. Gabbard, C. P., *Lifelong Motor Development,* 2nd ed., Benchmark, Indianapolis, IN, 1996.
30. Brunia, C. H. M., Woorn, F. J., and Berger, M. P. E., Movement related slow potentials: a contrast between finger and foot movements in left-handed subjects, *Electroencephalogr. Clin. Neurophysiol.*, 60(2), 135–142, 1985.
31. Bastings, E. P. et al., Co-registration of cortical magnetic stimulation and functional magnetic resonance imaging, *NeuroReport,* 9, 9, 1998.
32. Peters, M., Neuropsychological identification of motor problems: can we learn something from the feet and legs that hands and arms will not tell us? *Neuropsychol. Rev.*, 1(2), 165–183, 1990.
33. Manchester, D. et al., Visual, vestibular and somatosensory contributions to balance control in the older adult, *J. Gerontol.*, 44(4), M118–M127, 1989.
34. Hageman, P. A., Leibowitz, J. M., and Blanke, D., Age and gender effects on postural control measures, *Arch. Phys. Med. Rehabil.*, 76, 10, 1995.
35. Hageman, P. A., Gait characteristics on healthy elderly: a literature review, *Section of Geriatrics, American Physical Therapy Association*, 18, 2, 1995.
36. Murray, M. P., Sepic, S. B., and Barnard, E. J., Patterns of sagittal rotation of the upper limbs in walking, *Phys. Ther.,* 47, 1967.
37. Blanke, D. J. and Hageman, P. A., Comparison of gait of young men and elderly men, *Phys. Ther.*, 69, 2, 1989.
38. Waters, R. L. et al., Energy-speed relationship of walking: standard tables, *J. Orthop. Res.*, 6(2), 215–222, 1988.
39. Chen, H. et al., Stepping over obstacles: gait patterns of healthy young and old adults, *J. Gerontol.,* 46, 6, M196–203, 1991.
40. Hirasaki, J. E. et al., Analysis of head and body movements of elderly people during locomotion, *Acta Otolaryngol.*, Suppl. 501, 25–30, 1993.
41. Hageman, P. A. and Blanke, D. J., Comparison of gait of young women and elderly women, *Phys. Ther.*, 66, 9, 1986.
42. Fucile, S. et al., Functional oral-motor skills: do they change with age? *Dysphagia*, 13(4), 195–201, 1998.
43. Bloem, B. et al., Prevalence of subjective dysphagia in community residents aged over 87, *Br. Med. J.*, 300(6726), 721–722, 1990.
44. Siebens, H. et al., Correlates and eating dependency in institutionalized elderly, *J. Am. Geriat. Soc.,* 34(3), 192–198, 1986.
45. Fozo, M. S. and Watson, B. C., Task complexity effect on vocal reaction time in aged speakers, *J. Voice*, 12, 4, 1998.
46. Caruso, A. J., McClowry, M. T., and Max, L., Age-related effects on speech fluency, *Semin. Speech Language*, 18, 2, 1997.
47. Desrosiers, J. et al., Upper extremity performance test for the elderly (TEMPA): normative data and correlates with sensorimotor parameters, *Arch. Phys. Med. Rehabil.,* 76, 1125–1129, 1995.
48. Desrosiers, J. et al., Age-related changes in upper extremity performance of elderly people: a longitudinal study, *Exp. Gerontol.,* 34, 393–405, 1999.

49. Kluger, A. et al., Patterns of motor impairment in normal aging, mild cognitive decline, and early Alzheimer's disease, *J. Gerontol. B Psychol. Sci. Soc. Sci.*, 52, 1, 1997.

50. Wishart, L. R. and Lee, T. D., Effects of aging and reduced relative frequency of knowledge of results on learning a motor skill, *Percept. Mot. Skills*, 84, 3, 1997.

51. Swinnen, S. P. et al., Age-related deficits in motor learning and differences in feedback processing during the production of bimanual coordination pattern, *Cogn. Neuropsychol.*, 15, 5, 1998.

52. Rubia, K. et al., Functional frontalisation with age: mapping neurodevelopmental trajectories with fMRI, *Neurosci. Biobehav. Rev.*, 24, 1, 2000.

53. Hecaen, H., Apraxias, in *Handbook of Clinical Neuropsychology*, Filsko, S. B. and Boll, T. L., Eds., Senis, New York, 1981, chap. 8.

54. Gonzalez Rothi, L. J., Ochipa, C., and Heilman, K. M., A cognitive neuropsychological model of limb praxis and apraxia, in *Apraxia, the Neuropsychology of Action*, Rothi, L. J. G. and Heilman, K. M., Eds., Psychology Press, Hove, East Sussex, U.K., 1997, chap. 4.

55. De Renzi, E., Apraxia, in *Handbook of Neuropsychology*, Vol. 2. Boller, F. and Grafman, J., Eds., Elsevier Science, Amsterdam, 1989, chap. 13.

56. Heilman, K. M. and Gonzalez Rothi, L. J., Limb apraxia: a look back, in *Apraxia, the Neuropsychology of Action*, Rothi, L. J. G. and Heilman, K. M., Eds., Psychology Press, Hove, East Sussex, U.K., 1997, chap. 2.

57. Mozaz, M. J., Ideational and ideomotor apraxia: a qualitative analysis, *Behav. Neurol.*, 5, 1, 1992.

58. Berges, J. and Lezine, I., *Test d'imitation de gestes,* Masson, Paris, 1963.

59. Mozaz, M. J., Praxias gestuales in la exploración neuropsicológica, in *Congreso de la Sociedad Española de Neurología*, VII, Peña, J., Ed., MCR, Barcelona, 1987, chap. 10.

60. Christense, A. L., *El diagnostico neuropsicologico de Luria,* Visor, Madrid, 1979.

61. De Renzi, E., Moti, F., and Nichelli, D., Imitating gestures, *Arch. Neurol.*, 37, 6–10, 1980.

62. Watson, T. R. et al., Apraxia and the supplementary motor area, *Arch. Neurol.*, 43(8), 787–792, 1986.

63. De Renzi, E. Methods of limb apraxia examination and their bearing on the interpretation of the disorder, in *Neuropsychological Studies of Apraxia and Related Disorders,* Roy, E. A., Ed., Elsevier Science, New York, 1985, 2.

64. De Renzi, E. and Lucchelli, F., Ideational apraxia, *Brain*, 111, 1988.

65. Mozaz, M. et al., Use of body part as object in brain-damaged patients, *Clin. Neuropsychol.*, 7,1, 1993.

66. Mozaz, M., Espinal, J. B., and Formica, A., Diferencias en la imitacion de diferentes tipos de movimientos en pacientes con probable enfermedad de Alzheimer, *Rev. Esp. de Neuropsicol.*, 1, 1, 1999.

67. Gonzalez Rothi, L. J., Raymer, A. M., and Heilman, K. M., Limb Praxis assessment, in *Apraxia, the Neuropsychology of Action*, Rothi, L. J. G. and Heilman, K. M., Eds., Psychology Press, Hove, East Sussex, U.K., 1997, chap. 6.

68. Mozaz, M., et al., A Test of Action Knowledge for Use with Aphasic, Apraxic Patients, Poster Presentation, International Neuropsychological Society, Denver, February, 2000.

69. Folstein, M. F., Folstein, S. E., and McHugh, P. R., "Mini Mental State": a practical method for grading the cognitive state of patients for the clinician, *J. Psychatr. Res.*, 12, 189–198, 1975.

70. Folstein, M. F., The Mini-Mental State Examination, in *Assessment in Geriatric Psychopharmacology*, Crook, T. H., Ed., Mark Powley, CT, 1983.

71. Lobo, A. and Gomez, F., El "Minoiexamen cognoscitivo" en pacientes geriatricos, *Folia. Neuropsiquiatr.*, 14(4), 244–251, 1979.

72. Racpsak, S., Croswell, S., and Rubens, A., Apraxia in Alzheimer's disease, *Neurology*, 39, 1989.

73. Ochipa, C., Gonzalez Rothi, L. J., and Heilman, K. M., Conceptual apraxia in Alzheimer's disease, *Brain*, 115, 1061–1071, 1992.

74. Heilman, K. et al., Conceptual apraxia from lateralized lesions, *Neurology*, 49(2), 457–464, 1997.

75. Gonzalez Rothi, L. J. et al., Ideomotor Apraxia: error pattern analysis, *Aphasiology*, 2, 3–4, 1988.

76. Raymer, A. M. et al., Differences between transitive and intransitive gestures in limb apraxia, Poster Presentation, International Neuropsychological Society, Orlando, FL, February, 2000.

77. Mozaz, M. et al., *Postural Knowledge*, in preparation.

78. Roy, E. A. and Square, P. A., Control mechanisms in limb praxis: the conceptual-production system, in *Neuropsychological Studies of Apraxia and Related Disorders*, Rot, E. A., Ed., Elsevier Science Publishers, Amsterdam, 1985, chap. 6.

79. Lehmkuhl, G., Poeck, K., and Willmes, K., Ideomotor apraxia and aphasia: an examination of types of manifestations of apraxics symptoms, *Neuropsychologia*, 21, 199–212, 1983.

80. Ferro, J. M. et al., CT scan correlates off gesture recognition, *J. Neurol. Neurosurg. Psychiatr.*, 46(49), 943–952, 1983.

81. Haaland, K. Y. and Flaherty, D., The different types of limb apraxia errors made by patients with left vs. right hemisphere damage, *Brain Cogn.*, 3, 370–384, 1984.

82. Basso, A. and Della Salla, S., Ideomotor apraxia arising from a purely deep lesion, *J. Neurol. Neurosurg. Psychiatr.,* 49, 1986.

83. McDonald, S., Tate, R. L., and Rigby, J., Error types in ideomotor apraxia: a qualitative analysis, *Brain Cogn.*, 25, 458–465, 1994.

84. Poole, J. L. et al., The mechanisms for adult-onset apraxia and developmental dyspraxia: an examination and comparison of errors patterns, *Am. J. Occup. Ther.,* 51, 5, 1997.

85. Duffy, R. J. and Duffy, J. R., An investigation of body part as object (BPO) responses in normal and brain-damaged adults, *Brain Cogn.*, 10, 220–236, 1989.

86. Ska, B. and Nespoulus, J. L., Pantomimes and aging, *J. Clin. Exp. Neuropsychol.,* 9, 754–766, 1987.

87. Mozaz, M. J., *Aspectos Semiológicos de las Apraxias de los Miembros Superiores,* Publicacions Universitat de Barcelona, Baracelona, 1992.

88. Denny-Brown, D., The nature of apraxia, *J. Nerv. Mental Disorders*, 126, 1958.

89. Roy, E. A., Apraxia: a new look at an old syndrome, *J. Hum. Movement Stud.*, 4, 1978.

90. Piaget, J., *Play, Dreams and Imitation in Childhood*, Rutledge and Kegan, London, 1962.

91. Bringuier, J. C., *Conversation with Piaget*, The University of Chicago Press, Chicago, 1980.

92. Schindler, R., Empowering the aged—a postmodern approach, *Int. J. Aging Hum. Dev.*, 49, 3, 1999.

8 Normal and Pathological Language in Elderly People

José Miguel Rodríguez Santos
and Javier García Orza

CONTENTS

8.1 Communication, Language, and Aging 152
8.2 Language within Other Cognitive Functions 154
    8.2.1 Visual and Auditory Perceptual Impairments 154
    8.2.2 Attention and Memory Impairments 155
    8.2.3 Motor Deficiencies 157
    8.2.4 Language within the Overall Context
        of Other Cognitive Functions 157
8.3 Aspects of Language Preserved during the Aging Process 161
    8.3.1 Semantic Memory 161
    8.3.2 Syntax 162
    8.3.3 Prosody 163
8.4 The Core Issue in Language Problems in Elderly People:
    Difficulties in Lexical Retrieval 163
    8.4.1 Retrieval of the Phonological Representations 163
        8.4.1.1 The Problems of Naming and Verbal Fluency
            in Older Adults 164
        8.4.1.2 The Tip-of-the-Tongue Phenomenon 166
    8.4.2 Retrieval of Orthographic Representations 167
8.5 Discourse Comprehension and Elderspeak 169
8.6 Discourse Production and Compensation Mechanisms 170
8.7 Pathological Evolution of Language in Alzheimer's Disease 173
    8.7.1 Alzheimer's Disease in the Context
        of Neuropsychological Pathology 173
    8.7.2 Brief Summary of the Characteristics of Language
        in Alzheimer's Disease 174
8.8 Summary 175
References 177

8.1 COMMUNICATION, LANGUAGE, AND AGING

Language skills — the ability to produce and understand language and use the information given in this way — are absolutely essential for the autonomous functioning of individuals during their lifetime, and especially during old age. For elderly people to be able to maintain self-sufficiency, they must be capable of understanding, remembering, and using the kind of information they receive every day. It is impossible to be self-sufficient if one cannot understand or remember instructions on how to use an appliance or when to take medication, or cannot remember personal agreements, or carry out any other of the typical communicative acts that occur in everyday life.

Considering where society is heading, these skills are becoming increasingly essential. We live in the Information Age, and are inundated by information; advances in technology demand we use of our communication skills properly. For example, consider the massive amount of oral or written instructions we encounter daily in our automated environment: automated switchboards that guide us from one service to another, ATMs, information points in supermarkets, ordering a hamburger in a fast-food restaurant, and so on. Such automated aids are effective, provided the person is capable of dealing with the communicative challenges they present. These familiar situations place significant demands on the processing and cognitive resources of language in general, and of oral language in particular.

With increasing age, a deterioration of all the cognitive functions takes place. Language is no exception and, thus, as the person gets older, language function undergoes some changes. Naturally, these usually take the form of a deterioration in functionality. However, language has an interesting peculiarity: like intelligence, it does not deteriorate as much as other cognitive functions as time goes by. Memory, on the other hand, represents the paradigm of a cognitive function negatively affected by age. Language is one of the best-preserved functions as people get older.

However, when language problems appear in elderly people, they occur within a set of circumstances that are particular to this stage of human life; the person is most likely experiencing the loss of loved ones, neighbors, and friends, as well as the loss of health and work, etc. Within this context it becomes crucial for older people not to lose their language skills to the same degree as they are losing other mental faculties. Language becomes a very precious treasure for elderly people, as most are still able to use it. In fact, most elderly people speak a great deal to others, or to themselves if they do not have anyone else to talk to. Speech is one of the best-preserved faculties in elderly people and one of the most influential in maintaining their self-esteem.

The changes observed in language production during old age are very influential at a theoretical as well as at a practical level. If aging affects production skills, this will have direct repercussions on interpersonal communication, which in turn will contribute to the increased social isolation so common in old age. In addition, it should not be forgotten that people consider language production an indicator of intellectual functioning, and so deficiencies in this area will negatively affect self-assessment of a person's cognitive abilities as well as evaluations by others.[1]

A negative self-evaluation may lead to a progressive retreat from social interactions, while a negative evaluation on the part of others may lead the older person to use a simplified communication style — elderspeak — which will also undermine the older person's self-esteem.[1,2]

On the other hand, language processing provides insights into some of the natural compensatory mechanisms elderly people use to counteract deficits attributed to age. These compensation mechanisms can serve professionals involved in human resources as a model to design environments and interventions to improve communication in elderly people.

Moreover, it is important to recall that, given the current demographic figures, the number of elderly people will increase considerably in the future, and so any related issue will become increasingly significant.

In addition, the evolution of language in elderly people presents a pattern, which enables us to differentiate between normal and pathological aging. This pattern is especially useful for establishing a differential diagnosis of pathological degenerative disease, such as Alzheimer's disease, during aging. Since the onset of this kind of dementia is very insidious, it is important to have available differential criteria to detect the early symptoms of the disease. Later on we will review some of the peculiarities of such developments.

As understanding and remembering oral language is a common daily activity, perhaps people tend to think of it as a very easy task, whereas in fact it is an extremely complex activity from the cognitive point of view. Indeed, it puts serious demands on the processing capabilities of the person: there is a high rate of data input; the speaking rate is also relatively high — between 100 and 180 words per minute (wpm), and can even reach as many as 210 wpm in some instances such as on the radio or TV. The speed at which new information is received is not controlled by the listener (contrary to what happens while reading, which is self-administered). The listener can control the input rate in interpersonal interactions, but there are many other occasions when this is not possible (listening to the radio, watching TV, conversing in a group, listening to a lecture or to instructions for a group, etc.). If we add to this the fact that very often speech is not fully intelligible, we begin to grasp better the difficulties elderly people often have to face. Correct and successful dealing with this task requires an "online" analysis of streams of fast speech, not always received under the best conditions. This analysis involves many tasks in itself: breaking down the speech stream into isolated words; having access to the meaning of words; analyzing sets of words in syntactic terms; carrying out semantic interpretations, etc. Moreover, all this is happening without the chance to "rewind" when we make an error of comprehension or simply experience difficulties in understanding the message.

According to current cognitive aging theories, it is reasonable to assume that most of the aspects we have just described — rapid speech rates, absence of control over speakers, demands for online processing, lack of precision — play an important role in the difficulties older people experience in comprehending spoken language.

8.2 LANGUAGE WITHIN OTHER COGNITIVE FUNCTIONS

Language does not exhibit its evolutionary pattern in isolation, but rather evolves together with the rest of the cognitive functions. Therefore, it will reflect the impact of the deterioration of other cognitive functions. Let us look into this question by reviewing some of the cognitive functions most relevant to the evolution of language.

8.2.1 VISUAL AND AUDITORY PERCEPTUAL IMPAIRMENTS

The processes of language comprehension involve much more than the activation of linguistic elements. Before this, some perceptual processes, of an auditory nature in the case of spoken language and visual when dealing with written material, take place. If the input is poor, these processes can hinder the functioning of the language-processing system. If they are not properly isolated, deficiencies in sensorial and perceptual mechanisms characteristic of old age might become a source of error in the study of cognitive deficiencies, and so it is essential to clarify the true role they play in the communicative difficulties of elderly people.

There is no doubt that the auditory deterioration typical of old age, e.g., presbycusis, is at least partly responsible for the difficulties elderly people experience in speech perception. During aging, there is a degeneration of the cochlea that diminishes the spectral and temporal resolution of the auditory system hindering the capacity to recognize words.[3] These sensorial impairments advance in a subtle way and do not destroy the auditory capacity of elderly people, so they are often unaware of them.

However, the more complicated the communication conditions become, the more conscious elderly people are of their difficulties in comprehending auditory signals. In noisy environments or when several people are involved in the same conversation, older people, compared with younger adults, usually experience, and claim to have, more difficulties in understanding. These difficulties can have a sensorial origin (i.e., difficulties in picking up the signal) or may be perceptual (i.e., problems in interpreting the signal). According to the results obtained by Schneider et al.,[4] the complaints about understanding spoken language that older adults express seem to be fundamentally due to problems with their auditory systems. Schneider et al. set young and old adults to the task of hearing a message both under conversational noise conditions and in quiet conditions, and then replying to some questions. When conditions were adjusted to the auditory differences in subjects, i.e., the condition at which the auditory capacity for pure tones was the same for everybody, and thus eliminating the influence of sensorial losses, the performance of young and older adults was practically identical. However, when the auditory conditions were standard and similar for everybody, the young adults responded better, especially under the conversational noise condition, as expected.

Although this study shows the influence of sensorial losses on understanding spoken language, it does not rule out the influence of perceptual difficulties. Since the measurement unit was the comprehension of a text, the equality between the groups when sensorial losses were eliminated could be due to a better use of context, which is characteristic of elderly people, and not to the absence of difficulties in recognizing the signal. This would make the data obtained in the experiment of Schneider et al. compatible with the findings of other studies. For example, Sommers[5] presents evidence that perceptual problems also appear with age. His study suggests that in spite of having equal auditory levels, older adults were less skilled than younger ones in the process of normalizing the acoustic signal. This normalization process is a process that takes place during speech perception by which the acoustic differences typical of the variation in the characteristics of speakers are adjusted by the listener to standardized representations. A plausible explanation of the differences observed in perception in relation to age is that of processing rate.[6] Given that the quality of the stimulus deteriorates with time, the representation of the acoustic stimulus becomes less stable, and so the process of phonetic categorization is more susceptible to error, which could explain why it is easier for older people to confuse some words for others, for example, *cat* for *cot.*

Most studies seem to suggest that the difficulties elderly people exhibit in oral language comprehension have their origin in auditory losses, to which we have to add normalization problems during the process of word recognition.

When analyzing the role of visual alterations on text comprehension, we find a similar pattern to those described for speech comprehension and auditory signals.[7] Using techniques such as evoked potentials (ERP), Kuegler[8] tried to study the impact of age on visual sharpness during the perception of stimuli. The results showed that, although age is the factor that better predicts the variability in potentials (P300), visual sensorial functions also explain this variability to some extent. In other words, neither sensorial deficiencies, on the one hand, nor perceptual deficiencies, on the other, could explain in isolation the difficulties, albeit mild, elderly people experience with visual comprehension.

To sum up, the data available are compatible with the idea that language comprehension in elderly people is hindered by both sensorial and perceptual problems. As we will see later on, we have to add to the influence these factors have on language comprehension the effects of deficits on other basic processes, such as attention and memory. Paradoxically, the factors that do not seem to have any special relevance for the presence of difficulties in auditory comprehension are specifically linguistic, as we will discuss further on.

8.2.2 ATTENTION AND MEMORY IMPAIRMENTS

The previous section explored the influence of sensorial and perceptual processes on the difficulties older people experience in language comprehension. Language production and comprehension require other cognitive devices such as attention and memory to support processing, and given that both seem to be affected by age, different theoretical approaches make them responsible for the difficulties elderly people experience with language. Given that the deterioration of the attention and memory processes we observe with age is dealt with in other chapters of this book, we will just outline those aspects relevant to the linguistic difficulties typical of aging.

Concerning memory, it is worth bearing in mind that the extended and popular idea that aging brings about a generalized decline in memory has not been empirically demonstrated and, in fact, was rejected by the scientific community some time ago. Currently, memory is envisaged as a set of complex, multidimensional systems, and so it is suggested that some memory systems might be selectively affected by aging deterioration, but that others can even improve with age.[9] Although no agreement has been reached regarding which memory system is fundamentally involved in the processes of language comprehension, so-called working memory seems to be the one more important for the development of these processes.[10,11] Among other processes, language comprehension requires signal encoding, parsing the structure of the sentence, or constructing the meaning of the sentence. Working memory is involved in all these processes, manipulating information and storing the intermediate products of processing. Contrary to what happens with typical measurements of short-term memory — where individuals have to remember the highest possible number of words or digits, and which are not susceptible to variations with age — the measurements of working memory simultaneously take into account processing and storing capacity, and show a clear decrease with age.[12,13] The consequences of this decline in processing capacity are clearly observed in comprehension. For example, studies that manipulated the complexity of sentences have shown that as complexity increased, and therefore the demands on the processing capacity or resources of working memory, the performance of elderly people strongly declined in comparison with young adults.[14,15]

Regarding attention processes, by means of which a communication task or relationship becomes our focus of interest, data obtained with different experimental paradigms seem to point to a deterioration of attention abilities with age, for example, decreasing the capacity to avoid distraction[16] or to switch tasks,[17] which evidently can have an influence on the quality of linguistic processes.

In the field of memory and attention, theoreticians have turned to energy analogies, using concepts such as capacity, resources, or inhibition, to describe the functioning of the processing systems. In fact, the cognitive and language difficulties observed in old age have been attributed to these elements. For example, from the point of view of some theoretical models, systems have a limited quantity of resources to carry out cognitive processes. In the event of a lack of resources, the system cannot process all the information properly and this will give rise to errors. According to some hypotheses,[18-20] the amount of resources available decrease during old age, and so certain processes, such as linking a pronoun to its antecedent, which could previously be carried out with no difficulty, cannot be done correctly because they exceed the capacity of the memory system of elderly people.

A similar position is adopted by the inhibition theory defended by Zacks and Hasher,[16] among others. These authors postulate the existence of some inhibition processes as an essential constituent of the attention systems whose functions are to avoid interference. According to these authors, this inhibiting capacity is progressively lost with age, which generates a greater amount of interference, and consequently, more difficulties in understanding.

Although the study of the influence of these processes is complex and the data contradictory, the results obtained by Van der Linden et al.,[21] after several regression analyses, seem to confirm that the factor responsible for the relationships between age and language is *working memory*. This mechanism seems to account for the differences in cognitive slowdown, and the loss of inhibiting capacity typical of older adults.

Thus, there is considerable evidence for believing that some of the deficiencies that appear with age in certain linguistic processes, such as sentence comprehension, have their origins in systems that are not language specific, such as working memory.

8.2.3 Motor Deficiencies

In the same way that perception is relevant to language comprehension processes, since it provides the input for the language system to process, motor processes are involved in language output in any of its modalities: written, oral, gestural, etc. Therefore, motor impairments can also affect the output of language production processes, an output that might already be undermined by perceptual and cognitive deficits.

Slowdown is without doubt the most significant motor change occurring with age. Speed of movement is one of the parameters that slows early on, around the age of 30 to 35, although beginning in an almost imperceptible way. However, this slowing greatly varies as a function of the tasks and the individual's characteristics and habits. It is fundamentally observed in tasks that demand quick and repetitive movements, and it is manifested more clearly in people with sedentary habits, in contrast to more active people where the decrease in the speed of movements is almost imperceptible.[22]

In language tasks, it has been observed that elderly people are slightly slower in writing and speaking, but this does not seem to cause serious difficulties, because they are still within the parameters of normality. The absence of specific problems in motor patterns in writing and speech seems to be related to the automatic character of these movements. We know that the decrease in speed and the ability to control movement more affects those motor processes that are controlled by the individual rather than automatic ones, and this would explain the absence of difficulties in motor speech and writing patterns.

Some of the difficulties observed in writing processes are associated with the integration of visual and proprioceptive information needed to coordinate movements on the paper. As Guan and Wade[23] have shown in a test where old people had to point to a target through a prism that distorted vision, the integration of visual and manual information seems to suffer deficiencies with aging. However, these deficiencies in coordination abilities do not seem to affect the process of writing in a visible way.

8.2.4 Language within the Overall Context of Other Cognitive Functions

Changes in language abilities throughout normal aging has been systematically studied by using neuropsychological standardized batteries such as the Wechsler Adult Intelligence Scale (WAIS). A classic discovery in the neuropsychological study of aging is that the scores in the manipulation scale of the WAIS intelligence test decrease in a more marked way than the verbal scale of the same test. Also, when the time factor is eliminated from the different tests in this scale or from the Raven Progressive Matrix test, in spite of a clear improvement in performance, the older people do not fully equal the younger people, and this suggests the existence of a deficit in spatiovisual processing. Spatiovisual alterations associated with aging have been found in several neuropsychological studies that explored the ability to perform tasks such as line orientation discrimination, face recognition, shape learning, spatial memory, image recognition modifying perspective, and ways of imagining space.

However, there is a methodological question worth raising. The information provided by these neuropsychological batteries comes from cross-sectional studies and, therefore, the effects of aging can be easily confused with environmental or cultural differences existing among different generations of subjects, as well as with nutritional and health differences. From a longitudinal point of view, there are three classic studies on aging: the Seattle study, the Baltimore study, and the Duke study.

In the Seattle study,[24] Raven's Progressive Matrices (PM) and the Primary Mental Abilities test (PMA) were used. The results showed that older people scored lower in all the scales. However, it is necessary to point out that the results of all the tests used are performance-time dependent.

The Baltimore study began in 1984 and was carried out with men in good health, who had a high socioeconomic and educational level. In this study, verbal memory was studied with a word pairs method, and nonverbal memory with Benton's Visual Retention test (VRT). The results showed that loss of memory begins at middle age and increases with age. On the other hand, vocabulary skills measured with the WAIS test remained the same until the last stages of life.

Finally, the Duke study revolved around people of advanced age (60 to 94 years). In this study, a marked decline in visual memory was observed, although it was preserved when the pairs of words were easy. Generally speaking, the changes observed in longitudinal studies do not differ much from the results provided by cross-sectional studies, as they also show differences in the evolution pattern on the different cognitive abilities. For example, these demonstrated visible deterioration in memory, motor and speed functions, visual–perceptual functions, and executive functions. On the other hand, no noticeable deterioration is observed in language functions. In fact, improvements have occasionally been found with age. Typically in the vocabulary tests, 40- and 70-year-old people do not differ substantially in their capacity to recognize the correct definition of a word. Longitudinal studies show evidence that the capacity to use vocabulary improves between the onset of middle-age and old age, and also suggest that verbal capacity is preserved until very late in life. In spite of the similarities, this aspect seems to have been underestimated by cross-sectional studies because of mistaking age-related changes for changes due to socioeconomic, cultural, and educational differences in the various stages of the lives of the people studied. A good example of this issue is the initial standard data of a very well-known test, i.e., the Boston Naming Test (BNT). Borod and colleagues[25] obtained lower scores in older adults than in young adults. This result was proved erroneous when the educational level of the older adults was controlled. The differences then disappeared.

By using different research methods, the conclusion has been reached that some functions decline in a slow and progressive way during the mature life span of the person, whereas others remain invariable until very late stages of life. In addition, rather than deteriorating, others actually improve with time, such as certain language functions.

The preservation of language throughout the life span of the individual, despite the decline of spatiovisual abilities, has led some authors to consider that the right hemisphere of the brain, which essentially deals with processing spatiovisual information, degenerates more than the left side, which mainly deals with language information processes.[26]

From an anatomical point of view this distinction does not make much sense, since no macroscopic or microscopic asymmetries have been found in the degeneration of the hemispheres. In our opinion, language is preserved because it involves cortico–cortical connections, while visual-perceptual functions require cortico–subcortical connections. This means that pathologies in the white matter, characteristic of aging, might affect the visual-perceptual functions to a large extent. We also have to take into account the role that basal ganglia play in spatiovisual functions, and the greater vulnerability of the basal nuclei to the passing of time and to various pathologies associated with aging.[27]

On the other hand, we must not forget possible linguistic deterioration during the natural course of aging. This issue necessarily leads to the need to establish boundaries between normal aging and pathological conditions that affect the nervous system of the individual in the advanced stages of life. In this sense, it is not uncommon to mistake specific cognitive changes associated with age for the first signs of pathological conditions. This can happen, for example, in memory impairment, which, on the one hand, is the first cognitive sign of the onset of normal aging, but, on the other hand, might be a symptom of the first stages of Alzheimer's disease, the most common of the degenerative diseases. An author such as Zarranz[28] wonders whether the boundaries between normal and pathological aging would dissolve if the presence of common lesions accepted as "normal" were in fact characteristic of pathological states. Another author, La Rue,[29] points out that it is possible to find older adults with neuropathological alterations but normal cognitive functioning.

In addition, we must bear in mind that aging itself does not mean the same for everybody. The passing of time does not affect everyone in the same way. Within the general pattern of aging, there are great individual variations, and not all cognitive functions deteriorate to the same degree. In fact, language is a good example of this. While cognitive functions such as memory and attention present deteriorating symptoms early on, language does not present them at all or they appear at the very late stages of aging. Only certain aspects of language seem to suffer alterations and, as we pointed out already, these are not critical changes. From a developmental point of view, it has been found that variability increases with age.[30] There seems to be no clear explanation for this observation. It has been suggested that this could be due to a phenotype expressing itself in the later decades of life. On the other hand, other researchers argue that these individual differences could well be the result of an accumulation of biological differences and personal experience. It is obvious that understanding the aging process necessarily involves the attempt to know a vast number of variables related to aspects such as individual variability, the limitations of the research designs, the effect of aging on different biological structures, lifestyle and nutrition during the ontogenic process, the interrelation between aging and clinical manifestations, the social component, personality factors, and earlier lifestyle (whether it was healthy or not), etc.

As we mentioned earlier, a key variable affected by aging is the processing rate. It is widely accepted that a basic feature of the aging process is a more or less generalized slowdown of the sensorial, motor, and cognitive functions.[6,31-34] Furthermore, studies based on evoked potentials have also verified that the slowing down takes place at the electroencephalographic level.[35,36] Although it has been suggested that the basis of this slowing down might be attention alterations or difficulties in inhibiting distracting stimuli, Salthouse's review[6] suggests that this hypothesis has received little empirical support. In this sense, a more plausible hypothesis suggests that the slowdown could be related to the difficulty or demands of the tasks.[34]

Slowing down is the evolutionary counterpart of response and processing speed and alters the computational efficiency of the system in a special way. It implies the involution of cognitive functions,[37] understood as the disorganization or destructuring of complex processes that have been built up during the course of development. This destructuring does not have to follow an *exactly* inverse pattern to its construction. The involution process can be diverse and refers to certain aspects of development, especially those related to processing efficiency. The language system has been evolving during development, creating and perfecting very complex and hierarchical subsystems. During the involution process the system progressively loses, and in an inverse direction, the complexity previously acquired. Thus, the more complex and sophisticated aspects of the system deteriorate first, while the less complex and simpler aspects remain intact.

It is an open question whether this slowing down is a cause or an effect of the differences observed in other cognitive functions during aging. In this sense, Salthouse[6] points out that the processing rate could significantly affect the remaining cognitive processes as a consequence of a less effective coding of stimuli. Thus, the greater the processing rate, the greater the capacity to process information.[38] During aging, this means that the execution of the last stages of a task are carried out with less processing capacity because most of the time available is used to perform the earlier ones.[6]

On the other hand, there is still a question to be resolved: Does this slowing down process affect all the functions as a whole, or are some more prone than others to suffer from its effect? Currently, there is a model that seeks to explain the slowing down state observed with age. It is called the *general slowing model*. This model postulates that all cognitive processes present the same degree of slowing down during aging. However, variations on this model have been suggested. For example, one such model points out that the difference in the response time of elderly people in tasks and domains is a function of young people's response time.[34]

An extension of the general model has given rise to a *specific domain model*, which proposes that the slowing down function is the same for all the tasks dependent on that domain (for example, the verbal domain), but will vary from one domain to another. Finally, in 1993, Fisher suggested a third model called the *specific process model*. According to this model, different processes are controlled by different slowing mathematical functions, which can differ or not in the different domains. Fisher also predicted that the slowing function for a specific process does not vary between tasks and domains, but it does vary from one cognitive process to another.[32]

8.3 ASPECTS OF LANGUAGE PRESERVED DURING THE AGING PROCESS

The stereotypes of deterioration of cognitive abilities as we age might lead us to think that language is one of the many cognitive areas affected by aging. However, as we pointed out earlier, the presence of genuine language disorders in the elderly, that is, those not produced by problems in perceptual processes (e.g., audition), attention, or memory, has turned out to be an issue that is very difficult to test empirically.[39,40] Most of the difficulties we encounter when searching for language alterations can be attributed to the complexity of the cognitive–linguistic system: language production and comprehension processes are highly complex and imply the coordinated working of a great number of systems, some of which are exclusively linguistic and others not.

The cognitive aspects directly related to linguistic knowledge seem to be safe from the cognitive changes taking place during the aging process. In other words, it seems to be proved that age does not directly affect the preservation of semantic representations, syntactic rules, prosodic patterns or pragmatic components from which language processes are structured. However, this does not mean, for example, that in the process of understanding a sentence an elderly person might be free from experiencing difficulties with aspects transparent to younger people. Language comprehension and production require the use of linguistic knowledge, but also the correct manipulation of information. The distinction between processes and knowledge so common in language literature can help us understand the problem. Indeed, it seems that semantic representations from which production begins are preserved during old age, but there are difficulties in activating such representations. As another example, we have to distinguish between the knowledge needed to build the syntactic structure of a sentence, i.e., the syntactic rules of the actual language, which are preserved, and the actual process of building the syntactic structure, for which the processing systems have to manipulate the necessary syntactic rules.

8.3.1 Semantic Memory

Undoubtedly, semantic-conceptual representations, i.e., semantic memory, where the production and comprehension processes begin and conclude, seem to be one of the components of the cognitive system less affected by aging. This has been proved by asking elderly people to perform vocabulary tasks, semantic priming tasks (see Light,[41] for a review), or naming tasks.[42] The same has been found in fluency tasks where subjects had to say as quickly as possible all the items they could remember from a given semantic category. Although in some of these tasks their performance is worse than that of younger adults, the difference seems to be related to the nonsemantic components of the tasks, as we will explain later.[43] In some longitudinal[44] and cross-sectional studies,[40] especially in vocabulary tasks, older people performed better as they exhibited a richer lexicon, probably due to their greater linguistic and experiential knowledge.

8.3.2 SYNTAX

Regarding syntactic abilities, there is a certain controversy about whether these are preserved or not. While some authors maintain that there are no specific difficulties in sentence comprehension,[39,45] other authors argue that elderly people suffer deficits in syntactic processing.[46,47] The fact is that despite results showing greater difficulties in the elderly in comprehending complex sentences, it seems that the locus of the deficit is not linguistic, but is related, once again, to memory difficulties.[12] We must remember that most studies on sentence comprehension use tasks such as grammaticality judgment,[46] sentence repetition,[48] and sentence recall,[49] in which, besides correct syntactic processing, it is necessary to store the structure of the sentence in memory in order to give the correct answer. Therefore, it is likely that the difficulties elderly people seem to exhibit for processing complex structures are more apparent than real.[45]

To find out if there really is a deficit specific to syntax, other studies have been designed to avoid demands on memory that are not involved in the comprehension process. Among these studies we can mention those which use *cross modal priming*. In this experimental paradigm subjects have to listen to a sentence. At a critical moment participants are presented with a string of letters on a computer screen that can be related to the sentence heard or not, and the subject must decide as quickly as possible if this is a word or not. The analysis of the response times to the words reveals the knowledge subjects have developed about the sentence. By using such a task, Zurif et al.,[45] reached the conclusion that elderly people do not seem to present a specific deficit in the construction of syntactic structures. In other words, aging does not involve the loss of the ability to build the syntactic structures of sentences. The study, however, also showed that, on occasions, the construction of the syntactic structure on the part of older adults can be hindered in those structures where syntactic processing makes strong demands on memory, i.e., in syntactically complex sentences. Therefore, we can state that although there is no specific deficit in the syntax, some problems with sentence comprehension in older adults are related to memory difficulties.

Although the laboratory experiments show that elderly people have greater difficulties in sentence comprehension, these problems do not seem very visible on a day-to-day basis; at least, that is how it is perceived by the elderly people themselves. This perception of preserving their capacity for syntactic processing claimed by older people could be related to the great capacity elderly people seem to have of taking advantage of the discursive context during the comprehension process. In this way, some authors argue that the semantic representations of sentences and discourse that older people build up while the comprehension process takes place are robust enough to facilitate the processing of incoming information.[47]

Regarding sentence production, several experimental studies seem to show that the difficulties elderly people experience in producing complex syntactic structures is also related to memory. Although the sentences of young and elderly persons are the same regarding the number of words, the latter build sentences that are syntactically less complex.[50] The data also show that the mean number of clauses per utterance in all adults, which is a measure of the complexity of the language, correlates with the measurements of working memory and the age of subjects. This seems to confirm the hypothesis that limitations in working memory might affect the production of syntactically complex structures in elderly people.

8.3.3 Prosody

Another aspect that seems to be perfectly preserved in old age is prosody.[39] Elderly people vocalize their utterances with clarity and precision, making the pauses and variations needed for the listener to capture the differences these introduce to the message, for example, an ironic comment. It is even argued that, through an almost theatrical use of prosody, elderly people are able both to keep the listener's attention and to indicate in a clear way the delimitation of clauses, facilitating in this way comprehension of complex sentences.

Neither do they seem to have problems in comprehension of prosodic patterns. In a recent investigation, Kjelgaard et al.[51] used temporarily ambiguous sentences that could be disambiguated via prosodic patterns. In the task of completing sentences, although they were a bit slower, the older adults were as capable as the younger ones of integrating prosodic information to interpret the sentence properly. This is a clear indication of sensitivity toward this type of information. Other research[52] has shown that the manipulation of prosodic characteristics hinders comprehension in elderly people, which is also an indication that this population makes great use of their prosodic abilities in normal speech to really understand the discourse.

8.4 THE CORE ISSUE IN LANGUAGE PROBLEMS IN ELDERLY PEOPLE: DIFFICULTIES IN LEXICAL RETRIEVAL

The aspects of language that seem to be the ones most altered in elderly people, whether in speech or writing, are the processes in charge of word retrieval. Elderly people know what they want to say or write, the concept is clear in their minds, and so they do not have semantic problems. Rather, the difficulty seems to arise in the lexical retrieval of the orthographic or phonological representation of the word. Interestingly, this problem is found even in older people with a very rich vocabulary.

8.4.1 Retrieval of the Phonological Representations

In the opinion of many authors,[53] lexical production is the core issue in language problems related to old age. This view coincides with the actual experience of elderly people who report the increasing difficulties they experience in the retrieval of words. Indeed, there is considerable empirical evidence that the processes of word production are altered in older adults. These processes manifest themselves in three typical symptoms: (1) a greater failure rate to retrieve the appropriate words; (2) a larger rate of spontaneous errors during speech; and (3) less fluency in speech.

8.4.1.1 The Problems of Naming and Verbal Fluency in Older Adults

Elderly people seem to present specific problems with word retrieval in the area of naming tasks. In a classic study, Ballots and Duchek,[54] while measuring reaction times, found that older adults achieved worse results than young adults in naming tasks. Older adults did not present greater error rates, but they showed considerable slowdown while uttering the words they were presented with. This general phenomenon of slowing down affects word retrieval in a more critical way. However, it is important to note that this slowdown did not affect the 'quality' of the task. This variant was studied by Madden,[55] who concluded that the tasks showed a clear decline in some, but not all, of the components. The aspects of the task related to the semantic and conceptual components of language did not show any decline whatsoever when compared with younger adults. Therefore, this is proof that semantic factors are not sensitive to age, while the linguistic components linked to task performance, i.e., the phonological aspects, are sensitive to age.

The importance of distinguishing between the language components sensitive to age and those which are not led Nicholas et al.[56] to carry out a study in which they used a picture naming task. As usual, noticeable differences were found in the naming rate of objects or actions by young adults in comparison with older people. However, errors due to semantic mistakes did not only show little difference, but they even decreased with age. This confirms the idea that the conceptual and semantic components of language remain intact with age. In spite of all this, it is necessary to note that the researchers found more *circumlocutions* in the older people, who used them as a strategy to compensate for the deficit they noticed in their speed in naming an object or action.

In the use of spontaneous language, we can also detect these kinds of problems. Once again, we observe the same pattern: while some components are preserved, others, on the contrary, are impaired.[57] Concerning lexical wealth, although older adults do not show signs of deterioration caused by aging, an increase in difficulties with lexical performance has been found. For example, we notice the presence of phonemic paraphases; the use of ambiguous or imprecise terms increases; a difficulty specific to accessing proper nouns appears; the number of function words increases; the number of empty pauses and especially of filled pauses (lots of "hmms," "errs" between one word and the next) also increases, showing both a fluency problem as well as a problem in avoiding such pauses, since the target word should appear in their place. These pauses are a very common feature in the speech of elderly people. They give the impression of hesitation, but cannot strictly be considered a problem of fluency; rather, they signal difficulty in accessing words. Elderly people know perfectly well what words they are looking for, but have problems retrieving them. The lexical problem relates to accessing the form of the word, not its content.

This kind of problem in accessing words overloads the memory and attention capabilities of elderly people, which translates into an overall higher cognitive load. The consequence of such a cognitive load is greater difficulty in maintaining the discursive reference. This is why, after the hesitations, older adults can lose the thread of the narrative of what they were saying. The problem is not in itself a direct loss of the discursive capacity, characteristic of other pathologies, but rather an impairment at the lexical level that has repercussions at the discursive level of language.

A cross-linguistic study carried out by Juncos and Iglesias,[58] showed the great difficulty older adults experience in carrying out the language tasks proposed: retrieval of synonyms or antonyms. It also gave evidence of the discursive phenomena we have mentioned.

Another way of studying lexical access difficulties is by using verbal fluency tasks. Tests on verbal fluency, which also reflect the ability to retrieve a word, show even worse results in longitudinal studies. In typical fluency tasks, subjects are asked either to produce lots of examples (words) from a semantic category (for example, names of pieces of furniture or flowers or animals) or to provide as many words as possible beginning with a given letter or syllable in a limited set time.

These tests show the capacity to maintain attention, the speed of cognitive processing, the capacity to produce oral language, as well as the ability to inhibit dominant answers with the purpose of producing more additional answers. Dysfluencies, such as filled pauses, repetitions, and hesitations, increase with age and may indicate difficulties in retrieving words.[59]

Dysfluencies express a difference between what subjects want to say and the way they say it during language production. This is the reason dysfluencies seem to affect the capacity to plan language, as observed in people who stutter, although the nature of the symptom in older people is much less acute. The classic indicators for language planning problems (hesitations, false beginnings, word repetitions, empty pauses, etc.) increase with age.[50] This issue becomes more relevant when we bear in mind that both old and young adults place great importance on fluency as an indicator of the intellectual and linguistic competence of people.[50]

Although the explanation just offered about dysfluencies is the most widely accepted one, it reflects only one of the aspects implied in language planning. We cannot overlook the importance of other factors. Indeed, this increase of indicators for planning problems could reflect a natural decline in the ability of older adults to code new information. Research on story recall highlights this aspect. Recalling stories involves the retrieval of new information, i.e., it demands the establishment of new connections in memory, and we already know this is a problematic area in elderly people.[60] Consequently, this deficit in recalling stories might reflect a general deficit in the formation of new skills rather than a specific deficit in linguistic or communication skills.

When language-free tasks were used,[61] there arose many methodological problems in controlling the variables, and this led to confusing and, on occasions, contradictory results. Thus, it is difficult to attribute the results of the tasks to age because this cannot be separated from the results of communicative strategies, language compensation strategies, and the greater experience of elderly people, i.e., they are more educated and cultured.

However, in relation to age, the differences observed between naming tasks of the BNT kind and verbal fluency tasks can be explained by the fact that during fluency tasks the subject is provided with some help in finding the words in the lexical-semantic memory, whereas in the visually presented naming tasks, the actual picture has to facilitate the retrieval of the word. Therefore, it could be postulated that when the word retrieval task involves an automatic lexical process, there are no differences ascribed to age, whereas when the process has a controlled or voluntary nature, i.e., it is not automatic, then there are differences that can be attributed to age. This distinction between automatic and controlled processes may account for the greater effect of age on verbal fluency tasks when compared with BNT-like naming tasks.[44]

A modality of a naming task that allows the evaluation of the capacity to retrieve words, and which is related to the difference between automatic and controlled processes, is a naming task as a reply to a linguistic definition. In this task a decreased performance attributed to age is observed, although this reduction does not seem to be as important as the one observed in verbal fluency tasks.

The distinction between automatic and controlled processes is broadly accepted in cognitive psychology and can be an important way to differentiate between those language functions that deteriorate with age and those that are preserved. Goodglass[62] has already suggested a distinction of this kind when studying performance in naming tasks with patients with localized cerebral injuries. This difference is also useful in describing the breakdown of language in patients with Alzheimer's disease.

8.4.1.2 The Tip-of-the-Tongue Phenomenon

One of the difficulties often encountered by old people regarding word retrieval, and one they are fully aware of, is that sometimes they cannot retrieve from their lexical repertoire a given word despite having it on the "tip of the tongue." This is specifically known as the tip-of-the-tongue (TOT) phenomenon. It consists of occasional breaks of fluency in the speech, because the word we want to use does not "pop up" in our minds, although we know it. It is necessary to point out that this state is the result of a temporary and partial problem in accessing the phonological and orthographic information of the lexicon. Generally speaking, people know perfectly well the initial letter and the number of syllables of the word they are looking for. It also frequently occurs that other words semantically or phonologically close to the target word come to mind. The certainty of the person regarding knowledge of the word makes the person reject the other words. When these blockages take place, people use retrieval strategies, but it is not known whether the actual blockages are responsible for not finding the target word. When subjects are asked about the strategies used in such cases, they talk about either using an inner code, for example, an alphabetical search in their memory, or an external one, like a dictionary (when this option is available). The doubts are often resolved because the word finally pops up in an unexpected way, when attention is not focused directly on the search (when the subject is more relaxed). Although these TOT phenomena cannot be easily verified, they take place at any age, but they become more frequent in elderly persons.

Some authors[63] studied TOT difficulties within the context of daily life by using subjects' structured diaries. In the study by Burke et al.[64] some significant differences in the emergence rate of TOTs were found between younger and older adults, as well as differences in the type of strategies used to resolve them. Most TOT phenomena were resolved in the two groups, although they used different strategies: the older adults had more unexpected resolutions; i.e., the target word came without a conscious effort, while the younger group used external and internal codes. However, both groups reached the same percentage of resolutions, although the elderly adults used fewer strategies. The older group had less information regarding the word they were looking for (e.g., they often did not know how it sounded), while the younger group often had more information of this kind. Finally, these authors found significant differences in the type of words: the TOT phenomena in the elderly were most of the time proper and "concrete" common nouns (names of everyday objects), while in the young adults group, the TOTs took place with proper nouns, but also with abstract common nouns (fewer words of everyday objects).

Elderly people report a greater rate of TOTs in their daily life than younger adults.[63] The same thing is found in laboratory conditions when using definitions of rare words.[63,65] In a typical task of filling in the names of a family tree, older adults made many more spontaneous errors, or TOTs, than young adults. However, there was an important detail — the older adults offered a significantly smaller number of alternative words, that is, possible candidate words, than young adults.

8.4.2 RETRIEVAL OF ORTHOGRAPHIC REPRESENTATIONS

In the same way that difficulties in retrieving phonological representation have been found, other works have more recently pointed to the existence of similar problems in the retrieval of the orthographic representation of the word. Although initially it might be thought that such problems derive from the perceptual and usage differences elderly and younger people have regarding writing, it seems obvious that the difficulties encountered in spelling retrieval are not exclusively due to these factors.[40,66]

The retrieval of orthographic representations is fundamental to the production of writing, whether spontaneous or from dictation. Writing cannot be done exclusively via the use of phoneme–grapheme conversion rules because these do not always coincide, and this forces subjects to make use of the orthographic lexicon where the orthographic representations of the words we know are stored.[67] If access to these representations has deteriorated with age, we should find, once perceptual errors and differences in vocabulary are controlled, a greater number of spelling errors by elderly people. This seems to be the pattern found in several studies, but there are peculiarities that we believe should be pointed out.

The lexical frequency of the words with which elderly people make more mistakes seems to be relevant. There are more errors with low-frequency words than with high-frequency words, and when the scores in vocabulary are factored out, elderly people show more errors with both high- and low-frequency words than younger groups, with the difference greater with high-frequency words.

The difficulties elderly people seem to encounter in dictation are more persistent with phonologically irregular words [BUSH], which demand retrieval from the orthographic lexicon, than with regular ones [BUNT], which normally only require the use of phoneme–grapheme conversion rules. Only the group of oldest people (from 73 to 88 years old) make more errors with regular spelling words, but there are no differences between the group of less elderly persons (60 to 71 years old) and the younger group (17 to 23 years old).[40] The most common error in elderly people is the regularization of the spelling of phonologically irregular words. For example, a word like [STREET] can also be spelled [STREAT] by applying the phoneme to grapheme conversion rules. Following dual route models, the presence of differences derived from the regularity–irregularity of a word enable us to draw certain conclusions about the kind of age impairments found in systems involved in writing: the retrieval from the lexical store seems to be hindered earlier, between the ages of 60 and 70, than the use of conversion rules, where no problems are detected until after the age of 70.

Although some studies have shown the difficulties elderly people have in dictation and spelling, the analysis of their spontaneous writing does not seem to show a prominent number of orthographic errors. This absence of differences in spontaneous writing does not necessarily contradict other findings. The words subjects had to write down in the studies already reviewed, fundamentally that of MacKay and Abrams,[40] were more difficult and rare than those used commonly. It is also likely that due to their richer vocabulary and awareness of their difficulties while writing, elderly people might deliberately look for synonymous or grammatical expressions to replace those words they are unsure how to spell for others that are easier to spell. It seems that elderly people develop strategies to compensate for the difficulties they experience in retrieving the correct spelling of words.

Contrary to findings in other investigations[68] and certainly counterintuitive, the data obtained by MacKay and Abrams[40] do not show any relationship between the number of hours subjects spend writing weekly and their performance in the dictation task. This finding does not match at all the so-called *practice hypothesis*, which tries to explain performance in dictation by taking into account the differences in the writing habits of younger and older people. Although it is true that for academic reasons young people spend more time writing than do elderly people, the low correlation with performance in writing tasks in both groups seems to indicate that practice is not a relevant variable to explain the decline in the retrieval of orthographic representations that takes place with age. In the light of the data and the pattern of errors found in elderly peoples, the *practice hypothesis* has to be rejected in the same way that other hypotheses have to be rejected that try to explain writing deficiencies in elderly people by perceptual and/or attention difficulties. In a recent study, MacKay et al.[69] found a similar performance in elderly and young people while detecting spelling errors, which seems to eliminate perceptual and attention deficiencies as responsible for the increase in orthographic errors with age. Other hypotheses that do not score much better are those that attribute language deficiencies in elderly people to a general process of slowing in cognitive functions which, ultimately, would be responsible for the difficulties in retrieving orthographic representations. If this were the case, the linguistic impairments should be more pronounced as the cognitive processes became more complex, e.g., discourse production, and not in those specifically linguistic and comparatively simpler, such as the retrieval of orthographic representations.

Bearing in mind the data available, those explanations that defend the existence of deficits on the strength of the connections in charge of activating orthographic and phonological representations, such as those offered by MacKay et al., or those that defend the existence of difficulties in the inhibition process, like those of Hasher and Zacks, seem more plausible.[70]

8.5 DISCOURSE COMPREHENSION AND ELDERSPEAK

Regarding discourse comprehension, we must point out that once perceptual difficulties, fundamentally auditory problems, are isolated, elderly people do not seem to show special difficulties of a linguistic character.[71] A typical way of studying elderly persons' comprehension skills in discourse is to analyze their capacity to carry out inferences. This task demands comprehending the message and its connection to previous information, providing a measure of the older adults' comprehension abilities and possible differences with younger adults. Although some results indicate that the inferential processes carried out by older adults are similar to those of younger adults,[72] others seem to indicate the opposite.[18]

It is likely that given the preservation of the semantic and syntactic aspects of language, we are once again facing cognitive rather than linguistic alterations as responsible for the mild difficulties elderly people experience in comprehension of discourse. This seems to be the conclusion reached by research on production such as the study carried out by Light et al.,[73] who found that the problems older adults present in the comprehension of anaphors were not due to the lack of anaphoric strategies or to pragmatic issues, but to memory problems.

The properties of language, characterized by its redundancy, probably facilitates the setting up of mechanisms to compensate for the difficulties that appear in comprehension as a result of the decline in perceptual abilities and memory, and so make these almost imperceptible. The studies show that elderly people take greater advantage, in relation to their baseline, of syntactic and semantic structure than younger people. As we have pointed out, the prosodic pattern (pitch contour, stress pattern, and timing of natural speech) is of great support for the elderly person, because it facilitates syntax analysis and indicates the main topic of a sentence.[13] Elderly people also lean on the predictability of discourse to facilitate their understanding and storage in memory. This characteristic of language seems to help elderly people to remember the main aspects of the discourse, although not the details.[74]

When dealing with discourse comprehension, we need to refer to *elderspeak*. When interacting with elderly people, the rest of the population seems to make use of a way of speaking that is characterized by being slower, has a simplified syntax, vocabulary restrictions, and exaggerated prosody. It is repetitive and redundant speech, which we could consider to be the equivalent of *motherese*, the simplified speech mothers use with their infants. The origin of elderspeak is rooted in the perception of young adults that older people find it difficult to understand discourse, and its objective is to facilitate comprehension.

However, studies show that elderly people are not helped by all of the features of elderspeak. The data obtained by Kemper and Harden[75] suggest that only semantic elaborations, such as expansions, and the use of fewer subordinate sentences and embedded clauses, help comprehension as they diminish processing demands. Other features of elderspeak, such as shorter sentences, slow speaking rates, and exaggerated prosody on the part of the speaker, not only do not increase comprehension, but even seem to hinder it. It also appears that these latter features of elderspeak, which are the more visible ones, might trigger in elderly people a negative self-assessment of their communicative competence, as they are aware that the speaker is using a variant of baby talk with them. The perception of elderly people is indeed correct, because elderspeak, as we have already said, has its origin in the speaker's idea that the older person has impairments that hinder comprehension.

8.6 DISCOURSE PRODUCTION AND COMPENSATION MECHANISMS

In spite of the linguistic and cognitive deficits already described, the discourse of elderly people does not present severe problems. The assessment listeners make of elderly people's discourse is better on certain topics than the assessment they make of the discourse of young adults,[53] despite difficulties in the retrieval of phonological representations and in fluency. However, it is also true that in our daily contact with elderly people, we often perceive their discourse as very considerable, not very coherent, excessively detailed, and lacking in thematic structure. Frequently, the narration of a story by an elderly person becomes fairly difficult to follow because of the continuous insertion of not always relevant personal details and the existence of jumps in the thread of the discourse. These features of the discourse of older adults seem to be typical in the narration of personal stories, the famous "granddad's old stories," but there is no conclusive evidence regarding whether or not these impregnate all their discourse, even that furthest from the personal.[76,77]

Among the peculiarities of the discourse of older adults in the narration of personal stories, we can observe a greater use of multiple references and redundancies, greater predictability, and the use of exaggerated prosody. Although some of the features of this way of speaking can make the discourse tedious for the listener, not all of them are valued negatively by listeners. The prosodic emphasis seems to make it easier to follow the thread, as does the presence of redundancies. In general, the characteristics described seem to be present with a certain frequency, and this has led some authors to consider that elderly people make idiosyncratic use of language, which has been called Off Target Verbosity[77] or Off Topic Speech,[76] to emphasize the lack of focus in their discourse.

The reasons for the existence of such a discourse peculiar to elderly people are not very clear. Although some hypotheses speculate that this kind of speech is due to a change in the communicative intentions of elderly people, others consider that this way of speaking is the product of cognitive problems caused by aging. A third hypothesis, to which we subscribe, suggests that the discourse peculiar to elderly people emerges as the fruit of a compensation mechanism for discursive deficiencies (and possibly affective deficiencies, as well) that these people seem to experience, and it is also a consequence of the social stigma elderly people carry as communicatively challenged, which gives rise to their own communicative style.

Some authors have tried to explain the lack of focus on the topic and the talkativeness that seem to characterize the communicative style of the elderly people as a pragmatic change.[76] The pragmatic aspect of language makes reference to the speaker's communicative intentions during the act of speaking such that, in light of the *pragmatic change hypothesis*, it is understood that in certain situations, fundamentally when narrating personal experiences, elderly people would adopt a non-pathological communicative style that differs from younger adults and that emphasizes the meaning of their own experiences rather than the conciseness of the stories. Since they have fewer opportunities to relate to others, elderly people would more value the possibility of speaking and establishing social interactions, taking this opportunity to make themselves known through personal stories. To a certain extent this hypothesis uses variables of an affective kind to account for the discourse of elderly people, since these are the ones that originate the pragmatic change by setting the communicative goals.

The *inhibition deficit hypothesis*, on the contrary, argues that the deficits that appear with age in inhibition control are the ones responsible for the less coherent and wordier discourse characteristic of elderly people.[77] Such an inhibition deficit would prevent the subjects from being able to suppress irrelevant thoughts during speech production, and so they would include them in their discourse, making it less concise. In other words, according to this hypothesis, the lack of structure in the discourse of elderly people would reflect the cognitive deficiencies that appear with age.

The formulation of both hypotheses implies an important difference in the way of understanding the topic of the discourse. According to the hypothesis of pragmatic change, the discourse peculiar to elderly people should mainly take place when talking about autobiographical topics, whereas from point of view of the inhibition model, since this discourse is the fruit of cognitive deficiencies, the characteristics of the discourse should be independent of the topic. The studies carried out that have taken this parameter into account are contradictory, showing that the characteristics attributed to the discourse of elderly people do not always appear in non-autobiographical discourse.[77] This suggests that the peculiarities typical of elderly people's discourse are not inseparable, and thus they might be due to different factors and not exclusively to the existence of a pragmatic change or a cognitive deficit. This viewpoint is, in fact, the one we defend.

There is evidence to support the conclusion that inhibition mechanisms are unlikely to be the only ones responsible for the discursive style of elderly people. It would be striking if the stories valued as more entertaining by the listeners (which does not mean they are easiest to follow) were the result of inhibition problems.[76]

In our opinion, it is possible to hold an integrated viewpoint, with slight variations, of the two previous postures. Our view of the problem would be more complete if the peculiarities of the discourse of elderly people were conceived of as being generated by a set of variables: linguistic and cognitive deficits, affective deficits, and stereotypes about the weaker language capacity of this population. Such conditions would account for the generation of all the characteristics found in elderly people's discourse as a whole, but in a more specific way they would also account for the different peculiarities of such discourse. For example, circumlocutions could be basically provoked by deficits in phonological retrieval; the introduction of slightly irrelevant ideas may be due to executive problems; the use of multiple personal references by the need for self-affirmation, and the abundance of detail could be seen as a way to compensate for the difficulties that, according to the stereotype, the elderly experience when trying to communicate.

In recent years, the study of the discursive abilities of elderly people, and the possibility that they use a certain communicative style as a compensatory strategy,[13] have aroused great interest. In our opinion, the discourse of elderly people acquires its shape driven by the different determinants elderly people respond to by activating mechanisms to compensate for these deficiencies.

The use of compensation strategies to increase their communicative abilities seems something inherent to the linguistic processes of elderly people in the face of cognitive and linguistic difficulties. An example of this, although not directly visible, is the way they make use of their richer vocabulary in the discursive context to facilitate sentence processing and avoid any lexical (orthographic and phonological) retrieval problems they might suffer. Therefore, it is plausible that in the production of discourse, which requires a considerable cognitive and linguistic effort, compensatory strategies are being activated. Obviously, on occasions, no compensatory strategy will be able to overcome the cognitive deficits, and in such cases the deficiencies will be patent in the discourse. Light[73] has shown that during discourse, elderly people produce more ambiguous references than the younger population because of their difficulty in retrieving names and the scarcity of memory resources, which are not overcome by compensatory strategies.

It is also plausible, as the pragmatic change hypothesis states, that elderly people have different communicative goals that motivate them to focus on more personal aspects, as they have fewer opportunities for social and affective exchanges.

A novel element that we believe could be fundamental for understanding the peculiarities of elderly people's discourse is the perception they have of their communicative abilities, which is shared by the rest of the population. The difficulties in retrieving phonological representations and in motor programming, which promote an increase in the occurrence of hesitations, as well as the limitations in their memory, encourage the perception on the part of the listener and the actual speaker, the elderly person, that there is a deterioration in discursive abilities with age. Other evidence of their apparent communicative problems is the way we speak to elderly people (elderspeak) as we have already experienced. Elderspeak has the peculiarity of "reminding" elderly people of their communication difficulties, encouraging a negative self-assessment. In these circumstances it is very likely that older adults, aware of their limitations, will develop a way of speaking that allows them, through multiple redundancies and personal references, to maintain the discursive thread and facilitate the listener's comprehension.

Evidence leads us to suggest that elderly people develop a longer and more elaborate discursive style as a compensatory mechanism. By the use of multiple references, greater use of redundancies and predictability, as well as the use of more emphatic prosody, they compensate for their cognitive difficulties in the construction of discourse, which at the same time might help the listener to follow the thread, especially in those topics with personal implications, where they would be particularly inclined to include autobiographical details as an expression of their affective needs. Although it is necessary to confirm this hypothesis experimentally, current data seem to fit the model proposed.

8.7   PATHOLOGICAL EVOLUTION OF LANGUAGE IN ALZHEIMER'S DISEASE

8.7.1   ALZHEIMER'S DISEASE IN THE CONTEXT OF NEUROPSYCHOLOGICAL PATHOLOGY

The fact that language is one of the cognitive functions least affected by the normal process of aging, even though linguistic disorders are one of the first manifestations of Alzheimer's disease, gives language tremendous clinical value. The study of language enables us to make differential diagnoses between the deterioration of mental faculties associated with age and the onset of a pathological process such as dementia in Alzheimer's disease, and thus is a key element in detecting its insidious beginnings. The analysis of language facilitates the prognosis of Alzheimer's disease, because the presence of early and intense linguistic anomalies are a sign of this disease. Finally, the analysis of language allows us to distinguish between patients with an early onset of dementia and those whose pathology develops with greater speed.

One of the classic discussions in neuropsychological literature on Alzheimer's disease is elucidating whether we are dealing with the same process of cognitive deterioration, albeit accentuated, typical of normal aging, or whether we are dealing with a pathological process of a different character. Some authors[78–81] have argued that, indeed, Alzheimer's disease follows the same deterioration patterns that appear during normal aging, but with pathological acceleration, probably regulated by a genetic determinant, which leads to the progressive loss of cognitive capabilities. On the other hand, such authors as Gispen and Traber[82] defend the hypothesis that the two processes are of a different nature. They base their claim on the fact that, in Alzheimer's disease, the deficits that prevail during normal aging are not only magnified, but rather, from the onset, the alterations of neuropsychological functions that characterize them are different. This latter conception of the disease tends to prevail today.

A considerable number of investigations[83] have shown that language alterations are always present in patients with Alzheimer's disease who survive to the stage of medium severity of the pathology. This deterioration is the first symptom of dementia. The comparison between the relative prevalence of different cognitive deficits indicates that lexical and semantic language disorders appear immediately after alterations in the recent memory. Murdock et al.[83] have suggested that the collapse of language could be considered as a diagnostic criterion for Alzheimer's disease. This claim, however, is not very sound, since we can find patients with Alzheimer's disease with nonlinguistic deficits before they present linguistic deficits. We can also find patients with developmental aphasia who do not present with Alzheimer's disease.

Since dementia involves cognitive deterioration as well as deterioration of language, the use of the term *aphasia* to denote linguistic disorders in dementia presents some problems. In spite of this terminological issue, it seems that there is an overall consensus on the use of this term in Alzheimer's disease. Thus, comparison between language disorders in localized cerebral damage and diffuse damage have been useful to characterize those disorders found in Alzheimer's disease. The language collapse characteristic of Alzheimer's disease has been described in terms of aphasia-like symptoms: from anomic aphasia to sensorial transcortical aphasia, to Wernicke's aphasia and, finally, to global aphasia.

From the onset, the language disorders found in Alzheimer's disease manifest in the following symptoms: pauses during conversation to find the words, and greater difficulty to link ideas in the discourse. If we analyze this language formally, the breakdown of the discourse manifests as a lower fluency rate and the presence of perseveration of sentences.[84]

The tests of verbal fluency clearly reveal the deficits at the onset of linguistic deterioration. The reason for this is that they demand lexical-semantic processing, which is active and voluntary. It is well known that verbal fluency is greatly affected by injuries to the frontal lobe,[85] while the deterioration of language in patients with Alzheimer's disease reflect a much wider cerebral pathology. This pathology affects both semantic memory functions and attention functions.

8.7.2 Brief Summary of the Characteristics of Language in Alzheimer's Disease

Comprehension declines as the degree of dementia advances. The same happens with most of the other aspects of language. Oral comprehension is usually faulty in the sense that patients with Alzheimer's disease are able to understand and respond to specific problems and simple instructions, but not to complex conceptual material.

Concerning oral language, patients with Alzheimer's disease present an evident lack of initiative during speech as well as a much slower speech rate in their replies. In spontaneous language (conversation), they perform well regarding the length of sentences, are capable of uttering full sentences, and exhibit few paraphasias and anomias. On the other hand, we observe poor performance regarding information content. When analyzing language content, it is quite common to find incoherencies and perseveration (the simple repetition of syllables, words, and even a set of sentences or text).

Usually, one of the most frequent symptoms in Alzheimer's disease is the impoverishment of vocabulary, with a strong presence of semantic jargon (neologisms). This symptom depends greatly on the evolution of the disease, since in the first stages high scores are obtained in the kind of lexicon tests included in intelligence tests. Grammatical categories are differentially affected: nouns are more affected than adjectives, and adjectives more than verbs, while prepositions and conjunctions can remain relatively intact. In any case, the most common words are those that tend to be easily reproduced.

The highest level of preservation is usually found in repetition, which tends to be preserved in all areas, except in those where an important component of memory is involved.

People affected by Alzheimer's disease have difficulties with tasks that require access to semantic memory. Put in another words, they have problems in successfully completing tasks where lexical knowledge and the use of symbolic language are assessed. A clear indicator of the loss of semantic memory is the difficulty they encounter in finding words, a fact that is obvious in the early stages. Indeed, it is one of the earliest manifestations, which progresses along with the general deterioration of language. Over time their language becomes more and more telegraphic and poor in content.

Regarding naming, visual access to the lexicon is also affected, as this is active retrieval of the lexicon. Several researchers claim that these dysfunctions are not a consequence of the loss of vocabulary, but rather that they are due to the difficulty in accessing it. This difficulty would explain why they use far more circumlocutions and semantic paraphasias. Patients use these resources to compensate for their naming problems, but the result is the utterance of incoherent and content-empty language.

Another indicator of the deterioration of semantic memory is the loss of knowledge of concepts. Alzheimer's disease patients find it difficult to describe spontaneously the relevant attributes of objects (they also have problems in remembering the psychological or functional aspects of an object). In the earlier and moderate stages, these people preserve the ability to categorize stimuli within their semantic classes.

In the more advanced stages of Alzheimer's disease, a deeper deterioration in language production is observed as well as in language comprehension. Patients might end up mute, uttering echolalias, or producing a syntactic and phonologically correct discourse, but lacking any sense.

The great difference between normal aging and pathological aging of the cortical dementia kind (for example, Alzheimer's disease) is that in the first instance the problem is restricted to executive deficits but does not have a great impact on the conceptual aspects. On the other hand, in cortical dementia we witness a serious impairment of basic cognitive functions with special reference to semantic memory. In Alzheimer's disease we see a strong and overall cognitive deterioration, with great loss in the memory component. This leads to the fact that in the first stages, during the insidious onset of the disease, the symptoms of Alzheimer's disease and the symptoms of normal aging are very similar, because they seem to affect to the same components. However, the evolution of language in Alzheimer's disease is very different from the evolution of language in normal aging. This characteristic makes language a very useful diagnostic tool because it allows us to distinguish very early on between the two manifestations we mentioned: normal aging and pathological aging.

8.8 SUMMARY

Given the importance of verbal communication in our society, the impairment of language processes causes problems in the development and adjustment of people to their environment. This chapter has analyzed the changes that occur in language with age, reaching the conclusion that, contrary to what happens with other cognitive abilities, e.g., spatio-visual skills, language is preserved to all practical extents. Elderly people's language does not seem to present an overall deficit. Although linguistic competence remains intact, the difficulties seem to occur in the processes in charge of manipulation and storage (execution). With age, some key cognitive systems, such as attention, storage, and control mechanisms, suffer from deterioration and this generates problems in the selection, inhibition, planning, and control processes. These problems, apart from the sensorial and perceptual alterations that we usually encounter in elderly people, specifically affect access to the lexicon, and the comprehension and production of sentences and/or discourse of a certain complexity.

Given that language difficulties in elderly people basically revolve around the lexical aspect, although not exclusively, we have devoted this chapter to analyzing their main characteristics, which we now summarize:

- Passive vocabulary increases: Elderly people recognize and understand as many or more words than younger adults. In this case, the cultural level of the person is a critical variable.[86] Conceptual knowledge does not seem to deteriorate with age, but rather it seems to increase in elderly people.[50,87]
- The core issue regarding problems in accessing orthographic and phonological representations: This issue revolves around the following aspects: (1) problems in finding the right word to name objects with a decrease in reaction time; (2) an increase of TOT episodes;[62] (3) difficulty in finding the right word for a linguistic definition;[88] (4) specific difficulties when trying to retrieve proper nouns.[89]
- Important individual differences in the performance of language tasks.

Regarding the conversational peculiarities of elderly people, we pointed out that the perception of linguistic difficulties in the language of elderly people, albeit mild, has brought about the use of elderspeak by the younger population. This discursive style, characterized by a slower speaking rate, syntactic simplicity, the use of a limited vocabulary, and exaggerated prosody accentuates in elderly people the self-perception of reduced communicative abilities. We believe that this negative self-assessment, together with communicative and affective difficulties, is the basis for the discursive style that characterizes elderly people, and which has received the name Off Topic Speech. This very talkative style, with little focus on the topic, could play the role of not only compensating for cognitive deficits, but also explain the paucity of social interactions many elderly people suffer.

The study of language during aging has stressed its value for the diagnosis of Alzheimer's disease. Contrary to what happens during the normal process of aging, in Alzheimer's disease language comprehension as well as production are severely impaired, and, therefore, the appropriate analysis of language enables a differential diagnosis.

Although the study of language impairment in elderly people still has a long way to go, there is no doubt that, from the point of view of psycholinguistic research, it is an exemplary field for allowing the observation of the interaction between impaired and healthy processes and systems. The application of this knowledge should benefit a population that is increasing and that will continue to do so in the coming years.

REFERENCES

1. Ryan, E. B., See, S. K., Meneer, W. B., and Trovato, D., Age-based perceptions of conversational skills among younger and older adults, in *Interpersonal Communication in Older Adulthood,* Hummert, M. L., Wiemann, J. M., and Nussbaum, J. N., Eds., Sage Publications, Thousand Oaks, CA, 1994, 15.
2. Cohen, G., Age-related problems in the use of proper names in communication, in *Interpersonal Communication in Older Adulthood,* Hummert, M. L., Wiemann, J. M., and Nussbaum, J. N., Eds., Sage Publications, Thousand Oaks, CA, 1994, 40.
3. Schneider, B. A., Psychoacoustics and aging: implications for everyday listening, *J. Speech-Lang. Pathol. Audiol.*, 21, 111, 1997.
4. Schneider, B. A., Speranza, F., and Pichora-Fuller, M. K., Age related changes in temporal resolution: envelope and intensity effects, *Can. J. Exp. Psychol.*, 52, 184, 1998.
5. Sommers, M. S., Stimulus variability and spoken word recognition II: the effects of age and hearing impairment, *J. Acoust. Soc. Am.*, 101, 2278, 1997.
6. Salthouse, T. A., The processing-speed theory of adult age differences in cognition, *Psychol. Rev.*, 103, 403, 1996.
7. Schneider, B. A. and Pichora-Fuller, M. K., Implications of perceptual deterioration for cognitive aging research, in *The Handbook of Aging and Cognition*, 2nd ed., Craik, F. I. M. and Salthouse, T. A., Eds., Lawrence Erlbaum Associates, Mahwah, NJ, 2000, 155.
8. Kuegler, C. F. A., Interrelations of age, sensory functions, and human brain signal processing, *J. Gerontol. Biol. Sci. Med. Sci.*, 54A, 231, 1999.
9. Howard, J. H. and Howard, D. V., Learning and memory, in *Handbook of Human Factors and the Older Adult*, Fisk, A. D. and Rogers, W. A., Eds., Academic Press, San Diego, CA, 1997, 7.
10. Just, M. A. and Carpenter P. A., A capacity theory of comprehension: individual differences in working memory, *Psychol. Rev.*, 99, 122, 1992.
11. Waters, G. and Caplan, D., The capacity theory of sentence comprehension: a critique of Just and Carpenter (1992), *Psychol. Rev.*, 103, 761, 1996.
12. Carpenter, P. A., Miyake, A., and Just, M. A., Working memory constraints in comprehension: evidence from individual differences, aphasia and aging, in *Handbook of Psycholinguistics*, Gernsbacher, M. A., Ed., Academic Press, San Diego, CA, 1994, 1075.
13. Tun, P. A. and Wingfield, A., Language and communication: fundamentals of speech communication and language processing in old age, in *Handbook of Human Factors and the Older Adult*, Fisk, A. D. and Rogers, W. A., Eds., Academic Press, San Diego, CA, 1997, 125.
14. Norman, S., Kemper, S., and Kynette, D., Adults' reading comprehension: effects of syntactic complexity and working memory, *J. Gerontol. Psychol. Sci. Soc. Sci.,* 47B, 258, 1992.
15. Obler, L. K., Fein, D., Nicholas, M., and Albert, M. L., Auditory comprehension and aging: decline in syntactic processing, *Appl. Psycholinguistics*, 12, 433, 1991.

16. Zacks, R. and Hasher, L., Cognitive gerontology and attentional inhibition: a reply to Burke and McDowd, *J. Gerontol. Psychol. Sci. Soc. Sci.*, 52B, 274, 1997.

17. Hernandez, A. E. and Kohnert, K. J., Aging and language switching in bilinguals, *Aging Neuropsychol. Cogn.*, 2, 69, 1999.

18. Light, L. L., Memory and aging: four hypotheses in search of data, *Annu. Rev. Psychol.*, 42, 333, 1991.

19. Wingfield, A. and Stine-Morrow, E., Language and speech, in *The Handbook of Aging and Cognition,* Craik, F. I. M. and Salthouse, T. A. et al., Eds., Lawrence Erlbaum Associates, Mahwah, NJ, 2000, 359.

20. Zacks, R. T. and Hasher, L., Capacity theory and the processing of inferences, in *Language, Memory, and Aging*, Light, L. L. and Burke, D. M., Eds., Cambridge University Press, New York, 154, 1988.

21. Van der Linden, M. et al., Cognitive mediators of age-related differences in language comprehension and verbal memory performance, *Aging Neuropsychol. Cogn.*, 6, 32, 1999.

22. Vercruysen, M., Movement control and speed of behavior, in *Handbook of Human Factors and the Older Adult*, Fisk, A. D. and Rogers, W. A., Eds., Academic Press, San Diego, CA, 1997, 55.

23. Guan, J. and Wade, M. G., The effect of aging on adaptative eye-hand coordination, *J. Gerontol. Psychol. Sci. Soc. Sci.*, 55B, 151, 2000.

24. Schaie, K. W., Cognitive development in aging, in *Language and Communication in the Elderly,* Obler, L. K. and Albert, M. D., Eds., Lexington Books, Lexington, KY, 1980.

25. Borod, J. D., Goodglass, H., and Kaplan, E., Normative data on the Boston Diagnostic Aphasia Examination. Parietal Lobe Battery, and the Boston Naming Test, *J. Clin. Neuropsychol.*, 2, 209, 1980.

26. Goldstein, G. and Shelly, C., Does the right hemisphere age more rapidly than the left? *J. Clin. Neuropsychol.*, 3, 65, 1981.

27. Drayer, B. P., Imaging the aging brain. Part I. Normal findings, *Radiology*, 166, 785, 1988.

28. Zarranz, J., Antiguedad, A. et al., *Neurología*, Harcourt Brace, Madrid, 1998.

29. La-Rue, A., Adult development and aging, in *Handbook of Neuropsychological Assessment: A Biopsychosocial Perspective. Critical Issues in Neuropsychology,* Puente, A. E., McCaffrey, III, R. J. et al., Eds., Plenum Press, New York, 1992, 526.

30. Gallagher, M. and Rapp, P. R., The use of animal models to study the effects of aging on cognition, *Annu. Rev. Psychol.*, 48, 339, 1997.

31. Fisher, D. L. and Glaser, R. A., Molar and latent models of cognitive slowing: implications for aging, dementia, depression, development, and intelligence, *Psychonomic Bull. Rev.*, 3, 458, 1996.

32. Fisk, A. D. and Fisher, D. L., Brinley plots and theories of aging: the explicit, muddled, and implicit debates, *J. Gerontol.*, 49, 81, 1994.

33. Sliwinski, M., Aging and counting speed: evidence for process-specific slowing. *Psychol. Aging*, 12, 38, 1997

34. Swearer, J. M. and Kane, K. J., Behavioral slowing with age: boundary conditions of the generalized slowing model, *J. Gerontol. Ser. B Psychol. Sci. Soc. Sci.*, 51B, 189, 1996.

35. Bashore, Th. R., Osman, A., and Heffley, E. F., Mental slowing in elderly persons: a cognitive psychophysiological analysis, *Psychol. Aging,* 4, 235, 1989.

36. O'Donnell, B. F., Friedman, S., Swearer, J. M., and Drachman, D. A., Active and passive P3 latency and psychometric performance: influence of age and individual differences, *Int. J. Psychophysiol.*, 12, 187, 1992.

37. Birren, J. E. and Fisher, L. M., Aging and slowing of behavior: consequences for cognition and survival, in *Nebraska Symposium on Motivation 1991: Psychology and Aging. Current Theory and Research in Motivation*, Sonderegger, T. B. et. al., Eds., University of Nebraska Press, Lincoln, 1992, 1.

38. Salthouse, T. A., Letz, R., and Hooisma, J., Causes and consequences of age-related slowing in speeded substitution performance, *Dev. Neuropsychol.*, 10, 203, 1994.

39. Tun, P. A. and Wingfield, A., Is speech special? Perception and recall of spoken language in complex environments, in *Adult Information Processing: Limits on Loss*, Cerella, J., Hoyer, W., Rybash, J., and Commons, M. L., Eds., Academic Press, San Diego, CA, 1993, 425.

40. MacKay, D. A. and Abrams, L., Age-linked declines in retrieving orthographic knowledge: empirical, practical, and theoretical implications, *Psychol. Aging*, 13, 647, 1998.

41. Light, L. L., The organization of memory in old age, in *The Handbook of Aging and Cognition*, Craik, F. I. M. and Salthouse, T. A., Eds., Lawrence Erlbaum Associates, Hillsdale, NJ, 1992, 111.

42. Nicholas, M., Barth, Ch., Obler, L. K., Au, Rh., and Albert, M. L., Naming in normal aging and dementia of the Alzheimer's type, in *Anomia: Neuroanatomical and cog-Nitive Correlates. Foundations of Neuropsychology*, Goodglass, H., Wingfield, A. et al., Eds., Academic Press, San Diego, CA, 1997, 166.

43. Mayr, U. and Kliegl, R., Complex semantic processing in old age: does it stay or does it go? *Psychol. Aging*, 15, 29, 2000.

44. Huff, J., Language in normal aging and age-related neurological diseases, in *Handbook of Neuropsychology*, Nebes, R. D., Corkin, S. et al., Eds., Elsevier Science Publishing, Amsterdam, 1990, 251.

45. Zurif, W., Swinney, D., Porather, P., Wingfield, A., and Browell, H., The allocation of memory resources during sentence comprehension: evidence from the elderly, *J. Psycholinguistic Res.*, 24, 165, 1995.

46. Kemper, S., Geriatric psycholinguistics, in *Language, Memory and Aging*, Light, L. L. and Burke, D. M., Eds., Cambridge University Press, New York, 1988, 58.

47. Kemper, S. and Anagnopoulos, Ch., Adult use of discourse constraints on syntactic processing, in *Adult Information Processing: Limits on Loss*, Cerella, J., Rybash, J. M. et al., Eds., Academic Press, San Diego, CA, 1993, 489.

48. Kemper, S., Imitation of complex syntactic constructions by elderly adults, *Appl. Psycholinguistics*, 7, 277, 1986

49. Norman, S., Kemper, S., Kynette, D., Cheung, H., and Anagnapoulos, C., Syntatic complexity and adults' running memory span, *J. Gerontol. Psychol. Sci.*, 46, 346, 1991.

50. Kemper, S., Language and aging, in *The Handbook of Aging and Cognition*, Craik, F. I. M. and Salthouse, T. A., Eds., Lawrence Erlbaum Associates, Hillsdale, NJ, 1992, 213.

51. Kjelgaard, M. M., Titone, D. A., and Wingfield, A., The influence of prosodic structure on the interpretation of temporary syntactic ambiguity by young and elderly listeners, *Exp. Aging Res.*, 25, 187, 1999.

52. Wingfield, A., Wayland, S. C., and Stine, E. A., Adult age differences in the use of prosody for syntactic parsing and recall of spoken sentences, *J. Gerontol. Psychol. Sci. Soc. Sci.*, 47B, 350, 1992.

53. Burke, D., Language production and aging, in *Constraints on Language: Aging, Grammar, and Memory,* Kemper, S. and Kliegl, R., Eds., Kluwer Academic Publishers, Boston, 1999.

54. Balota, D. and Duchek, J., Age-related differences in lexical access, spreading activation, and simple pronunciation, *Psychol. Aging,* 3, 84, 1988.

55. Madden, D. J., Selective attention and visual search: revision of an allocation model and application to age differences, *J. Exp. Psychol. Hum. Percept. Performance,* 18, 821, 1992.

56. Nicholas, M., Obler, L. K., Albert, M. L., and Helm-Estabrooks, N., Empty speech in Alzheimer's disease and fluente aphasia, *J. Speech Hearing Res.,* 28, 405, 1985

57. Kemper, S., Kynette, D., and Norman, S., Age differences in spoken language, in *Everyday Memory and Aging. Current Research and Methodology,* West, R. and Sinnot, J., Eds., Springer-Verlag, New York, 1992.

58. Juncos, A. and Iglesias, F., Decline in the elderly's language: evidence from a cross-linguistic data, *J. Neurolinguistics,* 8, 183, 1994.

59. Cooper, P. V., Discourse production and normal aging: performance on oral picture description tasks, *J. Gerontol. Psychol. Sci.,* 45, 210, 1990

60. MacKay, D. G. and Burke, D. M., Cognition and aging: new learning and the use of old connections, in *Aging and Cognition: Knowledge Organization and Utilization,* Hess, T. M., Ed., North-Holland, Amsterdam, 1990, 213–263.

61. Glosser, G. and Deser, T., A comparison of changes in macrolinguistic and microlinguistic aspects of discourse production in normal aging, *J. Gerontol. Psychol. Sci.,* 47, 266, 1992.

62. Goodglass, H., Disorders of naming follosing brain injury, *Am. Sci.,* 68, 647, 1980.

63. Burke, D. M., MacKay, D. G., Worthley, J. S., and Wade, E., On the tip of the tongue: what causes word finding failures in young and older adults, *J. Mem. Language,* 30, 542, 1991.

64. Burke, D. M., Whorthey, J., and Martin, J., I'll never forget what's-her-name: aging and tip of the tongue experiences in everyday life, in *Practical Aspects of Memory: Current Research and Issues,* Vol. 2. *Clinical and Educational Implications,* Gruneberg, M. M., Moris, P. E., and Sykes, R. N., John Wiley & Sons, Chichester, U.K., 1988, 113.

65. Rastle, K. G. and Burke, D. M., Priming the tip of the tongue: effects of prior processing on word retrieval in young and older adults, *J. Mem. Language,* 35, 586, 1996.

66. Stadtlander, L. M., Age differences in orthographic and frequency neighborhoods, in *Age Differences in Word and Language Processes,* Allen, P. A. and Bashore, T. R., Eds., North-Holland, Amsterdam, 1995, 72.

67. Coltheart, M. et al., Models of reading aloud: dual-route and parallel-distributed-processing approaches, *Psychol. Rev.,* 100, 598, 1993.

68. Manly, J. J. et al., Effect of literacy on neuropsychological test performance in nondemented, education-matched elders, *J. Int. Neuropsychol. Soc.,* 5, 191, 1999.

69. MacKay, D. G., Abrams, L., and Pedroza, M. J., Aging in the output versus the output side: theoretical implications of age-linked asymmetries between detecting versus retrieving orthographic information, *Psychol. Aging,* 14, 3, 1999.

70. Hasher, L. and Zacks, R. T., Working memory, comprehension, and aging: a review and a new view, in *The Psychology of Learning and Motivation,* Vol. 22, Bower, G. H., Ed., Academic Press, San Diego, CA, 1988, 193.

71. Schneider, B. A., Daneman, M., Murphy, D. R., and Kwong See, S., Listening to discourse in distracting settings: the effects of aging, *Psychol. Aging,* 15, 110, 2000.

72. Burke, D. M. and Yee, P. L., Semantic priming during sentence processing by young and old adults, *Dev. Psychol.*, 20, 903, 1984.

73. Light, L. L. et al., Comprehension and use of anaphoric devices in young and older adults, *Discourse Processes*, 18, 77, 1994.

74. Tun, P. A. and Wingfield, A., Speech recall under heavy load conditions: age, predictability and limits on a dual task interference, *Aging Cogn.*, 2, 39, 1994.

75. Kemper, S. and Harden, T., Experimentally disentangling what's beneficial about elderspeak from what's not, *Psychol. Aging*, 14, 656, 1999.

76. James, L. E., Burke, D. M., Austin, A., and Hulme, E., Production and perception of "verbosity" in young and older adults, *Psychol. Aging,* 13, 355, 1998.

77. Arbuckle, T. Y., Nohara-LeClair, M., and Pushkar, D., Effect of off-target verbosity on communication efficiency in a Referential Communication task, *Psychol. Aging*, 15, 65, 2000.

78. Dorken, H., Psychometric differences between senile dementia and normal senescent decline, *Can. J. Psychol.*, 8, 187, 1984.

79. Miller, E., Impaired recall and the memory disturbance in presenile dementia, *Br. J. Soc. Clin. Psychol.*, 14, 73, 1975.

80. Obusek, C. J. and Warren, R. M., A comparison of speech perception in senile and well-preserved aged by means of the transformation effect, *J. Gerontol.*, 28, 184, 1973.

81. Wilson, R. S., Baker, L. D., Fox, J. H., and Kazniak, A., Primary memory and secondary memory in dementia of the Alzheimer type, *J. Clin. Neuropsychol.*, 5, 337, 1983.

82. Gispen, W. H. and Traber, J., *Aging Brain*, Elsevier, New York, 1983.

83. Murdoch, B. E., Chenery, H. J., Wilks, V., and Boyle, R. S., Language disorders in dementia of the Alzheimer type, *Brain Language,* 31, 122, 1987.

84. Hier, D. B., Hagenlocker, K., and Shindler, A. G., Language disintegration in dementia: effects of etiology and severity, *Brain Language,* 25, 117, 1985.

85. Jorm, A. F., Controlled and automatic information processing in senile dementia: a review, *Psychol. Med.*, 16, 77, 1986.

86. Wingfield, A., Aberdeen, J., and Stine-Morrow, E., Word onset gating and linguistic context in spoken word recognition by young and elderly adults, *J. Gerontol.*, 46, 127, 1991.

87. Bayles, K. A. and Kazniak, A. W., *Communication and Cognition in Normal Aging and Dementia*, Little, Brown, Boston, 1987.

88. Bowles, N. L., Age and semantic inhibition in word retrieval, *J. Gerontol.*, 44, 88, 1989.

89. Crook, T. and West, R. L., Name recall performance across the adult life-span, *Br. J. Psychol.*, 81, 335, 1990.

9 Emotional Disorders in the Neurologically Deteriorating Older Adult

Inés Monguió

CONTENTS

9.1 Introduction 184
9.2 Organic Etiology: Co-Morbid Conditions 184
    9.2.1 Depression 185
    9.2.2 Mania 186
    9.2.3 Anxiety 186
    9.2.4 Aggression 187
9.3 Psychosocial Etiology 187
    9.3.1 Preexisting Conditions 189
        9.3.1.1 Exacerbation of Symptoms 189
        9.3.1.2 Expression of Psychopathology 190
    9.3.2 Reactive Conditions 191
        9.3.2.1 Awareness of Deterioration of Functions 191
        9.3.2.2 Social Isolation 193
        9.3.2.3 Breakdown of Social Support 194
        9.2.3.4 Changes in Lifestyle 196
9.4 Conclusions 197
Acknowledgment 197
References 198

It's a strange sensation to pick up a book you enjoyed just a few months ago and discover you don't remember it.... I've got to try to hold on to some of it. Some of the things I've learned. Oh, God, please don't take it all away.

*— **D. Keyes**,*
***Flowers for Algernon**[1]*

9.1 INTRODUCTION

The incidence of diagnosis of psychiatric disorders among elderly people is high[2–5] and of various etiology.[6] There are changes in general health, status, lifestyle, and social support that are commonly associated with emotional disorders.[7–9] Among the older adults with neurological disorders there are also changes in the function of neurotransmitters and deterioration of brain tissue associated with mood, anxiety, and behavior disorders. The cognitive and behavioral correlates of the psychiatric condition are further complicated by physical and biochemical changes in the brain that are specific to the organic condition causing the neurological symptoms, although these two classes of events may occur independently of each other.[10] Of themselves, the symptoms specific to neurological disorders can present an especially frightening reality to the patient, causing further deterioration of mood and thought.[11,12] Deteriorating mood in turn can interact with the symptoms of dementia, aggravating cognitive deficits.[11,13,14] In fact, when assessing the mental status of elderly patients, care must be exercised to distinguish reversible pseudodementia from diseases of the central nervous system, since the cognitive and behavioral breakdown due to mood deterioration can be so marked that it appears due to an organic disorder.[15] Nonorganic causes for deteriorating cognition and behavior, whether due to endogenous or reactive conditions, can respond quite readily to the successful treatment of the psychiatric disorder,[16–18] and therefore it is imperative that reversible conditions be diagnosed accurately. Yet the identification of psychiatric symptoms in the geriatric population is often missed by medical personnel,[3] or, if identified, referrals to mental health care are not routinely made.[19] Because of the interaction of functional and neurological symptoms in elderly people with neurological conditions, it is important to separate organic from functional problems so that adequate treatment can be provided to the patient. As diagnosticians and clinicians, the professionals involved with elderly people suffering from neurological problems can significantly impact the general well-being of the patients by acknowledging the multiple sources that can have an impact on the development of psychiatric symptoms in this population.[18] Sensitivity to nonorganic factors that can affect everyday functioning affords the clinician the possibility of identifying and intervening effectively. This chapter is a review of organic and psychosocial causal factors for emotional changes among geriatric patients.

9.2 ORGANIC ETIOLOGY: CO-MORBID CONDITIONS

The changes in brain tissue that cause the symptoms of cognitive, motor, and behavioral disturbances in neurologically deteriorating elderly people may also result in psychiatric symptoms that are at least partially independent of external or premorbid factors. For example, frontotemporal dementia often presents with neuropsychiatric disturbances as the primary symptoms.[20] The following is a review of emotional disorders common to central nervous system deterioration. Thought disorders and behavioral problems due to disinhibition and impulsivity will not be reviewed as they are beyond the scope of this chapter. However, it can be just as useful to consider psychosocial antecedents and triggers for those problems for successful intervention as it is for emotional symptoms.

9.2.1 Depression

The neurological disorder most often associated with concomitant depression is Parkinson's disease (PD).[11,21] A review by Jeffrey Cummings in 1992[22] estimated the incidence of depression in patients with PD at 40%. Although biochemical changes and deterioration of brain structures appear related to the development of depressive symptoms, there are nonorganic risk factors in the development of mood disorders that can be identified as well, for example, a preexisting depression and more disability in conducting daily activities. According to Cumming's review,[22] the constellation of depressive symptoms in patients with PD was somewhat different from those of other depressed patients, including more agitation and fewer self-critical thoughts. The lower levels of serotonin found in the cerebrospinal fluid of depressed patients with PD[21] is congruent with the characterization of the depression as agitated. Other researchers consider dopamine the neurotransmitter most responsible for the development of depression among patients with PD.[23,23] It appears that the frontal lobes are highly involved in the modulation of affect through the rich connections with the limbic system, and disruption in the functioning or interactions of this system could result in the development of psychiatric symptoms, including mood disorders. Dopaminergic neurons in the ventral tegmentum enervate mesocorticolimbic structures, and the loss of cell bodies in this area has been documented in some patients with PD,[26] lending support to the dopamine hypothesis for the depression in these patients.

Degenerative brain changes, in general, predispose elderly people to the development of depression,[27] and this alone may account for the presence of mood disorders among patients with Alzheimer's disease. However, some affected individuals experience symptoms of depression as early as 2 years prior to the diagnosis of dementia,[28] before the deterioration of brain tissue is sufficient to cause the significant behavioral and cognitive disturbances that prompt the individual to seek diagnosis and treatment. It is possible that in the early stages of cortical dementia of the Alzheimer's type (DAT) the pathways connecting subcortical structures to the frontal lobes begin to deteriorate.[27] In the early stages of DAT the cognitive and behavioral changes may be too subtle to be recognized as the symptoms of incipient dementia, but the tissue degeneration may be sufficient to result in mood disorders. However, it is also possible that in the early stages, the individual is able to maintain enough contact with reality and engage in self-assessment, therefore accurately assessing the deterioration of functions. In contrast, with more advanced deterioration of central nervous systems as dementia advances, insight and accurate assessment of situations and consequences diminish. With less self-awareness the patient perceives fewer obstacles and difficulties in his or her daily functioning, and therefore has fewer problems that require adjustment. It is known that in the later stages of the disease, agitation and delusional thinking are more common than affective disturbances.[28] If the depressive symptoms often seen in patients in the early and middle stages of DAT were dependent on self-awareness, then initially one would expect a higher frequency of failures in adjustment rather than the full clinical syndrome of depression. A review of 30 studies on depression and psychosis in Alzheimer's disease[29] found that isolated psychiatric symptoms rather than the full diagnostic constellation were present in 30 to 40% of patients with dementia. More recent research using the Mattis Dementia Rating Scale and the Mini-Mental Status examination to identify dementia found that no major affective disorder could be diagnosed in the subjects, although symptoms of anxiety and depression were more common in subjects with dementia than in control subjects, but less than in depressed individuals.[30]

At the time of assessing the presence of mood disorders in elderly people with neurological deterioration it may be important to distinguish between observed and reported symptoms that may cluster into two separate categories of events. Forsell and others[31] applied the DSM-III-R criteria for major depressive episode to 643 elderly individuals. They found that the symptoms could be clustered into those signaling mood and motivation disturbances. Individuals with mild dementia most often displayed or complained of symptoms of mood disturbance, whereas individuals with more severe dementia had symptoms of motivation disturbances.

9.2.2 MANIA

The presence of cognitive deterioration has been associated with the presence of manic symptoms.[32] There is sufficient information in the literature to wonder if agitation, perseveration, and disinhibition may be misdiagnosed as symptoms of mania, given the significant difference between the incidence of the diagnosis among the hospitalized elderly population and the general population.[10] Neurological lesions in the right hemisphere are commonly associated with maniclike symptoms,[33] as are damages to areas of the orbitofrontal-limbic system.[34] It bears considering that the possibility that "manic" behaviors observed in elderly people with neurological deterioration may be more consistent with agitation, disorientation, disruption of thought processes, and disinhibition than with the psychiatric diagnosis of mania. If this were the case, then the high incidence of hospital admission rate for mania in elderly people reported by Shulman and Herrmann[10] could be accounted for by misdiagnosing neurological symptoms as psychiatric ones.

9.2.3 ANXIETY

It has been said before that anxiety or agitation is a psychological state that often coexists with some types of depression, particularly those in which a decrease of serotonin is a likely cause. The incidence of anxiety symptoms in the general elderly population has been estimated as high as 17% in males and 21% in females.[3] The presence of dementia is a factor in the development of anxiety,[35] as are factors common to younger populations such as prior exposure to important stressors.[2,36,37] The possibility that aggressive behavior in the elderly people with dementia may be due to anxiety or poor modulation of affect, which responds to carbamazepine in this population,[38] suggests that some of the behaviors identified with anxiety in elderly people suffering neurological deterioration may be a misinterpretation of agitation and restlessness as anxiety. Nevertheless, damage to more posterior areas of the right hemisphere often results in anxiety and agitation, often reminiscent of obsessive–compulsive disorder, rather than the anosognosia more often associated with anterior right hemisphere damage. In some elderly people with dementia the agitation may indeed be a behavioral manifestation of anxiety[11] and may be a direct consequence of the deterioration of the connections between the frontal lobes and the limbic system, which is responsible for a major portion of affect regulation.[34,39]

9.2.4 AGGRESSION

Other common psychiatric symptoms believed due to the effects of progressing brain deterioration are aggressive behaviors in patients with Huntington's disease[40] and advanced Alzheimer's disease.[28] Aggressive behavior in patients with dementia may respond to treatment with carbamazepine,[38] suggesting that in some cases aggression may be related to unmodulated arousal or anxiety. The paranoid ideation seen in some subcortical and traumatic dementia as well as in Alzheimer's dementia[28,29] may be due to disruption of dopamine production[40] or deterioration of brain tissue.[37,41] However, the nature and extent of neurological changes alone seem insufficient for the presence of psychiatric symptoms in affected elderly people, at least in patients with ADT.[29]

9.3 PSYCHOSOCIAL ETIOLOGY

Regardless of the systemic processes at the level of the central nervous system that result in the manifestation of psychiatric symptoms, the effect of psychosocial factors on mood, behavior, and thought deterioration in elderly patients cannot be minimized or ignored by individuals involved in the diagnosis and management of neurological disease. Human beings are an open-system ecology that reacts to and interacts with the environment. One cannot look at a patient independently of the internal and external environment in which he or she exists and expect to understand diagnostic and treatment issues.

When dealing with patients with dementia the clinician often seems to approach treatment as if from a sense of helplessness that perhaps grows from the knowledge of the inevitable likely course of the neurological disorder. But as LeDoux[42] has eloquently formulated, the brain/mind is not only a "processor of [cognitive] information" but of emotional information as well. Our Western culture has prized intellectual over emotional information since Aristotle, a stance that is reflected in the paradigms used in medicine and the neurosciences. In the author's own experience as a neuropsychologist, it seems that most colleagues, as brilliant as they might be as evaluators and diagnosticians, appear ill prepared to deal with the emotional reactions to brain injury. A favorite example is the one involving a patient with a preexisting dissociative disorder well under control for 40 years who decompensated after a motor vehicle accident that resulted in traumatic brain injury. The neuropsychologist assessed her and wrote an accurate and elegant report that suggested psychotherapy. As the patient began trusting the neuropsychologist she confided that there were some little children in her who were speaking to her. My colleague, without missing a beat, counseled the patient to tell them to shut up. Of course, the patient did not return for further treatment.

Cultural bias notwithstanding, the brain likely evolved into increasing complexity to evaluate approach–avoidance information to external and internal stimuli. For example, hunger is felt by a conscious living being, motivating it to seek food. Genetic makeup and prior learning leads to an appropriate food source. But even the hungriest rabbit will not venture outside the burrow if a predator is nearby. But what if the predator is smarter than the rabbit and knows to sit quietly, hidden, and downwind so its scent is not carried to the prey? The predator wins. A brain that allows integrating sensory information with the cognitive and emotional meaning of that event is able to appraise environmental conditions that are conducive to well-being, or detrimental to it, and therefore is able to develop a wide range of behaviors adaptive to a variety of situations and environments. Evaluation of one's self, actions, and relationship to the world is of paramount importance to adaptation, but also to well-being and therefore quality of life. Aesthetics, as a paramount result of self-in-the-world-evaluation product, has been discussed by Premack[43] with tenderness and insightful respect across species. Human beings range in habitat from the equator to the Arctic circle, from the deserts to the jungles. In all habitats cultures have developed, with songs, art, and games; rules, rewards, and punishment. Without our ability to process emotional information and meaning, adaptation to harsh conditions would have been quite difficult if not impossible. It may be that as our knowledge of emotional functioning grows with the current interest in the area, we may come to wonder if intellectual functions are not there to interpret, integrate, deal with, and act on emotional information. The elderly patient with neurological disease continues receiving/perceiving emotional information that deteriorating cognitive abilities cannot accurately interpret, or painful emotions that limited problem solving and flexibility cannot ease. Adjustment disorders are common among this population; and since the medical condition, which often is the proximal stressor, will only continue, the patient's affect will deteriorate further.

Neurological disorders usually first come to the attention of the general practitioner, who then may or may not refer to neurology. The physician may note the deteriorating mental health of the patient and attribute it to the inevitability of changes in mood or thought due to the organic disorder, which overtly or covertly sets up a paradigm of carelessness or hopelessness that limits the range of options that the physician may consider at the time of setting treatment goals.[44] There is plentiful evidence to suggest, as reviewed above, that deterioration of neurotransmitter availability or functions and changes in brain tissue account for a portion of the cause in the onset of psychiatric symptoms observed in the elderly individual with a neurological disease. Although the symptoms may be as responsive to medication treatment as in younger populations, geriatric patients are often taking multiple medications because of multiple health problems, which makes management of psychiatric symptoms a challenge because of adverse side effects and possibly even delirium.[45,46] However, there are other, nonorganic factors in a elderly patient's emotional status that, if successfully managed, can result in significant improvement of symptoms, and of quality of life.

9.3.1 PREEXISTING CONDITIONS

9.3.1.1 Exacerbation of Symptoms

Few if any psychiatric diagnoses truly result in a complete permanent remission of symptoms, or "cure." Rather, ongoing or periodic treatment is necessary for management when the disorder is not in remission. Given the social stigma of mental illness present in society even today, it is likely that many of the individuals born in the first quarter of the 20th century did not come to the attention of the mental health professional unless severely disabled by the psychiatric disorder. Therefore, the now-elderly population may be composed of a portion of individuals whose mental condition was not diagnosed while the patient was younger because he or she was able to hide the distress, or to cope with it by means other than psychiatric diagnosis and treatment. It is likely that the *Zeitgeist* of the 1930s and 1940s expected bouts of psychiatric symptoms to be "toughed out," handled through prayer, or hidden when all else failed. Obsessive–compulsive disorders may have been ascribed to "eccentricity," while anxiety and somatization disorders were treated by the medical profession then as they are now.[3]

Among elderly people with neurological disorders, mild to moderate emotional problems that existed prior to the diagnosis of central nervous system deterioration may become expressed in exacerbated symptoms as brain functioning deteriorates. A compromised central nervous system, particularly if frontal lobes and/or limbic system are involved, leads to a more limited repertoire of behaviors, decreased problem-solving ability, and more inflexible behaviors.[47] The individual who earlier may have been able to control a preexisting condition successfully through effective self-management could find himself or herself unable to engage in the coping mechanisms that allowed the preexisting disorder to stay in remission or under control. The following case illustrates this possible cause for the development of psychiatric symptoms in this population.

> C.S. is a 64-year-old female with a positive history for depression and alcohol abuse under control for 20 years. She had sought psychotherapy in her 30s for her psychiatric symptoms and had been functioning well until 2 years prior to consultation with this author. She was referred for a neuropsychological evaluation because of memory problems that were interfering with her work as an executive administrator at a school. The results of the battery were consistent with the presence of Alzheimer's disease. Executive functions in particular were significantly impaired in a bright and educated woman. The session scheduled for feedback on the results of testing was attended by the patient's daughter. She revealed that her mother, contrary to C.S.'s report, had become very depressed of late and had been abusing alcohol again. The patient herself described how scared and lonely she felt at night after returning from work, and how going out and drinking allowed her to "feel normal." She was able to verbalize her knowledge of the dangers of alcohol both to her depression and to her cognitive functioning.

9.3.1.2 Expression of Psychopathology

The presence of a neurological disorder can also result in the expression of a preexisting subclinical condition that may not have caused enough distress or functional impairment to come to the attention of the mental health professional even as a personality disorder. In individuals with a high intellectual capacity, a simple life, or a highly supportive social milieu, pathological adaptation may not significantly interfere with activities of daily living. The individual may have been described as "moody," "mercurial," "perfectionist," "set-in-his-ways," or a host of other red flags in clinical interviews. As the central nervous system deteriorates, cognitive and behavioral resources decrease and elderly people with beginning symptoms of a dementing disorder are vulnerable to decompensation[13] as resources dwindle. Loss of nonspecific tissue in the brain may result in limited available resources for overall functioning that is related to the amount of brain tissue affected. Support for this hypothesis is seen in the effects of traumatic brain injury in behavior and emotional adaptation.[48] Alternatively, the expression of subclinical psychiatric disorders in the neurologically impaired older adult may be specifically related to the preponderance of specific frontal and limbic lobe deterioration in many of the dementias.[11] As has been reviewed earlier, disruption of mesocorticolimbic connections has been implicated in the emergence of depression symptoms in neurological patients, since the frontal lobes are major contributors to the modulation of affect through higher-level cognitive processes and through the rich connections to the limbic system.[25,34] But if we can look beyond the physical reality of the brain and into the epiphenomenon of consciousness, impairment in executive functions may lead to decreased problem solving and a diminished sense of mastery in the affected patient. As the "master program" for behavior and emotional modulation deteriorates, the individual may find fewer resources to manage the subclinical preexisting condition, much like the patient in a stable remission of a preexisting condition may suffer an exacerbation of symptoms after the onset of dementia. In addition, the failure to inhibit impulses often associated with deterioration of frontal lobe functioning[47] may result in a diminished ability to manage eccentric or marginally acceptable behaviors. As the patient fails to manage the "quirks" in character, he or she may feel overwhelmed by the internal needs that the patient can no longer satisfy through actions or thoughts. The case of A.G. is illustrative.

> A.G. is a 62-year-old male who was being treated for depression by a psychiatrist and social worker team. A neuropsychological consult was requested because of persistent complaints of word-finding difficulties. The patient had no history of psychiatric diagnosis prior to beginning treatment with the referring psychiatrist. A.G. was a university graduate and had taught high-school English for almost 30 years. He was interviewed in the presence of his quiet, submissive wife. The patient gave an extremely detailed history of health problems with a lot of emphasis on the correct dates and sequence of events. He interrupted his wife's input with corrections for minimal differences. The writer began suspecting the presence of a psychiatric disorder instead of or in addition to

a neurological problem. A.G. denied any preexisting psychiatric conditions. His wife, however, related that he had always been "rigid" in his habits, and could become quite upset if things did not go his way. After interviewing both spouses it became apparent that A.G. had had a subclinical obsessive–compulsive disorder that he had managed because of his significant intellectual capacity, which had allowed him to structure his life in a manner that made allowances for his "rigidity" without impairing functioning. The neuropsychological battery revealed clear signs of the early stages of cortical dementia. In the opinion of this author the depression for which he was being treated was the common concomitant in obsessive–compulsive disorder when the patient feels over-whelmed by the demands of the obsessions that compulsive behaviors are not able to satisfy.

9.3.2 Reactive Conditions

There is a dearth of writing on the phenomenology of neurological deterioration. The fields in the neurosciences seem to have divorced themselves from the exploration of the effects that progressive alterations in consciousness have on patients. Detailed case studies seem to be relegated to the empathic writings of the neurologist Oliver Sacks in the popular press. In contrast, articles in most respected scientific journals do not usually allow the clinician to describe the richness of the individual experience of the subjects in the study, although there are notable exceptions.[45] However, book chapters afford the writer the ability to select topics for discussion from a wider field of experience. In this author's opinion this lack of appreciation for or interest in case studies apparent in scientific journals short-changes the consumer of research, the practitioner, by withholding information potentially crucial for understanding important issues relevant to assessment and treatment. In addition, neglecting small studies with detailed case histories in favor of large-scale studies with statistical conclusions robs the field of neuropsychology of much that is humanly valuable from the subjects and from the researchers themselves. Nelson Butters, as prolific and valuable a researcher as he was, did not reveal as a journal writer or editor the wealth of clinical sensitivity that his case presentations demonstrated.[50] We will not be able to hear Dr. Butters speak any more. His legacy in research will remain, but his humanity, the dignity and gentleness with which he approached evaluation and diagnosis, will be lost for future generations of neuropsychologists.

9.3.2.1 Awareness of Deterioration of Functions

The author is not alone in being aware that many patients with a progressively deteriorating neurological condition are acutely aware of the differences between former and current functioning.[51] Individuals with early-onset dementia are at high risk for psychiatric symptoms of depression and anxiety concomitant with the neurological disorder.[30,52] Particularly in the middle stages, patients worry about what will happen to them, to their families, to their relationships with loved ones, and to their independence[52] as their ability to function independently diminishes. It is likely that the patient's reaction to the deterioration or to the diagnosis itself has a bearing on the development of emotional symptoms in neurological disease, since the deterioration of brain tissue itself seems insufficient to account for the incidence of psychiatric symptoms in this population.[29] A review of depression and psychosis in patients with Alzheimer's disease[28] suggested that the common incidence of both dementia and psychiatric symptoms in geriatric patients was not sufficient to account for the prevalence of affective and thought disorder among patients with DAT. Sometimes the clinician in charge of diagnosis and management of elderly patients fails to recognize that, in addition to cognitive deterioration, many neurological disorders result in physical changes that affect mobility and independence,[53] as well as general well-being. Chronic illness in general has an impact on the life satisfaction of the individual,[54–57] and therefore the presence of a neurological condition likely facilitates the development of depression and anxiety symptoms. It is known that impairment in functional ability is related to depression in elderly people,[7,53] and physical illness of itself can lead to depressed mood.[54] Among the systemic illnesses and neurological disorders, gait slowing due to neurological conditions was the factor most associated with depression and life dissatisfaction among elderly people, together with heart disease and chronic pulmonary problems.[55] Some patients who begin to experience the early symptoms of neurological deterioration may opt to cope with the difficulties through denial, and thus seek diagnosis only when coping mechanisms are insufficient. For example, Josts and Grossberg[28] found that some patients had had symptoms of depression as early as 2 years prior to the diagnosis of dementia. As has been reviewed earlier in this chapter, some of the psychiatric symptoms may be due to the degeneration of brain tissue.[11,56,57] Parenchymal degeneration may be the primary cause of the development of psychiatric disorders in neurological disorders disrupting the functions of subcortical structures, such as Parkinson's disease[21] and Huntington's disease.[40] But particularly in DAT, subcortical deterioration comes after cortical problems become quite obvious to the family, co-workers, or primary physician. Therefore, it is likely that depressive symptoms preceding diagnosis of DAT in individuals with and without preexisting psychiatric conditions may be due to the individual's awareness of the beginning of deteriorating functions, the feared consequences on their lives, and other psychosocial variables. The case of C.S. given earlier likely combines elements of poor adjustment to her awareness of developing cognitive problems, and an exacerbation of a preexisting condition because of decreased internal coping resources. Her work had deteriorated greatly, and she was mortified that her employers had began joking about her being a "scatterbrain." From someone who enjoyed reading cutting-edge literature, she turned into someone who could hardly get through the newspaper. The following case further illustrates how awareness of deterioration of functions affects the patient's emotions.

> D.M. is a 53-year-old male who is a high-power executive in the finance world. Financially affluent, he had high expenses to cover, including house mortgage, car payments, and children's school. D.M. was referred for an evaluation by his physician because of persistent complaints of sudden onset of episodes of confusion. He

was getting lost for hours at a time, and had had to resort to carrying a cellular phone at all times so he could call home for directions on how to return from wherever he was. He was very frightened by these episodes. The results of the evaluation revealed language and memory deficits strongly suggestive of dementia. When he was given feedback on the diagnostic impressions, D.M. broke down, explaining that he had suspected that "something bad was happening." He begged the author to change her opinion regarding the prognosis of his being able to return to work. He added that he would not be able to cope with his failure to fulfill his obligations to his family.

9.3.2.2 Social Isolation

As frontal lobes deteriorate, the complex task of perceiving, understanding, and responding to subtle but crucial social behavioral cues can become impaired. If there is disinhibition or poor judgment, the individual may tell inappropriate jokes, or make comments in poor taste. The response of the listeners, often embarrassment, disgust, or offense, are not perceived or processed by the patient, who merrily carries on oblivious to the effect he or she is having on others. At social gatherings, the affected individual may become inappropriate in speech or behavior, or tiresome because of stories told *ad nauseam* due to perseveration or memory deficits. This often results in embarrassment or disgust in family and friends, and the opportunities for social interactions diminish or they become disagreeable. The affected individual, and often the caretaker, are invited to visit less and less often. The spouse may limit social contact on his or her own to avoid confrontation or embarrassment. For example, the wife of a patient complained to this author in front of the patient that her husband had begun to address all females as "honey" regardless of the situation, and that this was mortifying to her, a traditional and quite staid lady. The husband, of course, was confused about her discomfort. Further examples became clear that session: making sexual innuendoes to his attendant, whom he professed to respect; addressing the ethnicity of an in-law at a party in less than "politically correct terms"; and others.

Among patients with Parkinson's disease the problems in social functioning are often on the opposite end of the spectrum from those exhibited by patients with cortical deterioration. Facial expressions are often absent with Parkinson's. Individuals with this condition are often described as "wooden" and unfeeling, and if this is a newly developed behavior, friends and family may respond with criticism instead of understanding.

> The wife of E.L., a 69-year-old patient diagnosed with Parkinson's disease for 3 years, complained that her husband was no fun and more like a "bump on a log" than a mate. At home, the wife had been making a life of her own, leaving the husband at home more often than not. The daughters interacted with the mother but not with the father. Their oldest son, the pride of the family, was a graduate student at an out-of-state university. When the family attended his graduation, the husband was left at the hotel except

for the actual diploma award because "he does not enjoy those
things." Mr. E.L. told this author that he did get tired but enjoyed
people's company very much. He eventually said he was looking
forward to dying so that his family would no longer be embarrassed
by him.

Sometimes the social isolation of patients with neurological deterioration may
be due to problems communicating and perceiving affect, or the behavioral expression of mood. Human beings as social animals need to be able to communicate and
perceive social cues[58] to respond to the social environment. Neurological deterioration results, although not always,[59] in deficits either in expressing[60] or perceiving[61,62]
the emotional content of environmental cues. Although at least in the ability to
comprehend prosody there is too much individual variability for statistical association between deficit and depression,[62] clinical experience supports the hypothesis
that without the perception of subtle (or even obvious) clues about how the social
environment reacts to the individual, many neurologically impaired adults often find
themselves in the uncomfortable and confusing situation of ostracism but unable to
identify the cause.

K.W. was in her late 50s when she began developing signs of
cortical dementia. When 61, she lost her balance and fell, hitting
her head. Her functioning deteriorated further, with agitation and
perseveration. She had been a popular woman in her circle, a
feminist pioneer as a newspaper reporter. Since her deterioration,
she had become increasingly more isolated. Friends stopped invit-
ing her to dinner parties and eventually stopped visiting altogether.
She complained of loneliness and boredom. Symptoms of depression and anger became predominant and aggravated her neurological symptoms. Her husband confided to the author that K.W. had
become quite unpleasant in her social interactions, criticizing and
offering unwelcome opinions that "turned everybody off." The
patient herself was unaware of this. The way she understood her
increasing social isolation was that "people are becoming more
stupid every year."

9.3.2.3   Breakdown of Social Support

Particularly in the early stages of neurological deterioration family and friends are
bound to ascribe the changes in the patient as being due to a willful, uncaring, or
malicious disposition. Families often report that the patient's memory problems
cause more serious problems than would physical violence, matching only the
patient's catastrophic reactions for level of disturbance of symptoms in the family's
functioning.[63] Forgetfulness may be interpreted as not paying enough attention, or
not wanting to do the tasks assigned. The patient himself may contribute to this
misperception by overreacting when challenged or criticized. Resentment builds in
the members of the family, and the relationships suffer. When the neurological
deterioration causes or results in confusion/psychotic states, such as in Alzheimer's

dementia,[64] the problems become even more severe. For example, patients with memory deficits may become suspicious to the point of paranoia when they "become aware" of situations whose antecedents they have forgotten. They may blame lost or misplaced items on family members "stealing" them, or may interpret the actions of family members with suspicion. In turn, the patient's behavior causes a great deal of stress in the family.

> A.M. is a 61-year-old male who suffered a traumatic brain injury 6 years prior to referral to this author. Among many other difficult family issues, A.M. had recently excluded his wife from the bank account where his disability checks were deposited. This was the only source of income for the couple. Apparently, he had seen a bank statement showing withdrawals for which he had no explanation. He accused his wife of withdrawing money without his permission for jewelry and unnecessary expenses. In spite of the wife's repeated attempts at explaining that he had been with her when those withdrawals had been made for funds needed for household repairs, the patient remained adamant that she was stealing money from him. He believed he was being betrayed. His wife and adult children became angry and critical of the patient. Premorbid alcoholism became worse following the incident.

Sometimes the family members themselves have problems adjusting to the changes in the patient. Denial, anger, depression, and even an exacerbation of maladaptive family dynamics can become evident as the patient deteriorates.

> J.V. had been a liked and respected figure in his small town. In his middle 60s he began to deteriorate and at 68 he was diagnosed with dementia, Alzheimer's type. He complained that the only people who visited him any more were his children, and not that often. Mr. J.V. mourned his former social activity and wondered if the only reason his children visited was out of duty, since "he was no good any more." One of the daughters expressed terrible sadness when seeing the changes in her father. She said that visiting her parents had become a very difficult thing to do, and she tried to find "reasons" why she could not spend time with her parents. The other daughter felt the other siblings were putting too much responsibility on her. She was angry and very critical of her father. She resisted the diagnosis, and refused to read the literature on Alzheimer's disease that was provided for family education.

The toll on the family of a neurologically deteriorating spouse or parent can be huge.[63] Even in healthy families, the stress of coping and adapting to the changes in the loved one can result in maladaptive reactions of anger and blaming, or deterioration of psychological well-being.[65] The families of individuals with dementing illnesses require support,[66] which is not always available in the community. If the family was dysfunctional prior to the onset of the neurological disease in the affected member, as in the case of E.L., dynamics may become even more maladaptive and noxious[67] when they need to confront and adapt to the changes that are required in the family members' roles. The following case is an example.

> J.V. is a 61-year-old male who had acquired significant assets in his life as an investment banking official. He had gone through an ugly divorce 12 years prior to evaluation. He had two daughters from the marriage. The relationships between the eldest daughter and the patient had been strained for years as the young woman sided with her mother during and after the divorce. The eldest and youngest daughter had had a feud of years. The patient was diagnosed with Parkinson's disease and within 2 years he needed nursing care around the clock, which eventually necessitated his moving into a long-term care facility. The daughters began suing and countersuing each other for control over the decision-making rights regarding their father's care and financial affairs. When evaluated for mental status and competency in making legal decisions, the patient very clearly (although with moderate to severe dysarthria) articulated his distress over his daughters' fighting, and attributed much of his psychological distress to the frustration and sadness when seeing the animosity in his daughters' interactions.

9.2.3.4 Changes in Lifestyle

The neurologically deteriorating adult often has to face dramatic changes in leisure and social activities that would present significant adaptation challenges to anyone. One patient who had been a widow for 3 years had begun to manage her bereavement through involvement in volunteering activities and a bridge club. She began noticing forgetfulness, disorganization of daily activities, and difficulty with alternating the focus of her attention. As her cognitive functions began to deteriorate, her bridge partner became critical of the patient's failures in the game, and the coordinator for volunteer activities began changing the tasks assigned to the patient. As her ability to perform these activities decreased, the patient lost a significant source of positive social interactions and leisure activities. She became quite depressed and had to be hospitalized.

Cognitive changes in sustained attention and speed of processing are common in neurological conditions, even in the early stages. For many of the elderly people, driving, and therefore independence in some communities, becomes hazardous or impossible.[68] Spouses may become primary caretakers, which may result in significant changes in the dynamics of the relationship, adding stress to the patient and to the caretaker. Adult children unaware (or in denial) of the patient's deterioration may become critical of the patient who is failing to perform up to their expectations, reducing the amount and quality of time spent with the parent. The following case is illustrative.

M.B. is a 69-year-old female whose husband has been diagnosed with brittle diabetes for over 10 years. She has been in charge of monitoring diet and medication all that time. Recently, she has become depressed and sought psychological treatment. Imaging studies at the suggestion of the psychologist revealed large areas of periventricular damage. The patient expressed feeling over-whelmed with her household responsibilities, in particular, toward her ill husband. Her children had become increasingly critical of her failing abilities to manage her household, and this had added a great deal of stress to the patient.

Elderly adults with neurological deterioration have a higher incidence of trans-ference to an inpatient facility than their cohort matched for other demographic characteristics.[69] When the deteriorating health of the affected individual requires that he or she leave the home for assisted living, the consequences for mental health can be dramatic. Not only do the patients have to confront decisions such as what personal possessions to take and what to give up, but also loss of privacy and independence as well as having to face their deteriorating condition. In addition, they have to cope with standard of care in the particular institution that may or may not be optimal. The quality of care that a patient receives is related to his or her mental health.[70] Unfortunately, the elderly neurologically deteriorating adult rarely has the means or the opportunity to be able to choose or change the facility that provides assistance. Dissatisfaction with the quality of care adds to a sense of helplessness that can further alter mood and thought.

9.4 CONCLUSIONS

When assessing and treating elderly people with neurological problems the clinician must consider nonorganic factors in addition to the organic causes to understand and address the emotional, cognitive, and behavioral symptoms that the patient presents.[71] These patients face a number of important and sometimes overwhelming adaptation tasks that a compromised central nervous system is ill-equipped to handle. Although the deterioration of brain tissue that is intrinsic to the neurological disorder can of itself cause emotional disorders, it is important for diagnostic and treatment purposes that nonorganic potential causes for psychiatric symptoms be identified. Mood disorders, in particular, aggravate symptoms of dementia. Because psychiatric symptoms are as amenable to treatment in elderly people as in other populations, the clinician's sensitivity to psychosocial factors affecting mental status is important. Awareness of and sensitivity to nonorganic factors in the etiology of psychiatric symptoms in elderly people with a deteriorating central nervous system allows the clinician a broader range of management issues,[72] which if addressed appropriately[73] can result in an improvement of neurological symptoms if not the cause of them, in addition to the improvement in the quality of life of the patient.

ACKNOWLEDGMENT

The author thanks Susan Hellman, M.S., for her help with the preparation of this manuscript.

REFERENCES

1. Keyes, D., *Flowers for Algernon*, in *The Hugo Winners*, Vol. I and II, Asimov, I., Ed., Doubleday, New York, 1962, chap. 8.
2. Beekman, A. T. F., Bremer, M. A., Deeg, D. J. H. et al., Anxiety disorders in later life: a report from the longitudinal aging study in Amsterdam, *Int. J. Geriatr. Psychiatr.*, 13, 717, 1998.
3. Himmelfarb, S. and Murrell, S. A., The prevalence and correlates of anxiety symptoms in older adults, *J. Psychol.*, 116, 159, 1984.
4. Koenig, H. G., Meador, K. G., Cohen, H. J. et al., Depression in elderly hospitalized patients with medical illness, *Arch. Int. Med.*, 148, 1929, 1988.
5. Shah, A. K., Phongsathorn, V., Bielawska, C. et al., Screening for depression among geriatric inpatients with short versions of the Geriatric Depression Scale, *Int. J. Geriatr. Psychiatr.*, 11, 915, 1996.
6. Garland, B. J. and Cross, P. S., Epidemiology of psychopathology in old age: some implications for clinical services, *Psychiatr. Clin. North Am.*, 5, 11, 1982.
7. Dent, O. F., Waite, L. M., Bennet, H. P. et al., A longitudinal study of chronic disease and depressive symptoms in a community sample of older people, *Aging Ment. Health*, 3, 351, 1999.
8. Safford, F., Differential assessment of dementia and depression in elderly people, in *Gerontology for the Health Professional: A Practice Guide*, 2nd ed., Stafford, F. and Krell, G. I., Eds., National Association of Social Workers, Washington, D.C., 1997, chap. 5.
9. Valvanne, J., Juva, K., Edman, A., and Mansson, J., Major depression in the elderly: a population study in the Helsinki, *Int. Psychogeriatr.*, 8, 437, 1996.
10. Shulman, K. I., and Hermann N., The nature and management of mania in old age, *Psychiatr. Clin. North Am.*, 22, 649, 1999.
11. Cummings, J. L. and Benson, D. F., *Dementia: A Clinical Approach*, Butterworths, Boston, 1983.
12. Ritchie, K., Touchon, J., and Ledesert, B., Progressive disability in senile dementia is accelerated in the presence of depression, *Int. J. Geriatr. Psychiatr.*, 13, 459, 1998.
13. Hoch, C. C. and Reynolds, III, C. F., Psychiatric symptoms in dementia: interaction of affect and cognition, in *Handbook of Neuropsychology*, Vol. 4, Bolier, F. and Grafman, J., Eds., Elsevier, New York, 1990, 325.
14. Delis, D. C. and Lucas, J. A., Memory, in *Neuropsychiatry*, Fogel, B. S., Schiffer, R. B., and Rao, S. M., Eds., Williams & Wilkins, Baltimore, 1996, chap. 17.
15. La Rue, A., Memory loss and aging: distinguishing dementia from benign senescent forgetfulness and depressive pseudodementia, *Psychiatr. Clin. North Am.*, 5, 89, 1982.
16. Wells, C. E. and Whitehouse, P. J., Cortical dementia, in *Neuropsychiatry*, Fogel, B. S., Schiffer, R. B., and Rao, S. M., Eds., Williams & Wilkins, Baltimore, 1996, chap. 36.
17. Friedel, R. O., Affective disorders in the geriatric patient, in *Psychiatric Update: The American Psychiatric Association Annual Review*, Vol. II, Grinspoon, L., Ed., American Psychiatric Association, New York, 1983, chap. 9.

18. Charatam, F. B., Depression in the elderly: diagnosis and treatment, *Psychiatr. Ann.*, 15, 313, 1985.
19. Shah, A. K. and De, T., Documented evidence of depression in medical and nursing case-notes and its implications in acutely ill geriatric patients, *Int. Geriatr.*, 10, 163, 1998.
20. Mendez, M. F., Perryman, K. M., Miller, B. L. et al., Behavioral differences between frontotemporal dementia and Alzheimer's disease: a comparison on the BEHAVE-AD Rating Scale, *Int. Psychogeriatr.*, 10, 155, 1998.
21. Kostic, V. S., Lecic, D., Filipovic, S. R., and Stojanovic, M., Depression and Parkinson's disease, *Psychiatriki*, 6, 125, 1995.
22. Cummings, J. L., Depression and Parkinson's disease: a review, *Am. J. Psychiatr,*, 149, 443, 1992.
23. Grassi, G., Depression and Parkinson's disease: II. Biochemical and pharmacological aspects, *R. Sperimentale Freniatria Med. A. Ment.*, 111, 105, 1987.
24. Mayeux, R., Williams, J. B. W., and Stern, Y., Clinical and biochemical features of depression in Parkinson's disease, *Am. J. Psychiatr.*, 143, 756, 1986.
25. Kaufer, D. I. and Lewis, D. A., Frontal lobe anatomy and cortical connectivity, in *The Human Frontal Lobes: Functions and Disorders*, Miller, B. L. and Cummings, J. L., Eds., Guilford, New York, 1999, chap. 2.
26. Torack, R. M. and Morris, J. C., The association of ventral tegmental area histopathology with adult dementia, *Arch. Neurol.*, 45, 211, 1988.
27. Kalaayam, B., Editorial: evoked potential in geriatric depression, *Int. J. Geriatr. Psychiatr.*, 12, 3, 1997.
28. Jost, B. C. and Grossberg, G. T., The evolution of psychiatric symptoms in Alzheimer's disease: a natural history study, *J. Am. Geriatr. Soc.*, 44, 1078, 1996.
29. Wragg, R. E. and Jeste, D. V., Overview of depression and psychosis in Alzheimer's disease, *Am. J. Psychiatr.*, 146, 577, 1989.
30. Bungener, C., Jouvent, R., and Derouesne, C., Affective disturbance in Alzheimer's disease, *J. Am. Geriatr. Soc.*, 44, 1066, 1996.
31. Forsell, Y., Jorm, A. F., Fratiglioni, L. et al., Application of DSM-III-R criteria for major depressive episode to elderly subjects with and without dementia, *Am. J. Psychiatr.*, 150, 1199, 1993.
32. Shulman, K. I., Neurologic co-morbidity and mania in old age, *Clin. Neurosci.*, 4, 37, 1997.
33. Fawcet, R. G., Cerebral infarct presenting as mania, *J. Clin. Psychiatr.*, 52, 352, 1991.
34. Cummings, J. L., Frontal-subcortical circuits and human behavior, *Arch. Neurol.*, 50, 873, 1993.
35. Fisher, J. E. and Noll, J. P., Anxiety disorders, in *The Practical Handbook of Clinical Gerontology*, Eldstein, B. E. et al., Eds., Sage, Thousand Oaks, CA, 1996, 304.
36. Beekman, A. T. F., Bremmer, M. A., Deeg, D. J. H. et al., Anxiety disorders in later life: a report from the longitudinal aging study in Amsterdam, *Int. J. Geriatr. Psychiatr.*, 13, 717, 1998.
37. Charney, D. S., Nagy, L. M., Bremner, J. D. et al., Neurobiological mechanisms of human anxiety, in *Neuropsychiatry*, Fogel, B. S., Schiffer, R. B., and Rao, S. M., Eds., Williams & Wilkins, Baltimore, 1996, chap. 12.
38. Cooney, C., Mortimer, A., Smith, A. et al., Carbamazepine use in aggressive behavior associated with senile dementia, *Int. J. Geriatr. Psychiatr.*, 11, 901, 1996.
39. Swartz, J. R., Dopamine projections and frontal systems function, in *The Human Frontal Lobes: Functions and Disorders*, Miller, B. L. and Cummings, J. L., Eds., Guilford, New York, 1999, chap. 9.

40. Burns, A., Folstein, S., Brandt, J. et al., Clinical assessment of irritability, aggression, and apathy in Huntington and Alzheimer disease, *J. Nerv. Ment. Dis.*, 178, 20, 1990.

41. Chow, T. F. and Cummings, J. L., Frontal-subcortical circuits, in *The Human Frontal Lobes: Functions and Disorders*, Miller, B. L. and Cummings, J. L., Eds., Guilford, New York, 1999, chap. 1.

42. LeDoux, J. E., Cognition and emotion: processing functions and brain systems, in *Handbook of Cognitive Neuroscience*, Gazzaniga, M. S., Ed., Plenum Press, New York, 1984, chap. 17.

43. Premack, D., Pedagogy and aesthetics as sources of culture, in *Handbook of Cognitive Neuroscience*, Gazzaniga, M. S., Ed., Plenum Press, New York, 1984, chap. 2.

44. Wells, C. E., Diagnosis of dementia: a reassessment, *Psychosomatics*, 25, 183, 1984.

45. Ruegg, R. G., Zisook, S., and Swerdlow, N. R., Depression in the aged: an overview, *Psychiatr. Clin. North Am.*, 11, 83, 1988.

46. Liston, E. H., Delirium in the aged, *Psychiatr. Clin. North Am.*, 5, 49, 1982.

47. Lezak, M. D., *Neuropsychological Assessment*, 3rd ed., Oxford University Press, New York, 1995, chaps. 1, 16.

48. Groom, K. N., Shaw, T. G., O'Connor, M. E. et al., Neurobehavioral symptoms and family functioning in traumatically brain-injured adults, *Arch. Clin. Neuropsychol.*, 13, 683, 1998.

49. Parker, R. S., A taxonomy of neurobehavioral functions applied to neuropsychological assessment after brain injury, *Neuropsychol. Rev.*, 6, 135, 1996.

50. Butters, N., Memory disorders. Presentation at the X Meeting, Annual National Academy of Neuropsychology, Reno, Nevada, 1990.

51. LaBarge, E. and Wilcox, S., Emotional effects of cognitive testing in demented versus non-demented healthy older people, *J. Am. Geriatr. Soc.*, 43, 838, 1995.

52. Brink, T. L., Depression in the aged: dynamics and treatment, *J. Natl. Med. Assoc.*, 69, 891, 1977.

53. Cahn, D. A., Sullivan, E. V., Shear, P. K. et al., Differential contributions of cognitive and motor components processes to physical and instrumental activities of daily living in Parkinson's disease, *Arch. Clin. Neuropsychol.*, 13, 575, 1998.

54. Cohen-Cole, S. A. and Stoudermire, A., Major depression and clinical illness: special considerations in diagnosis and biologic treatment, *Psychiatr. Clin. North Am.*, 10, 1, 1987.

55. Kivela, S. L., Kongas-Saviaro, P., Kimmo, P. et al., Health, health behavior and functional ability predicting depression in old age: a longitudinal study, *Int. J. Geriatr. Psychiatr.*, 11, 871, 1996.

56. Broe, G. A., Jorm, A. F., Creasy, H. et al., Impact of chronic systemic and neurologic disorder on disability, depression and life satisfaction, *Int. J. Geriatr. Psychiatr.*, 13, 667, 1998.

57. von Ammon Cavanaugh, S., Depression in the medically ill: critical issues in diagnostic assessment, *Psychosomatics*, 36, 48, 1995.

58. Darwin, C., *The Expression of the Emotions in Man and Animals*, University of Chicago Press, Chicago, 1965.

59. Magai, C., Cohen, C., Gombetrg, D. et al., Emotional expression during mid- to late-stage dementia, *Int. Psychogeriatr.*, 8, 383, 1996.

60. Asplund, K., Norberg, A., Adolfsson, R. et al., Facial expression in severely demented patients: a stimulus response study of four patients of the Alzheimer's type, *Int. J. Geriatr. Psychiatr.*, 6, 599, 1991.

61. Rapsack, S. Z., Galper, S. R., Comer, J. F. et al., Fear recognition deficits after focal brain damage: a cautionary note, *Neurology*, 54, 575, 2000.

62. Starkstein, S. E., Federoff, J. P., Price, T. R. et al., Neuropsychological and neuroradiologic correlates of emotional prosody comprehension, *Neurology*, 44, 515, 1994.

63. Rabins, P. V., Mace, N. L., and Lucas, M. J., The impact of dementia on the family, *JAMA*, 248, 333, 1982.

64. Wragg, R. E. and Jeste, D. V., Overview of depression and psychosis in Alzheimer's disease, *Am. J. Psychiatr.*, 146, 577, 1989.

65. Deniham, A., Bruce, I., Coakley, D. et al., Psychiatric morbidity in cohabitants of community-dwelling elderly depressives, *Int. J. Geriatr. Psychiatr.*, 13, 691, 1998.

66. Jansson, W., Almberg, B., Grafstrom, M. et al., The Circle Model: support for relatives of people with dementia, *Int. J. Geriatr. Psychiatr.*, 13, 674, 1998.

67. Groom, K. N., Shaw, T. G., O'Connor, D. W. et al., Neurologic symptoms and family functioning in traumatically brain-injured adults, *Arch. Clin. Neuropsychol.*, 13, 695, 1998.

68. Warner, J. P., The older driver and mental illness, *Int. J. Geriatr. Psychiatr.*, 11, 859, 1996.

69. Pasternak, R., Rosenweig, A., Booth, B. et al., Morbidity of homebound versus inpatient elderly psychiatric patients, *Int. Psychogeriatr.*, 10, 117, 1998.

70. Challiner, Y. and Julious, S., Quality of care, quality of life and the relationship between them in long-term care institutions for the elderly, *Int. J. Geriatr. Psychiatr.*, 11, 883, 1996.

71. Sherman, A. G., Shaw, T. G., and Glidden, H., Emotional behavior as an agenda in neuropsychological evaluation, *Neuropsychol. Rev.*, 4, 45, 1994.

72. Cummings, J. L., Neuropsychiatric assessment and intervention in Alzheimer's disease, *Int. Psychogeriatr.*, 8, Suppl. 1, 25, 1996.

73. Klausner, E. J., Clarkin, J. F., Spielman, L. et al., Late depression and functional disability: the role of goal-focused group psychotherapy, *Int. J. Geriatr. Psychiatr.*, 13, 707, 1998.

10 Aging, Sleep, and Neuropsychological Functioning Outcomes

*María José Ramos-Platón
and Antonio Benetó-Pascual*

CONTENTS

10.1 Introduction 204
10.2 Physiological Changes in Sleep Due to Aging 204
    10.2.1 Cerebral Bioelectric Activity Variations 205
    10.2.2 Changes in Sleep Stages and Cycles.......................................205
    10.2.3 Sleep–Wake Circadian Rhythm Modifications.........................205
10.3 Sleep Disorders in Elderly People...206
    10.3.1 Dyssomnias 207
        10.3.1.1 Initiating or Maintaining Sleep
                  Difficulties (Insomnias) 207
        10.2.1.2 Excessive Daytime Sleepiness
                  Disorders (Hypersomnias)......................................210
        10.3.1.3 Circadian Rhythm Sleep Disorders 211
    10.3.2 Parasomnias..212
    10.3.3 Sleep Disorders Associated with Psychiatric
        and Medical Diseases..212
        10.3.3.1 Sleep Disorders Associated
                  with Psychiatric Alterations....................................212
        10.3.3.2 Sleep Disorders Associated
                  with Organic Diseases 213
        10.3.3.3 Sleep Disorders Associated
                  with Neurological Diseases 213
10.4 Changes in Cognitive Functioning with Normal Aging 215
    10.4.1 Cognitive Performance Pattern 215
        10.4.1.1 Executive Functions..218
        10.4.1.2 Memory Processes 219
    10.4.2 Neural Basis of Cognitive Dysfunction....................................220
        10.4.2.1 Cerebral Changes...220
        10.4.2.2 Aging Effects on Cognitive Functioning 221

0-8493-2066-/01/$0.00+$1.50
© 2001 by CRC Press LLC

10.5   Sleep Disorders and Cognitive Functioning 223
      10.5.1   Insomnia 224
      10.5.2   Hypersomnias (EDS) 226
           10.5.2.1   Sleep Apnea Syndrome 227
           10.5.2.2   Narcolepsy–Cataplexy Syndrome 229
10.6   Sleep Disorders and Affective Disorders 231
10.7   Conclusions 233
References 234

10.1   INTRODUCTION

Various sleep disorders, in particular, insomnia, sleep breathing disorders and sleep apnea, periodic limb movements, and phase advance of the sleep–wake cycle are frequent during the aging process. On the other hand, certain neurological illnesses, which are very prevalent in elderly people, such as Alzheimer's and Parkinson's disease, often provoke sleep disturbances. The subjective complaints of low-quality sleep of elderly subjects usually involve both daytime and nocturnal symptoms and are associated with affective disorders and cognitive deficits. Sleep is so intimately related to cognitive function that sleep disturbances affect both cognitive performance and the emotional state during the waking state. By the same token, emotional problems can cause sleep disturbances.

In this chapter the physiological changes found with age in sleep and cognition are reviewed. Also analyzed are the effects of the most frequent primary sleep disturbances, such as insomnia and daytime sleepiness, on the neuropsychological functioning of elderly people.

10.2   PHYSIOLOGICAL CHANGES IN SLEEP DUE TO AGING

Age may be the factor that has the greatest influence on the physiology and physiopathology of sleep and, as occurs in other organic and psychophysiological functions, some changes that affect both its amount and quality become evident in the sleep of elderly people. These changes can result from a predetermined involutive and individualized biological program or be due to the aging of the neural structures that regulate sleep. It has been demonstrated that there is neuronal loss with aging in the brain; however, this loss is not uniform but rather affects the frontal and temporal areas more than the parietal, brain stem, and cerebellum regions.[1] This loss produces functional deficits that are not always relevant from the clinical point of view, which would explain the lack of significant alterations in some elderly people.

In regard to sleep, some changes occur during aging that principally alter the cerebral bioelectric activity, the sleep architecture (phases and cycles that make it up), and its circadian rhythm.

10.2.1 Cerebral Bioelectric Activity Variations

With aging, progressive desynchronization, decrease in amplitude, and fragmentation of the cerebral rhythms are observed in the electroencephalographic (EEG)
recording. The temporal distribution of rapid-eye-movement (REM) sleep within the
nocturnal sleep, but not its amount, is modified, and a significant decrease in some
of its phasic events (rapid eye movements, twitches) is observed. Similarly, there is
a decrease in the amount of EEG phasic phenomena (sleep spindles, K-complexes,
and vertex sharp transients) in the non-REM (NREM) sleep,[2] which comprises stages
1, 2, 3, and 4. The amplitude and duration of the spindles (sinusoidal waves at 12
to 14 Hz, which are characteristic of stage 2) decrease in elderly people, whereas
their mean frequency continues to be similar to that of younger adults.[3] The global
decrease in the amplitude of the bioelectric activity also leads to a decrease in the
number of delta waves with a voltage >70 μV and, consequently, in the amount of
deep NREM sleep (stages 3 and 4 or delta sleep). This is more accentuated in males
than in females and has been related to the progressive increase in brain ventricle
size during aging, an increase that occurs in greater proportion in males.

10.2.2 Changes in Sleep Stages and Cycles

Even though the elderly people spend many hours in bed, their nocturnal sleep is
shorter and less consolidated than that of younger adults.[4] Delta sleep is the first to
be affected: the amount of stage 4 sleep decreases after 40 years of age and can
even disappear after 70 years of age.[5] This decrease in the amount of the deep NREM
sleep results in a shorter duration of the first sleep cycle (the regular alternation
between NREM and REM sleep every 90 min during nocturnal sleep), together with
a shortening of the latency of the first REM period. Although the proportion of REM
sleep in the total sleep time is not significantly reduced, its distribution changes
during the night. The durations of the different REM periods become equivalent,
thus masking the difference between the first half of the night, in which delta sleep
normally predominates, and the second half, in which REM sleep and the lighter
NREM sleep (stage 2) prevail. There are also more stage shifts or rapid stage changes
during sleep.

Sleep onset latency is usually normal in old age. Sleep fragmentation and
disruption of sleep stages due to the increase in both number and duration of
nocturnal awakenings, which can occupy from 12 to 25% of the sleep period, are
characteristic of elderly people.[6] This could be one of the reasons why elderly people
spend more hours in bed to obtain the necessary amount of sleep. Furthermore, with
aging, the arousal threshold decreases while difficulty falling back to sleep increases.

10.2.3 Sleep–Wake Circadian Rhythm Modifications

Changes in sleep, which are observed in most elderly people, suggest that the
circadian timing regulation is altered. It is possible that the biphasic sleep–wake
cycle tends to acquire a polyphasic rhythm and that an advanced sleep phase is

produced. The studies dedicated to investigating this question are recent and have not yet reached a final conclusion (for review, see Reference 7).

Under normal conditions (light–dark daily cycle), there is a reduction in the sleep–wake rhythm amplitude in elderly people, which could explain the frequent nocturnal awakenings they experience. The studies carried out in experimental conditions (temporal isolation, constant routine, etc.), in which the *Zeitgebers* (time cues or synchronizers) are suppressed and then the free-running rhythms are manifested, have shown that an internal desynchronization between the sleep–wake rhythm and the body temperature rhythm (which under normal conditions are closely synchronized) is produced in a high percentage of elderly people. These studies indicate that there is a phase advance of the temperature rhythm and that its duration is shorter; nevertheless, the sleep–wake cycle period is still normal. The early morning awakening would be related with the phase advance of the temperature rhythm, while the increase in nocturnal awakenings would be partially due to the lower amplitude of this rhythm.[8] In elderly people, synchronization between the melatonin and cortisol rhythms, hormones whose release is related to sleep, is also altered. Besides shortening the cortisol rhythm, the limited exposure to daylight, which influences the release of melatonin, can worsen the desynchronization of the sleep–wake rhythm.

Although existing data indicate that there are important changes in the circadian system with aging, these, by themselves, do not justify that the modification of the biological rhythms is the cause of the tendency observed in elderly people for an advanced sleep phase. In this sense, it has been suggested that social and environmental factors, together with physical limitations, increase leisure time and boredom, which generally lead to an earlier bedtime. In experiments carried out in young adults, the phase of the temperature rhythm was advanced by exposure to intense light in the morning to reproduce the alterations described in elderly people. Sleep abnormalities similar to those that usually occur in elderly people, but whose intensity was different, were recorded, which suggests that other factors exist.

10.3 SLEEP DISORDERS IN ELDERLY PEOPLE

Sleep alterations are frequent in aged adults. It has been estimated that half the individuals over 65 years of age who live in their own homes and 60% of those who live in social institutions suffer some sleep disorder.[9] Difficulties initiating and/or maintaining sleep and daytime somnolence are more frequent complaints in elderly subjects than in other age groups.[10,11] It is significant that some studies have found a relationship between the sleep alterations and a greater risk of death, above all in elderly males,[12] although this finding has not been confirmed by other studies.

Sleep alterations are much less frequent in healthy elderly individuals who have no relevant psychiatric or physical disorders. Because of this, there is a certain controversy regarding whether the low-quality sleep and daytime somnolence that elderly people complain of is due to the effects of aging itself or are secondary to illnesses associated with aging.[13] A recent study comparing the self-reported sleeping patterns and degree of sleepiness (estimated by sleepiness scales) of young adults with those of healthy elderly subjects found that the quality of sleep of the latter did not differ significantly from that of the younger subjects.[14] Other studies point out that subjective sleep complaints, confirmed by polysomnographic recordings, of healthy subjects over age 60 include an increase in the number as well as the duration of nocturnal awakenings. Other complaints include difficulties in going back to sleep, especially in the second part of the nocturnal sleep period, and a lowering of the awakening threshold. This indicates that even healthy elderly people experience sleep disturbances when compared with young subjects, as well as a lower degree of efficiency.

There have recently been reports of age-related differences in the sleep stage from which spontaneous awakenings occur: elderly people, in contrast to young adults, do not ordinarily awaken from REM sleep, especially when their sleep has been interrupted often by periods of wakefulness. The authors of the study attribute this to differences in the quality of the period of sleep preceding the final awakening. They suggest that the difficulties in maintaining sleep in old age facilitate the transition from sleep to the waking state from any phase of sleep.[15]

In accordance with the *International Classification of Sleep Disorders* (ICSD),[16] the following sections distinguish among dyssomnias, parasomnias, and sleep disorders associated with medical or psychiatric diseases. Of the different disorders, specific mention is given to those that are most prominent in elderly people.

10.3.1 Dyssomnias

Dyssomnias are disorders characterized either by difficulties in the onset or maintenance of sleep (insomnias) or by excessive daytime sleepiness (EDS) (hypersomnias).

10.3.1.1 Initiating or Maintaining Sleep Difficulties (Insomnias)

Problems of insomnia are very frequent in elderly people. In addition to nocturnal problems (poor and nonrestorative sleep and/or lack of capacity to remain asleep), insomnia also entails the difficulty of satisfactorily carrying out common daytime tasks. This is the most common disorder in the elderly subjects, not so much as a primary sleep alteration but rather as a disorder secondary to other factors. In fact, when the latter are eliminated, the greater prevalence of primary insomnia in this age group tends to disappear.[17] The prevalence of transient insomnia also increases with age, although not as significantly as chronic insomnia.[11] Elderly women complain more about sleeping difficulties than elderly men.[18] The most frequent complaint about insomnia is difficulty maintaining nocturnal sleep.[13] There is a correlation between complaints of insomnia in elderly people and their subjective perception of their state of health, degree of anxiety, and the amount of medication taken. Elderly people who visit the doctor more frequently and who take more drugs complain the most of insomnia.

It is possible to distinguish between insomnia originated by intrinsic alterations and that caused by extrinsic factors. Psychophysiological insomnia, produced by an excessive arousal state, is an intrinsic alteration. This state is incompatible with sleep and is generally accompanied by inadequate behaviors, erroneous beliefs, and false expectations in regard to sleep, due to a nonadaptive learning. In clinical practice, it is diagnosed by exclusion, after verifying that it is not due to medical or psychiatric causes, to drug effects, or to other sleep-specific disorders. Another intrinsic alteration is the sensation of insufficient or unsatisfying sleep, a very frequent complaint in elderly people that is not justified by any objective sleep abnormality.

There are also certain extrinsic factors that can give rise to insomnia problems; a few principal ones are as follows:

- Inadequate sleep hygiene (habits and style of life that are detrimental to sleep);
- Consumption of hypnotic drugs;
- Consumption of stimulants (drugs and substances) and alcohol intake.

These factors are analyzed in greater detail below.

Elderly people frequently develop habits inconducive to sleep, which lead to deficient sleep hygiene. For example, going to bed and getting up at irregular hours, remaining in bed for a long time without sleeping, taking daytime naps, etc. are behaviors that make it difficult to fall to sleep at night. It must also be considered that elderly people are very vulnerable to any change in the environment in which they usually sleep (room, bed, noises, temperature, etc.), changes that can significantly alter their sleep.

The high usage of medication by elderly people is a known fact.[19] A determining criterion in prescribing a drug, besides its specific therapeutic effect, is its possible side effects. Among these, the influence of the drug on sleep, especially when the drugs are nonpsychotropic, is not generally considered.

In general, there are three types of alterations observed in sleep: insomnia, parasomnias, and excessive daytime somnolence. Insomnia can be produced by a central stimulant effect, by a decrease in the amounts of REM sleep and of the deep NREM sleep within nocturnal sleep, and by an increase in nocturnal awakenings (and, consequently, in light NREM sleep). The parasomnias are related to an alteration of either the REM or the NREM sleep, and the daytime somnolence can be due to a direct hypnotic action or be secondary to insomnia provoked by stimulant substances.

It is well known that psychotropic drugs modify the sleep architecture. Their consumption has been widely documented and, in spite of the different methods used for the different studies, it is agreed that this consumption is greater in women, that it increases with age, and that there is a close relationship between the existence of depressive symptoms and sleep alterations.[20]

Hypnotics stand out among the principal types of drugs that produce adverse reactions in elderly people, and their common use is related to a deterioration of the quality of life.[21] In the United States, 25 million prescriptions are written for hypnotic agents, 40% of which are used by elderly people.[22] In Spain, 58% of those who take hypnotics are elderly and, as has been verified in other countries, they do not correctly follow the usage recommendations since intermediate-acting and long-acting agents are inadequately used and the doses that are indicated for adults and for elderly adults are not differentiated.[23,24]

Regarding nonpsychotropic drugs, cardiovascular, antineoplastic, asthma, and antiparkinsonian agents are used to great extent by older subjects.

Some of the most frequent adverse effects of antihypertensive agents are sleep disturbances, such as insomnia, nightmares, and hypnagogic hallucinations, disorders that affect the REM sleep.[25] The effect on sleep exerted by the ß-blockers depends on the liposolubility of the substances, although it has been suggested that their interaction with some neurotransmitters, such as serotonin, also plays a prominent role.[26] These effects are not very intense when therapeutic doses are administered and vary from one substance to another, with the effect on sleep the greatest with pindolol and propanolol.[27]

Very few antineoplastic drugs have been reported as a cause of sleep alterations. The study of the influence of this type of medication on sleep has been limited, but many of them produce gastrointestinal adverse effects, depression, and muscular and osteoarticular pain; which disturb the sleep quality secondarily.[28] To this question, investigation of antineoplastic chronotherapy is very interesting, given the interaction that exists between sleep and the immune system and considering that the adverse effects of chemotherapy decrease (without decreasing its efficacy) when it is administered in hours related to the sleep period.[29]

Regarding asthma medications, their effect on sleep is complex since, on the one hand, the patient's sleep can be benefited when respiratory symptoms are improved, but, on the other hand, most of these drugs have a direct action on sleep, some affecting it and others improving it. Exacerbation of nocturnal asthma can be due to several factors: supine posture, circadian variation of the plasma levels of epinephrine, histamine, and cortisol, and gastroesophageal reflux; even REM sleep can favor the appearance of an episode.[30] Theophylline induces gastroesophageal reflux.[31] Contradictory data are found on its effect on sleep: it seems to affect sleep in patients with asthma;[32,33] however, in healthy subjects, some studies have found that it has no influence on sleep[34] and others that it does have an influence on it.[35] In contrast to theophylline, salmeterol (a ß$_2$-adrenergic agent) clearly improves the quality of sleep in these patients.[36]

Regularly the antiparkinsonian drugs, the involvement of L-dopa and the dopaminergic agonists in the fragmentation of sleep is controversial since its administration improves the continuity of sleep, especially when administered at low doses,[37,38] while high doses and continued use fragment sleep.[39] Selegiline is an MAO-B inhibitor that does not exert intense adverse effects on sleep; in fact, these are more significant in healthy patients than in patients with Parkinson's disease.[40,41] The anticholinergic drugs can also alter the sleep structure, reducing the amount of REM sleep and increasing the deep NREM sleep.[42]

Finally, drinking coffee, tea, or other drinks with a stimulating effect that contain caffeine or other methylxanthines also interferes with sleep continuity and quality. Alcohol, although it facilitates induction of sleep, affects its continuity (above all in the second half of the night because it decreases REM sleep) and does not increase the total amount of sleep. In addition, it worsens the respiratory alterations associated with sleep, as it increases the atonia of the upper respiratory airways.

10.3.1.2 Excessive Daytime Sleepiness Disorders (Hypersomnias)

Idiopathic hypersomnias or excessive daytime sleepiness disorders (EDS) are usually manifested in the adolescent or middle-aged period of life and, although they can persist for a long time, they are not generally one of the reasons leading to a medical visit by aged people. In this stage of life, the most frequent hypersomnias are the secondary ones, whether of organic or psychogenic cause. The most prevalent organic hypersomnias in elderly people are those associated with sleep apnea syndrome (SAS) and to periodic leg movements syndrome (PLMS). The latter can also provoke severe insomnia.

SAS. SAS is very frequent in elderly people, both in men and in women.[43,44] However, its clinical significance is still being discussed. Several studies have manifested that "normal" elderly subjects have more respiratory abnormalities during sleep than middle-aged control subjects. One of these studies analyzed the diagnostic criterion of SAS as an apnea index (number of apneas + hypopneas/hour of sleep) (AHI) ≥ 5 and found that 12.1% of subjects 70 years old and 18.9% of the 80-year-old subjects fulfilled it.[45] In another study, it was found that the SAS prevalence in an large sample of the elderly population was 24% and that 62% of the sample had an AHI ≥ 10.[46] Contrary to most of the existing data, some authors have reported that there does not appear to be any significant cognitive impairment in these subjects, in spite of their increase in daytime somnolence, and that even the cardiovascular morbidity in the SAS is debatable.[47] Thus, the exact clinical meaning of SAS in elderly people, in which an AHI ≥ 10 can be within the "normality" limits, is questioned. On the other hand, although the SAS provokes EDS, it has been observed that between 0 to 20% of the patients with insomnia fulfill the SAS criteria, although without clinical significance, and that the determinant factors of SAS are age, obesity, and masculine sex.[48,49]

PLMS. PLMS is a neuromuscular dysfunction whose incidence and severity increase with age, rising in each decade of life, in particular after age 40.[50] It is estimated that its prevalence is 5% in normal subjects between 30 and 50 years of age, 29% between 50 and 65 years, and 44% after 65 years of age.[51,52] It is frequently associated with SAS in the aged population.[53] The syndrome consists of muscular contractions of the lower limbs with dorsiflexion of the big toe or the entire limb, and there can also be flexion of the knee and the hip. It has been related with several organic diseases, such as uremia, diabetes mellitus, myelopathies, peripheral neuropathies, rheumatoid arthritis, and fibromyositis; however, the etiology of PLMS is still unknown. The limb movements are periodic and preferentially occur during NREM sleep. They may or may not be accompanied by EEG arousals, which suggests the possibility that the same generator emits dual asynchronic stimuli, ascendant for the arousal system and descendent for motor control.[54] An index ≥ 10 of periodic leg movements with arousal per hour of sleep is considered pathological. This syndrome can be the cause of severe insomnia, especially when the movements disrupt sleep so that it is not very restorative; however, if the patient is not aware of the partial awakenings produced by the movements and the disorder is chronic, the presenting symptom can be diurnal somnolence.[55] The fact that the incidence of the disorder is not greater in patients with insomnia than in normal subjects makes its etiological role in insomnia questionable.[56] In a study of patients with PLMS, those who suffered insomnia had more prolonged awakenings and fewer bursts of movements than did the EDS subjects, who, in turn, presented a greater number of arousals.[56] However, in another study in a group of elderly people with PLMS who lived in social institutions, it was not possible to predict the type of symptom (insomnia or hypersomnia) presented by the patients based on the polysomnographic findings.[57]

10.3.1.3 Circadian Rhythm Sleep Disorders

Age is a key factor in adaptation to changes in the sleep schedule. After 50 years of age, the individual's tolerance of and adaptive capacity to time changes decrease. The reduction in the amplitude and length of the sleep–wake rhythm, as well as the tendency to advanced body temperature rhythm in old age, is involved in these alterations. This sleep disturbance becomes clear in transmeridian flights, where it has been observed that elderly people have less sleep efficiency and greater decrease in the degree of daytime alertness than younger adults. Furthermore, it has been observed that night-shift workers have a greater tendency toward an advanced sleep phase and growing reductions in amplitude of the temperature and of melatonin rhythms with aging, which is reflected in a decreased capacity to sleep after a night of work. Consequently, they have less ability to handle working with rotating shifts, which, in the long term, produces significant sleep problems accompanied by organic disorders, mostly gastrointestinal problems (for review, see Reference 7).

As has been previously mentioned, during aging there is a tendency to an advanced sleep phase as well as to a disruption of the temporal organization of the sleep–wake cycle, with intrusion of wake in sleep, and vice versa. When these circadian alterations are intense, they can produce an irregular pattern in the sleep–wake cycle.

With regard to the effect on sleep of the shiftwork experience, a recent report points out that subjects who currently work shifts as well as those who have worked shifts in the past claim to experience more trouble getting to sleep and with early awakening than individuals who have worked during normal hours.[58] Contrary to the hypothesis that having at some time worked shifts permanently alters sleep, in this study no defined effect of the duration or the recentness of the experience was found on sleep. It was, however, observed that women, especially older women, related more sleep problems to changes in work shifts than did men. The bulk of the research carried out in this regard coincides in that difficulties in initiating and/or maintaining sleep are closely associated with aging and the use of hypnotics but that work schedules have little influence on these difficulties. Even retirement, which allows for a more adaptive sleep–wake schedule, does not lead to a decrease in difficulties in falling to sleep nor does it reduce the use of hypnotics.

10.3.2 Parasomnias

Of the parasomnias associated with the NREM sleep, the arousal disorders (confusional arousals, sleepwalking, and sleep terrors) are characteristic of childhood and rarely occur in younger adults and elderly people. In old age, sleepwalking is usually manifested as "nocturnal wandering" and is generally due to an organic syndrome. A differential diagnosis is necessary to distinguish it from nocturnal delirium, which is described further on.

With respect to the parasomnias associated with REM sleep, nightmares are usually due to psychopathological causes, although they can also be produced by certain drugs, such as antihypertensive agents, neuroleptics, tricyclic antidepressants and benzodiazepines, which are frequently used in elderly people.

REM behavior disorder (RBD), or REM sleep without atonia, is one of the few parasomnias that occur preferentially in aged persons. It consists of increased activity of the different skeletal muscles in varying intensity, which is manifested by screaming, hand waving, kicking, wandering, and aggressive behavior. It is generally related to a dream setting whose content is threatening and violent, and can produce injuries to the patient and/or to his or her bed-partner. The objective data that make it possible to diagnose this problem are absence of muscle atonia as well as increase of phasic muscular activity in REM sleep. The physiopathology of RBD is not well known. In 1965, Jouvet carried out the first experimental observation in cats; he produced selective bilateral lesions in the pontomesencephalic area in the cats and observed that an absence of muscle atonia was produced during REM sleep. However, the different degrees of intensity of locomotor behavior observed in this syndrome suggest that other brain structures that participate in the motor control are affected and that there is probably an excess of activity in the brain stem locomotor centers.[58]

RBD is rarely seen in clinical practice, although it is possible that some cases have been confused with other sleep behavior disorders when diagnosed. In fact, age is a predisposing factor and the disorder is much more frequent in men than in women. The acute cases have a metabolic origin: intake of tricyclic antidepressants and selective serotonin uptake inhibitors, alcohol abstinence syndrome, etc. About half of the chronic cases are associated with degenerative neurological diseases and the other half are idiopathic. The neurological diseases that are generally associated with this syndrome are basically degenerative. Among these, Parkinson's disease stands out: it has been suggested that RBD could be a previous manifestation of the development of this disease.[58] In a series of 11 patients with Parkinson's disease and with clinical symptoms of RBD studied in the authors' laboratory, all had developed the syndrome some time after the onset of Parkinson's disease.[59]

10.3.3 Sleep Disorders Associated with Psychiatric and Medical Diseases

10.3.3.1 Sleep Disorders Associated with Psychiatric Alterations

With regard to psychiatric alterations, affective disorders have a high prevalence in elderly people. Their importance as an etiological factor of insomnia is generally

underestimated since the accumulation of frustrating experiences as well as organic problems in the aged individual can produce insomnia as a consequence of an emotional and depressive disturbance.[44,60] Several polysomnographic abnormalities, such as a decrease in sleep continuity and efficiency, a reduction in deep NREM sleep in the first sleep cycle, and, in particular, shortening of REM latency and increase of the total REM sleep time, have been described in subjects who presented major depressive episodes. These abnormalities are more frequent in elderly people than in young adults and adolescents.[61] On the other hand, it is known that anxiety disorders affect sleep continuity, and it must be kept in mind that fear of dying while asleep is frequently manifested in elderly people.[62]

10.3.3.2 Sleep Disorders Associated with Organic Diseases

Many organic diseases can lead to deterioration of sleep quality, either because they produce symptoms that, by themselves, wake the patient up and make sleeping difficult or because they are neurological diseases that affect (due to any pathogenic mechanism) the central nervous system (CNS) structures responsible for regulating sleep and wakefulness. In the first case and regardless of the causal disease, the factors that disturb sleep are pruritus, respiratory disorders, nocturia, abnormal motor activity, immobility, and, above all, pain of any type. Special emphasis should be given to headaches, some of which generally occur during the night and are related to REM sleep. Recently, a variety of headaches characteristic of elderly people, called "hypnic headache," has been described. This is rare and consists of short, recurrent episodes, whose duration ranges from 5 to 60 min, that wake the patient up with a diffuse and throbbing type of pain that generally always occurs at the same time (between 1 and 3 A.M.), several times a week, and is linked with REM sleep.[63,64]

10.3.3.3 Sleep Disorders Associated with Neurological Diseases

Concerning the neurological diseases, several CNS degenerative disorders with a limited prevalence and especially, Parkinson's disease and dementia, stand out in the elderly population.

Parkinson's Disease. In Parkinson's disease, sleep alterations such as onset difficulties, fragmentation, early morning awakening, and parasomnias are frequently observed. These symptoms have been verified by polysomnographic studies that have shown a prolonged sleep latency, numerous nocturnal awakenings (which increase the amount of wakefulness during the sleep period up to 30 to 40% of the total sleep recording time), and an increase in light NREM sleep together with a reduction in deep NREM and REM sleep. The etiology for these abnormalities is complex. They are partially due to an degenerative process that affects the neurophysiological and neurochemical systems involved in sleep regulation, and partially to aging and dementia processes.[39] The effects of dopaminergic drugs used in treatment[65] as well as the discomfort produced by the motor disorders and joint pains characteristic of Parkinson's disease[37] must be added to this.

On the other hand, the parasomnias presented by those patients in which the disease is sufficiently developed and who have been treated for a long time with L-dopa are attributed to a dopaminergic hyperactivity phenomenon[66] and could be one of the early symptoms of drug-induced psychosis. In a series of patients with Parkinson's studied in the authors' sleep unit, 67% perceived their sleep as altered vs. 35% in the control group. That study found that the factors that determined the changes in sleep habits and the appearance of the sleep alterations were years of evolution of the disease and its stage, and that sleep fragmentation, decrease in the total time of nocturnal sleep, and parasomnias were the most frequent disorders.[67]

Dementia.   The dementias represent a significant health problem, given the demographic profile of society. It has been estimated that 10% of the aged population suffers a clinically significant cognitive impairment[68] and that more than half of the subjects affected suffer Alzheimer's disease (AD).[69] Sleep is generally altered in the dementias. These alterations have been studied especially in AD, in which alterations similar to, although more intense than, the changes associated with aging in healthy control subjects of an equivalent age have been observed.[70] The sleep disturbances become worse during the course of the disease and, in general, consist of a disorganization of the sleep–wake rhythm, with reciprocal intrusions between both states and an increase in nocturnal awakenings, which produces EDS. Sleep behavior disorders that vary from simple psychomotor restlessness to agitation episodes and wandering and even delirium are also very frequent (20 to 50% of cases).[44] In regard to the polysomnographic abnormalities, given the slowing observed in the EEG recordings of some patients, difficulties can occur when trying to differentiate the different sleep stages and even to distinguish wake from sleep. An increase of arousals and stage 1 of NREM sleep together with a decrease in stages 3 and 4 of NREM sleep and of the REM sleep have been reported. In addition, there is an elevated incidence of such disorders as SAS and nocturnal myoclonus in these patients (for review, see Reference 44).

Nocturnal agitation, or delirium, is a frequent problem that patients with dementia can present during the nocturnal period or at nightfall. When the onset of this agitation is sudden, it is generally provoked by variations in the environmental conditions (changes in the bedroom, admission to an institution, etc.) although it can be produced by other causes such as infection (especially urinary), myocardial infarct, pulmonary thromboembolism, electrolytic alterations, and anticholinergic drugs. Recurrent nocturnal agitation is observed more frequently in elderly people with AD and can be precipitated by factors such as chronic pain, nocturnal enuresis, noises or voices of nearby persons, inadequate bedtime due to remaining in bed for a long time without sleeping, fear of the dark, etc.

The sundowning syndrome, or acute confusional state, is similar to that of nocturnal agitation, but occurs at nightfall, both before and after dinner. The changes in the sleep–wake circadian rhythm observed in many of the patients with dementia or with depression significantly influence its occurrence. Its origin seems to be related to postprandial changes in blood pressure or to cerebral oxygenation or glucose level deficits. Certain environmental factors (e.g., sensorial deprivation, inadequate lighting) or emotional factors (aggressiveness due to a delayed dinner time) can also contribute to its precipitation.[71]

10.4 CHANGES IN COGNITIVE FUNCTIONING WITH NORMAL AGING

10.4.1 COGNITIVE PERFORMANCE PATTERN

Normal aging is accompanied by slow and continuous changes in most cognitive functions. These changes are obviously related to the underlying changes in cerebral structure and function. Nonetheless, all cerebral systems are not equally sensitive to aging. Each type of behavior involves different cerebral systems, some clearly delimited and restricted to certain brain areas whereas others involve diverse regions of the brain. Consequently, cognitive functions vary in their degree of stability or decline through the aging process. The pattern of cognitive deficits common to aging (as shown in Table 10.1) is characterized by a slowing of different aspects of behavior. This is chiefly due to slower cognitive processing and in part to an increase in response time, and especially affects the performance of complex tasks.

TABLE 10.1
Main Cognitive Deficits in Normal Aging

Slowed mental processing and response speed
Alteration of complex attentional processes with disturbances of divided attention, sustained attention, and concentration
Decrease of learning and memory abilities, mainly of short-term and long-term memory and of visual memory
Progressive impairment of executive functions and of mental and behavioral flexibility

These cognitive deficits consist mainly of the following (for review, see References 73 through 75):

- *Decrease of attentional functions.* Particularly affected is divided attention, the capacity to manage various elements of a complex task simultaneously. Sustained attention (vigilance) and concentration are also diminished, while distractibility increases.
- *Alteration of certain learning and memory processes.* Aging affects different aspects of learning and memory in different ways, depending on the complexity of the information processing required by the given task. Performance in tasks involving difficult processes such as categorization, organization, and data association is decreased while performance remains stable in simple tasks, well-learned or automatic responses. Short-term memory starts to diminish sometime between 30 and 50 years of age, especially when complex cognitive processing is

required. The same occurs with the ability to store information, the visual memory, and the long-term memory. However, immediate memory of simple information and remote memory (knowledge acquired in early stages of life) remain stable.

- *Progressive impairment of abstract thinking abilities, concept formation, and mental and behavioral flexibility.* This impairment starts around age 60 and becomes more marked at 70 to 80 years of age. Generally, this is indicative of an alteration of the so-called executive functions (discussed below). Symptoms are similar to those of frontal dysfunction (perseveration of inappropriate responses, attention/concentration deficits, loss of immediate memory, and so forth), which become more severe during the last decades of life.

As can be observed in Table 10.2, certain cognitive functions are affected with aging whereas other remain relatively unchanged as the years pass. This has been verified by applying diverse neuropsychological tests that evaluate different verbal functions and varied aspects of motor performance, such as the classic Wechsler Intelligence Scale for Adults (WAIS). Other tests, such as the Wechsler Memory Scale—Revised and the Rey Auditory–Verbal Learning Test, which specifically evaluate memory processes, and the Wisconsin Card Sorting Test, the Stroop Test, and the Trail Making Test, which assess abstract reasoning abilities and frontal functions, have been likewise utilized.

TABLE 10.2
Aging Effects on Cognitive Functions

Impaired Cognitive Functions	Preserved Cognitive Functions
Visuospatial and constructional skills	Verbal skills
Capacity to retain new information	Early learnings
Short-term and long-term memory	Remote memory
Visual perception	
Motor performance	
Visuomotor coordination	
Perceptual organization	
Span and speed of information processing	
Motor performance	
Mental and behavioral flexibility	

The selective decline of certain functions beginning around 55 to 60 years of age can be seen on the WAIS as an increase in the difference normally found between the Verbal and Performance Intelligence Quotients (VIQ and PIQ) in middle-high sociocultural subjects (for review, see Reference 76). As age progresses throughout adulthood, there is a considerable decrease in visuoperceptual, visuospatial, and visuomotor coordination skills, functions that are predominately mediated by the right hemisphere. In contrast, most verbal skills (which depend predominantly on the left hemisphere, particularly verbal fluency) remain stable up to very advanced ages. As will be explained later, this led to formulation of the hypothesis that the right hemisphere "ages" earlier than the left. With regard to the cerebral asymmetry in cognitive processing, hemispheric specialization in verbal and visuospatial functions do not change with age.[77,78]

Aside from the variable changes produced in the different cognitive functions with age, the global cognitive performance of healthy elderly people is generally within the normal range until 80 years of age.[79]

To better understand this set of cognitive changes, the now classic distinction between "fluid" intelligence (the ability to confront a new situation) and "crystallized" intelligence (skills learned in early stages of development) can prove to be useful. The first is more vulnerable to the effects of aging than the second. Crystallized intelligence remains operative until the decade of 70 to 80 years, whereas functions requiring fluid intelligence begin to decline between 50 and 70 years of age, after which there is a sharper decline.[77]

In short, these changes indicate that there are two types of cognitive decline with age, depending on the type of function under consideration. The decrease in cognitive performance affects mainly the capacity to process, store, and retrieve new information, especially when this information is complex, and also the response speed (comprising functions requiring a relatively high degree of cerebral activation). Meanwhile, functions based on old information and well-established learning are conserved.

The decline of cerebral function in old age affects 55% of healthy individuals over age 60 and markedly impairs their quality of life.[73] Nonetheless, there is a wide intersubject variability with regard to the age at which symptoms manifest, as well as to the intensity of the symptoms. Cognitive performance in the last decades of life therefore greatly varies from one person to the next. For example, although learning and memory abilities tend to diminish through the course of normal aging, many individuals at an advanced age suffer very little loss of memory (for review, see Reference 80). These individual differences have led to questioning of the idea that normal aging is inevitably accompanied by significant cognitive impairment.[81]

The difference between the patterns of "normal aging" and "successful aging,"[82] as well as the concept of age-associated memory impairment (see References 83 and 84 for diagnostic criteria and Reference 85 for review) are of interest both to clinicians and researchers in the field of gerontology. Successful aging can be defined as that in which organic and cognitive functions are maintained at a level comparable with that of younger adults. Interindividual variability in the manner of aging is influenced by such factors as genetic inheritance, educational level, and the degree of each individual's physical and mental activity.

With regard to the differences between normal and pathological aging, since Kral, in the 1960s, proposed to distinguish between the "benign" and the "malignant" ways to age, various diagnostic categories have been developed. These are used to define cognitive deficits, especially in memory, of elderly people who, in spite of their impairments, do not meet the diagnostic criteria for dementia. These nosological categories include Age Associated Memory Impairment (AAMI), Mild Cognitive Impairment (MCI), Aging Associated Cognitive Decline (AACD), Mild Cognitive

Disorder (MCD), Age Related Cognitive Decline (ARCD), and Cognitively Impaired, Not Demented (CIND).

AAMI is one of the best defined and validated categories. It includes people over 50 years of age who do not suffer psychiatric, neurological, or medical problems but who present a significant age-related loss of memory that affects their daily life. The prevalence of AAMI has been estimated at 39% of the adult population between the ages of 50 and 59, rising to 85% in the over-85 group.[86] It seems to be more frequent in individuals with affective disorders from low sociocultural levels, both variables that have an influence on reduced memory performance.[87] Although the neurocognitive alterations of AAMI refer primarily to memory, they also involve impairment of other cognitive functions, in particular frontal functions.[88] It has even been suggested that, more than a pathology characteristic to normal aging, AAMI is a monosymptomatic stage that evolves toward AD.[89] As yet, there are no conclusive data concerning the evolution of this disorder, although several longitudinal studies have found it to be a stable set of symptoms that does not progress toward the cognitive deterioration characteristic of the dementias.[90,91]

According to the updated review of the nosology of cognitive disturbances in normal aging,[92] current research indicates that, although several of the aforementioned clinical categories overlap, some of the proposed diagnostic criteria, particularly those of AAMI and ARCD, can help to distinguish whether subjects present a cognitive state nearer to that of normal aging or to that of dementia. On the other hand, subjects who meet criteria of MCI or of MCD seem to be at a high risk of developing a dementia.

In the following section the most relevant cognitive changes associated with aging, those affecting executive function and memory processes, are analyzed.

10.4.1.1 Executive Functions

Executive functions are a group of mental abilities that are essential for the performance and control of purposeful, goal-directed behavior. It is a set of cognitive processes such as distraction-resistant attention directed simultaneously toward various elements, decision making, devising a plan of action, inhibition of automatic responses, sequential organization and performance of responses, verification of achieved results, and, finally, the ability to alter cognitive/behavioral strategies. These functions represent the highest level of cognitive functioning. They are closely related to other mental activity variables (consciousness, activity rate) and cognitive functions, in particular to attention, memory, and language. The difference is that, whereas cognitive functions can be defined as "what" or "how much" is known, executive functions consist of knowing "how" or "when" something is to be done (for review, see Reference 76).

Thus, executive functions are basically integrating functions involving the coordination of various cognitive functions. They constitute a functional entity. For the most part, the prefrontal areas mediate these functions, although they also depend on other cerebral regions. Executive functions should not be confused with frontal functions, although there is a close relationship between the two. Therefore, they can be preserved in the case of a frontal lesion but be affected by lesions in other cerebral regions. Executive function disorders will generally manifest globally, with effects on varied aspects of behavior given that the disorders can interfere with cognitive strategies essential to the planning and performance of tasks. They can similarly cause a deficiency in the control of behavior itself.

A progressive decrement in the executive functions of elderly subjects can be observed[93] and is more marked in patients with AD.[94] Although this cognitive decline undoubtedly reflects an impairment that also affects diverse cognitive functions, especially memory processes, it represents a direct alteration of executive functions.

10.4.1.2 Memory Processes

Memory function is one of the most sensitive to aging and is affected both in normal and pathological aging. Nonetheless, the memory deficits in these two circumstances are different. In normal subjects, there is a slow and progressive loss of memory abilities through the course of adulthood, affecting different types of memory in different ways. In neurophysiological terms, each cerebral system that makes up the "memory networks" is affected to a different degree. A representative example of these types of deficits is the difficulty that elderly people generally confront in acquiring new knowledge, especially when it is complex. Other examples are the difficulties in learning new names or in evoking infrequently used words; in retaining information not relevant to the individual; and, very frequently, in remembering, following a distraction, what it was they were intending to do. Memory problems, whether subjective or objectified through neuropsychological testing, are very frequent in the elderly population.[95]

In normal aging, what is the makeup of these decrements in memory? Light,[96] in a review, highlights four main hypotheses:

1. Failures of "meta-memory" (memory cognitions and self-management of memory ability)
2. Defective semantic encoding
3. Failures of deliberate recollection (access to stored information)
4. Diminished cognitive processing resources

Light concludes that these hypotheses, as a group or separately, are not enough to explain the pattern of preserved and altered memory functions characteristic of aging. Nonetheless, Light points out that most of the data suggest that the specific problem encountered by elderly people is in the retrieval of recently acquired information, particularly when deliberate, not automatic, recollection is required. It remains to be determined what the underlying neurocognitive mechanism to this deficit may be and if, in elderly people, one memory system is selectively affected while other systems are preserved.

Another highly important question, as yet to be resolved in spite of numerous studies, is whether there is a physiopathological *continuum* between the memory loss experienced during adulthood/old age and that of dementia or if they are two different processes.

10.4.2 NEURAL BASIS OF COGNITIVE DYSFUNCTION

10.4.2.1 Cerebral Changes

One of the main objectives of current research on aging is to define the neural basis of cognitive dysfunction with which aging is generally associated. Research proposes to identify structural alterations and, above all, changes in the cerebral function most directly related to the changes in cognitive performance observed in elderly subjects. Moreover, it is essential to distinguish between the cerebral and the consequential behavioral changes characteristic of normal aging and the changes that arise from pathological aging or dementia.

Normal aging is accompanied by marked degenerative cerebral changes affecting both the cerebral cortex and subcortical structures. Affected subcortical structures include the basal ganglia and the intrahemispheric white matter (for review, see Reference 97). This could explain the slowing of responses and cognitive processing observed in elderly people. There are data indicating that with age there is a slowing of reaction time (related to perception and decision-making time and to response performance time) as well as of cognitive processing itself. It could be that this cognitive slowing is related to the degenerative changes observed in the white matter (leukoaraiosis) and in the basal ganglia. Age-associated leukoaraiosis has thereby been related to several of the neurocognitive and affective symptoms present in elderly subjects: decrease of complex cognitive processing speed, reduction of the PIQ, alteration of visual memory and certain motor skills (sequencing, rhythm reproduction, and motor learning), symptoms of frontal dysfunction (inhibited or disinhibited behavior), apathy, lack of behavioral flexibility, and social maladjustment.[98]

As a whole, existing data indicate that the cerebral systems most affected with age are those that mediate executive functions and certain memory processes. These systems are for the most part localized in prefrontal and temporal areas of the brain as well as in other regions of the associative cortex. The results of studies relating data on cerebral metabolism (regional cerebral blood flow, or rCBF, and positron emission tomography, or PET, techniques) to those of the cognitive performance of elderly people are inconsistent. Nonetheless, most of these studies suggest that the degree of activity of the frontotemporal areas progressively decreases with old age. It seems therefore that the associative cortex areas, in charge of controlling the most complex cognitive, emotional, and behavioral aspects, are the most vulnerable to the aging process of the brain.

On the other hand, certain systemic diseases that frequently present in old age (hypertension, diabetes, cerebrovascular pathologies, and so forth) have an effect on cognitive performance. Cardiovascular failure is an important factor influencing the decreased performance on tasks requiring abstract thinking and mental flexibility.[99] By the same token, a poor diet coupled with the metabolic changes that occur in old age can provoke a deficiency in cerebral substances, such as vitamins B_6 and B_{12}, that are essential for correct cognitive functioning.[100]

10.4.2.2   Aging Effects on Cognitive Functioning

Various hypotheses have been formulated to explain the effects of aging on cognitive functioning (for review, see References 73, 76, and 101). The main hypotheses are listed in Table 10.3 and can be analyzed as follows.

TABLE 10.3
Hypotheses of Aging Effects on Cognitive Functioning

Hypothesis	Authors
Main deterioration of right hemisphere, which processes visuospatial information	Klisz, 1978; Schaie and Schaie, 1977
Reduction of available cognitive resources	Craick and Byrd, 1982
Dysfunction of prefrontal areas, which mediate the higher cognitive functions	Hochanadel and Kaplan,1984; Mittenberg et al., 1989
Impairment of cognitive processing system, due either to attentional deficits or to reduced working memory capacity	Hasher and Zacks, 1988
Global slowing of cognitive processing, which affects the majority of cognitive functions, especially complex ones	Salthouse, 1985, Storandt, 1990; Van Gorp et al., 1990
Pattern of cognitive deterioration similar to the subcortical dementias	Van Gorp and Mahler, 1990

One of the first hypotheses suggests that the right hemisphere is more vulnerable to aging than the left.[102,103] This is based on the fact that the reduced performance observed with aging is more severe in tasks that have a visuospatial component, such as manipulative tasks, which are preferentially controlled by the right hemisphere. In evaluating this hypothesis it must be taken into account that it is based on results obtained on intelligence scales such as the WAIS, tests that were not designed to compare the respective functions of each cerebral hemisphere. On the contrary, when using tests that specifically evaluate lateralization of cognitive functions, no selective dysfunction of the right hemisphere has been found. In fact, it seems that the two cerebral hemispheres have a similar rate of decline.[77,104]

Another more general theory proposes that in old age there is a decrease in the amount of available cognitive resources needed for processing information.[80] From this point of view, the cognitive changes associated with aging are not interpreted as an alteration of the specific cerebral systems that mediate each of the cognitive functions, such as memory, learning, and so forth. Rather, these changes are interpreted as a lessening of the availability of intellectual resources. This focus led to the development of the idea of "environmental support," which defends the idea that the decreased efficiency of mental processes is not an inevitable consequence of aging. In keeping with this idea, an adequate environmental context can reduce the limitations on performance encountered by elderly people, at least in tasks that are not overly complicated.

The hypothesis that suggests there is a dysfunction or lower degree of activation of certain areas of the frontal lobe,[77,104] in particular the prefrontal lobes (involved in the control of both executive functions and the higher cognitive functions), seems to be one of the most solid and could explain many of the cognitive changes associated with aging. Favoring this hypothesis are data resulting from PET studies conducted in the 1980s. These point to a more pronounced decrease in cerebral activity in the frontal region and to the similarities in the symptoms observed in elderly subjects and patients with frontal lesions. However, subsequent neuroimaging studies have found that the reduced cerebral blood flow found with age affects the cingulate cortex and the superior temporal parahippocampal region more than the frontal lobe.[105] On the other hand, the kind of cognitive dysfunction associated with aging cannot be sufficiently explained by an exclusive alteration of the prefrontal areas. This is because executive functions cannot be reduced to frontal functions. The role of executive functions is to integrate, which necessitates the coordination of a varied array of cognitive functions.

Focusing on how the brain processes information, Hasher and Zacks[106] suggested that aging alters the cognitive processing system, either through a decrease in attentional capacity or in working memory span, which in turn have repercussions on global cognitive performance. This supposition, corroborated in subsequent research, implies that aging reduces the ability to inhibit automatic responses. The inhibition of automatic responses is essential toward solving new problems and maintaining flexible, adaptive behavior.

One of the theories most strongly supported by current data upholds that the cognitive decline that manifests with aging is due to a general slowing of cognitive processing, affecting most functions and in particular those that are complex.[107–109] This progressive cognitive slowdown could account for a large part of the decrease in cognitive performance of elderly people. Complex cognitive tasks, those that require the integration of diverse types of information, would be the most affected, especially when there is a limited response performance time.

It has been suggested that there is a physiopathological *continuum* between the cognitive changes associated with normal aging and the pattern of cognitive deterioration characteristic of subcortical dementias.[110] It is true that a similarity can be found between the neuropsychological changes observed in normal aging and certain cognitive (difficulties in concentrating, problems in performing two tasks at the same time, decrease of immediate memory, difficulties in remembering information acquired some time in the past, reduced motor learning and behavior planning abilities, loss of flexibility in changing cognitive/behavioral strategies) and motor (slowed motor response, difficulties in initiating movements, rigidity, etc.) deficits characteristic of subcortical dementias. Nonetheless, both patterns seem to be different with regard to their intensity as well as to the development of the symptoms. There are also differential signs distinguishing the two. For example, aging with associated vascular alterations can be distinguished from vascular dementia in that the latter is characterized by disartria, aphasia, apraxia and agnosia, severe cognitive deficits, amnesia, and a decrease in IQ or a marked slowing of mental processes. In spite of this it is as yet to be determined whether these two patterns can be distinguished simply by the degree of the alterations or if they are qualitatively different patterns.

With the currently available data, it is still difficult to integrate the clinical observations of the cognitive/behavioral changes that occur during normal aging with the neurobiological data coming mainly from neuroimaging studies. An acceptable neuropsychological model of the cognitive changes in aging would have to take into account the complexity of the cognitive functions and the specific nature of the alterations that arise. Such a model must assume the possibility that the very complexity of the cognitive functions may allow for a compensation of deficits owing to the still existent neural plasticity in elderly subjects.

The observation that neurocognitive impairment is not an inevitable consequence of aging and that there are marked individual differences with regard both to the age at which it appears and to the intensity of the cognitive deficits have led to the development of preventive measures that would favor successful aging. There are reasons to believe that the neuropsychological decline is in part due to a lack of use of certain abilities as well as to a lack of external stimulation. In this sense, it has been shown that the functions of the CNS in elderly people can be optimized through activation procedures such as physical exercise. Exercise has been found to improve neuropsychological functioning as well as mood and outlook, possibly due to increased oxygenation improving neural function.[111] Certain nonaerobic exercises, such as playing video games, have also been found to improve cognitive performance, supposedly because they cause a more efficient degree of activation of the neural centers stimulated by the visuomotor task.[112]

The principal conclusion stemming from the preceding and other related psychobiological data is that the CNS retains its plasticity in old age and its functioning can therefore be improved with the appropriate stimulation. Appropriate physical activity and intellectual and social activities are aids to successful aging and counteract the effects of aging of the brain.

10.5 SLEEP DISORDERS AND COGNITIVE FUNCTIONING

There exists a close relationship between sleep and cognitive processes that has been documented in recent years by extensive research. One focus is on the study of the effects that age-related sleep disturbances have on cognitive/behavioral functioning when awake. According to a thorough review by Bliwise[113] concerning the correlation between polysomnographic measures and psychometrics in both subjects with dementia and normal subjects over the age of 50, initial studies focused on examining the following:

1. *The relationship between specific polysomnographic variables and cognitive performance.* Although the results of cross-sectional studies conducted during the seventies were inconsistent, most found a limited relationship between the decline in cognitive functioning and alterations in sleep architecture (percentage of REM vs. NREM sleep, nocturnal sleep, sleep efficiency, etc.), until a very advanced age. This agrees with the hypothesis that there is gap in the relationship between neurophysiological and cognitive measures, suggesting that such a relationship

would only appear after exceeding a set threshold of deterioration of the neurobiological substratum. A decrease in cognitive performance (specifically, of the PIQ and the Associative-learning WMS subscale score) associated with a reduced amount of REM sleep in elderly subjects was observed in only one longitudinal study.[114] As a whole, these studies suggest that the polysomnographic variables most closely related to cognitive impairment with aging are the number of nocturnal awakenings and the proportion of phase 1 and of REM sleep in nocturnal sleep. As a result, Bliwise concludes that what affects cognitive performance in elderly people is the general alteration of sleep pattern with age, rather than a decrease in any specific sleep phase.

2. *How sleep-related respiratory disturbances (SRRD) affect cognitive functioning.* The results of this second focus revealed that SSRD are associated with an increase of EDS and a decrease in cognitive performance. Nonetheless, it seems that the association between SRRD and EDS tends to diminish with age, particularly after the age of 65, which supports the idea that sleep apnea and its cognitive effects are more severe in young adults than in older individuals. Elderly people tend to experience specific alterations in their sleep pattern such as an increase in nocturnal awakening and a reduction of both delta sleep and REM sleep (see Section 10.1.2), as well as decreased cognitive performance and a high prevalence of SRRD.[115] In light of this, current research has attempted to determine what the relative contributions of disturbances in sleep patterns (with particular regard to sleep fragmentation), EDS, nocturnal hypoxemia, and aging are to the overall set of neuropsychological alterations (cognitive deficits, affective disorders, and behavioral disorders) observed in elderly people.

Sleep fragmentation in elderly people impairs their cognitive performance.[115-117] Not only the duration of the nocturnal sleep period, but also the continuity of the sleep period, contributes to the restorative function of sleep.[118] When the continuity is repeatedly interrupted, either by means of external (noises, extreme temperatures, etc.) or internal (pain, SRRD or apneas, PLMS, maintenance insomnia, etc.) stimuli, cognitive performance is altered.

The following sections analyze the most frequently found cognitive/emotional effects of primary sleep disorders in elderly people. These include insomnia and the hypersomnias, centering on SAS, a highly prevalent disorder in elderly subjects with serious psychosocial repercussions.

10.5.1 INSOMNIA

Insomnia due to difficulties in maintaining sleep is the most frequent type of insomnia found in old age. It is important to distinguish between prolonged awakenings and intermittent, but brief, awakenings, after which sleep is easily achieved. Intermittent awakenings are characteristic of physiological disturbances (e.g., apneas, periodic limb movements) that interrupt the continuity of sleep, whereas prolonged

awakenings suggest the presence of a circadian rhythm sleep–wake disorder or an affective disorder. Difficulties in maintaining sleep are the most common subjective sleep complaints in elderly people (65% of subjects over 60 years of age).

The fact that insomnia is more prevalent in old age than in younger ages can be accounted for by age-associated physiological changes in sleep as well as by the increased incidence in elderly people of illnesses that provoke insomnia. In addition, anxious-depressive feelings favor the development of insomnia. In elderly people, these can be caused by a stressful life event (retirement, bereavement), fear of dying while sleeping, or psychopathological disturbances. Psychopathological distur-bances are known to play an important role in the development of insomnia, espe-cially in chronic insomnia. In this regard, analysis of the MMPI personality profile of patients with chronic insomnia showed they were characterized by signs of neurotic depression, chronic anxiety, brooding and difficulties in outwardly express-ing negative emotions such as anger.[119] Although middle-aged people with insomnia tend to display a personality profile with elevations in the "neurotic triad" (hypo-chondriasis, depression, and hysteria scales), this has not been observed in elderly people with insomnia.[120] Although these data must be replicated, they suggest that the association between insomnia and psychopathology is weaker in old age. Elderly people with insomnia display fewer psychopathological signals than younger patients. However, a high percentage of them, as well as of elderly women with subjective complaints of "poor" or unsatisfactory sleep, display psychopathological disturbances. It been found that sleep disturbances are associated with depressive mood and anxiety traits in older poor sleepers. On the other hand, it must be taken into account that elderly people with poor sleep may remain bedridden for long periods of time and tend to display feelings of depression and anxiety (for review, see Reference 121).

Holding in or internalizing emotions is one of the most characteristic personality traits in patients with psychophysiological insomnia. This is related to certain affec-tive and personality disorders and has been considered the underlying trait in the psychophysiological mechanisms that initiate and maintain chronic insomnia.[119,122] This hypothesis maintains that holding in emotions leads to a state of emotional arousal, which in turn provokes somatic arousal, which leads to insomnia.

In this same sense, the neurocognitive model of psychophysiological insomnia[123] holds that acute insomnia tends to present in psychologically vulnerable subjects undergoing a stressful event. When these subjects confront these events with inap-propriate strategies (brooding, somatization of stress, excessive worry about the insomnia, increased time in bed), they develop persistent insomnia. Chronic insom-nia stems from cognitive-cortical and somatic hyperarousal resulting from a condi-tioned response to key stimuli (visual or temporal) that are usually associated with sleep (bed, bedroom, bedtime, etc.). This state of hyperarousal provokes a succession of cognitive disturbances that could account for insomnia complaints and the dis-crepancy between the subjective perception and the objective sleep data of patients with insomnia. It has been known for some time that subjective sleep complaints do not tend to coincide with the results of polysomnographic recordings, as a result of either under- or overestimation. Nonetheless, the subjective perception of the quality of sleep is a useful criterion and is ultimately the decisive criterion determining whether sleep is satisfactory or not.

Regarding daytime cognitive functioning in patients with insomnia, these patients tend to complain of sleepiness, concentration difficulties, tiredness upon awakening (while normal subjects tend to feel more tired in the afternoon), and decreased cognitive performance. It is difficult to determine whether these cognitive deficits are due to insufficient sleep, to the effect of medication, or to associated psychiatric or organic disorders. Most studies on nonmedicated patients with insomnia have not found a significant lowering of cognitive performance. A semantic memory deficit (declarative-type memory, such as knowing the meaning of a word) was seen in only one study. On the other hand, both subjective and objective measures of somnolence indicate that patients with insomnia, perhaps partly due to the generally present hyperarousal state, do not display more daytime somnolence than normal subjects (for review, see Reference 124).

Given the importance of emotional, cognitive, and behavioral factors in the development of psychophysiological insomnia, psychological therapies, including behavioral-cognitive technique, are an essential part of treatment. The behavior therapies are oriented toward extinguishing conditioned responses that are incompatible with sleep (cognitive, emotional, and physiological activation), modifying incorrect sleep habits, and reinforcing the association between certain stimuli and the sleep state. These therapies include relaxation, sleep restriction, and stimulus-control techniques. The cognitive treatments for insomnia are focused on modifying cognitive-emotional processes underlying nonadaptive behavior of patients faced with insomnia, aiding the patient in identifying erroneous beliefs and negative attitudes regarding sleep and substituting them with other, more adaptive beliefs. At the same time patients are taught stress management strategies and ways to express their emotions in a more appropriate way, as well as reinforcing their ability to control their own sleep themselves. These cognitive treatments include the cognitive change methods, the self-control procedures, and the paradoxical intention technique (for review, see Reference 125).

The medications traditionally used in the pharmacological treatment of insomnia are hypnotics and anxiolytics (benzodiazepines) to relieve sleep disorder, and anxiolytics, antidepressants, and neuroleptics when an underlying psychiatric disorder is detected, frequently a disthymic disorder. Aside from taking great care when prescribing hypnotic medication for elderly people, the adverse effects of some of these medications on cognitive functioning must be taken into account. Benzodiazepines can produce anterograde amnesia immediately following administration; hypnotic drugs that are quickly eliminated can provoke amnesia the day following their administration; trycyclic antidepressant sedatives and neuroleptic sedatives can cause difficulties in attention and concentration, slowness in thinking, and memory problems (for review, see Reference 124).

10.5.2 Hypersomnias (EDS)

EDS is not a single phenomenon that only varies in intensity in the different hypersomnias. EDS presents in qualitatively different states, based on different physiopathological mechanisms depending upon the etiology of the disorder. These qualitative differences can be established through polysomnographic recording, which determines the sleep latency (Multiple Sleep Latency Test), or by subjective evaluation of the degree of daytime sleepiness, either usually (Epworth Sleepiness Scale) or at the present moment (Stanford Sleepiness Scale). These differences in vigilance are also manifested in cognitive performance.

It is interesting to compare the neuropsychological performance of patients with different EDS disorders in order to determine the effects of sleepiness on cognitive functioning. The results of the authors' research indicates that in different hypersomnias there is a different pattern of neuropsychological disturbances. These seem to be related to the nature of the EDS as well as to other etiological factors of the specific illness. Patients with SAS display more intense cognitive deficits than patients with narcolepsy or those with psychiatric hypersomnia, and, in turn, the performance of patients with narcolepsy is worse than that of those with psychiatric hypersomnia. The emotional disturbances found in these three types of hypersomnia are also different. In SAS and narcolepsy (organic hypersomnias) are a consequence of the illness, whereas emotional disturbances are a causal factor of psychiatric hypersomnia. Psychopathological disturbances are more serious in SAS than in narcolepsy, and, in spite of the fact that both reflect a neurotic-anxious reaction to the illness, there are differential signs between them.[126]

10.5.2.1 Sleep Apnea Syndrome

Patients with SAS display diverse cognitive deficits that reduce their global intellectual performance, chiefly affecting attention capacity, memory and learning abilities, and visuomotor skills.

In SAS, sleep is interrupted by frequent EEG arousals, provoked by apneic episodes. The degree of hypoxemia during apneas is high in some patients. This sleep fragmentation, by inhibiting deepening of sleep, produces a reduced proportion of delta sleep and, to a lesser degree, of REM sleep. The alteration of the sleep pattern, which provokes partial sleep deprivation, and, in like manner, the hypoxemia, which impairs cerebral activity, both contribute to EDS. This impairment of vigilance provokes a global reduction of cerebral activity with repercussions on cognitive performance, especially on attention and memory processes. On the other hand, hypoxemia seems predominantly to affect the more complex cognitive functions such as the executive functions, manipulative abilities (including motor dexterity), and verbal fluency. These functions are mediated mainly by the frontal lobes.

As the severity of the syndrome increases, the deficits of moderate SAS intensify and other more serious deficits appear. It has been suggested that patients with severe SAS suffer cognitive impairment similar to that of patients with frontal dysfunction, such as problems in the inhibition of automatic mental processes and initiating new ones, a tendency toward perseveration, and decreased attentional and learning-memory abilities.

Upon summarizing data from various studies, the correlation found between the different physiopathological factors and the different cognitive deficits found in SAS (for review and references, see Reference 127) indicate that:

1. *Sleep fragmentation*, due to the arousals caused by the apneas, plays an important part in the pathogenesis of EDS. However, it is not the only factor given that the normalization of the sleep pattern after treatment does not completely restore a normal level of vigilance. This residual sleepiness could account for the fact that patients do not totally recover attentional and memory functions following treatment.
2. *AHI* is related to memory deficits.
3. The severity of *nocturnal hypoxemia* closely correlates with that of *EDS* (evaluated objectively with the Maintenance of Wakefulness test) and with frontal function disturbances. In addition, apnea-related changes in cerebral blood flow can contribute to altered cerebral/cognitive functions.
4. *Partial sleep deprivation,* caused by interruption of sleep from arousals, mainly affects mood, but also has repercussions on cognitive and complex motor functions. The subsequent decrease in the percentage of delta sleep, and occasionally REM sleep, reduces the restorative function of sleep and affects cognitive functioning. It is known that both types of sleep are involved in cognitive performance and that REM sleep, especially, favors consolidation of memory and learning. Impairments in different types of learning, in particular more complex learning, could be largely due to this factor.

Treatment with nasal continuous positive airway pressure (nasal CPAP) results in an overall, although incomplete, improvement in the deficits attributed to EDS. On the contrary, there is a persistence of deficits supposedly due to hypoxemia, or partial remission.[128,129] These deficits include problems with planning and carrying out behavior, scant ability to change mental strategies ("shifting"), and problems with short-term memory.

The cognitive deficits displayed in SAS that have been described are accompanied by psychopathological disturbances, especially symptoms of depression. Some data indicate that there is a close relationship between SAS and either major depression or a subclinical depressive syndrome. When evaluating patients with the MMPI it has been found that those with severe SAS display a characteristic personality profile that differentiates them from patients with other EDS disorders, in which the predominant signs are hypochondriasis, depression, and social withdrawal.[130] Other studies have shown elevations on the hypochondriasis, hysteria, social introversion, and psychasthenia MMPI scales, a pattern that indicates a moderately chronic dysthymic disorder in which depressive symptoms predominate.[131] It is clear, then, that in addition to depression other types of psychopathological symptoms are also observed in SAS. These disturbances seem to be interrelated and progress according to the severity of the syndrome. It has been suggested that a depressive pathology predominates in patients with moderate hypoxemia, whereas in patients with a greater desaturation of O_2 the pathology is more diverse.[131]

As a result of the cognitive deficits and psychopathological disturbances, SAS patients have serious problems with psychosocial adjustment. These mainly affect their social relationships and work performance.[130] Oddly enough, they encounter less trouble in their family circles than patients with narcolepsy,[126] whose somnolence is more sudden and intense. The psychosocial repercussions of the syndrome are manifested in a high incidence of work and social maladjustment and an increased risk of traffic accidents.[130] The cognitive deficits and psychopathological disturbances of patients treated with nasal CPAP or uvulopalatopharingoplasty (UPPP) are improved, as is their quality of life.[128–130]

Table 10.4 shows the course of cognitive deficits and affective disorders of patients with SAS from the first appearance of snoring to moderate and then to severe apnea syndrome. In this last stage, the intensity of EDS, and especially the nocturnal hypoxemia, can reach the point of provoking irreversible cognitive impairment. Given the severity of the consequences of SAS, it is important to evaluate the cognitive-executive functions of patients as well as their emotional state with specific tests. Treatment should be commenced in the initial stages of the illness to avoid the risk of cognitive decline.

TABLE 10.4
Evolution of Neuropsychological Alterations in Patients with SAS

	Snoring/Light Apnea	Moderate Apnea	Severe Apnea
Cognitive deficits	Complaints of loss of cognitive performance: concentration and memory difficulties	EDS: Decrease in vigilance, attention, and memory	Severe deficits of cognitive–executive functions
		Hypoxemia: Decrease in executive functions and fine motor skills	Cognitive impairment
Affective and personality disorders	Irritability Emotional unstableness Depressive feelings	Depression Psychosocial adjustment difficulties Social withdrawal	Neurotic–anxious reaction (depression, hypochondriasis, and social withdrawal) Social and laboral maladjustment

10.5.2.2 Narcolepsy–Cataplexy Syndrome

Narcolepsy–cataplexy syndrome is an organic type of hypersomnia affecting between 0.06 and 1.6% of the population. It is a chronic illness that generally appears during adolescence and that, if not treated or if treated inadequately, can have serious consequences on patients' cognitive performance, mental health, and family, social, and professional adjustment. At the present time, narcolepsy is considered to be a disorder of the cerebral mechanisms that regulate the maintenance of the waking and sleep states and the transition between the states. It is believed that both genetic and environmental factors play a decisive role in the development of the illness (for review, see Reference 132). This illness is not a frequent cause of complaint in elderly people; however, it is advisable to be familiar with its cognitive–behavioral consequences given that many patients are not diagnosed until well into adulthood, many years following the appearance of the syndrome.

Experimental research on the effects of narcolepsy–cataplexy syndrome on cognitive functioning and psychosocial adjustment (for review and references, see References 133 and 134) began in the 1980s, when Broughton's team reported that 40% of patients complained of memory problems from the outset of the illness. It was subsequently found that the circadian variations of performance in patients with narcolepsy are more accentuated than in normal subjects and are associated with attacks of daytime drowsiness and increased fatigue. Frequent falls in the level of daytime vigilance can interrupt the continuity of attentional processes, impairing learning and memory. This in turn impairs planning, execution, and behavior control processes. Automatic behavior episodes and memory lapses are characteristic symptoms of narcolepsy. It therefore seems that, rather than at the functional level, there is a disturbance of the temporal maintenance of the cognitive processes in patients with narcolepsy.

The most recent research has afforded data that have been instrumental in understanding the nature of disturbance in the cognitive processes of patients with narcolepsy and what kind of functions are affected by the kind of drowsiness that they experience. It has been demonstrated that in a state of high arousal, these patients show normal performance in automatic tasks, but that this specifically diminishes in complex cognitive tasks when they swing to a state of low arousal. This means that the functions most affected by narcolepsy are higher cognitive functions and tasks requiring high-speed cognitive processing, perceptual–motor coordination, as well as speed and precision in motor response. Naps have a beneficial effect on the overall cognitive performance of patients with narcolepsy, in spite of the effect of "sleep inertia," which diminishes their cognitive performance immediately after awakening. These data support the theory that the reduced performance found in patients with narcolepsy is essentially due to the effects of somnolence and partially confirm their subjective complaints of cognitive dysfunction. Another important factor influencing the cognitive performance of these patients affects their meta-memory processes. They show little confidence in their own cognitive ability, especially with regard to memory, which adversely affects their performance. In regard to the emotional well-being of patients with narcolepsy–cataplexy, the syndrome is associated with psychopathological disorders that have generally been interpreted as a consequence of the illness. Nonetheless, some authors have suggested that they may be a constituent part, or biological predisposition, of these patients. The most frequent symptoms are depression, anxiety, inhibition, low self-esteem, and social withdrawal. It is interesting to point out the high prevalence of depression and anxiety found in several studies. According to the authors' data, the MMPI personality profile of patients with narcolepsy is of the neurotic type, although within the normal range (T score <70), with significant elevations with regard to normal controls on the hypochondriasis, psychasthenia and schizophrenia scales, and a moderate elevation ($T > 60$) in the depression scale.[126] This personality profile is different from those of patients with SAS and, when comparing the two profiles, significant elevations are observed in patients with narcolepsy on the psychasthenia and schizophrenia scales (which are part of the so-called "psychotic" scales). This is worthy of note given that it can be interpreted as a sign of organicity. There have also been reports that there is no significant remission in the depression, symptoms

of fatigue, and lack of motivation in these patients with the use of various medications that control EDS. These symptoms seem to be independent of the presence of cataplexy and the degree of the effects of the syndrome on the patient's work and social life. Such anomalies could thus be more endogenous in nature than secondary to the illness.

The authors' data on the neuropsychological profile of narcolepsy–cataplexy patients suggest that: (1) the cognitive deficits of patients with narcolepsy are moderate and particularly affect the maintenance of attention and information processing speed; (2) the psychopathological disturbances displayed in these patients consist primarily of a neurotic reaction to the illness, in which distinctive personality traits are observed; and (3) the psychosocial consequences of the syndrome are serious and especially damaging to the social, emotional, and professional adjustment of the patients.[126,133]

10.6 SLEEP DISORDERS AND AFFECTIVE DISORDERS

Psychological factors play an important role in the quality of sleep, and this is perhaps even more evident in old age. The older adult is especially vulnerable to major life events or stressful situations, such as retirement, changes of residence, financial difficulties, the death of friends, and so forth. All of these situations can remarkably alter sleep in old age. An important cause of disturbed sleep at this age is bereavement following the death of a loved one, provoking depression in 10 to 20% of older people. Recent major life events and social and emotional instability stand out among the psychosocial factors influencing sleep disturbances in healthy elderly people.[135]

It has been found that, when these subjects suffer a "subsyndromal" depression (a depressive disorder that does not conform with all required criteria for a specific depressive disorder diagnosis, but which nonetheless can be equally serious), they present sleep fragmentation together with an elevation of the percentage of phase 1 sleep[136] as well as some of the alterations of REM sleep found in major depression (elevated REM density).[61] This can persist 23 months after bereavement.[137] In the case that a major depressive episode develops, polysomnographic anomalies can be observed that are somewhat similar to the characteristics of major depression (shortening of REM latency, increase of REM sleep, early morning awakening).[61] Consequently, it has been suggested that changes in sleep originating in bereavement in old age can foretell the development of a major depressive episode.[121]

Depression is one of the most frequent disorders found in old age. There are reports that neurotic depression is more prevalent in women than in men and in young-old (65 to 74 years) than in old-old (75 years or over) subjects. It is generally associated with organic illness (cardiovascular disease and diabetes mellitus), and a high percentage of these patients (40%) suffer sleep disturbances.[138]

In a recent prospective epidemiological study concerning the prevalence of sleep disorders and major depression done with a large sample of subjects over 50 years old, it was found that 23.1% had insomnia and 6.7% had hypersomnia. In addition, these disorders were important predictors of future depression. The data of this study indicate that gender, mood disturbance, and chronic health problems predict insomnia, while major life events, mood disturbances, and chronic conditions forecast hypersomnia. Age in itself, however, does not seem to be an important risk factor in either insomnia or hypersomnia.[139] The authors consider that the association between sleep problems and aging are primarily due to a depressive mood and health problems, and uphold the importance of these psychobiological factors in the genesis of sleep disorders in old age.

With regard to the characteristics of the sleep of institutionalized elderly people, there are reports that, although there is a high rate of sleep problems found in this population, it is no higher than in age-matched noninstitutionalized controls. Nonetheless, subjects in nursing homes present a phase advanced sleep–wake pattern, spend more time in bed, and consume more hypnotics.[140] Such variables as the effects of imposed sleep–wake schedules, the decrease in daily activity, the presence of affective disorders, and the increase of sleep disturbances as age advances can influence these findings. A high rate of SRRD and high levels of EDS,[141,142] problems that are interrelated, have also been observed in nursing home populations.

Sleep problems are also frequent in aged women who are caregivers of a family member with dementia. These subjects suffer the physical and psychological consequences of caring for a demented patient. It has been found that their sleep is more disturbed than that of normal controls of the same age. This is specifically due to difficulties in getting to sleep, frequent nocturnal awakenings, early morning awakening, and interruptions of sleep due to the need for visits to the toilet. The subjective complaints of the decline in the quality of sleep is quite similar to those of depressed subjects and proved to be associated to low levels of education, inappropriate management of negative emotions, the need to attend to the patient, and psychological stress.[143] Other studies report that certain behavioral techniques (sleep hygiene habits, stimulus control procedure, stress management techniques to reduce patient disruptive behaviors, etc.) prove useful in these cases, producing a significant improvement of sleep alterations.[144]

In spite of the clinical impression that the depressive symptoms suffered by many elderly people are due to their cognitive deficits, currently the following questions are being considered.

On the one hand, the affective disorders of normal older adults are different from classic major depression, both phenomenologically and in their effects on cognitive performance. Thus, it is seen that the outstanding effects of major depression are alterations of the level of arousal and psychomotor activation, memory coding deficits, and decreased cognitive performance. However, age-associated "depression" has minimal cognitive repercussions. When geriatric patients experience cognitive difficulties, these seem to be due to organic factors or to other illnesses that they have, and not to the effects of the pseudo-depressive state. If there is a history of major depression, with a nuclear symptom of loss of self-esteem, and the cognitive deficits have a depressive component, then treatment of the depression can improve cognitive functioning.[145]

On the other hand, depressed patients tend to complain of a loss of memory and poor concentration, which at times are objectified through neuropsychological assessment. In most cases, however, the cognitive deficits are less relevant than the dysphoric mood or other depressive symptoms. Even so, one out of five elderly patients with major depression suffers serious cognitive impairment ("depressive pseudodementia"). Patients with moderate depression generally do not display significant cognitive deficits, whereas severely depressed patients show more signs of cognitive impairment. Although the overall mental performance of the latter is usually within the normal range, it could be that certain characteristic symptoms of depression have an influence on these cognitive changes. Lack of energy and motivation, difficulties in concentrating, memory and meta-memory defects, and so on probably increase the cognitive difficulties of depressed older people. In short, most studies concur in that the relationship between the subjective complaints of cognitive deficits (particularly, memory problems) and the real cognitive performance of these subjects is weak (for review, see Reference 74).

10.7 CONCLUSIONS

In elderly people, complaints of sleep disturbances are generally accompanied by difficulties in cognitive performance, especially memory problems, and by affective disorders such as depressive states and anxiety. The alteration of the nocturnal sleep pattern that has the greatest effect on cognitive performance is sleep fragmentation, given that it reduces the sleep efficiency and its restorative function. It must also be taken into account that with aging the duration of the period of nocturnal sleep is reduced and at the same time the tendency to take daytime naps increases. These physiological changes have cognitive repercussions.

In examining the cognitive functioning of older people, the changes normally found in cognitive performance with aging as well as individual differences and the different patterns of aging must be considered. Normal aging brings with it a certain decline in cognitive performance and is characterized by a slowing of the brain's processing of higher functions and behavior. The cognitive functions most affected by normal aging are visuospatial abilities, short-term memory, and complex attentional processes. The decline in these processes is gradual and is not generally relevant until very advanced ages. A good state of health and physical and mental activity, as well as emotional and social support, all help to alleviate the damaging cognitive effects of neurobiological aging and to reinforce cognitive performance.

Sleep alterations are frequent in aged adults, especially in those with physical or psychiatric disorders. The most prevalent subjective sleep complaints in old age concern difficulties in staying asleep, or sleep maintenance, followed to a lesser degree by difficulties in getting to sleep. This trouble with initiating sleep is usually the consequence of a hyperarousal state due to psychopathological disturbances. Psychophysiological insomnia can become chronic if the patient uses inappropriate cognitive–behavioral strategies in confronting it; cognitive–behavioral therapy can therefore be a useful treatment. In spite of the subjective impression of the patient with insomnia, psychophysiological insomnia does not have a significant effect on cognitive performance.

EDS, one of the most frequent complaints of elderly people, can be due to nocturnal sleep fragmentation, which occurs both in SRRD and SAS, as well as in PLMS and maintenance insomnia. It can also be due to an advanced sleep phase syndrome, a circadian rhythm disorder often found with aging. Of the sleep disorders that develop with EDS, SAS is highly prevalent in middle-aged and elderly subjects and can cause irreversible cognitive impairment, mainly as a result of the effects of hypoxemia on cerebral functioning. Treatment with CPAP or UPPP, by controlling the apnea, reestablishes the sleep pattern and reduces EDS, thus improving cognitive performance.

REFERENCES

1. Katzman, R. and Terry, R., Normal aging of the nervous system, in *The Neurology of Aging*, Katzman, R. and Terry, R., Eds., F. A. Davies, Philadelphia, 1983, 15.
2. Kubicki, S. et al., Der Einfluss des Alters auf die Schlafspindel und K-Komplex-Dichte, *Z. EEG-EMG*, 20, 59, 1989.
3. Goldenberg, F., Sleep in normal aging, *Neurophysiol. Clin.*, 21, 267, 1991.
4. Mazzoni, G. and Gori, S., Word recall correlates with sleep cycles in elderly subjects, *J. Sleep Res.*, 8, 185, 1999.
5. Foret, J. and Webb, W. B., Évolution de l'organisation temporelle des stades de sommeil chez l'homme de 20 à 70 ans, *Rev. EEG Neurophysiol.*, 10, 171, 1980.
6. Culebras, A., El sueño en la vejez, in *La medicina del sueño*, Culebras, A., Ed., Ancora, Barcelona, 1994, 79.
7. Billiard, M., Modificaciones del ritmo circadiano durante el envejecimiento, in *Trastornos del sueño e insomnio en el anciano*, Albarede, J. L., Morley, J. E., Roth, T., and Vellas, B. J., Eds., Glosa, Barcelona, 1998, 59.
8. Dumont, M., Richardson, G. S., and Czeisler, C. A., Endogenous circadian phase and amplitude in elderly patients with a complaint of insomnia, *Sleep Res.*, 19, 217, 1990.
9. National Institute of Health Consensus Development Conference Statement, *The Treatment of Sleep Disorders in Older People*, Association of Professional Sleep Societies, 14, 169, 1990.
10. Bixler, E. O. et al., Prevalence of sleep disorders: a survey of the Los Angeles metropolitan area, *Am. J. Psychiatr.*, 136, 1257, 1979.
11. Mellinger, G. D., Blater, M. B., and Uhlenhuth, E. H., Insomnia and its treatment: prevalence and correlates, *Arch. Gen. Psychiatry*, 42, 225, 1985.
12. Pollack, C. P. et al., Sleep problems in the community elderly as predictors of death and nursing home placement, *J. Commun. Health*, 15, 123, 1990.
13. Ford, D. E. and Kamerow, D. B., Epidemiological study of sleep disturbances and psychiatric disorders, *JAMA*, 262, 1479, 1989.
14. Crowley, K. and Colrain, I. M., Self-reported sleep patterns and daytime sleepiness in the neurologically healthy aged [Letter], *J. Sleep Res.*, 9, 97, 2000.
15. Murphy, P. J., Rogers, N. L., and Campbell, S. S., Age differences in the spontaneous termination of sleep, *J. Sleep Res.*, 9, 27, 2000.
16. American Sleep Disorders Association (ASDA), *International Classification of Sleep Disorders (ICSD)*, revised, Diagnostic and Coding Manual, ASDA, Rochester, MN, 1997.
17. Espinar-Sierra, J., Trastornos del sueño en el envejecimiento normal y en las demencias, in *Sueño y Procesos Cognitivos*, Ramos-Platón, M. J., Ed., Síntesis Psicobiología, Madrid, 1996, 263.
18. Miles, L. and Dement, W. C., Sleep and aging, *Sleep*, 3, 119, 1980.
19. Aguilera, C. and Capella, H., Uso de fármacos en geriatría, *Medicine*, 7, 5811, 1999.

20. De Alberto, M. J. et al., Factors related to current and subsequent psychotropic drug use in an elderly cohort, *J. Clin. Epidemiol.*, 50, 357, 1997.
21. Ray, W. A., Psychotropic drugs and injuries among the elderly: a review, *J. Clin. Psychopharmacol.*, 12, 386, 1992.
22. Monane, M., Insomnia in the elderly, *J. Clin. Psychiatr.*, 53(Suppl. 6), 23, 1992.
23. Rayon, P. et al., Hypnotic drug use in Spain: a cross-sectional study based on a network of community pharmacies, *Ann. Pharmacother.*, 30, 1092, 1996.
24. Mullan, E., Katona, C., and Bellew, M., Patterns of sleep disorders and sedative hypnotic use in seniors, *Drugs Aging*, 5, 49, 1994.
25. Monti, J. M., Disturbances of sleep and wakefulness associated with the use of antihypertensive agents, *Life Sci.*, 41, 1979, 1987.
26. Ongini, E. et al., Effects of selected beta-adrenergic blocking agents on sleep stages in spontaneously hypertensive rats, *J. Pharmacol. Exp. Ther.*, 257, 114, 1991.
27. McAinish, J. and Cruickshank, J. M., Beta-blockers and central nervous system side effects, *Pharmacol. Ther.*, 46, 163, 1990.
28. Silferfarb, P. M. et al., Assessment of sleep in patients with lung cancer and breast cancer, *J. Clin. Oncol.*, 11, 997, 1993.
29. Hrushensky, W. J. M. and Bjarnason, G. A., Circadian cancer therapy, *J. Clin. Oncol.*, 11, 1403, 1993.
30. Douglas, N. J., Asthma, in *Principles and Practice of Sleep Medicine*, 2nd ed., Kryger, M. H., Roth, T. and Dement, W. C., Eds., W. B. Saunders, Philadelphia, 1994, 748.
31. Martin, J. R., Cicutto, L. C., and Ballard, R. D., Factors related to the nocturnal worsening in asthma, *Am. Rev. Respir. Dis.*, 141, 33, 1990.
32. Fitzpatrick, M. F. et al., Morbidity in nocturnal asthma: sleep quality and daytime cognitive performance, *Thorax*, 46, 569, 1991.
33. Janson, C. M. et al., Theophylline disturbs sleep mainly in caffeine-sensitive persons, *Pulm. Pharmacol.*, 1989, 2, 125, 1989.
34. Fitzpatrick, M. F. et al., Effect of therapeutic theophylline levels on the sleep quality and daytime cognitive performance of normal subjects, *Am. Rev. Respir. Dis.*, 145, 1355, 1992.
35. Kaplan, J. et al., Theophylline effect on sleep in normal subjects, *Chest*, 103, 193, 1993.
36. Fitzpatrick, M. F. et al., Salmeterol in nocturnal asthma: a double blind, placebo controlled trial of a long acting inhaled beta-2 agonist, *Br. Med. J.*, 301, 1365, 1990.
37. Askenasy, J. J. M. and Yahr, M. D., Reversal of sleep disturbance in Parkinson's disease by antiparkinsonian therapy: a preliminary study, *Neurology*, 35, 527, 1985.
38. Van den Kerchove, M. et al., Sustained-release in parkinsonian patients with nocturnal disabilities, *Acta Neurol. Belg.*, 93, 32, 1993.
39. Nausieda, P. A., Sleep in Parkinson's disease, in *Handbook of Parkinson's Disease*, Koller, W. C., Ed., Marcel Dekker, New York, 1992, 451.
40. Lavie, P., Wajsbort, J., and Youdim, M. B. H., Deprenyl does not causes insomnia in parkinsonian patients, *Commun. Psychopharmacol.*, 4, 303, 1980.
41. Stern, G. M., Lees, A. J., and Sandler, M., Recent observations on the clinical pharmacology of deprenyl. *J. Neural Transm.*, 43, 245, 1978.
42. Buysse, D. J., Drugs affecting sleep, sleepiness and performance, in *Sleep, Sleepiness and Performance*, Monk, T. H., Ed., John Wiley & Sons, New York, 1991, 250.
43. Ancoli-Israel, S. and Coy, T., Are breathing disturbances in elderly equivalent to sleep apnea syndrome? *Sleep*, 17, 77, 1994.
44. Bliwise, D. L., Sleep in normal aging and dementia, *Sleep*, 16, 40, 1993.

45. Hoch, C. et al., Comparison of sleep-disordered breathing among elderly in the seventh, eighth and ninth decades of life, *Sleep*, 13, 502, 1990.

46. Ancoli-Israel, S. et al., Sleep-disordered breathing in community-dwelling elderly, *Sleep*, 14, 486, 1991.

47. Phillips, B. A., Berry, D. T. R., and Lipke-Molby, T. C., Sleep-disordered breathing in healthy aged persons. Fifth and final year follow-up, *Chest*, 110, 654, 1996.

48. Ancoli-Israel, S. et al., Sleep apnea and nocturnal myoclonus in a senior population, *Sleep*, 4, 349, 1981.

49. Kales, A. et al., Biopsychobehavioral correlates of insomnia. I: Role of sleep apnea and nocturnal myoclonus, *Psychosomatics*, 23, 589, 1982.

50. Coleman, R. et al., Sleep-wake disorders in the elderly: a polysomnographic analysis, *J. Am. Geriatr. Soc.*, 29, 289, 1981.

51. Ancoli-Israel, S. et al., Periodic limb movements in sleep in community-dwelling elderly, *Sleep*, 14, 496, 1991.

52. Bixler, E. O. et al., Nocturnal myoclonus and nocturnal myoclonic activity in a normal population, *Res. Commun. Chem. Pathol. Pharmacol.*, 36, 129, 1989.

53. Ancoli-Israel, S. et al., Sleep apnea and periodic leg movements in sleep in a aging population, *J. Gerontol.*, 40: 419, 1985.

54. Lugaresi, E. et al., Nocturnal myoclonus and restless legs syndrome, in *Advances in Neurology*, Vol. 43, Fahn, S., Ed., Raven Press, New York, 1986, 295.

55. Coleman, R. M. et al., Epidemiology of periodic movements during sleep, in *Sleep-Wake Disorders: Natural History, Epidemiology and Long Term Evolution*, Guilleminault, C. and Lugaresi, E., Eds., Raven Press, New York, 1983, 217.

56. Rosenthal, L. et al., Periodic movements during sleep, sleep fragmentation and sleep-wake complaints, *Sleep*, 7, 326, 1984.

57. Dickel, M. and Mosko, S., Morbidity cut-offs for sleep apnea and periodic leg movements in predicting subjective complaints in seniors, *Sleep*, 13, 155, 1990.

58. Marquié, J. C. and Foret, J., Sleep, age, and shiftwork experience, *J. Sleep Res.*, 8, 297, 1999.

59. Schenck, Ch. and Mahowald, M. W., REM sleep parasomnias, *Neurol. Clin.*, 14, 697, 1996.

60. Rubio, P. et al., Enfermos de Parkinson con trastornos de conducta durante el sueño. Características clínicas y polisomnográficas, *Vigilia-Sueño*, 12, 97, 2000.

61. Reynolds, C. F. et al., Electroencephalographic sleep in spousal bereavement and bereavement related depression of late-life, *Biol. Psychiatr.*, 31, 69, 1992.

62. Benca, R. M. et al., Sleep and psychiatric disorders: a meta-analysis, *Arch. Gen. Psychiatr.*, 49, 651, 1992.

63. Berlin, R. M., Disturbed sleep in the elderly, *Am. J. Psychiatr.*, 146, 810, 1989.

64. Newman, L. C., Lipton, R. B., and Solomon, S., The hypnic headache syndrome: a benign headache disorder of the elderly, *Neurology*, 40, 1904, 1990.

65. Raskin, N. H., The hypnic headache syndrome, *Headache*, 28, 534, 1988.

66. Lees, A. J., Blackburn, N. A., and Campbell, V.L., The night-time problems of Parkinson's disease, *Clin. Neuropharmacol.*, 6, 512, 1988.

67. Factor, S. A. et al., Sleep disorders and sleep effect in Parkinson's disease, *Movement Disorders*, 5, 280, 1990.

68. Rubio, P. et al., Trastornos del sueño y enfermedad de Parkinson: estudio de una casuística, *Rev. Neurol.* (Barcelona), 23, 265, 1995.

69. Mortimer, J. and Hutton, J. T., Epidemiology and etiology of Alzheimer's disease, in *Senile Dementia of the Alzheimer Type*, Hutton, J. T. and Kenny, A. D., Eds., Alan R. Liss, New York, 1985, 177.

70. Terry, R. and Katzman, R., Senile dementia of the Alzheimer type, *Ann. Neurol.*, 14, 497, 1983.

71. Prinz, P. N. and Vitiello, M. V., Sleep in Alzheimer's disease, in *Sleep Disorders and Insomnia in the Elderly*, Vellas, B. and Albarede, J. L., Eds., Serdi Publisher, Paris, 1993, 33.

72. Morley, J. E., Nocturnal agitation, in *Sleep Disorders and Insomnia in the Elderly*, Vellas, B. and Albarede, J. L., Eds., Serdi Publisher, Paris, 1993, 109.

73. Boller, F., Marcie, P., and Traykov, L., La neuropsychologie du vieillissement normal, in *Neuropsychologie Clinique et Neurologie du Comportement*, 2nd ed., Botez, M. I., Ed., Les Presses de l'Université de Montréal, Masson, Paris, 1996, 527.

74. La Rue, A., Cognition in normal aging, in *Aging and Neuropsychological Assessment*, Plenum Press, New York, 1992, chap. 3.

75. Laursen, P., The impact of aging on cognitive functions, *Acta Neurol. Scand.*, 172 (Suppl.), 1997.

76. Lezak, M., *Neuropsychological Assessment*, 3rd. ed., Oxford University Press, New York, 1995.

77. Hochanadel, G. and Kaplan, E., Neuropsychology of normal aging, in *Clinical Neurology of Aging*, Albert, M. L., Ed., Lexington Books, Lexington, MA, 1984, 231.

78. Nebes, R. S., Hemispheric specialization in the aged brain, in *Brain Circuits and Functions of the Mind; Essays in Honor of Roger W. Sperry*, Trevarthen, C., Ed., Cambridge University Press, Cambridge, 1990.

79. Albert, M. S., Duffy, F. H., and Naeser, M., Non-linear changes in cognition with age and their neurosychological correlates, *Can. J. Psychol.*, 41, 141, 1987.

80. Craik, F. I. M. and Byrd, M., Aging and cognitive deficits. The role of attentional resources, in *Aging and Cognitive Processes. Advances in the Study of Communication and Affect*, Vol. 8, Craik, F. I. M. and Trehub, S., Eds., Plenum Press, New York, 1982, 191.

81. Rapp, P. R. and Amaral, D. G., Individual differences in the cognitive and neurobiological consequences of normal aging, *TINS*, 15, 340, 1992.

82. Rowe, J. W. and Kahn, R. L., Human aging: usual and succesful, *Science*, 237, 143, 1987.

83. Crook, T. H. et al., Age-associated memory impairment: proposed diagnostic criteria of clinical change (Report of a National Institute of Mental Health work group), *Dev. Neuropsychol.*, 2, 261, 1986.

84. Crook, T. H., Larrabee, G., and Youngjohn, J. R., Diagnosis and assessment of age-associated memory impairment, *Clin. Neuropharmacol.*, 13(Suppl. 3), S81, 1990.

85. Crook, T. H. and Ferris, S. H., Age associated memory impairment, *Br. Med. J.*, 304, 71, 1992.

86. Larrabee, G. J. and Crook, T. H., Estimated prevalence of age-associated memory impairment derived from standardized tests of memory function, *Int. Psychogeriatr.*, 6, 95, 1994.

87. Koivisto, K. et al., Prevalence of age-associated memory impairment in a randomly selected population from eastern Finland, *Neurology*, 45, 741, 1995.

88. Hänninen, T. et al., Decline of frontal lobe functions in subjects with age-associated memory impairment, *Neurology*, 48, 148, 1997.

89. Parnetti, L. et al., H-MRS, MRI-based hippocampal volumetry, and 99^{ml} Tc-HMPAO-SPECT in normal aging, age-associated memory impairment, and probable Alzheimer's disease, *J. Am. Geriatr. Soc.*, 4, 133, 1996.

90. Hänninen, T. et al., A follow-up study of age-associated memory impairment: neuropsychological predictors of dementia, *J. Am. Geriatr. Soc.*, 43, 1017, 1995.

91. Nielsen, H. et al., Age-associated memory impairment — pathological memory decline or normal aging, *Scand. J. Psychol.*, 39, 33, 1998.

92. Bartrés-Faz, D., Clemente, I., and Junqué, C., Alteración cognitiva en el envejecimiento normal: nosología y estado actual, *Rev. Neurol.*, 29, 64, 1999.

93. Daum, I. et al., Memory dysfunction of frontal type in normal ageing, *NeuroReport*, 7, 2625, 1996.

94. Patterson, M. B. et al., Executive functions and Alzheimer's disease: problems and reports, *Eur. J. Neurol.*, 3, 5, 1996.

95. Bolla, K. I. et al., Memory complaint in older adults. Fact or fiction? *Arch. Neurol.*, 48, 61, 1991.

96. Light, L. L., Memory and aging: four hypotheses in search of data, *Annu. Rev. Psychol.*, 42, 333, 1991.

97. La Rue, A., The aging brain, in *Aging and Neuropsychological Assessment*, Plenum Press, New York, 1992, chap. 2.

98. Junqué, C. et al., Leuko-araiosis on magnetic resonance imaging and speed of mental processing, *Arch. Neurol.*, 47, 151, 1990.

99. Dywan, J., Segalowitz, S. J., and Unsal, A., Speed of information processing, health, and cognitive performance in older adults, *Dev. Neuropsychol.*, 8, 473, 1992.

100. Rosenberg, I. H. and Miller, J. W., Nutritional factors in physical and cognitive functions of elderly people, *Am. J. Clin. Nutr.*, 55, 1237, 1992.

101. Salthouse, T. A., Initializing the formalization of theories of cognitive aging, *Psychol. Aging*, 3, 1, 1988.

102. Klisz, D., Neuropsychological evaluation in older persons, in *The Clinical Psychology of Aging*, Storandt, M., Stiegler, I. C., and Elias, M. F., Eds, Plenum Press, New York, 1978, 71.

103. Schaie, K. W. and Schaie, J. P., Clinical assessment and aging, in *Handbook of the Psychology of Aging*, Birren, J. E. and Schaie, K. W., Eds.,Van Nostrand Reinhold, New York, 1977, 92.

104. Mittenberg, W. et al., Changes in cerebral functioning associated with normal aging, *J. Clin. Exper. Neuropsychol.*, 11, 1989, 918.

105. Martin, A. J. et al., Decreases in regional cerebral flood flow with normal aging, *J. Cereb. Flow Metabol.*, 11, 684, 1991.

106. Hasher, L. and Zacks, R. T., Working memory, comprehension, and aging. A review and a new view, in *The Psychology of Learning and Motivation*, Vol. 8, Bower, G. H., Ed., Academic Press, New York, 1988, 193.

107. Salthouse, T. A., Speed of behavior and its implications for cognition, in *Handbook of the Psychology of Aging*, Birren, J. E. and Schaie, K. W., Eds., Van Nostrand Reinhold, New York, 1985, 400.

108. Storandt, M., Longitudinal studies of aging and age-associated dementias, in *Handbook of Neuropsychology*, Vol. 4, Boller, F. and Grafman, J., Eds., Elsevier, Amsterdam, 1990.

109. Van Gorp, W. G., Satz, P., and Mitrushina, M., Neuropsychological processes associated with normal aging, *Dev. Neuropsychol.*, 6, 279, 1990.

110. Van Gorp, W. G. and Mahler, M., Subcortical features of normal aging, in *Subcortical Dementia*, Cummings, J., Ed., Oxford University Press, New York, 1990.

111. Dustman, R. E., Emmerson, R. Y., and Shearer, D. E., Electrophysiology and aging: slowing, inhibition, and aerobic fitness, in *Cognitive and Behavioral Performance Factors in Atypical Aging*, Howe, M. L., Stones, M. J., and Brainerd, C. J., Eds., Springer-Verlag, New York, 1990.

112. Dustman, R. E. et al., The effects of videogame playing on neuropsychological performance of elderly individuals, *J. Gerontol.*, 47, 168, 1992.

113. Bliwise, D. L., Neuropsychological function and sleep, *Clin. Geriatr. Med.*, 5, 381, 1989.

114. Prinz, P. N., Sleep patterns in the healthy aged: relationship with intellectual function, *J. Gerontol.*, 32, 179, 1997.

115. Prinz, P. N. et al., Geriatrics: sleep disorders and aging, *N. Engl. J. Med.*, 323, 520, 1990.

116. Carskadon, M. A., Brown, E. D., and Dement, W. E., Sleep fragmentation in the elderly: relationship to possible daytime sleep tendency, *Neurobiol. Aging*, 3, 321, 1982.

117. Hayward, L. B. et al., Sleep disordered breathing and cognitive function in a retirement village population, *Age Ageing*, 21, 121, 1992.

118. Wesensten, N. J., Balkin, T. J., and Belenky, G., Does sleep fragmentation impact recuperation? A review and reanalysis, *J. Sleep Res.*, 8, 237, 1999.

119. Kales, J. D. et al., Biopsychobehavioral correlates of insomnia. V: clinical characteristics and behavioral correlates, *Am. J. Psychiatr.*, 141, 1371, 1984.

120. Roehrs, T. et al., Relationship of psychopathology to insomnia in the elderly, *J. Am. Geriatr. Soc.*, 30, 312, 1982.

121. Bliwise, D. L., Sleep and aging, in *Understanding Sleep*, Presman, M. R. and Orr, W. C., Eds., American Psychiatric Association, Washington, D.C., 1997, chap. 23.

122. Kales, A. and Vgontzas, A. N., Predisposition to and development and persistence of chronic insomnia: importance of psychobehavioral factors, *Arch. Intern. Medicine*, 152, 1570, 1992.

123. Perlis, M. L. et al., Psychophysiological insomnia: the behavioural model and a neurocognitive perspective, *J. Sleep Res.*, 6, 179, 1997.

124. Vela-Bueno, A., Insomnio y trastornos del ritmo circadiano vigilia-sueño, in *Sueño y procesos cognitivos*, Ramos-Platón, M. J., Ed., Síntesis Psicobiología, Madrid, 1996, chap. 9.

125. Morin, C. M. et al., Cognitive-behavior therapy for late-life insomnia, *J. Consult. Clin. Psychol.*, 61, 137, 1993.

126. Ramos-Platón, M. J. et al., Alteraciones neuropsicológicas diferenciales en los trastornos de excesiva somnolencia diurna, *Vigilia-Sueño*, 5, 13, 1994.

127. Ramos-Platón, M. J., Déficits cognitivos en el síndrome de apnea obstructiva del sueño, *Vigilia-Sueño*, 12, S41, 2000.

128. Bédard, M. A. et al., Persistent neuropsychological deficits and vigilance impairment in sleep apnea syndrome after treatment with continuous positive airway pressure (CPAP), *J. Clin. Exp. Neuropsychol.*, 15, 330, 1993.

129. Naëgelé, B. et al., Deficits of cognitive executive functions in patients with sleep apnea syndrome, *Sleep*, 18, 43, 1995.

130. Ramos-Platón, M. J. and Espinar-Sierra, J., Changes in psychopathological symptoms in sleep apnea patients after treatment with nasal continuous positive airway pressure, *Int. J. Neurosci.*, 62, 73, 1992.

131. Aikens, J. E. et al., MMPI correlates of sleep and respiratory disturbance in obstructive sleep apnea, *Sleep*, 22, 362, 1999.

132. Guilleminault, C., Narcolepsy syndrome, in *Principles and Practice of Sleep Medicine*, 2nd ed., Kryger, M. H., Roth, T., and Dement, W. C., Eds., W. B. Saunders, Philadelphia, 1994, 549.

133. Ramos-Platón, M. J., Procesos cognitivos y adaptación psicosocial en la narcolepsia, *Vigilia-Sueño*, 10, S63, 1998.

134. Schulz, H. and Wilde-Franz, J., The disturbance of cognitive processes in narcolepsy, *J. Sleep Res.*, 4, 10, 1995.

135. Dew, M. A. et al., Psychosocial correlates and sequelae of electroencephalographic sleep in healthy elders, *J. Gerontol.*, 49, 8, 1994.

136. Pasternak, R. E. et al., Sleep in spousally bereaved elders with subsyndromal depressive symptoms, *Psychiatr. Res.*, 43, 43, 1992.

137. Reynolds, C. F. et al., Sleep after spousal bereavement: a study of recovery from stress, *Biol. Psychiatr.*, 34, 791, 1993.

138. Ko, S. M., Neurotic depression in the elderly, *Ann. Acad. Med.*, 23, 367, 1994.

139. Roberts, R. E. et al., Sleep complaints in an aging cohort: a prospective study, *Am. J. Psychiatr.*, 157, 81, 2000.

140. Middelkoop, H. A. et al., Sleep and ageing: the effect of institutionalization on subjective and objective characteristics of sleep, *Age Ageing*, 23, 611, 1994.

141. Ancoli-Israel, S. and Kripke, D. F., Epidemiology of sleep apnea in three populations in the elderly, in *Sleep'88*, Horne, J., Ed., Fischer Verlag, Stuttgart, 1989, 258.

142. Meguro, K. et al., Disturbance in daily sleep/wake patterns in patients with cognitive impairment and decreased daily activity, *J. Am. Geriatr. Soc.*, 38, 1176, 1990.

143. Wilcox, S. and King, A. C., Sleep complaints in older women who are family caregivers, *J. Gerontol. B Psychol. Sci. Soc. Sci.*, 54, 189, 1999.

144. McCurry, S. M. et al., Successful behavioral treatment for reported sleep problems in elderly caregivers of dementia patients: a controlled study, *J. Gerontol. B Psychol. Sci. Soc. Sci.*, 53, 122, 1998.

145. Bieliauskas, L. A., Depressed or not depressed? that is the question, *J. Clin. Exp. Neuropsychol.*, 15, 119, 1993.

Part III

Neurobehavioral Assessment

Part III

Part III

Neurobehavioral Assessment

Part III

Neurobehavioral Assessment

11 Neuropsychological Assessment in Elderly People

José León-Carrión
and Juan Manuel Barroso y Martín

CONTENTS

11.1 Introduction 244
11.2 Assessment of Premorbid Cognitive and Behavioral Baseline 244
    11.2.1 Psychological and Health Biography 245
    11.2.2 Premorbid Intellectual Functioning 248
    11.2.3 Social and Work History of the Patient 249
11.3 Scientific Guarantee of Neuropsychological Evaluation
    in Elderly Adults 251
11.4 Assessment of Intellectual Functioning 251
    11.4.1 The Wechsler Adult Intelligence Scales 251
    11.4.2 Test of General Intelligence 253
11.5 Assessment of Attentional Processes 253
11.6 Assessment of Memory Processes 254
    11.6.1 Assessment of Memory Processes and Learning 254
    11.6.2 Functional Organic Memory Questionnaire 255
    11.6.3 Wechsler Memory Scales — Revised 256
11.7 Assessment of Language 257
    11.7.1 Verbal Fluency Measures 257
    11.7.2 Boston Naming Test 258
11.8 Assessment of Executive Functioning 259
    11.8.1 Assessment of Neurocognitive Interference;
        Stroop Effect 259
    11.8.2 Evaluation of Cognitive Functions Associated
        with the Frontal Lobe: The Tower of Hanoi–Seville 260
    11.8.3 Trail Making Test 261
    11.8.4 Digits Backward 262
11.9 Assessment of the Visuoperceptive and Visuoconstructive Processes 262
11.10 Assessment of Sensory and Motor Skills 263
11.11 Assessment of Affective, Emotional, and Personality Problems 265
11.12 Assessment of Dementing Processes 267

0-8493-2066-/01/$0.00+$1.50
© 2001 by CRC Press LLC

11.12.1 Cognitive Symptoms 268
11.12.2 Psychiatric and Behavioral Symptoms 268
11.12.3 Functional Alterations 269
11.13 Assessment of Cerebrovascular Disorders.................................271
11.14 Assessing Traumatic Brain Injury and Other Neurological Conditions ...272
11.15 Concluding Remarks 272
References...273

11.1 INTRODUCTION

It is well accepted that physiological aging has effects on cognitive functioning and on behavior, although not all functions and not all people are affected in the same way. The reality is that more and more elderly people are visiting geriatricians, psychologists, neurologists, psychiatrists, and general practitioners complaining of problems associated with psychological functions that affect their daily lives and activities, such as driving, having a sense of direction, cooking, managing finances, getting dressed, following television programs, reading, conducting personal hygiene, etc.

On the other hand, there is a great deal of information available to the public about the extent and consequences of Alzheimer's disease. This sometimes prodigious amount of information has caused many elderly patients or their family members to go to a specialist at the first symptoms of a problem with memory or behavior, seeking a diagnosis that discards the feared senile dementia and confirms that the cognitive changes that have begun to show themselves are a normal result of the natural effects of the aging process.

As a result, in recent years neuropsychological evaluation in geriatrics has become indispensable, especially when considering degenerative dementia, vascular dementia, medication side effects, and normal changes associated with aging. This evaluation concerns the application of neuropsychological tests that measure qualitatively and quantitatively the cognitive functioning in older people and analysis of the complaints and the reports given by the family or the caregivers of the patient.

11.2 ASSESSMENT OF PREMORBID COGNITIVE AND BEHAVIORAL BASELINE

The cognitive and behavioral changes about which patients and their families complain must be investigated to verify that these are indeed *changes* in the psychological functioning of the patient, as it could occur that what is observed as a "change" is merely an accentuation of the cognitive characteristics and the personality that the patient has possessed all his or her life. Some people tend to manifest in old age, more directly and clearly than before, their cognitive structure and their personality. On the other hand, it is essential to establish a cognitive and behavioral baseline to be able to monitor the possible alterations of behavior and cognitive functioning that could occur in the future. The evaluation of three aspects is imperative to obtain the premorbid baseline of the patient: psychological and health biography, premorbid intellectual functioning, and social and work history of the patient.

11.2.1 PSYCHOLOGICAL AND HEALTH BIOGRAPHY

The psychological biography of the patient offers important information with respect to the patient's premorbid cognitive and behavioral functioning. These data must be collected through an interview with the patient and the family, as well as through the patient's lifelong medical and psychological records.

The initial interview with the patient should be oriented toward firmly establishing, with the least amount of doubt possible, the lifelong psychological profile of the patient. This profile must include normal aspects as well as abnormal aspects. Furthermore, at least some data must be obtained regarding the following.

a. Consultations made with psychologists or psychiatrists, or clinical admissions, at any time in the past. This information is quite useful for determining the patient's vulnerability to mental disorders or if the complaint relates to the development of a previously existing chronic mental disturbance.

b. Psychological/psychiatric diagnoses received in the past. It is important to determine if a previously suffered disorder could influence the development of the problems that are currently at hand.

c. Educational background of the patient. The educational level affects the way in which cognitive deficits present themselves at all ages. A low level of education dramatically affects the scores that are obtained in the cognitive tests. It must be clearly determined which of the obtained scores are due to the cultural and educational level of the patient and which are due to a presumed neuropsychological disorder.

d. Personal and family socioeconomic background. Patients who have lived their whole lives in economically deprived families and environments tend to have had more psychiatric diagnoses. As well, the personal psychological resources available to face the normal cognitive deterioration that is present in aging are more limited for the person with a low socioeconomic background. The slight or moderate neurocognitive deficits of people with a high socioeconomic background tend to be more disguised because they have more social, family, and personal resources to fall back on when confronting these changes.

e. Family mental health background. A family case history of stroke, senility, cerebral vascular deformations, congenital diseases, or other factors can be very useful for establishing possible etiological diagnoses.

f. Affective history. The affective case history of a patient is important for determining his or her current neurological state. It is a question of determining what the patient's predominant emotional style has been throughout his or her lifetime. There are people who interpret the situations of their lives from an emotional standpoint, whereas there are others who take an intellectual approach. For those who have maintained an intellectual style, a cognitive or behavioral decline is more noticeable. However, in the patient who has maintained an emotional approach to life, it is more difficult and complicated to determine cognitive and behavioral deterioration, as these patients tend to mix intellectual and emotional aspects in their daily activities and in the way they solve problems.

On the other hand, during old age, many people are not capable of recognizing that they suffer from any emotional problem. They may be especially unaware of their needs and emotional reactiveness. This phenomenon[1] is referred to as *unawareness of deficit*, or *affective anosognosia*, which can be linked to alterations or damage to the frontal lobes[2] and in the right hemisphere.[3] In addition, a phenomenon that Heilman et al.[4] define as *pseudobulbar behavior* can appear. These are cases where patients display inappropriate tearfulness in reaction to a conversation or discussion that is seemingly devoid of emotional charge.

g. Language. The type and style of language that the patient uses are clear indicators of possible neurological alterations. Deterioration in the capacity to say what one wants to say or to understand what is said (expressive language vs. impressive language) indicates the possible existence of an underlying neurological disorder that in old age usually has a vascular, degenerative, or traumatic origin. Language clearly deteriorates in the Alzheimer's type of senility. In the initial phases of the illness it is common to detect an anomic problem, and the existence of aphasia, along with agnosia and apraxia. This is one of the essential requirements in the diagnosis of Alzheimer's disease. When a dysfunction in the structures of the sub-cortex associated with language exists, dysarthria appears, especially when the damage affects the cerebellum and the basal ganglia.[5,6]

Sensory or receptive aphasia appears when patients do not understand what is said to them. In these cases it must be determined that this is not due to hearing loss; therefore, a hearing test is indicated. In any event, when a deficit in language is observed, a neuropsychological evaluation of the language functions is recommended.

h. Memory. Memory is one of the cognitive functions whose deterioration is most commonly observed in elderly people, with or without neurological illness. Because memory is not a unitary concept, as different systems of memory exist, one must examine which of the systems of memory could be affected (see Chapter 12). It is common to observe important alterations both in episodic memory, with retrograde amnesia, and in working memory.[7] Different cerebral systems are implicated in memory deficits, especially in the temporal lobe and in the hippocampus. The frontal lobe plays a relevant role in the organization and planning of the functions of memory, as well.

Additionally, the neuropsychological evaluation of memory should differentiate between memory for verbal vs. memory for visual-spatial stimuli, recent vs. remote memory, and recall vs. recognition.

i. Personal case history of consumption of toxic substances (alcohol, heroin, cocaine, etc.). The use and abuse of substances considered toxic (alcohol, cocaine, etc.) produce a series of significant alterations in the cognitive functioning of people who consume them. Alcohol and medications are the drug substances most commonly used by the geriatric population. Estimates of the rate of alcoholism among older adults are generally comparable with those established for younger groups.[8]

Ingesting alcohol in large quantities over a period of years will unleash various clinical symptoms, among which are encephalopathies. The severity of the associated specific deficits is related to the quantity and duration of the drinking problem. As a direct consequence of these encephalopathies, the appearance of neurocognitive alterations will be detected; the most important are Korsakoff's disease and Gayet–Wernike's disease, among others. The cognitive effects that are derived from these disturbances can range from the appearance of *delirium tremens*, with agitation, hallucinations, etc., to important and devastating memory problems that are observed in Korsakoff's disease. The traditional diagnostic criteria for alcoholism typically include specific impairments in physical, psychological, and social/occupational functioning.

Ethanol acts in the nervous system as a depressant with effects similar to tranquilizing and hypnotic drugs.[9] Alcohol is itself a drug, and even a small intake can contribute to serious difficulties when interacting with other substances such as medications. This is a very serious problem in geriatric patients because they often take more medication than do younger people, and at the same time they may consume alcohol. Even a substance that by itself would not create difficulties when interacting with alcohol may become a serious problem when other medications are added. It is very important for physicians to know the total amount and the configuration of substances (prescribed and not) that the patient is using to anticipate possible alcohol-related problems and potential consequences on behavior in general and on cognitive functioning in particular.

With the use of drugs (depressants, stimulants) that distort the central nervous system (CNS), different characteristics with different pathological manifestations and different consequent effects on the cognitive functioning of the mature adult will be observed. These effects, depending upon the type of toxic substance consumed, will encompass a large variety of symptoms, but in general some effect, in greater or lesser measure, will be observed on almost all of the neurocognitive functioning of the patient (attention, orientation, language, memory, executive functioning, daily living activities, etc.).

Brust[10] found personality changes in heavy users of marijuana or hashish. The most commonly described characteristics for long-term marijuana smokers are affective blunting, mental and physical sluggishness, apathy, restlessness, memory problems, and others.

Cocaine is a stimulant. It increases alertness, arousal levels, and motor activation. Long-term users of this drug develop physical symptoms such as acute hypertension and other CNS symptoms of overstimulation, which can lead to stroke or death from respiratory or cardiac failure. Cognitive effects of chronic use are concentration deficits along with memory impairment (reduced retrieval efficiency and storage).[11]

j. Chronic use of medication. It is well known that a wide variety of medications have the potential to cause different cognitive impairments. The *Physician's Desk Reference*[12] contains a list of prescription medications that possibly produce neuropsychological effects. Elderly patients are particularly susceptible to drug reactions that can affect several areas of their cognitive functioning, such as alertness or general activity levels.[13] The routine use of prescribed medicines, especially those that treat alterations of the CNS, is implicated in some of the alterations that can be observed on a cognitive level. In general, the medications used for neurological effects are implicated in some deficits detected in the area of memory.[14] By the same token, some medications used to improve cardiac functioning will also have a detrimental effect on memory.[15] Some antihypertension medications may contribute to slowed reaction time.[16]

Cognitive side effects can also be observed with the use of medications such as antihistamines, gastrointestinal medication, nonsteroidal anti-inflammatory medication, antiparkinson drugs (anticholinergics), antidepressives, and anticonvulsive medication. These medications may interfere with memory functioning or create the impression of a low level of cognitive functioning in an "intact" elderly person (without cognitive deficits).[17]

Phenytoin, carbamazepine, and sodium valproate affect cognitive functions. Phenobarbital and phenytoin tend to depress performance in tests of motor speed, attention, and memory.[18] Phenytoin, especially, produces the most adverse effects on memory performance when compared with other drugs.[14] In addition, it is common for elderly people to be under pharmacotherapy composed of many different types of drugs to treat the various afflictions. The different drugs interact in such a way that in many cases cognitive functioning is impaired with many limitations. The elderly population is at increased risk for substance-related disorders with the use of prescription medications. People over 60 consume more than 30% of all prescription medicines.[19]

11.2.2 PREMORBID INTELLECTUAL FUNCTIONING

One of the main problems that appears when examining an elderly patient who has experienced severe deterioration is knowing his or her premorbid intellectual level. At times it is not easy to determine what intellectual capacity the patient had before the neurological deterioration occurred. Situating the patient within a premorbid intellectual category can help assess the extension of the cognitive deterioration that is now present. Normally, this is done through information given by the family or significant others, which situates the patient as a person with a normal intellectual capacity (or subnormal capacity). However, it is not always possible to obtain this information and in many cases the information that is obtained is not reliable.

Taking all this into account, formulas for determining the premorbid intellectual level of the patient have been developed that can predict with some reliability the level of intellectual functioning of the patient prior to the appearance of the neurological condition. Table 11.1 describes one of the most commonly used formulas to determine the premorbid intellectual quotient (IQ) of the patient via common objective data. The formula is taken from Barona et al.,[20] with the adaptation for elderly people from Helmes.[21] The estimation of premorbid IQ is a regression equation with education, race, and occupation as the most powerful predictors (Table 11.1).

TABLE 11.1
Barona Estimation of Premorbid IQ

Estimated VIQ = 54.23 + 0.49 (age) + 1.92 (sex) + 4.24 (race) + 5.25 (education) + 1.89 (occupation) + 1.24 (urban–rural residence). Standard error of estimate of VIQ = 11.79; R = 0.62.

Estimated PIQ = 61.58 + 0.31 (age) + 1.09 (sex) + 4.95 (race) + 3.75 (education) + 1.54 (occupation) + 0.82 (region). Standard error of estimate of PIQ = 13.23; R = .49.

Estimated FSIQ = 54.96 + 0.47 (age) + 1.76 (sex) + 4.71 (race) + 5.02 (education) + 1.89 (occupation) + 0.59 (region). Standard error of estimate of FSIQ = 12.14; R = 0.60.

Variables take the following values:

Sex

Female = 1   Male = 2

Race

White = 3   Black = 2   Other = 1

Region (U.S.)

Southern = 1   North central = 2

Western = 3   Northeast = 4

Residence

Rural (<2500) = 1   Urban (>2500) = 2

Occupation

Professional/Technical = 6

Managerial/Official/Clerical/Sales = 5

Craftsmen/Foremen (Skilled labor) = 4

Not in labor force = 3

Operatives/Service workers/Farmers and Farm managers (Semiskilled labor) = 2

Farm laborers, Farm foremen, and Laborers (Unskilled labor) = 1

Age

16–17 = 1	25–34 = 4	55–64 = 7	75–79 = 10	90–94 = 13
18–19 = 2	35–44 = 5	65–69 = 8	80–84 = 11	95–99 = 14
20–24 = 3	45–54 = 6	70–74 = 9	85–89 = 12	>100 = 15

Education (years of school)

0–7 = 1	12 = 4
8 = 2	13–15 = 5
9–11 = 3	16+ = 6

Note: **VIQ** = Verbal IQ; **PIQ** = Performance IQ; **FSIQ** = Full Scale IQ

Sources: Barona et al.[20] and Helmes;[21] extended age coding for use with persons over 74.

11.2.3 SOCIAL AND WORK HISTORY OF THE PATIENT

Another important aspect to take into account for choosing the relevant information that will permit establishment of a premorbid baseline of patients is information about their social, educational, family, and work history. Unfortunately, data on these aspects of the patient's life have generally been paltry and badly collected.

It is important to collect data regarding the patient's education (elementary school, high school, university, etc.) because this information can be useful in estimating the patient's characteristic level of functioning. Information concerning the characteristics of the physical environment that surrounds the patient can also become very relevant for providing clear data to explain, and even describe, the reasons subjects present the neurocognitive functioning that they show. These social data are important because determined alterations and/or manners of functioning have a greater incidence in one or another group of the population. Lifestyle differs depending upon the social environment in which a person has developed. In general, people who come from lower socioeconomic backgrounds are more likely to practice activities that put their health at risk than are people who come from higher socio-economic backgrounds. This has its consequences in terms of cognitive deterioration. Thus, the level of cognitive development is influenced as well by the social environment from which a person comes, with variables such as a rural or urban living environment (in the past or currently), characteristics of the dwelling, the number of people who live there together, and the type of relationship that they maintain with the patient, socioeconomic status of the family, siblings, etc.

By the same token, it is important to know if there is a family history of certain neurodegenerative disorders, because this can increase the risk for developing these disorders. Patients with a history of Alzheimer's disease in their families have an increased risk for developing this disorder.[22]

Work history is another of the factors that must be studied in detail. Daily exposure to certain toxic products (toluene, tricholoethylene, mercury, etc.) over a long period of time may produce significant cognitive impairments. Exposure can result in memory dysfunctions and other important deficits in cognitive functioning as part of a toxic encephalopathy syndrome, which is manifested in workers exposed to organic solvents.[23,24] Similar memory deficits were found by Iregren[25] in painters and/or workers exposed to solvents in the paint industry. Arlien-Soborg et al.[26] reported memory impairment in 50% of all subjects (housepainters) referred to their study because organic solvent intoxication or dementia was suspected.

A similar relationship has been found between mercury levels and memory performance. The work of Williamson et al.[27] demonstrates that impairments on tests of verbal paired associated learning have been found in subjects with long-term exposure to mercury. In the same way, Uzzell and Oler[28] found evidence of impairment on visual nonverbal memory tasks in a group of dental workers with elevated mercury levels.

Some neurotoxic effects may take time to evolve and can exacerbate preexisting nervous system dysfunction.[29] With long-term exposure to toxic substances, memory and concentration problems with diminished attention level and slow responses,[30] emotional liability, depression, sleep disturbances, and sensory/motor symptoms,[31] along with reasoning and problem-solving abilities impairment,[32] may be observed.

An exact localization of these personal, social, environmental, and labor variables of patients will permit placing them within a precise frame of reference, which at the same time will allow formulation of an adequate evaluation and, later, an individualized program of treatment.

11.3 SCIENTIFIC GUARANTEE OF NEUROPSYCHOLOGICAL EVALUATION IN ELDERLY ADULTS

Neuropsychological evaluation in elderly people should be conducted with scientific methods and procedures to guarantee the validity and reliability of the results that are obtained. The classic instruments of evaluation are tests, questionnaires, or specific techniques, relative to behavior, cognition, emotions and feelings, and the capacity for communication. The instruments of measure are systematic procedures for observing behavior and describing it with scientific guarantees that each instrument must possess to be reliable and valid. To guarantee the tests and the techniques that are used during the process of psychological and neuropsychological evaluation, standards for the construction of tests and instruments have been established.[33] The two main properties that the tests and the techniques of neuropsychological measure must possess are reliability and validity.

Reliability is an attempt to estimate the percentage of error, and refers to some form of consistency or stability in the values of the scores obtained in the tests. Reliability is an attempt to know the proportion of variance that is due to extraneous and unstable influences. Reliability can be defined as the ability of a test to elicit a stable performance from the subject in the absence of outside influences.[34]

Validity in clinical neuropsychological research is related to findings that scores derived from a test can accurately distinguish brain-impaired individuals from non-impaired individuals as well as a statistical relation found between scores on a neuropsychological test and the results of a medical neurodiagnostic procedure such as postmortem surgery or computed tomography (CT) scans.[34]

11.4 ASSESSMENT OF INTELLECTUAL FUNCTIONING

This section is fundamentally concerned with evaluation of IQ. In the later years of the 20th century the concept of IQ has been controversial, and it has been suggested that it is not very useful.[35,36] It is argued that evaluation of the intellectual processes and the concept of intelligence itself should be revised. However, it is a fact that intelligence is still evaluated with traditional concepts and instruments worldwide. Because of this, the following sections introduce the most widely used classic intruments for the evaluation of intelligence and its deterioration.

11.4.1 THE WECHSLER ADULT INTELLIGENCE SCALES

The Wechsler Adult Intelligence Scale (WAIS) is a classic and is one of the most widely used intelligence scales worldwide. It has the advantage that there is an ample amount of literature referring to elderly people included in this test. However, the first standardization sample[37] ranged only from age 17 to 64 years. Subsequently, these data have been amplified by different authors in samples older than 65.

This scale can be used with elderly patients except in cases of very severely impaired elderly people. The WAIS uses the IQ concept, with Verbal and Performance Scales, providing measures of Full-scale (FSIQ), Verbal (VIQ), and Performance (PIQ). The WAIS-R, WAIS-III, and WAIS use the same procedure. Some of these scales take into account age differentials in the computation of the IQ scores, although different authors have added age corrections for the range scores of different groups. WAIS-R norms have been developed for older adults and are available for ages 56 to 66 to 88+.[38]

Caution must be taken when interpreting the scores of subjects aged 65 and older, particularly in the Performance Scale tests because scores tend to run higher in this group than in those of other representative groups of elderly subjects.[39] WAIS and WAIS-R norms for the 55-and-over age groups were based on small population samples.

Heaton et al.[40] included the WAIS in a normative project that involved normative data, *T*-scores, presented by age group (20 to 34, 75 to 80) and other groupings (gender and education). Along the same lines, Ryan et al.[41] present an age-corrected WAIS-R score for persons age 80 and older.

Albert and Moss[42] suggested a *classic age pattern*, consisting of a selective decline on Performance Scales at the sixth decade, and a small decline on Verbal Scales until the eighth decade.

A new version of the Wechsler scale, the WAIS-III,[43] provides a comprehensive measure of general intellectual function and generates index scores reflecting Verbal Comprehension, Perceptual Organization, Working Memory, and Processing Speed.[44] This scale bases the scores obtained for older patients in population-based normative data.

Different abbreviated versions of the WAIS, made up of selected subtest/items to estimate FSIQ, have been developed. There is a Wechsler Abbreviated Scale of Intelligence,[45] designed to measure general intellectual functioning in limited testing time. It consists of four tests: Similarities, Vocabulary, Block Design, and Reasoning. The administration of all four tests, WAIS-4, allows for an estimation of the classical IQ (VIQ, PIS, and FSIQ), whereas the administration of the Vocabulary and Matrix Reasoning alone, WAIS-2, allows for an estimation of the FSIQ. Normative data are available ranging from the age 6 to 89.

This test must not be used alone. In older adults it can be used for detecting subtle changes in high functioning in subjects without obvious deficits. It is especially useful for tracking changes in general intellectual functions in the context of a more comprehensive evaluation.

There are different approaches to the interpretation of performance on the WAIS. The first is the comparison between subtest score levels; the second is the examination of the variability within a scale; and the third is determining Verbal and Performance IQ discrepancy. The first and second are known as intersubtest and intrasubtest scatters. Fuld[46] identified in older populations a score pattern that was characteristic of disorders affecting brain function (Alzheimer's disease, cholinergic deficits, etc). This author, using the age-corrected scale scores, identified a profile $A > B > C < D$. (*A* is determined by summing the scores for Information and Vocabulary then dividing by 2; *B* is determined by summing the scores for Similarities and Digit Span, then dividing by 2; *C* is determined by summing the scores for Digit Symbol and Block Design, then dividing by 2; and *D* is the score of Object Assembly.)

11.4.2 TEST OF GENERAL INTELLIGENCE

Another task widely used to assess intelligence is Raven's Progressive Matrices. This test does not require verbalization, skilled abilities, and is not timed. There are three different forms available: Standard, Colored, and Advanced. However, only the two first provide scores for elderly persons.

The Standard Progressive Matrices[47] consist of 60 different items divided in five forms (A to E) involving different principles of matrix transformation. The task consists of a set of visual patterns in which each item contains a pattern problem at the top with a part missing. Below each item are alternative solutions (6 for forms A and B, and 8 for forms C to E). The difficulty increases in each form from item 1 to item 12. Scores for ages ranging from 6.5 to 70 years are provided.

Spreen and Strauss[48] noted that very old people cannot solve more than the two first forms, and the first items (easier) on the others. Negative correlations between the scores for this task and age have been observed.[49]

The colored version[50] is the shortest and simplest. In this task there are 36 items divided into three forms. The task is similar to that of the standard version but is printed in color. Percentile scores are provided in the manual for persons aged 65 to 85.

11.5 ASSESSMENT OF ATTENTIONAL PROCESSES

The evaluation of attention processes is important to include in all of the neurological and neuropsychological explorations in elderly patients, because, when attentional problems exist, it is possible that other cognitive functions are affected as well. The attention span is one of the psychophysiological mechanisms essential to the operation of the rest of the cognitive functions.[51] For example, if attention capacity is compromised there is no normal memory.

There are few tests with normative data for evaluating attention. Among the ones available, the authors recommend those that their team usually uses: evaluation of the attention mechanisms (simple attention) and the evaluation of vigilance, two subtests of the Seville Neuropsychological Test Battery (BNS).[52]

The assessment of attention is fundamental because attention is one of the processes that affects neurologically damaged patients first. It plays an important role in all the cognitive processes given that psychological functions consume attention. Attentional deficits can affect the processes of memory, reasoning, language, executive functioning, among others. Thus, it is necessary to obtain data on the functioning of this mechanism in the course of neuropsychological assessment of neurological patients.

Attention tests should be simple. Attentional mechanisms are assessed in a series of tasks measuring alertness and vigilance through efficacy in perceptual and motor speed and reaction time. The tasks are a computerized version of classical letter cancellation, divided into subtest of simple attention (tonic alertness) and a subtest of conditioned attention (phasic alertness).

In the subtests, the task consists of the patient pressing the space bar on the keyboard each time the letter O, and no other letter, appears in the center of the computer screen. In the first subtest the patient only has to pay attention to the appearance of the letter O for a predetermined time. This subtest measures patients' capacity for simple attention or tonic alertness, their selective visual capacity, and their perceptive and motor speed. This task determines the minimum attention needed to carry out other cognitive processes.

The second subtest is basically similar to the first, with a simple modification. The patient is still to press the space bar when the letter O appears, but only when the O is immediately preceded by the letter X. This is a task of sustained attention and vigilance to a monotonous task. The capacity to attend requires the frontal use of the activation/inhibition mechanism.

Using both attention subtests, of the BNS, Tellado et al.[53] presented data on the evolution of attentional deficits in patients with different types of cerebral defects and found significant statistical differences ($p < 0.05$) in all the variables studied in the two tests except in response time for simple attention and number of errors of conditioned attention. These data indicated the sensitivity of these subtests for registering how attentional mechanisms are affected even when a short time (6 to 9 months) has passed between test and retest. In conclusion, these two subtests, together with the identification of color while ignoring the content, are the most sensitive for detecting defects in attentional mechanisms.

11.6 ASSESSMENT OF MEMORY PROCESSES

Memory is one of the cognitive functions that is most easily affected by neurological damage, and difficulty with memory is one of the indications that an older patient should be referred for neuropsychological examination. Given that memory is not a one-dimensional concept, during the process of neuropsychological evaluation the following aspects of memory, at a minimum, must be evaluated: working memory, capacity to consolidate and store new information; phenomenon of contamination and sources of memory; and memory for everyday activities.

The main tests usually employed for the evaluation of problems with memory in elderly people are evaluation of memory and learning processes, Functional Organic Memory Questionnaire, and the Wechsler Memory Scale–R.

11.6.1 ASSESSMENT OF MEMORY PROCESSES AND LEARNING

Most classical tests used for neuropsychological assessment of verbal memory and learning processes consisted of presenting to the patient an extensive list of words that they are required to store and later repeat using one or more trials. Based on this idea, Luria developed his "Memory Curve"[54] as a test to assess short-term memory. This test was later adapted by Christensen[55] for assessment of learning processes, and the BNS contains a revision of the "Memory Curve" test. In this version, new indexes on learning processes and different indexes on memory have been added. These are adapted to the computer for administration and correction, and can be interpreted qualitatively and quantitatively. Patients must remember a list of ten words that are spoken by the evaluator at a rhythm of one word per second. (Previously, patients have chosen the words they think they will be able to remember in each of the attempts so that, in the end, the degree of awareness patients have about their own mnesic functioning can be assessed.) This task is repeated 10 times, regardless of whether the patient is or is not able to remember all the words. At 30 min after finalizing the last attempt, patients are asked to say all the words they remember without the evaluator saying the words previously. In this way, information on the degree of consolidation of the patient's memory is obtained. Also, indexes are obtained on the effects of primacy and recency, mnesic contamination, memory volume, mnesic gain, and others (Table 11.2).

TABLE 11.2
Memory Processes Assessed by the Memory Curve in BNS

Index of Real Memory	Memory volume
Index of Total Memory	Memory of volume including confabulated and/or repeated material
Index of Contamination	Quantity of remembered material but not real
Index of Confabulations	Numbers of invented words
Index of Repetitions	Number of repeated words
Index of Adherence	Number of words repeated in two or more consecutive trials
Index of Aspiration	Volume of memory the subject esteems having
Index of Self-Knowledge	Difference between the Index of Aspiration and Real Memory
Index of Primacy	Better memory of the first words of the list
Index of Recency	Better memory of the first words of the list
Index of Learning 1	Difference of learning between the final and central part of the tests
Index of Learning 2	Difference of learning between the central and initial part of the test
Index of Learning 3	Difference of learning between the final and initial part of the test
Index of Consolidation	Percentage of equal words remembered in the last three trials
Index of Mnesic Gain	Difference between what one remembers in the last three trials and the first

11.6.2 FUNCTIONAL ORGANIC MEMORY QUESTIONNAIRE

The Functional Organic Memory Questionnaire (FOM)[56] is a brief questionnaire for evaluating functional organic memory disorders that is used in daily clinical neurological practice to detect patients with memory disorders easily and quickly.

The task introduces a new methodology for evaluating functional memory disorders that requires the tester to ask family members or close relatives about the activities of daily living of the patient in a natural context. The family member or close relative gives his or her opinion concerning the intensity or frequency with which a certain behavior is applicable to the patient.

The questionnaire contains 23 items requiring yes/no answers, and scored 1 or 0 (yes = 1 / no = 0). The sum of the positively scored items grouped in each factor gives the score for each factor. The authors observed six factors: (1) *working memory* (related to the volume of information the patient can process simultaneously), (2) *source memory* (related to the spatial-temporal context in which the information is acquired), (3) *recognition memory* (related to the capacity to identify people, places, and knowledge as familiar), (4) *prospective memory* (the capacity to carry out plans and preestablished programs of behavior), (5) *consolidation memory* (the capacity to form long-term memory), and (6) procedural memory (memory expressed by changes in performance or by acquisition of habits, actions, and skills as a result of previous experience). Age scores ranging from 18 to 85 are available.

11.6.3 WECHSLER MEMORY SCALES — REVISED

The use of the Wechsler Memory Scales (WMS-I, WMS-II, WMS-R, and WMS-III) permit the evaluation of memory via various indexes (in WMS-I and WMS-II only a Memory Quotient was obtained). Through the use of these indexes the level of deterioration can be determined.

In the first two versions (WMS-I and WMS-II), important slopes were observed (see Lezak[9]) that made publication of a new version of the test necessary. The main advantage of the WMS is the brief time needed for administration and the amount of data collected on performance relating to a variety of neurological conditions.

The revised version contains nine tests, of which six originated in prior versions. The nine tests are (1) Information and Orientation (I/O); (2) Mental Control; (3) Digit Span; (4) Logical Memory–Revised (LM-R); (5) Verbal Paired Associates (Verbal PA); (6) Visual Reproduction–Revised (VR-R); (7) Figural Memory; (8) Visual Paired Associates (Visual PA); and (9) Delayed Recall of some prior subtest.

The authors developed five indexes derived from two or more of the 12 raw scores from all of the tests generated and their delayed trials, with the exception of I/O. These indexes are Verbal Memory (VBMI); Visual Memory (VSMI); General Memory (GMI); Attention and Concentration (ACI); and Delayed Recall (DRI).

By using methods developed by Cullum et al.,[57] sensitivity to age effects was studied. Comparing two groups of people with different ages (young vs. old, 50 to 70; old vs. old, 70 to 90 years old), the authors found that forgetting increased greatly with age on immediate and delayed trials of Visual Reproduction, Logical Memory, Verbal Paired Associates, and delayed trials of Visual Paired Associates.

The recent revised and updated version of this test, the WMS-III,[58] consists of six primary tests — (1) Logical Memory, (2) Verbal Paired Associated, (3) Letter-Number Sequencing, (4) Faces, (5) Family Pictures, and (6) Spatial Span — and five optionals — (1) Information and Orientation, (2) Word List, (3) Mental Control, (4) Digit Span, and (5) Visual Reproduction. This new version includes population-based norms for ages from 16 to 89 presented for the index scores and for measures derived from the primary and optional tests, facilitating the evaluation of older adults.

With the publication of this revised version, which includes these new indexes and new normative data for elderly people, the study of different mechanisms of memory can be undertaken with more precision than could be done with previous versions.

11.7 ASSESSMENT OF LANGUAGE

Language functions seem unlikely to deteriorate with normal aging. After the age of 70 some aspects of language may be more vulnerable: naming, verbal fluency, and semantic organization. Aphasia and other language disorders may be observed in aged clinical populations. Some language problems may be related to deficits in memory, which makes it necessary, when examining elderly patients, to know their memory status. In general, a screening of the linguistic capacity of the patient must be done. To begin with, language expression ability must be assessed. This deals with knowing if the patient is capable of describing an object in detail, and his or her verbal fluency, and capacity for generative naming in a semantic category. As well, linguistic comprehension must be evaluated. It must be known if the patient is capable of following commands, responding to comparative questions, repetition, or reading comprehension.

Among the most important tests that can be used to evaluate language deficits in elderly people are the verbal fluency measures and the Boston Naming Test.

11.7.1 Verbal Fluency Measures

In general, these measures attempt to determine if the patient experiences changes in the speed of verbal production. Some aphasic alterations occur with a large decline in verbal production, especially in word generation, such as in the case of the patients diagnosed with a dementia, particularly one of a cortical origin. Age, among other variables (sex, education, etc.), has a marked influence on performance on these tests.[59]

In addition to speech, fluency in writing can also be affected, as well as fluency in reading, even though, normally, low verbal fluency affects all three areas. In general, writing fluency with aging tends to slow earlier than speech fluency.[60]

Verbal fluency is usually evaluated by counting the number of words that a patient is capable of saying in a given category within a determined interval of time. Generally, word-naming tests are used. Estes[61] noted that successful performance in these tasks depends in part on the ability to organize output in terms of clusters of words that are meaningfully related to each other. Performance also involves short-term memory (working memory) because it is necessary to remember what words have been said. Estes pointed out that these tests provide a good measure for surmising how the patient organizes his or her thinking.

The Controlled Oral Word Association Test (COWAT)/FAS is widely used; the authors' group uses the Spanish version, which is called PAC.[48] The test consists of six independent attempts, each of 1 min in duration, in which the patients must say as many words in a given category as they can without repeating any words or using the same word with a different suffix. The first three lists include words that begin with a given letter (F, A, and S, if in English; P, A, or C, if in Spanish); the last three should list things according to more specific categories (animals, fruits, and proper nouns). The score is determined by the total number of words generated, as well as the average score of all the mentioned words in the six attempts that are adjusted as a function of the age, gender, and years of formal education of the subject. In addition, the number and nature of the errors made during word fluency exercises can also be informative, particularly perseverative (repetitions of words or variations previously generated) and intrusion errors (beginning a trial correctly but generating one or several items outside of the specified criteria). The first case may reflect cognitive inflexibility and suggest a possible deficit in memory storage; the second may suggest that the patient has difficulty maintaining the response set appropriately, which may indicate an executive dysfunction.

Kozora and Cullum[62] have found that age changes are minimal in letter fluency, but age-related decline is higher for category fluency, fluctuating according to the specific category used. Lucas et al. [63] provide normative data for FAS letter fluency, with ranges for 55 to 97 years of age; for category fluency normative data are separated depending on the category used.

This technique of evaluation of verbal fluency by means of the FAS/PAC test is very sensitive to cerebral dysfunction in general. In all the processes related to the appearance of dementia, a reduction in the ability and fluency for producing words has been observed that reflects different etiologies. Thus, in some patients diagnosed with Parkinson's or Huntington's disease the problem in generating words depends on their low mental flexibility and has been related to deficiencies in memory retrieval mechanisms,[64] whereas in Alzheimer's disease it has been hypothesized that the problem reflects the breakdown and loss of semantic memory associated with this disorder.[65]

11.7.2 BOSTON NAMING TEST[66]

This instrument provides information concerning the ease and accuracy of word retrieval and indicates vocabulary and expressive speech levels. It is relatively brief and easily administered.

The test consists of 60 drawings of items ranging from common items at the beginning to uncommon ones at the end. The patient is encouraged to give the names of the objects. If the patient is incapable of naming an object within 20 s, the examiner gives a semantic cue; if patient is still unable to produce the name within another 20 s, then a phonetic cue is provided. The examiner must note how many cues are given (semantic or phonetic) and how many responses are correct. After six consecutive failures, the test is discontinued. The total raw score includes the correct responses plus correct responses after cues are provided. To compute the patient's total score it is important that the examiner analyze the nature of the effects of cueing to have a more complete view of the patient's deficit.

The scores obtained by Ross et al.[67] indicate no appreciable decline until the late 70s, but standard deviations increase steadily, indicating greater variability in the normal older population. Other authors[68] found different responses increasing with aging, such as comments about an item or the test, circumlocutions describing the picture, and responses to the dotted lines around the picture stimulus. The educational variable is important in older patients when using this test.

11.8 ASSESSMENT OF EXECUTIVE FUNCTIONING

Age-related declines in executive functioning have been extensively reported by different authors;[69–74] it has been noted that prefrontal (43%) and orbit frontal (25%) areas have greater reductions in volume than parietal (11%) and occipital (13%) areas. As expected, increased age is associated with poorer performance on all executive tasks. Although psychomotor speed may be involved in executive functioning in aged people, in a study by Keys and White[75] it was found that age accounted for a unique and significant proportion of variance in executive performance after controlling for psychomotor speed. Their work suggests that age has an effect on prefrontally mediated executive abilities that cannot be explained solely by psychomotor slowing.

Among the principal measures of executive functioning that the authors use are (1) The Stroop Test; (2) The Tower of Hanoi–Seville; and (3) The Trail Making Test; and (4) Digits Backward.

11.8.1 ASSESSMENT OF NEUROCOGNITIVE INTERFERENCE; STROOP EFFECT

Each of the functional cerebral systems contains a highly specialized neural network with a well-controlled system of balance between activation and inhibitory mechanisms that causes some of them to be active while others remain either deactivated or inhibited to maintain an optimal level of effectiveness and precision in the different cognitive functions allowing for proper functioning.[76] The mechanisms that are involved in this double process of activation/inhibition are various: the most important ones are the frontal lobe, which plays a central role in the inhibition of irrelevant information; the prefrontal dorsolateral area, which performs an important role in continuous maintenance of the information that recorded responses require; and the basal ganglia, which are implicated in the inhibition of some automatic processes.

The BNS, includes a computerized adaptation of the classic Stroop's Words and Colors Test,[77] which was originally designed to study perceptive interference. The specialists who have presented the most relevant research carried out with this task agree that it can be used to study mechanisms of divided attention, of functioning, of activation/inhibition mechanisms, and also the functioning of neurocognitive interference.

In this test, eight subtests are used to observe the described mechanisms:

1. Identification of monochromatic words
2. Identification of colored blocks
3. Identification of color ignoring the content (both eyes)
4. Identification of content ignoring the color (both eyes)
5. Identification of color ignoring the content (left eye)
6. Identification of content ignoring the color (left eye)
7. Identification of color ignoring the content (right eye)
8. Identification of content ignoring the color (right eye)

The first and second subtests introduce patients to the mechanics of this test and evaluate their visual capacity and minimum reading levels, necessary to performance of the rest of the subtests. The third and fourth subtests evaluate the Stroop effect; the patient only need respond to one of the stimulus characteristics (color of the writing or the word written), inhibiting the other. In the last four subtests, the same procedure is followed as for those previously mentioned, depending on whether the answer requested is the color in which the words are written, omitting their content, or the word itself, ignoring the color in which it is written. The only difference between these subtests is that they use monocular vision, the fifth and sixth covering the right eye, and the seventh and eighth covering the left eye.

The results obtained by Tellado et al.[53] in this subtest coincide with those described by León-Carrión and Barroso,[78] showing that, in cerebral lesions in the frontal area, a serious problem exists in the mechanisms of activation/inhibition observed in this test that are associated with the frontal lobe, which affects regulation of cognition and behavior.

11.8.2 EVALUATION OF COGNITIVE FUNCTIONS ASSOCIATED WITH THE FRONTAL LOBE: THE TOWER OF HANOI–SEVILLE

A review of the literature specializing in problem solving, planning, prospective, control, and executive functions associates these functions with the frontal lobe because of the way behavior is affected when these areas of the brain, especially the prefrontal areas, are injured.[9,78] The classical tests that have been used to assess these functions are classification tasks like the Wisconsin Card Sorting Test,[79] category tests like the Category Test,[80] or maze tasks like the Porteus Maze Test.[81] At present, specialized clinical neuropsychologists agree that very structured tests are not sensitive to the deficits observed when assessing behavior directed toward a goal; they defend the use of less-structured tests in which the subject must work actively to discover the rules and principles that regulate the task.[51]

In keeping with the principle of using less structure, together with ease of correction and interpretation, a computerized version of the Tower of Hanoi[82] has been developed for use within the BNS; thus computerized version is called the Tower of Hanoi/Seville.[51,83] The task consists of a transformation problem in which the subject has to reach a final goal through the execution of a series of nonroutine movements in which strategies of ordered planning and abilities of problem solving must be applied. Subjects should establish a plan to then execute and reach the correct solution. This plan should include a global solution that, at the same time, is broken down into various subsolutions that should be sequenced in time to reach the final goal. All the abilities of directed planning needed to solve a complex problem, which are seriously affected in lesions of the frontal lobe after suffering a traumatic brain injury (TBI), can be observed executing the Tower of Hanoi/Seville test.[84]

The test contains three parallel pegs numbered from left to right from 1 to 3. On peg 1 there are different disks of different size and color (from 3 to 5 disks depending on the examiner's choice) forming a pyramid with the largest at the bottom and the smallest on top. The objective of the task is to move the disks by pressing a key on the computer corresponding to the number appearing on the peg until a tower identical with the first is formed on peg 3. The Seville version of the Tower of Hanoi presents two types of administration: A and B. In B, the subject is told the principles and rules of the task. Administration A best describes the functioning of problem solving since the subject must discover the rules and principles of the task to solve it correctly.

Barroso Martín et al.,[84] using this subtest of BNS, have obtained significant statistical differences ($p > 0.05$) in the four variables studied when comparing the results of 20 patients affected with TBI to frontal lobe areas with those of another group that presented with damage to another cerebral area. This study showed that, as a group, subjects with frontal lesions have a more limited capacity to use problem-solving strategies, even at a much less sophisticated level, than patients with lesions not in the frontal area, which is translated in a greater deterioration of executive function and of frontal reasoning.

11.8.3 TRAIL MAKING TEST

Developed by the U.S. Army, this test has been widely used since its publication in 1944 because of its great simplicity of application and interpretation. Basically, with this test an attempt is made to evaluate visual, conceptual, and visuomotor tracking with a motor speed and agility component. However, the different tasks demonstrate that, to these abilities, this test is of great clinical value for providing information on how effectively a patient responds to a visual array of varied complexity, follows a sequence mentally, deals with more than one stimulus at a time, and/or has flexibility in shifting the course of an ongoing activity.

This test is divided in two parts, A and B. In part A, using a pencil and working as quickly as possible, the patient must connect, in ascending numerical order and without lifting the pencil from the paper, circles with numbers inside. In part B, the patient must connect, in the same manner, circles with both numbers and letters inside, alternating numbers and letters, in logical ascending order ($1 - A - 2 - B - 3 - C$, etc.). The examiner notes the time taken and errors made by the patient, pointing out to the patient when an error occurs, and encouraging the patient to work as quickly as possible. Separate measures are obtained in parts A and B, computing total errors and time consumed.

There is an oral Trail Making Test available for attention and mental tracking evaluation in patients with known vision or motor ability impairments.[85]

Both parts of the test are very sensitive to the cognitive deterioration that is observed in dementia processes. Further, the time necessary for doing part B of the test slows with age,[86] and depression interacts with the slowing effect in such a way that depressed elderly patients require a disproportionate amount of time to finish the task.

The Trail Making Test is a very sensitive instrument for assessing brain injury. Part B of this test is associated with a spatial component that requires logical and sequential thought in greater measure than part A; it also assesses the efficiency in the conceptual changes when alternating numbers and letters. The score obtained in part B of this test is also associated with attentional functioning mediated by the frontal lobe.

11.8.4 DIGITS BACKWARD

This task is part of the mental tracking test in which neuropsychologists try to assess how many bits of information a patient can attend to at the same time by repeating the sequence in reverse order. The test involves sequences of complex mental operations, and when a patient receives a low score, a general attention deficit may be implicated. The task involves simultaneous operation of memory and reversing operations, in which temporal ordering is operating under frontal lobe supervision. Deficits in mental flexibility and concrete thinking cause patients to be unable to understand the instructions, which is the first capacity that declines when mental deterioration occurs.

The Digits Backward number sequence from the Wechsler Memory Scale consists of two different sequences of digits, comprising two to eight and two to seven digits. The patient first hears the numbers read aloud, and subsequently has to repeat them in exactly reverse order. Working memory plays an important role in reverse digit span tasks given that a few bits of data must be retained during a brief interval of time as their order is being correctly reversed.

The scores in this test typically decrease about one point during the seventh decade of life.[9]

11.9 ASSESSMENT OF THE VISUOPERCEPTIVE AND VISUOCONSTRUCTIVE PROCESSES

The phenomenon of visual inattention or negligence implies omitting visual stimuli in the left visual field that depend directly on the lesions produced in the right hemisphere, which also tend to coincide with the lesions found in the posterior areas. Another type of alteration exists, called hemi-inattention, that is manifested as defects in some of the visual semifields, which is not necessarily classified as negligence. Another phenomenon is hemianopsia, which refers to a visual defect that causes blindness for half the visual field. These alterations are made evident when subjects are asked to focus their attention on a certain point while they are presented with stimuli in each of the existing visual quadrants/hemifields.[7]

For assessment of problems of inattention and hemianopsia, a letter cancellation test is administered with a tachistoscopic methodology adapted to the computer. In this task, patients must keep their eyes fixed on a white point that appears at the center of the monitor, while different letters appear in the center of each of the four quadrants into which the computer screen is divided. Patients should look at the white spot in the center without shifting their eyes, and should press the space bar only when the letter O appears in one of the quadrants. Three subtests make up this module:

1. Subtest of tachistoscopic attention for both eyes
2. Subtest of tachistoscopic attention of the right eye
3. Subtest of tachistoscopic attention of the left eye

The assessment procedure in these three tests is the same, with the exception of the type of vision used in each. In the first, subjects perform the test with binocular vision, whereas in the following two they can use only monocular vision. The results obtained in the study by Tellado et al.[53] showed a clear tendency in the patients studied to commit a greater number of errors and omissions and to identify a lower number of elements in the tachistoscopic tests than in the BNS.

11.10 ASSESSMENT OF SENSORY AND MOTOR SKILLS

In general, to assess the sense of touch, techniques can be employed that present simple recognition or discrimination tactile problems. Tactile sensation can be evaluated by asking patients, whose eyes are closed, to indicate where they feel sharp pressure when the pressure is applied to a point or simultaneously applied to two points.

One important part of this assessment is stereognosis or recognition of objects by touch. In this technique, patients are asked to close their eyes and then to recognize common objects by touch first in one hand, then in the other. The results obtained in the recognition of objects through this test should present no errors, since a single error could indicate that this function may be altered.

To obtain an adequate evaluation of this function and to ensure that it is intact, Luria[54] presents a procedure with four consecutive steps. In the first step an object is laid in the patient's hand. If the patient is unable to identify it, the second step then consists of moving the object in different positions in the patient's hand. The third step, if the patient still cannot identify the object, consists of choosing, by means of touch, an item that is similar to the one the patient cannot identify and distinguishing it from other items. In step four, if the patient continues to be unable to recognize the object, the same object is used, but it is placed in the other hand.

Another way used to obtain information regarding tactile recognition is the technique of writing letters or numbers on the palms of both of the patient's hands and/or on the fingertips.

The preceding tests form sections of batteries that permit a very precise and detailed neuropsychological evaluation of these functions. Similarly, the Halstead–Reintan battery contains independent tests for evaluation of both sensory and motor skills.

The Tactual Performance Test is included in this battery. In this test, subjects, eyes covered, are given ten geometric figures that they must fit into the appropriate hollows on a board (the Goddard–Segin board). This task begins with patients using the dominant hand, followed by the nondominant hand, and ending with both hands. Once finished, patients are asked to draw the figures that they remember, indicating their position on the board. The score obtained evaluates the time used for all three attempts and the number of correct figures recorded and drawn in the correct position. In this task, motor speed, tactile discrimination, coordination of movements, manual dexterity, spatial configuration, psychomotor coordination, and the ability to remember perceived objects by touch and localization are assessed.

The Seashore Rhythm Test is also included in the Halstead–Reintan battery of tests. It consists of 30 elements of sounds with two patterns in each. The patient listens and must distinguish whether the patterns are the same or different from each other. The primary focus of this task is to evaluate auditory (not verbal) perception and the capacity to discriminate between auditory sequences.

Also included is the Speech Sound Perception Test. This test is divided into six different parts, each of which is composed of ten elements. For each one of these elements, patients hear a nonsense word that they must pick out from the other four when these words are presented in written form. The primary focus of this task is to assess audioverbal perception.

The Finger Oscillation Test (Finger Tapping Test) is the primary test for the evaluation of motor skills. In this test, the motor speed and psychomotor coordination differential is evaluated in both hands using the index fingers. In this test, 10-s attempts with the dominant hand are made followed by the same with the non-dominant hand.

The Senso-Perceptive Examination entails four tests that have already been described in previous sections. These tests are used to assess finger agnosia, skin-writing recognition, sensory extinction in tactile, auditory, and visual modalities, and figure recognition by touch.

The last test in the Halstead–Reintan battery is the Lateral Dominance Examination, in which ocular, manual, and patellar dominance is examined. The abilities of the patient's dominant and nondominant sides are determined as well.

Age-graded norms and scores are available in Heaton et al.[40] and D'Elia et al.[38]

The Grooved Pegboard is one of the most commonly used tests for measuring manual dexterity. In this task, the patient inserts pegs into a 5×5 matrix of holes on a small board. The holes are angled in different directions. The score is determined by the time taken to complete the task with the dominant and then with the non-dominant hand. Heaton et al.[40] observed that age appears to have some effect on task performance.

Another test battery that includes tests for evaluating sensory and motor functioning are those of Luria/Christensen. Because this battery permits a far more flexible and personalized assessment, the qualitative approach of this test battery is particularly appropriate when evaluating elderly patients. The battery comprises a group of tasks that lead to a detailed qualitative assessment of higher psychological functions. It does not provide normative data in its publication, which allows for flexibility in its application and in results analysis.

The test is made up of ten sections.[87] The first is dedicated to the study of the motor functions. It begins with the praxes as an initial step toward the analysis of the most basic components of the motor act and ends with the more complex forms of praxia. Subsections are included that study the motor functions of the hands, oral praxes, and the verbal regulation of the motor act. Each of these subsections is divided into different parts to afford a detailed analysis of each grouped component.

The second section of this test is concerned with acoustic-motor organization, the investigation of which comprises two series of tasks. In the first series, concerning perception and reproduction of pitch relationships, the patient must discern whether the pairs of tones presented are identical or if there are differences between them. In the second series, concerned with the perception and reproduction of rhythmic patterns, an analysis is made of the measure to which the patient is capable of perceiving the groups of signals that are presented and the motor execution of rhythmic groups.

The third section evaluates the higher cutaneous functions and the kinestesic functions. This section is divided into three parts: cutaneous sensations, muscular and articulatory sensations, and stereognosis. All these tests are conducted with the patients' eyes covered. Some of the activities described in other sections (identifying numbers written in the palms of the hands, identifying by sense of touch objects that are placed in the hand, identifying where one has been touched, and so forth) are used.

The remaining sections of this test battery are dedicated to the evaluation of the higher visual functions, language (expressive and receptive), and memory, among others.

11.11 ASSESSMENT OF AFFECTIVE, EMOTIONAL, AND PERSONALITY PROBLEMS

Traditionally, the assessment of emotional aspects has not been included as part of neuropsychological evaluation, although currently it has become an essential part of rehabilitation programs. Therefore, BNS includes a specific test for the assessment of emotional changes presented by neurological patients: the neurological-related changes of emotions and personality inventory (NECHAPI).

NECHAPI is a clinical tool especially designed for observing emotional changes that appear most frequently in patients who have suffered TBI, cerebrovascular disease, brain tumors, and neurological alterations. This inventory contains 40 items that family members must rank from 1 to 5 depending on how they feel the item defines the patient (5 is indicative of high frequency of occurrence and 1 is the minimum frequency). Intermediate scores also exist. The family member should score each item twice, the first time referring to the patient before suffering the neurological problem, and the second time referring to the patient's present state.

The 40 items of this test are grouped into 5 factors that collect the scores observed by family members in the patient (Table 11.3).

According to a study done by Madrazo Lazcano et al. in 1999,[88] the changes observed in patients who have suffered severe TBI showed significant changes in emotional and behavioral aspects, according to the reference values of NECHAPI.[89] In this study, they observed that emotional vulnerability is the factor that most frequently showed changes in this type of patient; 75% of the patients become more emotionally vulnerable according to the reference values of the tests. It also found that the irritability factor changed in a high percentage of the patients, being significant in 56.25%. Data indicated that the factor of sensation seeking decreased by an average of 23% in these patients and was significant in 50% of them (Table 11.4).

TABLE 11.3
The Five Emotional Dimensions Assessed by NECHAPI

1. *Irritability*: High scores in this factor indicate a tendency to be more sensitive to offenses and therefore to interpret situations as threatening. It also indicates that reactions to apparently normal situations can be aggressive.
2. *Sensation seeking:* When high scores are seen in this factor, they usually refer to people who look to experience new feelings that may imply some type of danger. It has been observed that this factor was high in young people affected by TBI before suffering the accident.
3. *Emotional vulnerability*: People who have high scores in this factor tend to live their interpersonal relationships very intensely, are easily influenced, and have a tendency to get depressed and frustrated.
4. *Sociability*: This factor measures the number of social relationships the patient has. When scores are high they tend to be people with ease in social relations, who feel comfortable in situations when surrounded by people.
5. *Motivation:* A high score in this factor indicates difficulty in feeling motivation. Emotional coldness is also observed toward other people's proposals and thoughts.

TABLE 11.4
Neurologically Related Changes in Personality Inventory (NECHAPI)

Name: _____   Date: ____ / ____ / ____

Age: _____   Educational Level: _____   Sex: _____   Marital Status: _____

A B C D *

		LESS			MORE	
1.	Is usually a hot-blooded person	1	2	3	4	5
2.	Usually experiences everything very intensely	1	2	3	4	5
3.	Is difficult to calm down when he or she gets excited	1	2	3	4	5
4.	Has very strong emotions	1	2	3	4	5
5.	Sometimes behaves in a very cruel way	1	2	3	4	5
6.	Gets upset easily	1	2	3	4	5
7.	Is a violent person	1	2	3	4	5
8.	Normally engages in dangerous behavior	1	2	3	4	5
9.	Is usually in control of him or herself and his or her behavior	1	2	3	4	5
10.	Is easily annoyed	1	2	3	4	5
11.	Is a vulnerable person	1	2	3	4	5
12.	Is a very sensitive person	1	2	3	4	5
13.	Gets in a lot of trouble	1	2	3	4	5
14.	Is not afraid of anything	1	2	3	4	5
15.	Has a lot of friends	1	2	3	4	5
16.	Is involved in a lot of social activities	1	2	3	4	5
17.	In my opinion, drinks more than he or she should	1	2	3	4	5
18.	Probably takes drugs sometimes	1	2	3	4	5
19.	Likes to make other people suffer	1	2	3	4	5
20.	Is always on the lookout for new emotional experiences	1	2	3	4	5

TABLE 11.4 (CONTINUED)
Neurologically Related Changes in Personality Inventory (NECHAPI)

		LESS			MORE	
21.	Is fickle	1	2	3	4	5
22.	Doesn't offer explanations for what he/she does	1	2	3	4	5
23.	Is definitely shy	1	2	3	4	5
24.	Usually feels guilty about insignificant things	1	2	3	4	5
25.	Could be described as being on the sadistic side	1	2	3	4	5
26.	Does things as if he or she were fearless or unaware of danger	1	2	3	4	5
27.	Is always open to new experiences	1	2	3	4	5
28.	Is always looking for new sensations	1	2	3	4	5
29.	Never takes into account how his or her actions may have made other people feel	1	2	3	4	5
30.	Is not interested in very many things	1	2	3	4	5
31.	Is a hostile person	1	2	3	4	5
32.	Is a frustrated person	1	2	3	4	5
33.	Is a very negative person	1	2	3	4	5
34.	Is a depressive person	1	2	3	4	5
35.	Is capable of committing suicide	1	2	3	4	5
36.	Enjoys sex a lot	1	2	3	4	5
37.	Probably wouldn't mind any kind of sexual experience, no matter how strange	1	2	3	4	5
38.	Has a lot of sexual experience	1	2	3	4	5
39.	Is easily angered	1	2	3	4	5
40.	Has a strong desire to live	1	2	3	4	5

* A: Family members that live with the patient; B: Girl/boyfriend; committed relationship; C: Close friends; D: Neighbors, acquaintances, other: please specify.

Source: Courtesy of José León-Carrión, University of Seville, Spain, and Center for Brain Injury Rehabilitation (C.RE.CER).

11.12 ASSESSMENT OF DEMENTING PROCESSES

Between 10 to 15% of patients over the age of 65 experience at least mild dementia. Approximately 6% experience severe dementia,[90] and moderate to severe dementia occurs in 16% of individuals above the age of 79.[91] The concept of dementia is to be understood as a syndrome characterized by the decline, in relation to the patient's previous levels, of certain neurocognitive functions. The most frequent cause of dementia is Alzheimer's disease followed by cerebrovascular disease. The clinical situation of a patient suffering Alzheimer's disease must fit within certain characteristics. The patient should present a normal level of awareness; the dementia disorder must be acquired; it must persist over time; it must affect various cognitive functions; and finally, it should have noticeable repercussions (for review, see Chapter 15 on Dementia).

As few as 50% of dementia cases are diagnosed by physicians.[92] In the awareness phase, the family plays a key role in bringing the case to the physician's attention. The assessment phase carried out by physicians is another important step in the process, and it is very important to have complete criteria to make a correct first diagnosis. In the evaluation of a dementia process multiple symptoms will be observed. Nonetheless, the most common deficits are those of a neurocognitive nature. Generally, cognitive, psychological/behavioral, and functional symptoms are the three types of symptoms that will be observed in patients diagnosed with dementia.

11.12.1 COGNITIVE SYMPTOMS

Although not always blatant, cognitive symptoms are the first to appear. They are nonetheless the basis and the cause of both the functional disability and the subsequent deterioration of activities of daily living. Perhaps the most common and disabling symptoms are those that affect *memory*. The most useful tools for memory assessment have already been described in Section 11.6.

Another group of very characteristic symptoms, grouped under aphasic–apraxic–agnosic symptoms, affect *language*, *praxias*, and the *gnosias*. The principal strategies used in the evaluation of both language and gnosias have been described in the sections on language assessment and sensory and motor skills assessment. The praxes, the ability to carry out sequences of goal-oriented coordinated movements, are classified as follows:

Constructive praxias. Evaluated by means of copying from a simple model or figure.
Ideomotor praxias. Those movements made by means of orders or imitations, but in total absence of the imitated object.
Ideatory praxias. Actions that are carried out in an ordered sequence in the presence of the object to be imitated.

The praxia subtest from the Boston Battery of Tests[93] affords a very detailed assessment of both constructive and ideatory praxias.

Other functions that can be found to be altered are *orientation, attention, calculation, executive functioning*, and *thought capacity for judgment*. Specific tests have already been described in previous sections with regard to the evaluation of most of these alterations

11.12.2 PSYCHIATRIC AND BEHAVIORAL SYMPTOMS

This group of symptoms directly affects both the patients and their families. The quality of life of both will, to an important extent, be conditioned by these symptoms. Although the symptoms normally appear in the more advanced stages of the illness, they may also appear prematurely. These symptoms are very dysfunctional and are the primary cause for the hospitalization of affected patients.

Of the many symptoms that should be highlighted, delirium, hallucinations, personality changes, and, above all, depression are most important. Given that depression is the most frequent cause of confusion in disorders of a demential nature, its correct identification and etiology is paramount to achieving a differential diagnosis.

11.12.3 FUNCTIONAL ALTERATIONS

Functional alterations are derived from the interaction of the cognitive and behavioral alterations. The direct consequence of functional alterations is the inability to carry out everyday activities. The deficits in everyday activities are manifest from the onset of the dementia, first as small difficulties in the areas of work, social life, management of personal finances, and housework. These difficulties are easily compensated for. However, the alterations become more and more evident as the illness develops. The patient needs supervision and external help to carry out even the most basic daily activities. In the final stages, the patient becomes completely helpless and totally dependent on others.

There are several tests used to evaluate dementia symptoms. The Informant Interview,[94] known as the IQ CODE, provides general information regarding the patient's state in all areas in which some type of characteristic deterioration is anticipated. The test comprises 26 items with a possible score of 1 to 5 points each. The items seek to compare the patient's current state with that observed before deficits appeared. The maximum score, 5, represents maximum deterioration for each item.

The Barthel Index for Daily Living Activity is used to measure the degree of a patient's limitation in activities of daily living. Nine items are included that evaluate an array of abilities, including such activities as cooking and dressing to elimination and transfer. It is scored in a range of 0 to 10 points, where the maximum score coincides with the least incidence of symptoms.

The Blessed Scale of Deterioration[95] evaluates general deterioration in three areas. The first area concerns changes in activities of daily living and consists of eight point/no point items. This is followed by an evaluation of changes in habits in which eating and dressing habits and changes in bowel movements are taken into account. Items included in this area are scored from 0 to 3 points. Changes in personality and behavior is the third area evaluated in the Blessed Scale of Deterioration; 11 items are included in this area with a possible total of 28 points. As the score rises in this area, there is increasing certainty of deterioration.

Special mention should be made of the section that specifically evaluates for sadness and feeling dejected or discouraged, coming under the generic term of depression. The somatic symptoms (i.e., sleep problems, physical health concerns, etc.) and the cognitive symptoms (i.e., attention, memory, etc.) of depression are generally both present in older people. An accurate differential diagnosis must therefore be based on a multidimensional study.

There is certainly no lack of scales that can be used for this purpose. Two classic scales that stand out are the Beck Depression Inventory (BDI)[96] and the Hamilton Assessment of Mood Disorders (HAMD).[97] The BDI consists of 21 items evaluated by means of four alternatives, with special reference to the cognitive symptoms of depression (mood, pessimism, guilt). Outstanding among the advantages of this test are its capacity to detect changes in the intensity of the depression with the passage of time, its emphasis on cognitive changes, and the fact that it covers virtually all the diagnostic items of the DSM-IV. The format of the second scale mentioned, Hamilton's HAMD, includes two versions, which allow it to be either interviewer applied or used for self-evaluation. It also consists of 21 items, and it is easy to apply. The HAMD focuses more on somatic symptoms, which is a drawback when dealing with elderly patients. Developed especially for the elderly and extensively used is Yesavage's Geriatric Depression Scale.[98] This test consists of 30 point/no point items. The presence of depression is considered with a score of 11 points and up. Outstanding advantages of this test are the ease of application and the simplicity with which it differentiates between depressed and nondepressed elderly people.

The CAMDEX interview[99] is one of the most extensive tests used for multi-dimensional studies. This test is a diagnostic interview made up of eight (A to H) main sections. Section A is a structured interview consisting of questions concerning different areas: current mental state of the patient, family and medical antecedents, and personal history. These questions are in turn structured into specific sections within each area. Section B, a cognitive study, affords a very complete examination of different neurocognitive functions. These functions include orientation, language, memory, attention, reading, praxias, perception, math, abstract thought, visual perception, and the awareness of time. Section C presents a standardized table of the evaluator's observations concerning the patient's mental state, appearance, and behavior. Section D affords a detailed physical examination including a neurological exploration. Diverse complementary medical test results, such as blood tests and results of neuroimaging examinations, are included in Section E. Section F is a list of the specific medications required by the patient. Additional information is given in Section G, which is optional. The last section, Section H, is used to conduct a structured interview with a family member. This is designed to gather pertinent information on the patient's mental functioning, history, adaptation, and so forth. Following analysis of the data obtained in each area of the interview, both a clear view of the patient's symptoms and a possible diagnosis are achieved.

The ADAS Test[100] is another of the tests used in the field. This test is divided into two, *cognitive* and *noncognitive,* subtests.

The cognitive subtest is used to evaluate memory, language, praxias, and orientation. Immediate word recall, reasoning, and recall of the test instructions are used to assess memory. Language is assessed through the naming of the fingers, linking multiple commands, difficulties in finding the appropriate word, items in spoken language comprehension, and general language dysfunction. Constructive praxias are evaluated by copying geometric figures and ideatory praxias through the sequence of five consecutive commands. A score of 70 points is the highest possible score in the cognitive part of the test and indicates the highest degree of deficit. The cognitive part of the test is 60% of the total.

The noncognitive part of the test comprises nine items that evaluate the degree to which the emotional state is altered. Different aspects, such as the presence of crying, depression, or an altered appetite, are scored. Behavior is assessed by scoring concentration/distraction, lack of cooperation, hallucinations, psychomotor agitation, and shaking. This noncognitive part of the test is evaluated via an interview with the patient and a family member, scoring items with 0 to 5 points with regard to intensity. The maximum score is 115 points, which directly correlates to maximum severity.

11.13 ASSESSMENT OF CEREBROVASCULAR DISORDERS

Following heart disease and cancer, cerebrovascular disease is the third-ranking cause of death. This death rate due to the disease increases within older age groups. The disorder jeopardizes the blood supply to the brain, and high blood pressure is the most important variable in increased risk of its development.

A reduction or disruption of the blood supply to the brain can result in tissue death and lesions. When the blood supply is blocked, oxygen, glucose, and other necessary nutrients for metabolic activity cannot reach the tissues. Ischemia (reduction of the blood supply) and hemorrhage (abnormal bleeding into the tissues) are the most common etiologies of cerebrovascular disease. Some patients can develop transient ischemic attacks as a temporary vascular blockage and experience transient symptoms (i.e., dysarthria) without suffering significant tissue death.

Fundamental knowledge of the cerebrovascular system and the general organization of the brain is a necessary prerequisite to achieving a complete understanding of the neuropsychological sequelae found in cerebrovascular disease. Rarely will a cerebrovascular disease result in a single deficit. Usually, deficits will be the impairment of a concrete neuropsychological ability accompanied by less severe deficits in other abilities, depending on the location and quantity of the affected brain tissue.

Lesions located on the frontal lobe are associated with executive functioning impairments; the particular impairment will depend on the area affected within this lobe. Orbitofrontal lesions are associated with personality changes, disinhibited behavior, irritability, emotional lability, impulsiveness, poor judgment, and so forth. Lesions in dorsolateral frontal areas are associated with poor verbal fluency, abnormalities in motor programs, inflexibility, and a depressive component, among other manifestations. Lesions in medial areas can result in problems such as mutism, akinetic component, reduced motivation, and a lack of emotional response.

Lesions in the middle and anterior area of the temporal lobe are closely associated with amnesic syndromes, particularly concerning new information. Lesions located on temporal left hemisphere are associated with a verbal memory deficit, whereas lesions located on the right temporal hemisphere involve visual memory deficits. A lesion on a more posterior left location on this lobe would produce acalculia and/or apraxia, and sometimes alexia and agraphia.

Some aphasic problems, especially Broca's (expressive) and Wernicke's (receptive) aphasia, are associated with lesions in left frontotemporal areas. Lesions in the area of the angular gyrus (temporoparietal union) may produce acalculia, agraphia, finger agnosia, and right–left disorientation. The denomination of all of these symptoms shown together is Gerstman's syndrome.[101]

A cerebrovascular accident involving right parietal lobe impairs visuoconstructive and visuospatial abilities.[102] Neglect is also observed in lesions of right parietal areas. In contrast to this, left lesions cause loss of perception of details.

Lesions of the occipital lobe affect visual perception (anopsia). Lesions here can cause a wide variety of different impairments. Cortical blindness affects the capacity to distinguish forms; in hemianopsia, one of the visual hemifields cannot be perceived; quadrantanopsia is the defective perception of a quadrant of the visual field; in prosopagnosia, a patient cannot recognize faces; simultagnosia is a disturbance in which two stimuli cannot be simultaneously perceived; and the list goes on.

Lesions in subcortical zones may produce neuropsychological impairments similar to those described earlier. Lesions located in the corpus callosum may produce disconnection syndrome, characterized by the loss of communication between the two brain hemispheres. Other basal ganglia or thalamus infarcts can produce memory impairments.

11.14 ASSESSING TRAUMATIC BRAIN INJURY AND OTHER NEUROLOGICAL CONDITIONS

The elderly population ranks third as a risk group for TBI. Thus, TBI is not overly common in this group and, when it does occur, it is most frequently the result of a fall at home[103] and causes higher rates of mortality.[104] Elderly people are at a high risk for falls due to balance problems and movement disorders.

The outcome of elderly patients with TBI is complicated, especially because of their longer recovery times.[105] It is important to note that consequences are not immediately apparent after the accident, and the sequelae of TBI develop over the course of several days in elderly patients. After an older person suffers an accident, physicians and family members need to watch for and detect any change (dizziness, confusion, disorientation, and so forth).

The neuropsychological changes observed in elderly patients after TBI are not well established, and seem to be the same as those found in young adults.[106] However, the authors found that the neurobehavioral problems affecting older adults following TBI were more troublesome, persisted longer, and increased as time passed. Some of the post-TBI neuropsychological symptoms most frequently found in this population are fatigue, problems in processing information, depression, and dizziness.[107] Other authors found more emotional and behavioral problems than in younger people.[108]

In any case, the tests described earlier in this chapter can be used for evaluating any neurospsychological changes found following TBI in elderly patients.

11.15 CONCLUDING REMARKS

There are certain inherent difficulties in evaluation of elderly patients for which there is no easy solution. Continued research is necessary, with priority on clearly establishing the typical characteristics observed in normal aging. A differential diagnosis must be established that can discriminate as precisely as possible between physical disorders and dementia and the natural process deriving from normal aging.

The path taken in the neuropsychological evaluation of elderly patients should first be to observe those cognitive abilities that are most clearly intact and properly functioning. Once these criteria are established, the best strategy can be formulated to confront the physical, mental, and/or functional problems that have been detected.

REFERENCES

1. Prigatano, G. P. and Schachter, D. L., *Awareness of Deficit after Brain Injury*, Oxford University Press, New York, 1991.
2. Goldberg, E. S. and Barr, W., Three possible mechanisms of unawareness of deficits, in *Awareness of Deficit after Brain-Injury*, Prigatano, G. and Schacter, D., Eds., Oxford University Press, New York, 1992, 152.
3. Starktein, S. E. et al., A single-photon emission computed tomography study of ansognosia in Alzheimer diseases, *Arch. Neurol.*, 52, 415, 1995.
4. Hellman, K., Bowers, D., and Valenstein, E., Emotional disorders associated with neurological diseases, in *Clinical Neuropsychology*, 3rd ed., Heilman, K. and Valenstein, E., Eds., Oxford University Press, New York, 1993, 461.
5. Ackerman, H. S. and Hertzik, J., Voice onset time in ataxic dysartria, *Brain Language*, 156, 321, 1997.
6. Lechtenberg, R. S. and Gilman, S., Speech disorders in cerebellar disease, *Ann. Neurol.*, 3, 285, 1978.
7. León-Carrión, J., Rehabilitation of memory, in *Neuropsychological Rehabilitation: Fundamentals, Innovations, and Directions*, León-Carrión, J., Ed., St. Lucie Press, Delray Beach, FL, 1997, 371.
8. Stern, D. and Kastebaum, R., Alcohol use and abuse in old age, in *Geriatric Mental Health*, Abrahams, J. P. and Crooks, V., Eds., Grune & Stratton, Orlando, FL, 1984.
9. Lezak, M. D., *Neuropsychological Assessment*, 3rd ed., Oxford University Press, New York, 1995.
10. Brust, J., *Neuropsychological Aspects of Substance Abuse*, Butterworth-Heinemann, Boston, 1993.
11. Mittenberg, W. and Motta, S., Effects of chronic cocaine abuse on memory and learning, *Arch. Clin. Neuropsychol.*, 8, 477–483, 1993.
12. *Physician's Desk Reference*, Medical Economics Company, Montvale, NJ, 1999.
13. Godwin-Austen, R. and Bendall, J., *The Neuropsychology of the Elderly*, Springer-Verlag, New York, 1990.
14. Kapur, N., *Memory Disorders in Clinical Practice*, Lawrence Erlbaum Associates, Hillsdale, NJ, 1994.
15. Tucker, A. and Ng, K., Digoxin-related impairment of learning and memory in cardiac patients, *Psychopharmacology*, 81, 86–88, 1983.
16. Farmer, M., White, L., and Abbott, R., Blood pressure and cognitve performance. The Framingham study, *Am. J. Epidemiol.*, 126, 1103–1114, 1987.
17. Vollhardt, B., Bergener, M., and Hesse, C., Psychotropics in the elderly, in Bergener, M., Hasegawa, K., Finkel, S., and Nishimura, T., Eds., *Aging and Mental Disorders: International Perspectives*, Springer-Verlag, New York, 1992.
18. Dodrill, C. and Troupin, A., Neuropsychological effects of carbamacepine and pheny-toin: a reanalysis, *Neuropsychology*, 41, 141–143, 1991.
19. Baumm, C., Kennedy, P., and Forbes, M., Drug use in the United States in 1981, *JAMA*, 241, 1293, 1984.
20. Barona, A., Reynolds, C. R., and Chastain, R., A demographically based index of premorbid intelligence for the WAIS-R+D, *J. Consult. Clin. Psychol.*, 52, 885, 1984.

21. Helmes, E., Use of the Barona method to predict premorbid intelligence in the elderly, *Clin. Neuropsychol.*, 10, 255, 1996.

22. Mayeux, R., Sano, M., Chen, J., Tatemichi, T., and Stern, Y., Risk of dementia in first-degree relatives of patients with Alzheimer's disease and related disorders, *Arch. Neurol.*, 48, 269–273, 1991.

23. Lindstrom, K., Behavioral effects of long-term exposure to organic solvents, *Acta Neurol. Scand.*, 50, Suppl. 56, 1982.

24. León-Carrión, J., Cognitive and Behavioral Effects of Long Exposure to Organic Solvents by Workers, Unpublished research data, Consejeria de Trabajo, Junta de Andalucia, 1996.

25. Iregren, A., Effects on psychological test performance of workers exposed to a single solvent (toluene) — a comparison with effects of exposure to a mixture of organic solvents, *Neurobehav. Toxicol. Teratol.*, 4, 695–701, 1982.

26. Arlien-Soborg, P., Brhun, P., Glyndenstead, C., and Melgaard, B., Chronic painter's syndrome, *Acta Neurol. Scand.*, 60, 149–156, 1979.

27. Williamson, A., Teo, R., and Sanderson, J., Occupational mercury exposure and its consequences for behaviour, *Int. Arch. Occup. Environ. Health*, 50, 273–286, 1982.

28. Uzzell, B. and Oler, J., Chronic low-level mercury exposure and neuropsychological functioning, *J. Clin. Exp. Neuropsychol.*, 8, 581–593, 1986.

29. Arenzzo, J. and Schumburg, H., Screening for neurotoxic disease in humans, *J. Am. Coll. Toxicol.*, 8, 147–155, 1989.

30. Anger, W., Worksite behavioral research: results, sensitive methods, test batteries and the transition from laboratory data to human health, *Neurotoxicology*, 11, 629–720, 1990.

31. Bowler, R., Mergler, D., and Rauch, S., Affective and personality disturbances among female former microelectronics workers, *J. Clin. Psychol.*, 47, 41–52, 1991.

32. Linz, D., deGarmo, P., and Morton, W., Organic solvent-induced encephalopathy in an industry patient, *J. Occup. Med.*, 28, 119–25, 1986.

33. American Psychological Association, *Standards for Educational and Psychological Testing*, American Psychological Association, Washington, D.C., 1985.

34. Franzen, M. D., *Reliability and Validity in Neuropsychological Assessment*, New York, 1989.

35. León-Carrión, J., *Diagnóstico Clínico en Psicología*, Alfar Ed, Seville, 1985.

36. Lezak, M. D., IQ. R.I.P, *J. Clin. Exp. Neuropsychol.*, 10, 351, 1988.

37. Wechsler, D., *WAIS Manual*, The Psychological Corporation, New York, 1955.

38. D'elia, L., Boone, K., and Mitrushima, A., *Handbook of Normative Data for Neuropsychological Assessment*, Oxford University Press, New York, 1995.

39. Price, L., Fein, G., and Feinberg, I., Neuropsychological assessment of cognitive function in the elderly, in *Aging in the 1980's*, Poon, L., Ed., American Psychological Association, Washington, D.C., 1980.

40. Heaton, R., Grant, I., and Matthews, C., *Comprehensive Norms for an Expanded Halstead-Reitan Battery: Demographics Correction, Research Findings, and Clinical Applications*, Psychological Assessment Resources, Odessa, FL, 1991.

41. Ryan, A., Paolo, M., and Brungardt, T., Standardization of the Wechsler Adult Intelligence Scale-Revisited for persons 75 years and older, *Psychol. Assessment*, 2, 410, 1990.

42. Albert, M. and Moss, M., *Geriatric Neuropsychology*, Guilford, New York, 1988.

43. Wechsler, D., *WAIS-III. Administration and Scoring Manual*, The Psychological Corporation, San Antonio, TX, 1997.

44. Green, J., *Neuropsychological Evaluation of the Older Adult. A Clinician's Guidebook*, Academic Press, San Diego, CA, 2000.

45. *WAIS Manual*, The Psychological Corporation, San Antonio, TX, 1999.

46. Fuld, P., Test profile of cholinergic dysfunction and of Alzheimer-type dementia, *J. Clin. Neuropsychol.*, 6, 380–392, 1984.

47. Raven, J., Court, J., and Raven, J., *Manual for Raven's Progressive Matrices and Vocabulary Scales*, H. K. Lewis, London, 1976.

48. Spreen, O. and Strauss, E., *A Compendium of Neuropsychological Tests*, Oxford University Press, New York, 1991.

49. O'Leary, U., Rush, K., and Guastello, S., Estimating age-stratified WAIS-R IQs from scores on the Raven's Standard Progressive Matrices, *J. Clin. Pscychol.*, 47, 277, 1991.

50. Raven, J., *Guide to Using the Coloured Progressive Matrices*, H. K. Lewis, London, 1965.

51. León-Carrión, J., *Handbook of Human Neuropsychology*, Siglo XXI Ed., Madrid, 1995.

52. León-Carrión, J., *Seville Neuropsychological Test Battery*, TEA, Madrid, 1999.

53. Tellado, I., Perez, F., Pardo, J., and Forja, J., Evolución cognitiva de los enfermos de Alzheimer en pruebas neuropsicológicas frontales, *Rev. Esp. de Neuropsicol.*, 1, 2–3, 1999.

54. Luria, A. R., *Higher Cortical Function in Man*, Basic Books, New York, 1966.

55. Christensen, A., *Luria's Neuropsychological Investigation*, 2nd ed., Munksgaard, Copenhagen, 1997.

56. León-Carrión, J. and Morales-Ortiz, M., A brief questionnaire for the evaluation of functional organic memory disorders, *Rev. Esp. de Neuropsicol.*, 2(3), 37–43, 2000.

57. Cullum. C. M., Butters, N., Troster, A., and Salmon, D., Normal aging and forgetting rates on the Wechsler Memory Scale — Revised, *Arch. Clin. Neuropsychol.*, 5, 23–30, 1990.

58. Wechsler, D., *WMS-III Administration and Scoring Manual*, The Psychological Corporation, San Antonio, TX, 1997.

59. Benton, A., Hamsher, K., Varney, N., and Spreen, O., *Contributions to Neuropsychological Assessment*, Oxford University Press, New York, 1983.

60. Benton, A. and Sivan, A., Problems and conceptual issues in neuropsychological research in aging and dementia, *J. Clin. Neuropsychol.*, 6, 57–64, 1984.

61. Estes, W., Learning theory and intelligence, *Am. Psychol.*, 29, 740–749, 1974.

62. Kozora, E. and Cullum, C., Generative naming in normal aging: total output and qualitative changes using phonemic and semantic constraints, *Clin. Neuropsychol.*, 9, 313–320, 1995.

63. Lucas, J., Ivnik, R., Smith, G., Bohac, D., Tangalos, E., Graff-Radford, N., and Petersen, R., Mayo's older Americans normative studies: category fluency norms, *J. Clin. Exp. Neuropsychol.*, 20, 194–200, 1998.

64. Randolph, C., Braum, A., Cgoldberg, T., and Chase, T., Semantic fluency in Alzheimer's, Parkinson's and Huntington's disease: dissociation of storage and retrieval failures, *Neuropsychology*, 7, 82–88, 1993.

65. Monsh, A., Bondi, M., Salmon, D., Butters, N., Katzman, R., and Thal, L., Comparison of verbal fluency task in the detection of dementia of the Alzheimer type, *Arch. Neurol.*, 49, 1253–1258, 1995.

66. Kaplan, E., Goodglass, H., and Weintraub, S., *The Boston Naming Test*, 2nd ed., Lea & Febiger, Philadelphia, 1983.

67. Ross, R., Lichtemberg, P., and Christensen, K., Normative data on the Boston Naming Test for elderly adults in a demographically diverse medical sample, *Clin. Neuropsychol.*, 9, 321–325, 1995.

68. Obler, L. and Albert, M., Language skills across adulthood, in *The Psychology of Aging*, Birren, J. and Schaine, K. W., Eds., Van Nostrand Reinhold, New York, 1985.

69. Brennan, M., Welsh, M. C., and Fisher, C. B., Aging and executive functioning skills: an examination of a community dwelling older adult population, *Percept. Mot. Skills,* 84, 1187, 1997.

70. Fisk, J. E. and Warr, P., Age and working memory: the role of perceptual speed, the central executive, and the phonological loop, *Psychol. Aging,* 11, 316, 1996.

71. Corey-Bloom, J., Wiederholt, W. C., Edelstein, S. et al., Cognitive and functional status of the oldest old, *JAGS,* 44, 671, 1996.

72. West, R. L., An application of prefrontal cortex function theory to cognitive aging, *Psychol. Bull.,* 120, 272, 1996.

73. Daigneault, S. and Braun, C. M., Working memory and the Self-ordered Pointing Task: further evidence of early prefrontal decline in normal aging, *J. Clin. Exp. Psychol.,* 15, 881, 1993.

74. Haug, H. and Eggers, R., Morphometry of the human cortex cerebri and the corpus striatum during aging, *Neurobiol. Aging,* 12, 336, 1991.

75. Keys, B. A. and White, D., Exploring the relationship between age, executive abilities and psychomotor speed, *J. Neuropsychol. Soc.,* 6, 76, 2000.

76. Zacks, R. T. and Hasher, L., Directed ignoring: Inhibitory regulation of working memory, in *Inhibitory Processes in Attention, Memory, and Language,* Dagenbach, D. and Carr, T. H., Eds., Academic Press, New York, 1994, 241.

77. Stroop, J. R., Studies of interference in serial verbal reactions. *J. Exp. Psychol.,* 18, 643–662, 1935.

78. León-Carrión, J. and Barroso y Martín, J., *Neuropsicología del Pensamiento: Control Ejecutivo y Lóbulo Frontal,* Kronos, Seville, 1997.

79. Grant, P. B. and Berg, E. A., A behavioral analysis of degree of reinforcement and case of shifting to new response in a Weigl-type card-sorting problem, *J. Exp. Psychol.,* 38, 404, 1948.

80. Halstead, W. C., *Brain and Intelligence. A Quantitative Study of the Frontal Lobes,* University on Chicago Press, Chicago, 1947.

81. Porteus, S. D., *The Porteus Maze Test and Intelligence,* Pacific Books, Palo Alto, CA, 1950.

82. Gagnè, R. M. and Smith, E. C., A study of the effects of verbalization on problem solving, *J. Exp. Psychol.,* 63, 12–18, 1962.

83. León-Carrión, J., Morales, M., and Domínguez-Morales, M. R., The computerized Torre of Hanoi: a new form of administration and suggestion for interpretation, *Percept. Mot. Skills,* 73, 63, 1991.

84. Barroso y Martín, J. M., León-Carrión, J., Murillo, F., Domínguez, J. M., and Muñoz, M. A., Funcionamiento ejecutivo y capacidad para la resolucion de problemas en pacientes con TCE, *Rev. Esp. Neuropsicol.,* 1(1), 3–21, 1999.

85. Ricker, J., Axelrod, B., and Houtler, B., Clinical validation of the oral Trail Making Test, *Neuropsychiatr. Neuropsychol. Behav. Neurol.,* 9, 50–53, 1996.

86. Ivnick, R., Malec, J., Smith, G., Tangalpos, E., and Peterson, R., Neuropsychological test norms above age 55: COWAT, BNT, MAE Token, WRAT.R Reading, AMNART, Stroop, TMT, JLO, *Clin. Neuropsychol.,* 6, 1–30, 1996.

87. Christensen, A., *Diagnostico Neuropsicologico de Luria,* Pablo del Rio, Madrid, 1978.

88. Madrazo Lazcano, M., Machuca, F., Barroso, J. M., Dominguez, R., and León-Carrión, J., Cambios emocionales después de un TCE grave, *Rev. Esp. Neuropsicol.,* 1(4), 75–82, 1999.

89. León-Carrión, J., Neurologically-related changes in personality inventory (NECHAPI): a clinical tool addressed to neurorehabilitation planning and monitoring the effects of personality treatment, *Neurorehabilitation,* 11, 129, 1988.

90. Cummings, J. and Benson, D., *Dementia: A Clinical Approach*, Butterworth-Heinemann, Boston, 1992.

91. Alzheimer's Disease and Related Dementia Guideline Panel, Recognition and Initial Assessment of Alzheimer's Disease and Related Dementia, Vol. 19, U.S. Department of Health and Human Services. AHCPR Publication No. 97-0702, Rockville, MD, 1996.

92. Boise, L., Camicioli, R., Morgan, D., Rose, J., and Congleton, L., Diagnosis dementia: perspectives of primary care physicians, *Gerontologist*, 39, 457–464, 1999.

93. Goodglass, H. and Kaplan, E., *Boston Diagnostic Aphasia Examination (BDAE)*, Lea & Febiger, Philadelphia, 1983.

94. Jorm, P. and Korten, F., Informant interview (IQ CODE), 1988.

95. Blessed, G., Tomlinson, B., and Roth, M., The association between quantitative measure of dementia and of senile changes in the cerebral grey matter of the elderly subjects, *Br. J. Psychiatr.*, 114, 797–811, 1968.

96. Beck, A., Ward, C., Mendelson, M., Mock, J., and Erbaugh, J., An inventory for measuring depression, *Arch. Gen. Psychiatr.*, 4, 451–571, 1961.

97. Hamilton, M., Development of rating scale for primary depressive illness, *Br. J. Soc. Clini. Psychol.*, 6, 278–296, 1967.

98. Yesavage, J., Brink, T., Rose, T., Lum, O., Huang, V., Adeley, M., and Leirer, V., Development and validation of geriatric depresion screening scale: a preliminary report, *J. Psychiatr. Res.*, 17, 37–49, 1983.

99. Linas, R., Vilalta, J., and Lopez, S., *CAMDEX. Examen Cambridge para trastoros mentales en la vejez. Adaptación de la version Inglesa*, Ancora, Barcelona, 1991.

100. Mhos, R., Rasen, W., and Davis, K., The Alzheimer Disease Assessment Scale: an instrument for assessing treatment efficacy, *Psychopharmacol. Bull.*, 19, 448–450, 1983.

101. Benton, A., Gerstmann's syndrome, *Arch. Neurol.*, 49, 445–447, 1992.

102. Benton, A. and Tranel, D., Visuoperceptual, visuospatial and visuoconstructive disorders, in *Clinical Neuropsychology*, 3rd ed., Heilman, K. and Valenstein, E., Eds., Oxford University Press, New York, 1993.

103. Naugle, R., Epidemiology of TBI in adults, in *Traumatic Brain Injury*, Bigler, E. B., Ed., Pro-Ed, Austin, TX, 1990.

104. Goldstein, F. and Levin, H., Epidemiolgy of traumatic brain injury: incidence, clinical characteristics, and risk factors, in *Traumatic Brain Injury*, Bigler, E. B., Ed., Pro-Ed, Austin, TX, 1990.

105. Rothweiler, B., Temkin, N., and Dikmen, S., Aging effect on psychological outcome in TBI, *Arch. Phys. Med. Rehabil.*, 79, 881–887, 1998.

106. Fields, R., Geriatric head injury, in *Handbook of Neuropsychology and Aging*, Nussbaum, P., Ed., Plenum Press, New York, 1997.

107. Tailor, C., Fields, R., Starratt, G., Russo, B., and Diamond, D., Neuropsychiatric complaints following traumatic brain injury: head injured versus non-head-injured trauma patients, paper presented at the American Neuropsychiatric Association, San Antonio, TX, 1993.

108. Thomsen, I., Recognizing the development of behavior disorders, in Wood, R., Ed., *Neurobehavioral Sequelae of Traumatic Brain Injury*, Taylor & Francis, Bristol, PA, 1990.

12 Mild Cognitive Impairment

Luis Fornazzari

CONTENTS

12.1 Introduction 279
12.2 Diagnosis of MCI...280
12.3 Neuropathologic Correlation...282
12.4 Neuroimaging In MCI 283
12.5 Economic Impact of Early Diagnosis of AD 283
12.6 Early Detection of MCI 284
References...284

12.1 INTRODUCTION

There is clinical, neuropathological, and recent neuroimaging evidence of a transitional state between the normal physiological aging process and the development of Alzheimer's disease (AD).[1,2] During the last 15 years scholars have shown considerable interest in the diagnosis of this transitional condition. A variety of terms and concepts have been used in the past to define this stage. This variation in cognitive functioning in elderly people has been defined as "benign senescent forgetfulness" (1962), "limited dementia" (1982), "questionable dementia" (1972), "mild cognitive decline" (1982), "mild dementia" (1984), "age associated memory impairment" (1986), "minimal dementia" (1986), and "mild cognitive impairment" (1991).[3] Each of these expressions consists of a construct of diagnostic criteria differing in the age of onset, the degree of cognitive decline, and the subjective experience of memory impairment. The common and necessary denominator is a documented memory deficit.[4] The practical construct of the term mild cognitive impairment (MCI) is a relatively new concept that has been under intense investigation by academic groups in Canada and the United States (Columbia University, Mayo Clinic, Washington University in St. Louis, University of Toronto, University of Montreal) and in France, England, and Sweden. This construct, MCI, is so new that it still does not have a place as such in the DSM-IV. The diagnostic criterion of MCI refers to the preclinical state of AD as a stage of age-related cognitive decline.[5] Although the expression and concept of MCI has not yet been implemented widely, the urgent need for control of this not so "silent epidemic" is making the clinical use of the term quite valuable. MCI can be described as the "intermediate state of cognitive functioning in which the decline from a previously higher level has occurred which is not severe enough to fulfill the criteria of dementia." In an operational way, MCI has been characterized by memory impairment that is beyond that expected for normal aging, but that has not been diagnosed as dementia, particularly when other cognitive domains are believed to remain intact. The population with MCI can thus be differentiated from normal older people and those with mild AD. In agreement with J.C. Morris and R.C. Petersen from Washington University and the Mayo Clinic, respectively, the operational criteria to be used in MCI are as follows:

1. Self-reported memory complaints (preferably corroborated by a family member);
2. Age adjusted memory deficit (about 1.5 standard deviation below normative values on a quantitative test of episodic memory, such as paragraph recall);
3. Normal general cognitive abilities (other than memory);
4. Maintenance activities of daily living;
5. Absence of clinically diagnosed dementia.

It is important to delay the appearance of neurodegenerative dementias such as AD, because a few years of such delay could considerably decrease the human suffering and the economic burden of this pathological aging. It is of great interest to diagnose subjects who may develop AD at the earliest possible stage of the disorder, to try to decrease or slow the progression. One could visualize in the near future ways to deter or prevent the deterioration with more aggressive etiological types of treatment. In the meantime, the availability of symptomatic treatment with different cholinergic agents of the anticholinesterasic type, such as Donepezil, Rivastigmine, Galantamine, and others, mandates all clinicians to make a very early diagnosis of the pre-Alzheimer condition.[8]

12.2 DIAGNOSIS OF MCI

The general consensus in recent scholarship is that a healthy elderly adult will have an overall normal cognitive function that does not decline with the aging process.[9] These cognitive functions are more or less homogeneous, but there are certain areas that decline with age in a normal fashion and others that are totally well preserved.[10] The most important issue about this is that normal physiological aging is associated with a normal memory and other cognitive functions. Consequently, any cognitive decline in an elderly individual, after ruling out other possible neurological, psychiatric, and medical causes, may reflect an early dementia.

The aforementioned operational criteria for diagnosis are quite adequate as a working diagnosis. However, there are still some aspects surrounding these criteria that are far from consensus. For example, the European Community Consensus on Minimal Cognitive Impairment suggests the following diagnostic criteria for MCI:

1. There should be a report by the individual or an informant relative that memory or other cognitive functions have declined from previous performance.
2. Simple activities of daily living are preserved but complex activities are more or less impaired.
3. The score on a global screening tool such as the Mini Mental Status Examination, Cambridge Cognitive (CAMCOG), or other global screening tool indicates that the cognitive function is not sufficiently impaired, compared to age and education matched control to allow a diagnosis of dementia.
4. Impairment in memory or other cognitive abilities should be indicated by a score below the cutoff for age and education matched control in a memory or another cognitive test.
5. The cognitive impairment and its interference with activities of daily living are not of sufficient severity for a diagnosis of dementia to be made.
6. Exclusion criteria:
   a. Depression or major psychiatric disorder;
   b. Clouding of consciousness;
   c. Intake of central-acting drugs.

In spite of the differences in the diagnostic criteria, the outcome of patients with MCI who developed AD is more or less consistent. The European Community data suggest a range of change from MCI to AD of approximately 50 to 80% during the fifth to seventh year following the initial diagnosis of MCI. The data from Mayo Clinic suggest that individuals with the diagnosis of MCI may progress to AD at a rate of approximately 12% per year. After 4 years, approximately half of the MCI individuals were recognized as suffering from AD according to the National Institute of Neurological and Communicative Disorders and Stroke — Alzheimer's Disease and Related Dementias Association (NINCDS-ADRDA) and DSM-IV criteria. In contrast, normal elderly people without memory deficit may develop AD at a rate of 1 to 2%.[12] There is no consensus regarding the time of the decline in memory, but there are some studies that suggest the cognitive decline appears to start many years before the clinical onset of AD. Moreover, the progression of the impairment appears to be continuous, and this pattern of impaired performance is generalized across the different forms of AD, familiar or sporadic, early or late onset. This is also true regardless of the composition of the sample studied, either hospital or community-based and/or the method used for assessment.[13]

One of the unresolved questions is what type of memory impairment is the earliest manifestation of MCI. There is still no consensus, but different groups of investigators have suggested that in their own laboratories, particularly in Memory Clinics, there are combinations of neuropsychological assessments that are most sensitive and more specific for a very early diagnosis of AD and particularly very early MCI. The research group led by D. M. Jacobs and Mary Sano at Columbia University suggests that in its clinic, its most sensitive combination of tests corresponds to a poor word-finding ability, abstract reasoning, and decline in memory.[14] Another group describes a decline in verbal memory as the earliest sign in the preclinical stage and suggests that this might be a useful marker for diagnosing AD in the future.[15] A predictive study done by Mary Tierney in Toronto includes informal perception about patients' cognitive deficit, mental control subtests of the memory scale of the Weschler Memory Scale and the Rey Auditory Verbal learning test delayed recall. She suggests a valuable 2-year prediction time before the appearance of the clinical signs of dementia.[16] Researchers at the Mayo Clinic suggest that there was a marked difference between normal controls and patients with MCI and AD patients in all memory measures relative to learning and delayed recall using word lists, paragraphs, and nonverbal material. Interestingly, the differences were less dramatic between the subjects with MCI and the patients with AD. The Boston Naming test paralleled those of the memory domain, so these findings can be interpreted as indicating either that the linguistic function of naming is impaired early in the disease process or that this naming test actually assesses semantic memory and therefore should be considered with the other memory data.[17] In essence, regarding the group studying patients with dementia, almost all the actual evidence is based on tests that focus on hippocampus functions. The earliest pathological lesions recognized in AD are the entorhinal cortex, the perforant pathways, and hippocampal formation of the medial temporal lobe.[18]

12.3 NEUROPATHOLOGIC CORRELATION

It is accepted worldwide that neurofibrillary tangles and the β-amyloid plaques occur in aging individuals without AD. Both are the histological hallmarks of AD. However, in spite of this, when AD or other neurodegenerative disorders are carefully excluded in the prospective studies, aging itself may not result in any substantial cognitive or neuronal loss.[19–21] In concert with the above concept, sufficient amounts of plaques and tangles make the pathological diagnosis of the disease more possible.[22] It is highly suggested that a preclinical stage of AD, "where a neuropathological gradual involvement of the vulnerable areas like the entorhinal cortex and the medial temporal lobe are involved but have not yet produced any clinical detectable cognitive change."[23] In accordance with the two most important papers on this issue, there is a very attractive suggestion that the neuropathological deposition of abnormal elements in the brain may start very early in AD. According to Braak and Braak,[18] the neurofibrillary changes and the site of deposition may begin at a young age, even before the age of 30 and both markers increase with age. In the Price and Morris study[24] and also in other reports,[25] the neurofibrillary depository would begin virtually at birth and could reach 50% prevalence at the age of 50. In their calculation, it is suggested that the amyloid deposition reaches a 50% prevalence 25 years later at about 73 years of age. There were some discrepancies in the order of the appearance of the changes and, in one group, the neurofibrillary changes, occur before the earliest amyloid deposition. In addition to the time of the appearance of the neuropathological abnormalities in AD, which of the two markers is the first to appear is also debatable. In other words, are neurofibrillary tangles the earliest manifestation of AD or, as the study done on the familiar form of AD indicates, is it the β-amyloid deposition that accelerates not only the formation of plaque, but particularly the acceleration of the process associated with the formation of neurofibrillary tangles?

Other groups of investigators, particularly the team led by J. C. Troncoso at Johns Hopkins University, suggest that the amyloid deposition and endosomal-lysosomal changes are very early events, particularly in the sporadic late onset of AD and are, without question, the most common form of presentation of the disease.[26]

12.4 NEUROIMAGING IN MCI

There is evidence that magnetic resonance imaging (MRI) volumetric measurement of the hippocampal formation is able to differentiate normal aging subjects from patients with very mild AD.[27,28] Apart from the atrophy of the hippocampal formation, the suggestion is that a structure per se may be a "very early marker of incipient AD." Other studies (Solininen and Scheltens[29]) suggest that hippocampal atrophy demonstrated by MRI, with associated molecular genetic factors, and memory test scores would be sufficient to diagnose AD in its preclinical phase. The same research group has produced some very interesting results with respect to the use of functional MRI. They were able to visualize morphology and function in their pilot studies, during visual encoding tasks; patients with very mild AD show that hippocampal activation is greatly diminished compared with controls.[30]

12.5 ECONOMIC IMPACT
OF EARLY DIAGNOSIS OF AD

Higher health costs and a greater need for institutionalization are the result of an increase in the prevalence of dementias all over the world, particularly in developed countries. According to the Canadian Auditor-General's report in 1998, the changing demographics could mean that government spending on social security and health care could rise from 11.6% to between 14 and 20% of the gross domestic product by 2030. Based on the "Canadian Study on Health and Aging," an epidemological study, it is believed that over $3.9 billion (Canadian dollars) is currently spent annually for the treatment of dementia, which affects approximately 250 to 6000 Canadians. Among them, nearly 70% have AD.[31,32] Quite simply, the number of Canadians with AD will more than double by the year 2030.[33] Large costs of palliative care for AD and other dementias can be attributed to nursing-home care (formal services at least $21,924/year taking into consideration all severities of disease). But maintaining the patient at home (informal care) reduces the cost to less than $500/month, practically decreasing the amount of the total cost to almost one quarter. In all the international experiences, it has been suggested that delaying the onset of AD by 5 years would actually halve the number of patients.[34] With the advent of symptomatic treatment with anticholinesterasic agents and particularly the anticipated advent of treatment directed at the pathogenesis of the disease, for example, drugs currently under development to inhibit A β-amyloid production (Elan Pharmaceutical, Bristol-Myers-Squibb), NSAIDS, estrogen and estrogen analogues, vitamin E, etc., early diagnosis is at this moment imperative. Early detection, preferably during the preclinical stage, would yield the possibility of better outcomes and the maintenance of a greater quality of life for a longer duration.

12.6 EARLY DETECTION OF MCI

There are data suggesting that cognitive[35] and behavioral disorders[36] are under-diagnosed in primary care. In spite of the prominent role of geriatric medicine, memory difficulties and dementia are still considered to be a "natural' consequence of aging. This factor probably plays a role in the delay in referrals to a memory clinic, where patients frequently arrive with a mild to moderate degree of dementia, and, as mentioned before, the process may have already had years of development. A practical way to approach this delay in detecting and referring cases is to increase the knowledge of cognitive disorder in primary practice through theoretical and practical procedures, such as the use of screening instruments.

The author's group is using a different and novel approach, which involves going to the community with a brief, culturally and literacy-sensible battery of neuro-psychological tests to identify subjects at risk of MCI, and following them every 6 months for 36 months. These batteries include items that assess episodic memory, verbal and confrontation naming, attention and executive functions, and a very brief smell-identification test. Visuoconstructional abilities are also investigated.

Genetic and biochemical tests (Apoe gene, Beta APP, PS2, A Beta 42, CYP2D6B, etc.) are to be performed in each subject. These tests will permit dis-cernment of whether particular genetic profiles predispose toward one or more of the common causes of cognitive impairment in elderly people; further, prior knowl-edge of such genotypes could alert physicians to take appropriate action in those patients presenting with subtle cognitive problems.

Neuroimaging MRI, with special emphasis in entorhinal hippocampus measure-ments, either atrophy or dilatation, will be an important correlation to consider with neuropsychological and biological markers.

If the data collected show good sensitivity and specificity in diagnosing MCI, this brief battery could be useful to primary health-care professionals and particularly to the nonmedical community for awareness and intervention purposes.

Early detection and diagnosis of MCI could result in increased possibilities of independence and functionality, improved quality of life, and substantially decreased costs in the care of patients with AD.

REFERENCES

1. Almkvist, O. et al., Mild cognitive impairment: an early stage of Alzheimer's disease? *J. Neural Transm.*, Suppl. 54, 21–29, 1998.
2. Hulette, C. M. et al., Neuropathological and neuropsychological changes in "normal" aging: evidence for preclinical Alzheimer disease in cognitively normal individuals, *J. Neuropathol. Exp. Neurol.*, 57(2), 1168–1174, 1998.
3. Wolf, H. et al., The prognosis of mild cognitive impairment in the elderly, *J. Neural Transm.*, Suppl. 54, 31–50, 1998.
4. Morris, J. C. and Petersen, R. C., Is mild cognitive impairment simply incipient Alzheimer's disease? Education Program Syllabus, American Academy of Neurology 52nd Annual Meeting, San Diego, CA, April 29–May 6, 2000.

5. American Psychiatric Association, *Diagnostic and Statistical Manual of Mental Disorders*, 4th ed., American Psychiatric Association, Washington, D.C., 1994.

6. Petersen, R. C. et al., Mild cognitive impairment: clinical characterization and outcome, *Arch. Neurol.*, 56, 303–338, 1999.

7. Morris, J. C., Storandt, M., Miller, J. P., McKeel, D. W., Price, J. L., Rubin, E. H., and Berg, L., Mild cognitive impairment represents early-stage Alzheimer disease, *Arch. Neurol.*, 58(3), 397–405, 2001.

8. Ernst, R. L. and Hay, J. W., Economic research on Alzheimer's disease: a review of the literature, *Alzheimer Dis. Assoc. Disorders*, 11(Suppl. 6), 135–145, 1997.

9. Rubin, E. H. et al., A prospective study of cognitive function and onset of dementia in cognitively healthy elders, *Arch. Neurol.*, 55, 395–401, 1998.

10. Craik, F. I. M., Memory functions in normal aging, in *Memory Disorders, Research and Clinical Practice*, Yanagihara, T. and Petersen, R. C., Eds., Marcel Dekker, New York, 347–367, 1991.

11. Baro, F. et al., Consensus paper on mild cognitive impairment, European Parliament Document, 1998.

12. Petersen, R. C. et al., Mild cognitive impairment, *Arch. Neurol.*, 56, 303–308, 1999.

13. Almkvist, O. et al., Mild cognitive impairment: an early stage of Alzheimer's disease? *J. Neural Transm.*, Suppl. 54, 21–29, 1998.

14. Jacobs, D. M. et al., Neuropsychological detection and characterization of preclinical Alzheimer's disease, *Neurology*, 45, 957–962, 1995.

15. Howieson, D. B. et al., Cognitive markers preceding Alzheimer's dementia in the healthy oldest old, *J. Am. Geriatr. Soc.*, 45, 584–589, 1997.

16. Tierney, M. et al., The prediction of Alzheimer's disease, *Arch. Neurol.*, 53, 423–427, 1996.

17. Petersen, R. C. et al., Mild cognitive impairment, *Arch. Neurol.*, 56, 303–308, 1999.

18. Braak, H. and Braak, E., Neuropathological staging of Alzheimer-related changes, *Acta Neuropathol.*, 82, 239–259, 1991.

19. Tomlinson, B. E., Blessed, G., and Roth, M., Observations on the brains of non-demented old people, *J. Neurol. Sci.*, 7, 331–356, 1968.

20. West, M. J. et al., Differences in the pattern of hippocampal neuronal loss in normal aging and Alzheimer's disease, *Lancet*, 334, 769–772, 1994.

21. Morris, J. C. et al., Very mild Alzheimer's disease: informant-based clinical, psychometric, and pathological distinction from normal aging, *Neurology*, 41, 469–478, 1991.

22. Price, J. L. et al., The distribution of tangles, plaques and related immunohistochemical markers in healthy aging and Alzheimer's disease, *Neurobiol. Aging*, 12, 295–312, 1991.

23. Morris, J. C. et al., Cerebral amyloid deposition and diffuse palques in "normal" aging: evidence for presymptomatic and very mild Alzheimer's disease, *Neurology*, 46, 707–719, 1996.

24. Price, J. L. and Morris, J. C., Tangles and plaques in nondemented aging and "preclinical" Alzheimer's disease, *Ann. Neurol.*, 45, 358–368, 1999.

25. Duyckaerts, C. and Hauw, J. J., Prevalence, incidence and duration of Braak's stages in the general population: can we know? *Neurobiol. Aging*, 18, 362–369, 1997.

26. Troncoso, J. C. et al., Neuropathology of preclinical and clinical late-onset Alzheimer's disease, *Ann. Neurol.*, 43(5), 673–676, 1998.

27. De Leon, M. J. et al., Frequency of hippocampal formation atrophy in normal aging and Alzheimer's disease, *Neurbiol. Aging*, 18, 1–11, 1997.

28. Jack, C. R., Jr. et al., MR-based hippocampal volumetry in the diagnosis of Alzheimer's disease, *Neurology*, 42, 183–188, 1992.

29. Soininen, H. S. and Scheltens, P., Early diagnostic indices for the prevention of Alzheimer's disease, the Finnish Medical Society Duodecim, *Ann. Med.*, 30, 553–559, 1998.
30. Rombouts, S. A. R. B. et al., Visual association encoding activates the medial temporal lobe; a functional magnetic resonance imaging study, *Hippocampus*, 7, 594–601, 1997.
31. Bushke, L., Canada's greying population, *Can. Med. Assoc. J.*, 151(3), 239, 1999.
32. Ostbye, T. and Crosse, E., Net economic costs of dementia in Canada, *Can. Med. Assoc. J.*, 151(10), 1457–1464, 1994.
33. Hux, M. J. et al., Relation between severity of Alzheimer's disease and costs of caring, *Can. Med. Assoc. J.*, 159(5), 457–465, 1998.
34. Thal, L. J., Potential prevention strategies for Alzheimer's disease, *Alzheimer Dis. Assoc. Disorders*, 120, 6–8, 1996.
35. Henderson, A. S., Epidemiology of mental disorders and psychosocial problems, in *Dementia*, World Health Organization, Geneva, 1994.
36. Lecubier, Y., Is depression under-recognised and undertreated? *Int. Clin. Psychopharmacol.*, 13(Suppl. 5), S3–6, 1998.

13 Evaluation of Intervention Programs for Elderly People: Enhancing Validity

Salvador Chacón Moscoso,
José Antonio Pérez-Gil,
and Francisco Pablo Holgado Tello

CONTENTS

13.1 Introduction 288
13.2 Intervention Programs for Elderly People 288
13.3 Program Evaluation 289
13.4 Conceptual Foundations of Validity in the Evaluation of Programs
for Elderly People 290
    13.4.1 Elements Involved in the Concept of Global Validity 293
    13.4.2 Achieving Validity in Evaluation of Intervention Programs
for Elderly People 294
13.5 Design Issues for Improving the Evaluation of Programs 294
    13.5.1 State of the Art in Intervention Programs
for Elderly People 295
        13.5.1.1 Obtaining Information from Databases 295
        13.5.1.2 Description of Obtained Information 297
    13.5.2 Improving Evaluation of Intervention Programs
for Elderly People 299
13.6 Methodological Implications of Validity in the Evaluative Process
of Intervention Programs 302
13.7 Concluding Remarks 303
Acknowledgments 304
References 304

13.1 INTRODUCTION

The evaluation of intervention programs for elderly people, through adaptation to the needs arising from a modern and continually changing society, has a diversity of objectives. The purpose of this chapter is to analyze the major elements that enhance validity in the evaluation of intervention programs for elderly people. We introduce a methodological analysis of the evaluative process to specify the most relevant elements in achieving validity in evaluative data. We then give useful decision criteria for those involved in designing, implementing, and evaluating intervention programs for the elderly population.

To begin with, we will introduce a brief description of intervention programs for the elderly population and of program evaluation. This is followed by the analysis of the conceptual foundations of validity for these programs.[1] This analysis establishes the relevance of correspondence, theoretical coherence, and pragmatism as the dominant criteria in achieving evaluation validity.[2] The first part of the following section describes the state of the art for intervention programs for elderly people, and the second part describes design criteria for improving the evaluation of these programs. This is followed by a general discussion introducing the methodological implications of validity in the evaluative process of intervention programs.

13.2 INTERVENTION PROGRAMS FOR ELDERLY PEOPLE

Intervention programs for the elderly population have flourished in industrialized countries in recent years. Championed by both professional and social policies, the changes we are witnessing in the areas of support and care for physically and mentally disabled elderly people are part of a reform movement that began decades ago.[3]

These reforms have encompassed such endeavors as exposing the inhumane conditions found in many institutions, the creation of alternative residential and day care centers in communities, the passage of significant federal and state legislation supporting the rights of elderly people with disabilities, and the provision of support to families to allow elderly people with disabilities to remain in their communities. As each step of change has come about, the ideals of "normalization," "inclusion," and "participation" have become empowered with the ability to bring about further reform. It seems that the closer we think we are to achieving these ideals, the more they demand of our skills and creativity. These changes show a generalized and increasing interest in attaining a state of well-being for all.

This context of reform is related to the World Health Organization and the U.S. Public Health Service definition of health as the product of forces converging from four fields — environment, genetics, lifestyle, and medical care. Increasing longevity, the "squaring of the age pyramid" with all its transformative implications, which took place during the 20th century, has resulted largely from these fields.[4]

Federal agencies and professional groups are developing new intervention programs in the care system for elderly people.[5] These developments include proposals for the planning and carrying out of programs and for improving the training of professionals in the fields involved. This would give greater flexibility to the system of services in such aspects as interdisciplinary collaboration,[6,7] choice and self-determination, circles of support (friends, relations, visitors),[8] family support programs, educational and training programs,[9] and evaluation of the internal health of senior communities.[10,11]

Currently, most programs for older people are related to four general intervention types: objective-driven programs, intervention–treatment programs, satisfaction programs, and comparison of different intervention–treatment programs. These programs are principally oriented to improving psychological well-being, increasing the general health status, and reinforcing social networks for elderly people.

For example, the Iowan Elderly Outreach Program (EOP) is designed to identify and provide mental health services to elderly rural people.[12] The project integrates a variety of health, mental health, and human service agencies in the planning and delivery of services. Other programs, such as the Nurse Education Link to Aged (NELA) Wellness Center,[13] are oriented to satisfying physical and emotional health needs of clients (primary nursing care programs, consumer satisfaction, health promotion, health services for the aged) and also delivering programs for coping with depression and stress, alcoholism, and arthritis, and for increasing social interaction between men and women.

Another example can be found in the Arizona Long Term Care System (ALTCS), which combines Medicaid acute and long-term-care services.[14] ALTCS provides institutional, residential, and in-home services to elderly and disabled Medicaid recipients who meet the criteria for placement in a nursing facility.

The Mount Sinai Medical Center Geriatric Evaluation and Treatment Unit (GETU) is another typical service for elderly people. It is a 16-bed acute-care geriatric unit,[15] which provides acute geriatric care and geriatric assessment and is a site for education and clinical research. The GETU serves a targeted group of acutely ill, hospitalized, frail elderly people with complex, interdisciplinary needs.

Although there has been a major growth in the number of intervention programs for the elderly population, the growth has been very heterogeneous and scattered. Given this unsystematic development, a very important element within this range of activity is the ever-increasing concern in designing, implementing, and evaluating programs with systematic scientific rigor. Development in intervention strategies will come about only through the careful evaluation of currently used and newly presented models.[5]

13.3   PROGRAM EVALUATION

The need for program evaluation stems from the commonsense logic that interventions should offer demonstrable benefits.[16] This reasoning assumes that intervention programs have defined objectives, and that their success or failure will be assessed empirically.

We can find as many answers as there are people involved when we ask, "What is evaluation?" In spite of this, evaluators tend to assume that evaluation implies a systematic analysis of the worth of the implemented programs to bring about change in the areas of intervention.[17] Therefore, program evaluation is the scientific and systematic investigation of the effects, results, and objectives of a program and the subsequent practical decisions regarding the program.

Because of the diversity of intervention programs and theoretical models, there are many different types of evaluations. For example, we can talk about summative or formative evaluations depending on the consideration of evaluation results at the end of the intervention program or during its implementation, respectively. We can consider internal or external evaluations depending on where the evaluators come from (inside or outside the organization being evaluated). Prospective or retrospective evaluations are related to when the evaluation process is considered to begin, and so forth.

Program evaluation is undoubtedly complex, not only with regard to its content, but in its methodological aspects as well. The difficulties of program evaluation are conditioned by diverse factors, among which we would highlight the nature of the intervention program, the availability of appropriate measurement instruments, and resources and technological advancements.

As a result, the need for a methodological framework of analysis from which the systematic design and evaluation of intervention programs can be devised becomes manifest.

13.4 CONCEPTUAL FOUNDATIONS OF VALIDITY IN THE EVALUATION OF PROGRAMS FOR ELDERLY PEOPLE

In describing the conceptual foundations of the principal validity types we will refer to the different elements that intervene in intervention processes. These elements are as follows: units, treatments, outcomes, setting, and time.[1] The initials of these five elements comprise the acronym $utost_i$. According to the logic of Cronbach's original work,[18] we can differentiate three different levels in each one of these five elements. These three levels are known as: $UTOST_i$, the defined population of the five elements; $utost_i$, particular samples drawn from the defined population; and $*UTOST_i$, a different population of $UTOST_i$ to which study results are to be generalized.

By focusing on this framework of analysis, we find the following validity types.[1]

Statistical Conclusion Validity

Statistical conclusion validity refers to the study of the correlation between t (treatment) and o (outcome) in the $utost_i$. Its aim is to analyze if the treatment (in this case, the intervention program), as implemented, significantly correlates with the measured outcomes. For example, in a neuropsychological rehabilitation program intended to increase visuospatial coordination in older adults, the statistical conclusion validity seeks to answer the question of whether the increase in visuospatial coordination (outcome) significantly correlates with the implementation of the neuropsychological rehabilitation program (treatment).

Internal Validity

Internal validity refers to the question of a causal relationship between t (treatment) and o (outcome). Its aim is to analyze whether the observed outcomes would have been displayed in the absence of the program. In accord with the previous example, to study the internal validity means analyzing whether the implementation of the neuropsychological rehabilitation program (treatment) was the factor that caused an increase in the visuospatial coordination (outcome) in the patients. The question — "Would visuospatial coordination have increased (outcome) if the program had not been implemented? — is asked.

Construct Validity

Construct validity involves making inferences regarding the defined population (constructs), based on the particular sample of $utost_i$ used in the intervention program. It implies making inferences to $UTOST_i$ from sampling particular $utost_i$. Continuing with the example, in this case construct validity would be analyzed in terms of whether it is possible to make inferences to the population from which the sample was drawn.

Construct validity tries to answer the following question: Can we make inferences to a population from sampling the items listed below?

1. *Units*, e.g., the older adults with certain characteristics who were treated.
2. *Treatments*, e.g., a predetermined neuropsychological rehabilitation program that included intervention on predetermined variables, and not on others.
3. *Outcomes*, e.g., to observe, for example, the error frequency in a visuospatial coordination task and not record other possible alternative outcomes.
4. *Context*, e.g., to focus on certain rehabilitation centers and not on others.
5. *Time*, e.g., to carry out the study in a set time interval, such as during certain seasons of the year and/or at predetermined hours.

External Validity

External validity is conceptualized as the possibility of generalizing the causal relationship studied in the $utost_i$ to populations ($*UTOST_i$) different from those used in the intervention. External validity would analyze the possibility of extrapolating to populations different from that delimited in the program the conclusions obtained regarding the effects of the causal relationship between treatment (t), the rehabilitation program, and outcome (o), the decrease in the frequency of errors made in the visuospatial coordination task used, on particular units (u), patients who underwent treatment, and setting and time (s and t_i), predetermined spatial/temporal coordinates.

In the example, a possible external validity study would analyze the possibility of whether the same rehabilitation program could be used in different rehabilitation centers ($S*$), or on patients suffering traumatic brain injury of a nature different from those in the study ($U*$).

The object of this conceptualization of validity types is to give equal importance to external as to internal validity, thus avoiding the bias of earlier versions in favor of internal validity.[19] In so doing, external validity is based on the same principles thats justify making inferences (generalizing or extrapolating) in construct validity. Construct validity refers to the extrapolation to constructs from the sampling operations of implemented interventions. External validity analyzes the extrapolation to different constructs from those same sampling operations of implemented interventions. Therefore, in both cases we analyze the same principles underlying the study of constructs.

Figure 13.1 is a summary of different validity types, following the framework of analysis used based on the utost$_i$ acronym.

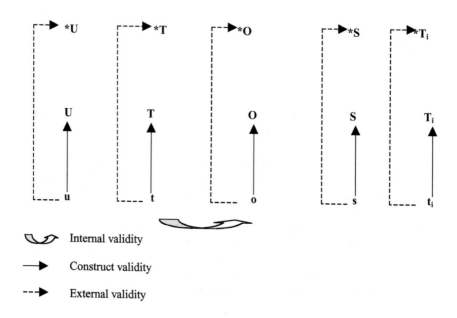

FIGURE 13.1   Validity types (following the model proposed by Cook et al.[20]).

Following this explanation, we must emphasize that it is unlikely that absolute certainty will be achieved with regard to validity of evaluation results. Therefore, whenever we refer to the validity of evaluation results we should use the term *approximation to validity*. In spite of this, as Campbell and Stanley[21] originally pointed out, the purpose of validity types and validity threats is to encourage scrutiny of the designs and their subsequent analysis with the aim of achieving an appropriate interpretation of studies.

The following section introduces the common elements implicit to validity types. Through these common elements we can approach the global concept of validity from which we can develop the evaluative process.

13.4.1   ELEMENTS INVOLVED IN THE CONCEPT OF GLOBAL VALIDITY

The concept of global validity refers to the extent to which there is a correspondence of similarity between the defined constructs and the data (observations) obtained on those constructs. It is what Schmitt[22] defines as theoretical correspondence. At the same time, evaluative results will be valid if they are coherent with a set of previously established constructs (theoretical models) and if they are useful to the parties involved in the intervention program. Through the course of the evaluative process these three criteria (Correspondence, Coherence, and Pragmatism) must be combined to enhance the achievement of the intended validity.

A valid evaluation of the efficacy of a rehabilitation program for patients with traumatic brain injury, would involve three steps:

1. Clearly define the constructs of the program (mainly implementers' constructs, as observations are related to the implemented program and not necessarily related to what was designed during the initial conceptualization of the program).
2. Make observations from said constructs.
3. Analyze the similarity correspondence between the observations and the defined construct.

At the same time we must analyze whether these results are coherent with previous studies (theoretical models) and whether they are useful to the different parties involved in the intervention program.

This global definition of validity sheds light on the common scientific recommendation that to obtain valid data, the object of study must be clearly defined. Nonetheless, given the complexity of most intervention programs, it is reasonable to acknowledge the improbability of achieving absolute validity in program evaluation because of the relative definition of the term. In addition, as authors such as Cronbach[18,23] propose, we are referring to a subjective judgment and dependent therefore on criteria used to make such an assessment. Similarly, Messick[24] defines validity as an integrating evaluative assessment of the degree to which empirical data and theoretical models justify inferences based on particular scores or other assessment models.

At this point we have come to a circular argument. We began by emphasizing the need to obtain valid information and finish by clarifying that a well-defined construct is needed to obtain that valid information. At the same time, the validity of the defined construct will depend on its correspondence with empirical data, previous theories and pragmatism (usefulness) of that construct to the different parties involved in the intervention program. All this directly relates to the conclusion that construct validity is the only validity, that is, the unifying concept that integrates the considerations of content and criteria within a common framework to test hypotheses regarding relevant theoretical relationships.[24] In the same sense, Cronbach[25] points out that the ultimate object of validation is explanation and comprehension and we are therefore made to consider that all validation is construct validation. Based on the development of these ideas, Shadish et al.[1] use the concept of construct validity as the foundation upon which the different proposed validity types are developed.

13.4.2 ACHIEVING VALIDITY IN EVALUATION OF INTERVENTION PROGRAMS FOR ELDERLY PEOPLE

To achieve approximation to validity in program evaluation, considering validity as the interrelation of the principles of correspondence between defined constructs and the obtained data, the coherence of said constructs with previous theories and with the usefulness (pragmatism) of the results obtained, the elements set forth as follows must be taken into account.

The operationalization of constructs (translation of constructs into an operative reality) is very complex, because of the multiplicity of variables and the relationship between them. It is conditioned and modulated in turn by an equally complex and unstable intervention context, while the constructs imply considering both the intervention program (u, t, o) and the context (s, t_i) in which it is set.

On the other hand, aside from operationalizing a construct as clearly as possible, we must ensure that it is implemented exactly as it was defined and in the context for which it was designed. This ensures that all parties involved in the intervention process accept and assume the defined constructs (UTOST$_i$). It would be difficult to expect implementers to carry out an intervention program without having first accepted it from their own construct criteria, or at least having participated in the definition.

In accord with this same line of reasoning, the need to promote the participation of the different parties involved in the development of the different stages of the intervention program is established. In the same way, it entails a process of consensus concerning the aspects that must be considered in the program and fulfilling the demands of the different parties involved in the intervention process.

This sequence supports the interrelationship of the principles of correspondence, coherence, and pragmatism. It establishes the need to analyze the different types of pragmatic uses assigned to the evaluative results. A given use involves meeting the different involved parties' demands from which to comprehend their role in the intervention program.

In conclusion, we propose that in promoting the pragmatic uses of the results of an evaluation program, its validity is improved. This follows from having met the demands of the parties involved in the intervention process that will contribute to the effective implementation of the program. All this implies obtaining valid information concerning the possible effects caused by the program.

13.5 DESIGN ISSUES FOR IMPROVING THE EVALUATION OF PROGRAMS

To this point, the chapter has emphasized the need to achieve validity in the evaluation of programs for elderly people. This present section has two objectives: (1) to describe the characteristics of programs currently under way and (2) to introduce design issues to improve their quality. The general aim of this section is to avoid the idea of design structures that can be applied in standard situations; we want to highlight the need to coordinate design issues for enhancing validity.[1,26]

We use the following topics to illustrate the state of the art of intervention programs for elderly people:

1. Theoretical models on which programs are based;
2. Operationalization of intervention variables (treatments);
3. Assignment procedure of units to program conditions;
4. Operationalization of outcome variables;
5. Outcome variables observations, before, during, and after program implementation;
6. Program follow-up;
7. Measurement scale and statistical analysis applied to outcome variables.

After beginning with a description of the state of the art in evaluation of the programs for elderly people, we will propose possible advances that can be introduced to improve the quality of these designs. We will endeavor to give a hierarchical description of design issues with regard to validity and the generalization of evaluative results.

13.5.1 STATE OF THE ART IN INTERVENTION PROGRAMS FOR ELDERLY PEOPLE

13.5.1.1 Obtaining Information from Databases

In researching the state of the art of evaluation programs for elderly people we used information from the following databases: *Current Contents, Sociological Abstract, Humanities Index*, Educational Resources Information Center (ERIC), FSTA Current, MEDLINE EXPRESS, *The MLA International Bibliography*, The National Technical Information Service (NTIS), and PsycINFO®.

Current Contents Search® editions provide access to more than 7000 of the world's leading scholarly research journals and books in the following disciplines: agriculture, biology and environmental sciences, arts and humanities, clinical medicine, engineering, computing and technology, life sciences, physical, chemical and earth sciences, social and behavioral sciences.

Sociological Abstracts provides access to the world's literature in sociology and related disciplines, both theoretical and applied. Approximately 2500 journals in 30 different languages from about 55 countries are scanned for inclusion, covering sociological topics in fields such as anthropology, economics, education, medicine, community development, philosophy, demography, political science, and social psychology. Journals published by sociological associations, groups, faculties, and institutes, and periodicals containing the term *sociology* in their titles are abstracted fully, irrespective of language or country of publication. Non-core journals are screened for articles by sociologists and/or articles of immediate interest or relevance to sociologists.

Humanities Index, produced by the H. W. Wilson Company, is a bibliographic database that cites articles from English-language periodicals. Periodical coverage includes some of the best-known scholarly journals and numerous lesser-known but important specialized magazines (archaeology, area studies, art, classical studies, communications, dance, film, folklore, gender studies, history, journalism, linguistics, literary and social criticism literature, music, performing arts, philosophy, religion and theology).

ERIC (Educational Resources Information Center), is an information system sponsored by the U.S. Department of Education that generates the U.S. national bibliographic database covering the literature of education. The ERIC database consists of two files: the Resources in Education (RIE) file of document citations and the Current Index to Journals in Education (CIJE) file of journal article citations from over 750 professional journals. In addition, ERIC now contains over 850 ERIC digest records that feature the full text of the original document.

The International Food Information Service (IFIS) produces *Food Science and Technology Abstracts* (FSTA), which contains over 500,000 references; annual updates add approximately 18,000 references per year. FSTA covers all areas of food science, food technology, and human nutrition, including basic food science, biotechnology, toxicology, packaging, and engineering. Some 1800 publications in over 40 languages are scanned regularly, including journals, reviews, standards, legislation, patents, books, theses, and conference proceedings. Abstracts with complete bibliographic details are produced from these original sources. Sources of all the materials abstracted are listed together with instructions for full-text document delivery. Available search aids include a thesaurus and lists of journals covered regularly.

MEDLINE EXPRESS® contains the complete MEDLINE database, including such topics as microbiology, delivery of health care, nutrition, pharmacology, and environmental health. The categories covered in the database include anatomy, organisms, diseases, chemicals and drugs, techniques and equipment, psychiatry and psychology, biological sciences, physical sciences, social sciences and education, technology, agriculture, food, industry, humanities, information science and communications, and health care.

The MLA International Bibliography, produced by the Modern Language Association of America, consists of bibliographic records pertaining to literature, language, linguistics, and folklore and includes coverage from 1963 to the present. *The MLA International Bibliography* provides access to scholarly research in nearly 4000 journals and series. It also covers relevant monographs, working papers, proceedings, bibliographies, and other formats.

The National Technical Information Service (NTIS), an agency of the U.S. Department of Commerce, is the central source for the public sale of U.S. Government–sponsored research, development, and engineering reports. The NTIS Bibliographic Database contains bibliographic citations and summaries of information products, including technical reports, software packages, and data files.

PsycINFO® contains citations and summaries of journal articles, book chapters, books, and technical reports, as well as citations to dissertations, all in the field of psychology and psychological aspects of related disciplines, such as medicine, psychiatry, nursing, sociology, education, pharmacology, physiology, linguistics, anthropology, business, and law. Journal coverage, spanning 1967 to the present, includes international material selected from more than 1300 periodicals written in over 25 languages. Current chapter and book coverage includes worldwide English-language material published from 1967 to the present. Over 55,000 references are added annually through regular updates.

The dates of article coverage in each of these databases is included in Table 13.1.

TABLE 13.1
Database Coverage

Database	From	To
CC Search 7 editions	1999	2000/11
Sociological Abstracts	1986	2000/06
Humanities Index	1984	2000/08
The ERIC database	1966	2000/06
FSTA current	1990	2000/11
MEDLINE EXPRESS	1966	2000/10
MLA directory of periodicals	1963	2000/08
NTIS	1983	2000/10
PsycINFO®	1967	2000/10

We obtained a total number of 827 articles following a very thorough criteria in our search for information. The key words used were *elderly, evaluation & programs.* Selection criteria from the 827 articles included articles with specific reference to program evaluation aimed at the elderly population explicitly stating as an objective the promotion of health and the prevention of disease from a bio-psycho-social point of view. We selected 83 articles, approximately 10% of the total population, after following the established criteria.

13.5.1.2 Description of Obtained Information

To begin with, rarely was reference made in the articles studied to the theoretical models on which program intervention or evaluation programs are based. The highest level of operationalization of constructs made reference to treatment variables (intervention), and to the outcome variables. Table 13.2 shows the frequency distribution of the main treatment (intervention) variables.

The treatment variables used in intervention programs for elderly people are mainly derived from the characteristics of the subjects themselves (sex, self-perception, incontinence, and so forth).[27–29] Following these would come those variables forming part of an overall treatment plan for the improvement or prevention of certain bio-psycho-social aspects, such as physical exercise and social skills training.[30,31] It is important to note that we find nonrandom assignment of units to program conditions in most analyzed studies (80%), and only 20% of studies with random assignment of units to program conditions.

TABLE 13.2
Treatment Variables

Treatment Variables	Articles Studied	Percent	Examples
Subject variables (units)	59	60	Sex, age, self control, degree of functional impairment, falls, incontinence, confusion, self-perception
Application of specific treatments	16	20	Physical exercise, music, memory therapy, social skills training, motivational
Types of programs to be implemented	8	10	Educational and training programs

Table 13.3 shows the frequency distribution of the main outcome variables.

TABLE 13.3
Outcome Variables

Outcome Variables	Articles	Percent	Examples
Efficiency	37	44.6	Monthly costs, cost differences, cost of services, client cost
Psychological well-being	21	25.3	Life satisfaction, self-sufficiency, self-concept, self-esteem, loneliness, measures of psychosocial well-being
General health status	19	22.9	Mental disorders (stress, depression), Alzheimer's disease, physical disorders (cholesterol, hypertension, arthritis, weight)
Social network	6	7.2	Friends, relations, telephone calls, visitors

Outcome variables are focused on program efficacy, on its capacity to improve the health and psychological well-being of the subjects (units).[32–34] To do this, the analyzed articles describe the questionnaire and the interview as the principal evaluation instruments. In this sense, most of the data found in the analyzed articles (80%) are qualitative. This is all related to the statistical techniques employed, generally descriptive analysis or means differences, and at times factor analysis.[35]

In Table 13.4 the frequency distribution of outcome observations are shown (post-test; pretest and post-test; or during program implementation).

TABLE 13.4
Outcome Observations

Outcome Observations	Articles	Percent	Examples
Post-tests	73	88.0	Response Bias Using Two-Stage Data Collection: A Study of Elderly Participants in a Program Evaluating the Internal Health of Senior Communities
Pretest and post-test	6	7.2	An impact evaluation of a falls prevention program The Impact of Alcoholism Education on Service Providers, Elders, and Their Family Members
During program implementation	4	4.8	Leisure Education Program Weight loss in Alzheimer disease

Outcome observations are usually made once the intervention program has ended (post-test).[36] Observations made during, before, or after the implementation of programs are rare.[37,38] This explains why we find summative evaluations vs. formative evaluations (20%) in most analyzed articles (80%).

Last, Table 13.5 describes the main evaluative constructs used in the different articles reviewed.

Table 13.5 shows that the principal evaluative constructs of intervention programs for elderly people are those that are aimed at achieving the objectives of the program, as well as those focused on improving units (subject) variables, such as memory and self-control.[39,40] This is followed by programs aimed at evaluating the degree of user satisfaction. Last, Table 13.5 describes articles referring to the evaluation of efficacy or alternative interventions.[41,42]

13.5.2 Improving Evaluation of Intervention Programs for Elderly People

This section establishes the different structural design dimensions based on which we can improve the design and evaluation of intervention programs for older people.

Rarely was reference made in the articles we studied to the theoretical models on which intervention or evaluation programs should be based. This is a serious problem because, as we have discussed in previous sections, theoretical models should support the reasons we choose to sample any given design elements (units, treatments, outcomes, settings, or time).

It is important to uphold the choice of a particular intervention program from different options, not only to validate the intervention model we use, but also to be able to introduce changes systematically to these interventions programs. In

TABLE 13.5
Evaluative Construct

Evaluative Construct	Articles	Percent	Examples
Objective-driven programs	37	44.44	Specification of Functional Goals Principles for Geriatric Health Promotion
Intervention–treatment programs	27	33.33	Internship Training Program Combining Practice and Theory Reminiscence as a Therapeutic Intervention
Satisfaction	10	12.11	Ohio's Options for Elders Initiative Clients and Bureaucracies: Evaluations of Public Service
Comparison of different intervention–treatment programs	9	10.11	Comparing medical centers treating hip fractures in the elderly Comparing the results of two of the study physical therapists

addition, if we design intervention programs without explicitly stating the theoretical model on which they are based, it is nearly impossible to generalize our results to different populations given that we do not really know which our previous defined population was.

With regard to unit assignment, we should try to assign units to program conditions randomly, to obtain an unbiased estimation of program effect size. If this is not possible the assignment procedure should be executed exactly as was intended in the design, to obtain comparable groups (as similar as possible).

To obtain comparable groups of units assigned to program conditions, we can use stable matching of comparison groups. We must have very clear matching criteria before matching subjects and then analyze the feasibility of the assignment procedure.

In summary, when we form comparison groups we want to have a valid control group to test what would have happened if we had not implemented our intervention program. The object is to obtain comparable, or similar, groups differentiated only by reception/nonreception of intervention. It is therefore better to use cohort groups than nonequivalent comparison groups (nonrandomly formed groups). Members of a cohort group (families, groups of classes, or members of a team) are more similar to each other than are members of a nonequivalent comparison group (participants, units, of the intervention program that do not have similar daily living contexts). Thus, the term *cohort* refers to a naturally formed group of subjects, e.g., members of a club or a school class.

In addition, in our endeavor to improve the quality of the information obtained from comparison groups, we can use multiple nonequivalent comparison groups and statistical adjustment techniques to control the influence of confounding variables

on the estimation of program effects. Although we may encounter serious representation and reliability problems, we can sometimes obtain comparison groups based
on data from regression extrapolation, normed groups of comparison, or by using
secondary data for comparison.

Regarding pretest observations, we found that the analyzed articles generally
had no pretest observations, and only one had a post-test observation. We can
improve evaluation designs by introducing multiple pretest observations. This is
useful in analyzing such validity threats as maturation effects, regression artifacts,
instrumentation, and testing.

Although sometimes it is not possible to obtain multiple pretest observations,
we should obtain at least one. If there is no pretest, we can use pretests from
independent samples, keeping in mind that this solution poses a problem as the
chosen sample may not represent the same population we are trying to evaluate. We
can also use retrospective pretests or proxy pretests, although these two solutions
are rarely used given their high risk of low reliability and the use of inadequate
variables if we develop a proxy measurement model.

With regard to the design of post-test observations, we found only one in most
of the articles. To improve the evaluation design, we should add multiple post-test
observations that would allow us to compare them with a substantive pattern of
evidence concerning the expected effects based on theoretical knowledge. This
follows the same logic as when we use special post-test observations that would
nonequivalent outcome variables, which require the post-test measurements of two
plausibly related constructs (e.g., two measures of health), one of which, the target
or outcome variable, is expected to change because of the intervention, while the
other, the nonequivalent outcome variable, is not predicted to change as an effect
of the intervention, although it is expected to respond to the same validity threats
in the same way as the target outcome.

With regard to program implementation, we rarely found in the analyzed articles
any observation during the course of program implementation. The following design
alternative (variations of implementation of program interventions) will improve
evaluations. The *switching replication method* replicates the intervention effect at a
later date in a group that originally served as a control (comparison) group but is
subsequently given the intervention. It is better to use multiple comparison groups
which will all receive intervention at different times. The *reversed treatment method*
can also be applied. In this case, the evaluator applies the intervention that is expected
to reverse the outcome when compared to the expected outcome in the intervention
condition. Also we can use the *removed treatment method*, which first presents and
then removes the intervention to demonstrate that the pattern of outcomes follows
the pattern of intervention application. We can also use the *repeated treatments
method*, which reintroduces the intervention after its removal, doing so as often as
is feasible (sometimes this design is called the ABAB design, with A standing for
absence of intervention and B for presence of intervention). Finally, the *dosage
variation method* varies the amount of intervention given to participants, under the
assumption that greater dosages should show greater effectiveness.

After analyzing different structural design dimensions for improving the evaluation process we have to stress that there is no perfect design. Evaluation designs

are conditioned by the objectives of the evaluation and successfully detecting different validity threats before designing the intervention program. These two points will be modulated by prior knowledge concerning the intervention field and the features of the context in which the intervention program is to be implemented. Different circumstances modulate the use of different structural design dimensions. In spite of these modulating conditions, our aim has been to describe useful design criteria to improve evaluation of intervention programs for older people. In summary, and after having analyzed the current situation, program evaluation can be improved principally by using multiple pretest and post-test observations, nonequivalent outcome variables, multiple comparison groups, increasing observations during implementation, and introducing variations to given interventions.

This section has stressed that, when not using random procedures, valid evaluations must be based on an appropriate selection of structural design dimensions to control as many validity threats as possible. This concerns obtaining as much data as possible with the highest possible quality (validity and reliability), thus enabling us to achieve higher-quality evaluation results.

13.6 METHODOLOGICAL IMPLICATIONS OF VALIDITY IN THE EVALUATIVE PROCESS OF INTERVENTION PROGRAMS

The experimental tradition that has dominated research in scientific methodology has conditioned program evaluation. The possibility of manipulating variables, analyzing their effects, and modifying the experimental context have made standardized experimental research designs possible. However, we find a different situation in the context of program evaluation. We have multiple interrelated variables, interrelated in different ways and at different times. In addition, the evaluator is not the only person in charge of deciding on the object of the evaluation; there are different parties involved in defining the object of the program evaluation, and sometimes these parties have different interests. At the same time, intervention programs are implemented in an unstable and continually changing context.

All these circumstances make it virtually impossible to achieve standardized design structures for evaluating intervention programs. Therefore, it is all the more important to emphasize validity of evaluative data. Validity, however, is not an absolute criterion. It is a relative criterion as it represents a global assessment of decisions made concerning the intervention program. This assessment depends on empirical evidence, theoretical constructs, and the utility of evaluative results. All this substantiates the need of the participation of all the different parties involved in the intervention program. The main objective is to achieve a global consensual evaluation,[43–46] coherent with existing theoretical models.[47–49] Thus, given that the evaluation results have to be useful in solving intervention problems in the particular context in which the program is developed, validity is directly related to pragmatic criteria.[50]

In short, we describe the conceptualization of the program developed by different parties involved in the intervention process, but we must emphasize that the conceptualization is not what is being implemented, it is just an approximation of the actual implemented program.[51] The convergence of the conceptualization of the different involved parties[52,53] will make it possible to triangulate different methods and subsequently analyze the convergent validity of obtained results,[54] using complementary techniques to analyze error variation in obtained data.[55]

This complex context justifies the need for an ongoing interrelationship between the intervention and evaluation processes. We cannot change intervention program designs without having evaluated their effects, and this in turn modulates the evaluation process. In light of this analysis we propose the implementation of formative evaluations, or at least approximations to them, whenever possible, with the object of promoting the participation of the different parties involved in the intervention and evaluation designs. This can reinforce timely effective feedback on designing and implementing intervention programs for elderly people.

13.7 CONCLUDING REMARKS

The following is a summary of the most salient conclusions of this chapter:

1. Validity of the intervention process is based on the interrelationship between intervention and evaluation.
2. The participation of the different parties involved in the intervention program must be encouraged in order to delimitate, as precisely as possible, the intervention–evaluation interrelationship.
3. We have to emphasize the usefulness of evaluative results.
4. The global validity of evaluation results depends on:
   a. Similarity correspondence between defined constructs and the data obtained on those constructs;
   b. Coherence of the evaluative results with a set of previously established constructs (theoretical models);
   c. The utility of evaluative results to those involved in the intervention program (pragmatism).
5. Validity of program evaluation depends on the interrelationship of the following structural design dimensions:
   a. Assignment procedure of units (subjects) to program conditions:
      • Assignment criteria should be clearly specified.
      • We must use similar comparison groups (using previous matching of units before assignment or using cohort groups).
   b. Pretest observations (observations previous to program implementation):
      • Multiple pretest observations should be used (as many as possible, but always within the boundaries of obtaining valid data).
      • We must have at least one pretest observation (to test effects of the intervention program).
      • We can use alternatives to pretest observations (pretests of independent samples, retrospective pretest, or proxy pretest of outcome variables).

c. Post-test observations:
- We will always have one post-test observation, but we should add multiple post-test observations whenever possible.
- We can combine post-test observations with nonequivalent outcome variables.

d. Comparison groups:
- It is better to use cohort groups than nonequivalent comparison groups.
- Multiple comparison groups should be used.
- In extreme cases we can obtain comparison groups based on data from regression extrapolation, normed groups of comparison, or by using secondary data for making comparisons.

e. Program implementation:
- We should implement what we have designed.
- Observations during program implementation should be made.
- We can introduce some variations to the implementation of program interventions to maximize detection of program effects (switching replication method, reversed treatment method, the removed treatment method, repeated treatments methods, the dosage variation method).

6. There is no ideal solution. Design depends on the interrelationship between previous described structural design dimensions, and this interrelationship is conditioned by:
   a. Object of program evaluation;
   b. Analysis and identification of potential validity threats;
   c. Previous knowledge of existing theoretical models;
   d. Features of the intervention context.

ACKNOWLEDGMENTS

The authors thank JoEllen Wheelock for her help in the English translation of this chapter and in particular for her patience when trying to understand this sometimes abstract matter of "validity."

REFERENCES

1. Shadish, W. R., Cook, T., and Campbell, D., *Experimental and Quasi-Experimental Design for Generalized Causal Inference*, Houghton Mifflin, Boston, 2001.
2. Chacón, S., Validez, in *Evaluación de Programas Sociales y Sanitarios: Un Abordaje Metodológico,* Anguera, M. T., Ed., Síntesis, Madrid, in press.
3. Belcher, J. R., Mental health and social policy: the emergency of managed care, *Health Soc. Work*, 25(1), 78, 2000.
4. Keigher, S. M., Reflecting on progress, health, and racism: 1900 to 2000, *Health Soc. Work*, 24(4), 243, 1999.

5. Bradley, V. J., Changes in services and supports for people with developmental disabilities: new challenges to established practice, *Health Soc. Work*, 25(3), 191, 2000.

6. Abramson, J. S. and Mizrahi, T., When social workers and physicians collaborate: positive and negative interdisciplinary experiences, *Soc. Work*, 41, 270, 1996.

7. Allen-Meares, P., The interdisciplinary movement, *J. Soc. Work Educ.*, 34, 2, 1998.

8. Davis, C., Leveille, S., Favaro, S., and LoGerfo, M., Benefits to volunteers in a community-based health promotion and chronic illness self-management program for the elderly, *J. Gerontol. Nurs.*, 24(10), 16, 1998.

9. Kagan, S. L. and Weissbourd, B., Eds., *Putting Families First: America's Family Support Movement and the Challenge of Change*, Jossey-Bass, San Francisco, 1994.

10. H. M. O. Workgroup on Care Management, Essential components of geriatric care provided through health maintenance organizations, *J. Am. Geriatr. Soc.*, 46(3), 303, 1998.

11. Buckwalter, K. C., Smith, M., Zevenbergen, P., and Russell, D., Mental health services of the rural elderly outreach program, *Gerontologist*, 31(3), 408, 1991.

12. Pulliam, L., Client satisfaction with a nurse managed clinic, *J. Commun. Health Nurs*, 8(2), 97, 1991.

13. Riley, T. and Mollica, R. L., The Arizona long term care system, *J. Case Managing*, 5(2), 78, 1996.

14. Fillit, H., Challenges for acute care geriatric impatient units under the present medicare prospective payment system, *J. Am. Geriatr. Soc.*, 42(5), 553, 1994.

15. Berkman, B., The emerging health care world: implications for social work practice and education, *Soc. Work*, 41, 541, 1996.

16. Berk, R. and Rossi, P. J., *Thinking about Program Evaluation*, Sage, Beverly Hills, CA, 1990.

17. Anguera, M. T. and Chacón, S., Aproximación conceptual, in *Evaluación de Programas Sociales y Sanitarios: Un abordaje Metodológico*, Anguera, M. T., Ed., Síntesis, Madrid, in press.

18. Cronbach, L. J., *Designing Evaluation of Educational and Social Programs,* Jossey-Bass, San Francisco, 1982.

19. Cook, T. and Campbell, D., *Quasi-Experimentation. Designs and Analyses Uses for Fields Settings*, Houghton Mifflin, Boston, 1979.

20. Cook, T., Campbell, D. T., and Peracchio, L., Quasi-experimentation, in *Handbook of Industrial and Organizational Psychology,* Dunnette, M. D. and Hough, L. M., Eds., Random House, New York, 1991, 491.

21. Campbell, D. and Stanley, J., *Experimental and Quasi-experimental Designs for Research,* Rand McNally, Chicago, 1966.

22. Schmitt, F. F., *Truth: A Primer,* Westview Press, Boulder, CO, 1995.

23. Cronbach, L., Construct validation after thirty years, in *Intelligence: Measurement, Theory and Public Policy*, Linn, R. L., Ed., University of Illinois Press, Urbana, 1989.

24. Messick, S., Validity, in *Educational Measurement,* Linn, R. E., Ed., National Council of Measurement in Education, Series on Higher Education, Oryx Press, Phoenix, AZ, 1989, 13.

25. Cronbach, L., *Essentials of Psychological Testing,* 4th ed., Harper & Row, New York, 1984.

26. Corrin, W. and Cook, T. D., Design elements of quasi-experiments, in *Advances in Educational Productivity,* Waldberg, H. J., Reynolds, A. J., and Walberg, H. J., Eds., 7, 35, 1998.

27. Lave, J. R., Ives, D. G., Traven, N. D., and Kuller, L. H., Participation in health promotion programs by the rural elderly, *Am. J. Prev. Med.*, 11(1), 46, 1995.

28. Di Carlo, A., Lamassa, M., Pracucci, G., Basile, A. M., Trefoloni, G., Vanni, P., Wolfe, C. D. A., Tilling, K., Ebrahim, S., and Inzitari, D., Stroke in the very old — clinical presentation and determinants of 3-month functional outcome: a European perspective, *Stroke*, 30(11), 2313, 1999.

29. Duffy, J. A., Duffy, M., and Kilbourne, W., Cross national study of perceived service quality in long-term care facilities, *J. Aging Stud.*, 11(4), 327, 1997.

30. Dubney, L., Working with the elderly: a one-year internship training program combining practice and theory, *J. Appl. Gerontol.*, 9(1), 118, 1990.

31. Husaini, B. A., Castor, R. S., Whitten, S. R., Moore, S. T., Neser, W., Linn, J. G., and Griffin, D., An evaluation of a therapeutic health program for the black elderly, *J. Health Soc. Policy*, 2(2), 67, 1990.

32. Kassner, E., The Older Americans Act: should participants share in the cost of services? *J. Aging Soc. Policy*, 4(1–2), 51, 1992.

33. Hashizume, Y. and Kanagawa, K., Correlates of participation in adult day care and quality of life in ambulatory frail elderly in Japan, *Publ. Health Nurs.*, 13(6), 404, 1996.

34. Kim, J. H., The influence of employment on older Korean-American economic self-sufficiency, psychological well-being, status, and social support: impact evaluation of the senior community service employment program (SC-SEP), *Humanities Soc. Sci.*, 59(8), 3210-A, 1999.

35. Chumbler, N. R., Beverly, C. J., and Beck, C. K., Rural older adults' likelihood of receiving a personal response system: the Arkansas medicaid waiver program, *Eval. Program Planning*, 20(2), 117, 1997.

36. Goodfellow, M., Response bias using two-stage data collection: a study of elderly participants in a program, *Eval. Rev.*, 12(6), 638, 1988.

37. Dunn, N. J. and Wilhite, B., The effects of a leisure education program on leisure participation and psychosocial well-being of two older women who are home centered, *Ther. Recreation J.*, 31(1), 53, 1997.

38. Coogle, C. L., Osgood, N. J., Pyles, M. A., and Wood, H. E., The impact of alcoholism education on service providers, elders, and their family members, *J. Appl. Gerontol.*, 14(3), 321, 1995.

39. Dubney, L., Working with the elderly: a one-year internship training progam combining practice and theory, *J. Appl. Gerontol.*, 9(1), 118, 1990.

40. Fielden, M. A., Reminiscence as a therapeutic intervention with sheltered housing residents: a comparative study, *Br. J. Soc. Work*, 20(1), 21, 1990.

41. Nelson, B. J., Clients and bureaucracies: applicant evaluations of public human service and benefit programs, paper presented at the Annual Meeting of the American Political Science Association, Washington, D.C., September 1, 1979.

42. Mozes, B., Maor, Y., Olmer, L., and Shabtai, E., Comparing medical centers treating hip fractures in the elderly: the importance of multi-outcome measurements, *Am. J. Med. Qual.*, 14(3), 117, 1999.

43. Carey, M. A. and Smith, M. W., Enhancement of validity through qualitative approaches: incorporating the patient's perspectives, *Eval. Health Prof.*, 15(4), 107, 1992.

44. Lobosco, A. F. and Newman, D. L., Stakeholder information needs. Implications for evaluation practice and policy development in early childhood special education, *Eval. Rev.*, 16(5), 443, 1992.

45. Brandon, P. R., Newton, B. J., and Harman, J. W., Enhancing validity through beneficiaries' equitable involvement in identifying and prioritizing homeless children's educational problems, *Eval. Program Planning*, 6, 287, 1993.

46. Camasso, M. J. and Dick, J., Using multiattribute utility theory as a priority-setting tool in human services planning, *Eval. Program Planning*, 16, 295, 1993.

47. Chen, H. and Rossi, P. H., Evaluating with sense: the theory-driven approach, *Eval. Rev.*, 7, 283, 1983.

48. Gottfredson, G. D., A theory-driven approach to program evaluation. A method of stimulating researcher-implementer collaboration, *Am. Psychol.*, 39(10), 1101, 1984.

49. Chen, H., *Theory-Driven Evaluations*, Sage, London, 1990.

50. Fishman, D. B., An introduction to the experimental versus the pragmatic paradigm in evaluation, *Eval. Program Planning,* 14, 353, 1991.

51. Shadish, W. R., The quantitative-qualitative debates: "DeKuhnifying" the conceptual context, *Eval. Program Planning*, 18, 47, 1995.

52. Guba, E. G. and Lincoln, Y. S., *Effective Evaluation: Improving the Usefulness of Evaluation Results through Responsive and Naturalistic Approaches*, Jossey-Bass, San Francisco, 1985.

53. Guba, E. G. and Lincoln, Y. S., *Fourth Generation Evaluation*, Sage, Beverly Hills, CA, 1989.

54. Fiske, D., Convergent-discriminant validation in measurements and research strategies, *in Forms of Validity Research*, Brinberg, D. and Kidder, L. H., Eds., Jossey-Bass, San Francisco, 1982, 77.

55. Sechrest, L. and Sidani, S., Quantitative and qualitative methods: is there an alternative? *Eval. Program Planning*, 18(1), 77, 1995.

Part IV

Advances in Treatment

14 Neuropharmacology for Older Adults

José León-Carrión,
María Rosario Domínguez-Morales,
and Manuel Murga Sierra

CONTENTS

14.1 Introduction 311
14.2 Neuroleptics for Confusion and Agitation...312
14.3 Antiparkinsonism Agents for Movement Control 313
14.4 Benzodiazepines for Anxiety and Sleep Disorders 314
14.5 Antidepressants 315
14.6 Nootropic (Cognition Enhancing) Drugs 318
14.7 Side Effects of Some Common Medications on Cognition
       and Behavior 318
14.8 Final Comments 319
References 320

14.1 INTRODUCTION

When using medication in the treatment of neurological and psychiatric problems it is important to be aware of the processes and events that occur once the drug is administered. This is especially true in the case of elderly people given that most older people use a combination of several different medications. The first step to be considered is the route of administration of a medication. The route will determine how quickly the drug takes effect. The most common route is *oral administration*, which in most cases can be self-administered and which is also both the safest and the most economical method. Nonetheless, oral administration is not the fastest route and, with the exception of sublingual administration, there may be difficulties in absorption. Absorption of medication is faster when administered through the route of *inhalation*. However, *intravenous injection*, given that the drug reaches the blood flow immediately and thus the site of action promptly, is the fastest route. *Intramuscular injection* is used when a slower absorption over a period of time is desired. Slow absorption is also attained with *subcutaneous administration*, with the rate of absorption dependent on the blood flow to the site. *Topical application* of the medication to membranes is used when it is preferable to achieve localized effects of a drug. Pharmacokinetics and pharmacodynamics must also be considered given

0-8493-2066-/01/$0.00+$1.50
© 2001 by CRC Press LLC

that both are altered in older people. This is due to several reasons, including physiological and structural age-related changes in the gastrointestinal tract.[3,6,7,19] This chapter considers the pharmacokinetic and pharmacodynamic effects of the different kinds of neurological and psychotropic drugs commonly prescribed for elderly people.

14.2 NEUROLEPTICS FOR CONFUSION AND AGITATION

Neuroleptics, most commonly phenothiazines, are widely used as antipsychotic drugs to control symptoms of schizophrenia, mania, or psychotic depression in older as well as younger adults. Their most common use in older persons is for controlling the behavioral problems and agitation associated with delirium in dementing processes and in Huntington's disease. The new class of neuroleptics, or atypical antipsychotics, is used in the treatment of Parkinson's disease. The dosage administered to older people is normally between one third to one half the amount administered to younger adults.

Neuroleptic drugs modify several neurotransmitter systems. They especially interfere with DA (dopamine) transmission by blocking DA receptors or by inhibiting DA release. In older people the pharmacokinetics of neuroleptics is altered, normally producing higher active blood levels and more prolonged drug effects. Tolerance is related to the sedative effects of phenothiazines and develops gradually. An acquired dependence on these drugs is very unusual because of the unpleasant effects they have on individuals who have no psychotic symptoms.

It is important to determine the adequate dosage when prescribing neuroleptics to older people. It generally takes 4 to 6 weeks or longer to achieve full therapeutic effectiveness.[17] Therefore, the decision whether or not to increase (tap) the dosage or increase the duration of treatment depends upon the observed effects of the drug on the patient. Higher effectiveness does not always correlate with a higher dosage. This depends on the patient. Some authors[39] have suggested that there is a therapeutic window of effectiveness in the use of haloperidol. Lower clinical effectiveness is produced by dosage above or below its therapeutic optimum. There is some controversy in finding the most effective neuroleptic, and there is no definitive answer. Because they notably decrease the tendency to produce extrapyramidal effects, some authors recommend the high-potency neuroleptics, such as haloperidol, or an atypical antipsychotic, such as risperidone or alanzapine, as a generally preferred treatment for psychotic and agitated states in elderly people.[23]

People become more sensitive to the side effects of neuroleptics as the brain ages. For this reason elderly patients receiving neuroleptic medication must be closely monitored.

Side effects involving the basal ganglia, such as parkinsonism, are among the most common and are known as extrapyramidal disorders. These mainly occur with the use of potent neuroleptics. In these cases the patient has problems controlling voluntary movements. The most common symptoms are tremors, spasticity, akinesia (slowing movements) and akathisia (patient cannot sit down). Most patients will develop these side effects and normally symptoms will not disappear until the treatment is ended.

Sedation is another common side effect in elderly people when using low-potency neuroleptics. Because of delayed metabolism and excretion there can be an accumulation of doses within the body. In these cases, sedation may be present for hours after administration, which seriously affects the level of arousal needed for carrying out activities of daily living. This kind of neuroleptic sedation may produce orthostatic hypotension, which is a serious problem for the older patient suffering motor problems.

Another common side effect associated with the prolonged use of neuroleptics is tardive dyskinesia. Older women seem to be more likely to suffer this side effect. The symptoms are stereotyped involuntary movements in the face and jaws such as lateral jaw movements and "fly-catching" darting of the tongue. Other possible symptoms are uncontrolled movements of the arms and legs. Whenever possible, treatment must be discontinued if these symptoms are observed. This side effect may persist even once the treatment with neuroleptics is suspended. There is no effective treatment for tardive dyskinesia and it may be irreversible in some patients.

Generally, psychotropic medication, including neuroleptics and benzodiazepine, must be carefully considered when prescribing them for elderly people. Elderly people are at an increased risk of dementia, visual impairment, postural hypotension, and neurological and musculoskeletal disability.[2]

14.3   ANTIPARKINSONISM AGENTS FOR MOVEMENT CONTROL

Parkinson's disease (PD) is a degenerative disorder, which causes a marked impairment of normal motor control. A loss of DA neurons in the *substantia nigra pars compacta* occurs in PD. Compensating for this DA neuronal loss is the objective of most antiparkinsonism medications. Given that the administration of DA is not possible because of the inability of DA to cross the blood–brain barrier, a DA precursor is normally administered. This precursor is levodopa (L-dopa) which penetrates the blood–brain barrier and is converted to DA by the enzyme aromatic L-amino acid decarboxylase.

Levodopa, when used in combination with a peripheral dopa decarboxylase inhibitor, such as carbidopa or benzeraside, produces a significant improvement of the clinical symptoms of the early stages of PD. This combination increases the availability of levodopa to the brain by reducing extracerebral metabolism while avoiding the side effects of levodopa such as nausea and orthostatic hypotension. Levodopa combined with carbidopa is produced under the trademark of Sinemet. levodopa combined with benzarazide is under the trademark of Madopar. PD symptoms may take 1 to 6 months to improve when using L-dopa.

Elderly patients show a sensitivity to the behavioral side effects of levodopa. These can include confusion, anxiety, fatigue, increased libido, depression, delusions, hallucinations, nightmares, insomnia, and agitation. Some authors[30,36] have suggested the possibility of an increase in the cognitive deterioration of mild dementia. Normally, levodopa therapy is effective for several years. Nonetheless, after a period of 3 to 5 years a large number of patients begin to notice, under the same treatment, an impairment in motor facilitation between one dose and the next (wearing-off effect). Later, patients begin to show an "on–off" effect not related to drug dose. They experience unpredictable tremors or rigidity alternating with periods of mobility. Some authors note that treatment with levodopa should be started as late as possible, especially in younger patients.[32] To improve levodopa therapy and reduce motor fluctuations, it is recommended that the diet of patients with PD contain a 7:1 ratio of carbohydrate to protein.[31]

Other drug treatments have been attempted with patients with PD. To reduce the "off" periods, some researchers[15,33] suggest a continuous dopaminergic stimulation through intravenous or intraduodenal infusion of levodopa. However, this methodology presents some practical problems. Sustained-release oral levodopa preparations such as Madopar CR, Madopar HBS, and Sinemet CR have been developed to resolve these problems. These preparations have better results at the onset of the "wearing–off" period than when a severe "on–off" effect has appeared. Some clinicians recommend bromocriptine as a supplementary therapy to L-dopa, especially at the onset of the "wearing-off" effect. A large number of patients receiving only bromocriptine benefit from it. Amantadine is another option occasionally used by clinicians, but tolerance soon develops and the drug can be toxic in elderly patients with impaired renal function. The use of anticholinergic drugs in the treatment of patients with PD is very limited because of side effects that include cardiovascular symptoms and orthostatic hypotension as well as ocular, gastrointestinal, urologic, and psychiatric symptoms.

Some authors have suggested that an early treatment with L-dopa combined with MAO-B inhibitors (seligiline or Deprenyl) may retard the development of PD.[27–29] Studies with animals suggest that Deprenyl saves damaged neurons and provides neural protection. It is recommended as the drug of choice for the initial treatment of PD. Another author, Bianchine,[4] considers the effects of deprenyl to be transient.

14.4 BENZODIAZEPINES FOR ANXIETY AND SLEEP DISORDERS

Benzodiazepines (BDZ) are widely used in the treatment of older adults. More than 40% of prescriptions for this drug are for patients over 65 years of age.[8] The main use of benzodiazepines is in the treatment of anxiety and sleep disorders. They are also used to calm agitated patients with dementia, although, paradoxically, the drug can exacerbate confusion and agitation during the night. They are also used in the treatment of epilepsy and as a preanesthetic sedative (midazolam induces rapid calming and deep sleep when using local anesthetics during brief surgical procedures) and alprazolam is sometimes used as an antidepressant.[38]

BDZ are also used to reduce anxiety and fear in patients with cancer, stroke, and cardiovascular diseases; in psychosomatic disorders such as asthma, angina pectoris, irritable colon, gastric ulcers, and skin diseases; in treating alcohol withdrawal; in the neuromuscular disorders associated with cerebral palsy, multiple sclerosis, hemiplegia, paraplegia, and bone fractures.[10] Because of such undesirable side effects as sedation, confusion, and coordination and memory problems in older adults, BDZ does not seem to be the most appropriate long-term treatment for insomnia. These side effects are sometimes misdiagnosed as normal age-related conditions in elderly people. Traffic accidents involving older people in the morning may be the results of the residual effects of BDZ hypnotics.[14] BDZ hypnotic drugs seem to be prescribed with minimal physician follow-up in older patients.

Normally, BDZ are well absorbed after oral administration; however, with the exception of lorazepam, intramuscular absorption is poor. BDZ are mainly metabolized by the liver. Depending on the drug used, the peak concentration in the blood plasma is achieved within 0.5 to 8 h. The behavioral effects of BDZ do not correlate with the elimination of the drug. For example, the active metabolite of flurazepam has a half-life of 50 h, whereas its blood plasma half-life is 2 to 3 h (Table 14.1). The long-acting BDZ, such as diazepam and flurazepam, have active metabolites with long half-lives, but in older persons these can cause somnolence and confusion due to accumulative effects. In elderly people, the use of short-acting BDZ such as triazolam and oxazepam is recommended given that the probability of producing accumulative and toxic effects is decreased. Between the long- and short-acting BDZ are lorazepam and temazepam.

Some studies suggest that BDZ may produce subtle to moderate cognitive impairment in older people and it must be carefully controlled when used in patients with dementia. BDZ can produce dependency and patients have difficulty in giving it up after prolonged use. Older people are more sensitive to the effect of BDZ on memory than are young people. During the first 6 weeks of treatment there is very little risk of developing dependence. The risk of developing a dependency on the medication increases after 3 to 8 months of treatment and increases even more beyond this time. Withdrawal symptoms include tremors, agitation, gastrointestinal problems, seizures, and idiosyncratic reactions. A paradoxical effect can sometimes be observed in some patients, especially those treated with diazepam, who may become more assertive and aggressive or even have suicide ideation. This paradoxical effect is usually resolved within a week after medication is withdrawn (Table 14.1).

14.5 ANTIDEPRESSANTS

Depression is an important health problem in elderly people. Some authors suggest that depression in older patients, when the patients are compliant and their symptoms have been recognized and are treated aggressively, is as treatable as depression in younger patients.

However, treatment resistance is observed in elderly patients. Depending on the definition, the prevalence of treatment resistance in elderly people could be as high as 33%.[18] Certain patients, with no clinical history of depression before age 60, can present a late-onset depression. To quote Kamholz and Mellow:[18]

> There may be a higher rate of delusional depression among these patients, necessitating adjunctive treatment with neuroleptic medication. Furthermore, these patients may have a higher relapse rate. The brains of late-onset depressive patients show significantly more subcortical and deep white matter lesions, referred to as leukoencephalopathy when observed with MR imaging. These MR imaging lesions are also associated with risk factors for cerebrovascular disease such as diabetes, cardiac disease and extracerebral carotid artery disease.

See Chapter 17 on depression.

Depression in older persons may be accompanied by cognitive impairment (mnesic, verbal, thinking, visuospatial) and may be the initial manifestation of a dementive process. Severe depression in older patients is sometimes mistaken for a dementia.

TABLE 14.1
Pharmacokinetic Summary of the Benzodiazepines

Administered Drug	Most Common Indication	Initial Biotransformation Pathway	Substances Present in Blood (with usual range of elimination half-life, hr)[a]
Diazepam	Anxiolytic	Oxidation	Diazepam (20–70)
			Desmethyldiazepam (36–96)
			Oxazepam*
			Temazepam*
Clorazepate[b]	Anxiolytic	Oxidation	Desmethyldiazepam (36–96)
Prazepam[b]	Anxiolytic	Oxidation	Desmethyldiazepam (36–96)
Oxazolam[b]	Anxiolytic	Oxidation	Desmethyldiazepam (36–96)
Alprazolam	Anxiolytic	Oxidation	Alprazolam (8–15)
Lorazepam	Anxiolytic	Conjugation	Lorazepam (10–20)
Oxazepam	Anxiolytic	Conjugation	Oxazepam (5–15)
Bromazepam	Anxiolytic	Oxidation	Bromazepam (20–30)
Clobazam	Anxiolytic	Oxidation	Clobazam (20–30)
Flurazepam	Hypnotic		Desmethylclobazam
		Oxidation	Desalkylflurazepam (36–120)
			Hydroxyethyl flurazepam (1–4)
			Flurazepam aldehyde
			Flurazepam*
Temazepam	Hypnotic	Conjugation	Temazepam (8–20)
Lormetazepam	Hypnotic	Conjugation	Lormetazepam (8–20)
Triazolam	Hypnotic	Oxidation	Triazolam (1.5–5)
Nitrazepam	Hypnotic	Nitroreduction	Nitrazepam (20–30)
Flunitrazepam	Hypnotic, perioperative	Oxidation, nitroreduction	Flunitrazepam (10–40)
			Desmethylflunitrazepam
Quazepam	Hypnotic	Oxidation	Quazepam (15–35)
			Oxoquazepam (25–35)
			Desalkylflurazepam (36–120)
Estazolam	Hypnotic	Oxidation	Estazolam (20–30)
Midazolam	Perioperative, hypnotic	Oxidation	Midazolam (1–4)
			1-Hydroxymethyl midazolam*
			4-Hydroxy midazolam*
Clonazepam	Antiseizure	Nitroreduction	Clonazepam (30–60)

[a] Asterisk (*) indicates compounds present in quantitatively minor amounts and/or those that have reduced pharmacological activity.

[b] Clorazepate, prazepam, and oxazolam all serve as desmethyldiazepam precursors.

Source: Principles of Neuropsychopharmacology, Feldman et al., Sinauer Associates, Sunderland, MA, 1997. With permission.

Monoamine oxidase (MAO) inhibitors, tricyclic antidepressants, and second-generation antidepressants (including the selective serotonin uptake blockers) are the three most important groups of antidepressants. Atypical antidepressants, electroconvulsive therapy, and lithium (mainly used in bipolar disorders) are also used in the treatment of depression. MAO inhibitors have been found to be useful in the treatment of the depressed older patient. Nonetheless, the use of MAO inhibitors in these patients is very complicated because of the possible side effects and the complexity of the diet and life of the elderly patient and is normally avoided. Common side effects are hypertension (under certain dietary conditions), orthostatic hypotension, agitation, confusion, and insomnia.

Tricyclic antidepressants (TCAs) were widely used in older patients before the arrival of the new generation of antidepressants. The different TCAs seem to be therapeutically equivalent to one other. Patients may respond better to one TCA than another. The selection of an individual agent is primarily based on the side effect profile rather than the differential therapeutic efficacy. The most important side effects of TCA are sedation, low blood pressure, and the anticholinergic side effects of the TCAs, which are orthostatic hypotension and effects on cardiac conduction. Older patients are sensitive to these side effects, but are even more so to the peripheral cholinergic side effects. These include dry mouth, constipation, blurred vision, and urinary retention. Central anticholinergic side effects such as agitation, confusion, hallucination, and impairment of concentration, attention, and memory[19] can also be present.

Given that they cause fewer side effects than TCA, the newer generation of antidepressants have been the drugs of choice for the treatment of depression in all ages (Figure 14.1). Probably the most popular are the selective serotonin reuptake inhibitors (SSRI) whose antidepressant effects are due both to the increase of the 5-HT neurotransmitter and to the fact that their side effects are better tolerated by elderly patients.

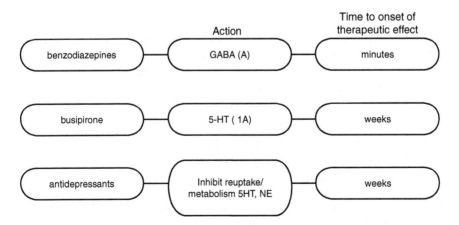

FIGURE 14.1 Presumed mechanism of action for drugs used to treat anxiety disorders. (From Smith, P. F. and Darlington, C. L., *Clinical Psychopharmacology*, Lawrence Erlbaum Associates, Mahwah, NJ, 1996. With permission.)

14.6   NOOTROPIC (COGNITION ENHANCING) DRUGS

The increasing level of life expectancy has facilitated the coming of nootropic drugs. These drugs increase the resistance of the central nervous system to damage associated with or related to the aging process. Studies have shown that these drugs improve learning and memory, increase cortical-subcortical control function, and improve the transfer of information in the telencephalon.[12] Positive results with the use of these drugs include a better quality of life, fewer neurobehavioral problems, increased cognitive capacity, and a considerable improvement in activities of daily living of elderly patients. The mechanisms of action of these drugs seem to be an improvement of microcerebral circulation, greater neural cell protection, and the facilitation of regeneration of damaged brain tissue.[35] From a chemical point of view, nootropic drugs are a very heterogeneous group and include several different kinds of agents.

Tacrine is a reversible tissue and plasma cholinesterese inhibitor used in treatment during the mild or moderate stage of Alzheimer's disease (AD). Although results are not conclusive, some studies have found a 50% reduction in the progress of AD when using tacrine. The most important side effects are nausea, vomiting, abdominal pain, diarrhea, and hepatoxicity. Most of these side effects are intolerable for many patients.

Nimodipine is a calcium channel blocker used for the treatment of neurological deficits associated with subarachnoidal hemorrhage and in the prevention of cerebral vasospasms. In some countries, it is used for the treatment of impaired organic cognitive functions, AD, and vascular dementias.[16] Further research is needed to demonstrate its beneficial effects on dementia as well as in stroke. The most common side effects are hypotension, dizziness, and light-headedness.

Ginko biloba leaf extract is widely used for the enhancement of cognition and behavior in elderly people as well as in the early stages of dementia. Most published studies show improvement of concentration and memory as well as reduced anxiety, dizziness, headache, and tinnitus.

Cerebrolysin is used in some countries in the treatment of vascular dementia, AD, acute stroke, traumatic brain injury, and cognitive and behavioral sequelae of neurosurgery. Although there is very little information concerning its peptide components and pharmacokinetics,[16] this drug seems to show neurotropic and neuroprotective activity.

14.7   SIDE EFFECTS OF SOME COMMON MEDICATIONS ON COGNITION AND BEHAVIOR

Possible iatrogenic neurological and cognitive complications must be considered when prescribing medication to elderly people. These complications seem to be relatively frequent[25] and most of them are potentially preventable.

Antihypertensive drugs are widely and frequently prescribed for older adults in the prevention of cerebrovascular disorders. The effects of antihypertensive drugs on cognition and behavior are not as yet well established. However, it is known that these drugs have diverse neuropsychological effects. The main effect of β-blockers is sedation. Calcium channel blockers can in some cases produce confusion, diuretics can produce subjective behavioral side effects, and methyldopa, when compared with other antihypertensives, has proved to cause more side effects (sedation and deterioration of mood and activities of daily living). The angiotensin-converting enzyme inhibitors seem to produce the fewest subjective side effects in the hypertensive patient.[5,11,22,26]

The indiscriminate use of analgesics should be avoided as they can affect memory and bring on delirium.[9] Antibiotics should be used with care given that penicillin, cephalosporines, and ciprofloxacin can affect memory and have been related to encephalopathy and seizures.[37] Steroids can produce memory problems, depression, psychosis, or delirium in some patients.[21] Patients undergoing immune suppression therapy may show motor problems, ataxia, hallucinations, confusion, and reversible white matter changes in neuroimaging.[22] A toxic encephalopathy can be observed in some patients with cancer treated with interferon,[24] although most of the neuropsychological manifestations of human leukocyte interferon therapy in patients with cancer are mild, even subtle, and normally will not be clinically detected.[1]

Meador's review[22] states that, at toxic levels, cardiac drugs such as digoxin can produce delirium, dementia, hallucinations, and other neuropsychiatric symptoms and that cognitive impairment is correlated with plasma levels even within therapeutic ranges. Quinidine and disopyramide can cause cognitive deterioration perhaps due to their antimuscarinic properties. Lidocaine, flecainide, and tocainide have been associated with delirium and other neuropsychiatric symptoms.

14.8 FINAL COMMENTS

Elderly people take an average of three different medications when treated for neurological or psychiatric symptoms. There is, however, a significant (57%) percentage of medical errors in treatment, with the subsequent potential for adverse outcomes. Errors in dosage seem to be the most common, followed by the prescription of medication inappropriate to the patient or to which the patient is allergic.[20] In light of this, precautionary measures should be taken when prescribing psychotropics or neurological medication. To begin with, the number of different medications should be reduced to a necessary minimum. Once the necessary medication is established, the lowest possible dosage for each must be determined. The best policy is to start at a low dosage and to monitor the effects continually to establish the most effective dosage. When a patient is under the care of more than one physician, the physicians should consult one other concerning the medication they prescribe to avoid the risk of adverse reactions or collateral effects of the different drugs. Anticipating and then controlling any possible side effects is a way of preventing an adverse outcome of treatment. It is the duty of neurologists and psychiatrists to set a standard in the pharmacological treatment of neurological and psychiatric patients.

REFERENCES

1. Adams, F., Quesada, J., and Gutterman, J., Neuropsychiatric manifestations of human leukocyte interferon therapy in patients with cancer, *JAMA*, 252, 938, 1984.
2. Baskys, A. and Remington, G., *Psychotropic Drugs*, CRC Press, Boca Raton, FL, 1996.
3. Benet, L. Z., Kroetz, D. L., and Sheiner, L. B., Pharmacokinetics: the dynamics of drug absorption, distribution, and elimination, in *Goldman and Gilman's: The Pharmacological Basis of Therapeutics*, 9th ed., Hardman, J. G. and Limbird, L. E., Eds., McGraw-Hill, New York, 1996, 3.
4. Bianchine, J. R., Drugs for Parkinson's disease, spasticity and acute muscle spasm, in *The Pharmacological Basis of Therapeutics*, Gilman, A. G., Goodman, L. S., Rall, T. W., and Murad, F., Eds., Macmillan, New York, 1985, 473.
5. Bulpitt, C. F. and Fletcher, A. E., Cognitive function and angiotension-converting enzyme inhibitors in comparison with other antihypertensive drugs, *J. Cardiovasc. Pharmacol.*, 19 (Suppl. 6), S100, 1992.
6. Cadieux, R. J., Drug interactions in the elderly: how multiple drug use increases risk exponentially, *Postgrad. Med.*, 86, 179, 1989
7. Chapron, D. J., Influence of advanced age on drug disposition and response, in *Therapeutics in the Elderly,* Delafuente, J. C. and Stewart, R. B., Eds., Williams & Williams, Baltimore, 1988, 107–120.
8. Creasey, H. and Rapoport, S. I., The ageing human brain, *Ann. Neurol.*, 17, 2, 1985.
9. Eisandrath, S. F. et al., Meperidine-induced delirium, *Am. J. Psychiatr.*, 13, 1062, 1987.
10. Feldman, R. S., Meyer, J. S., and Quenzer, L. F., *Principles of Neuropsychopharmacology*, Sinauer Associates, Sunderland, MA, 1997
11. Frcka, G. and Lader, M., Psychotropic effects of repeated doses of enalapril, propranolol and atenolol in normal subjects, *Br. J. Clin. Pharm.*, 25, 67, 1988.
12. Giurgea, C. E., *Fundamentals to a Pharmacology of the Mind*, Charles C Thomas, Springfield, IL, 1982.
13. Greenblatt, D. H. and Shader, R. I., Pharmacokinetics of anxiety agents, in *Psychopharmacology: The Third Generation of Progress*, Meltzer, H. Y., Ed., Raven Press, New York, 1987, 1377.
14. Harvey, S. C., Hypnotics and sedatives, in *The Pharmacological Basis of Therapeutics*, Gilman, A. G., Goodman, L. S., Rall, T. W., and Murad, F., Eds., Macmillan, New York, 1985, 339.
15. Hutton, J. T. and Morris, J. L., Therapeutic advantages of sustained release levadopa formulations in Parkinson's disease, *CNS Drugs*, 2, 110, 1994.
16. Jellinger, K., Fazekas, F., and Windish, M., *Aging and Dementia*, Springer-Verlag, New York, 1998.
17. Kane, J. M., Treatment of schizophrenia, *Schizophr. Bull.*, 3, 147, 1987.
18. Kalmholz, B. A. and Mellow, A. M., Management of treatment resistance in the depressed geriatric patient, *Psychiatr. Clin. North Am.*, 19(2), 269, 1996.
19. Kompoliti, K. and Goetz, C. G., Neuropharmacology in the elderly, *Neurol. Clin.*, 16(3), 599, 1998.
20. Lesar, T. S., Briceland, L., and Stein, D. S., Factors related to errors in medication prescribing, *JAMA*, 277, 312, 1997.
21. Lewis, D. A. and Smith, R. E., Steroid-induced psychiatric syndromes, *J. Affect. Disorders*, 5, 319, 1953.
22. Meador, K. J., Cognitive side effects of medications, *Neurol. Clin.*, 16(1), 141, 1998.
23. Menza, M. A. and Liberatore, B. J., Psychiatry in the geriatric neurology practice, *Neurol. Clin.*, 16(3), 611, 1998.

24. Morrison, R. L. and Katz, I. R., Drug-related cognitive impairment: current progress and recurrent problems, *Ann. Rev. Gerontol. Geriatr.*, 9, 232, 1989.
25. Moses, H. and Kanden, I., Neurolgic consultations in a general hospital. Spectrum of iatrogenic disease, *Am. J. Med.*, 81(6), 955, 1986.
26. Muldoon, M. F. et al., Neurobehavioral effects of antihypertensive medications, *J. Hypertens.*, 9, 549, 1991.
27. Myllylä, V. V. et al., Selegiline as initial treatment in *de novo* parkinsonian patients, *Neurology*, 42, 339, 1992.
28. Neal, M. J., *Medical Pharmacology at a Glance*, Blackwell Scientific, Oxford, 1988.
29. The Parkinson Study Group, Effects of tocopherol and deprenyl on the progression of disability in early Parkinson's disease, *N. Engl. J. Med.*, 328, 176, 1993.
30. Penny, J. B. and Young, A. B., Movement disorders, in *Principles of Drug Therapy in Neurology*, Johnston, M. V. and McDonald, R. L., Eds., F. A. Davis, Philadelphia, 1995, 50.
31. Pincus, J. H. and Barry, K., Influence of dietary proteins on motor fluctuations in Parkinson's disease, *Arch. Neurol.*, 44, 270, 1987.
32. Quinn, N., The modern management of Parkinson's disease, *J. Neurosurg. Psychiatr.*, 35(2), 93, 1990.
33. Schelosky, L. and Poewe, W., Current strategies in the advanced treatment of Parkinson's disease — new modes of dopamine substitution, *Acta Neurol.*, 87 (Suppl. 146), 46, 1993
34. Smith, P. F. and Darlington, C. L., *Clinical Psychopharmacology*, Lawrence Erlbaum Associates, Mahwah, NJ, 1996, 40.
35. Smith, R. J., Study finds sleeping pills overprescribed, *Science*, 204, 287. 1979.
36. Swonger, A. K. and Burbank, P. M., *Drug Therapy and the Elderly*, Jones & Bartlett, Sudbury, MA, 1995.
37. Thomas, R. F., Neurotoxicity of antibacterial therapy, *S. Med. J.*, 87, 869, 1994.
38. Tiller, J. and Schweitzer, I., Benzodiazepines: depressants or antidepressants? *Drugs*, 44, 165, 1992.
39. Van Putten, T. et al., Plasma levels of haloperidol and clinical response, *Psychopharmacol. Bull.*, 21, 69, 1985.

15 Dementia in Primary Care

Luis M. Iriarte, Amaya Castela, and Dolores Torrecillas

CONTENTS

15.1 Introduction 323
15.2 Definition 324
15.3 Etiology 324
15.4 Diagnostic Criteria 326
15.5 Differential Diagnosis: Is Dementia Present? 327
    15.5.1 Age-Related Cognitive Impairments 327
    15.5.2 Delirium 328
    15.5.3 Focal Cerebral Syndromes 328
    15.5.4 Depression 328
15.6 Clinical Assessment 329
    15.6.1 Clinical History 330
    15.6.2 Examination 331
    15.6.3 Mental Status Examination 331
    15.6.4 Additional Tests 332
        15.6.4.1 Additional Analysis and Tests 332
        15.6.4.2 Lumbar Puncture 332
        15.6.4.3 Electroencephalogram 332
        15.6.4.4 Brain Imaging 333
        15.6.4.5 Positron Emission Tomography 333
        15.6.4.6 Brain Biopsy 333
        15.6.4.7 Other Additional Tests 333
References 334

15.1 INTRODUCTION

Dementia is defined as a cognitive "decline" in a patient's previous level of functioning. This decline is usually associated with behavioral changes and with an impairment of social and professional activities.[1] About 5% of the populations over 65 years of age suffers a type of dementia. Dementia includes a wide variety of symptoms that may be responsible for more than 100 disorders. Among these, more than 50% are dementias with a degenerative element disorder, of which the most common is Alzheimer's disease (AD).[2]

The diagnosis of the specific disorder producing dementia is of paramount concern for the physician. This should be based on a clinical diagnosis and a careful examination of both the patient and his or her clinical history. Evidence obtained by diagnostic testing such as a computerized tomography (CT) and laboratory tests are essential to rule out specific etiologies.[3]

15.2 DEFINITION

Dementia is due to an acquired, global, cognitive, memory, and personality impairment, which involves the clouding of consciousness and leads to abnormalities in several aspects of behavior.[4] The elements in the definition of dementia as it is understood it today include the following. Dementia is a condition that:

1. Is acquired, i.e., it is not congenital. There is also an implied differentiation from mental subnormality.
2. Is global, i.e., it is not just a series of focal deficits.
3. Involves impairment of memory, intellectual capacity, and personality changes.
4. Does not affect the level of consciousness.

15.3 ETIOLOGY

The main causes of cognitive decline can be summarized in the following categories (Table 15.1):[5,6]

1. Systemic diseases
2. Psychiatric diseases
3. Neurological diseases with secondary dementia, e.g., brain tumors, subdural hematomas, and vascular diseases
4. Primary degenerative dementias, of which the most common is Alzheimer's dementia

It is useful to identify in which category the patient should be included, as the first three categories are very likely to be associated with treatable causes. It can also be helpful to determine whether the patient presents a predominantly cortical, subcortical, or mixed pattern of cognitive decline. A cortical dementia will manifest itself in the form of memory, language, praxis, and gnosis impairment (known as aphaso-apraxo-agnosic syndrome).[7] By contrast, the main characteristic of subcortical dementia is a marked cognitive slowing, which is often associated with personality or behavior abnormalities, speech difficulties, and motor deficits such as bradykinesia and gait disorders.[8] However, it is clear that AD (50 to 80%) and vascular dementia (5 to 15%) are the most common causes of dementia, with AD being the main therapeutic target.

TABLE 15.1
Etiology of Dementia

Degenerative Diseases
Alzheimer's disease
Pick's disease
Parkinson's disease
Huntington's disease
Wilson's disease
Supranuclear progressive palsy
Hallervordam–Spatz disease
Striatonigral degeneration
Cortical-basal ganglia degeneration
Fahr's disease
Atrophy of the cerebellum
Down's syndrome
Dementia with Lewy bodies

Vascular Dementias
Multi-infarction
Binswanger's disease
Vasculitis
Hematomas
Vascular malformations

Infectious Diseases
Neurosyphilis
Creutzfeldt–Jakob's disease
Subacute sclerosing panencephalitis
Multifocal progressive leukoencephalopaty
Herpetic encephalitis
Whipple disease
Brucellar meningoencephalitis
Tuberculous meningoencephalitis
Cysticercosis
Brain abscess

Hydrocephaly
Obstructive
Communicanting

Tumors of the Central Nervous System
Primary tumors
Metastatic tumors
Carcinomatous meningitis
Paraneoplastic syndromes

Dementia Caused by Metabolism Disorders
Liver complaints
Hypo/hyperthyroidism
Hypo/hyperparathyroidism
Metabollic failures in the nervous system

Deficiency-Related Dementias
Folic acid deficiency dementia
Vitamin B_{12} deficiency
Pellagra
Thiamine deficiency

Toxic Dementias
Alcohol
Drugs
Metals
Drug abuse

Traumatic Dementias
Subdural hematoma
Post-traumatic dementia

Demyelinating Diseases
Multiple sclerosis
Others

Psychiatric Disorders
Depression

15.4 DIAGNOSTIC CRITERIA

The criteria for the diagnosis of dementia described in the fourth edition of the *Diagnostic and Statistical Manual of the American Psychiatric Association* (DSM-IV) have been widely accepted.[9] The DSM-IV defines dementia as a syndrome characterized by the development of multiple cognitive deficits, including memory impairment and at least one of the following cognitive disturbances: aphasia, apraxia, agnosia, or a disturbance in executive functioning. The deficit must be sufficiently severe to cause impairment in the patient's professional or social activities and must represent a decline from a previously higher level of functioning (Table 15.2).[10]

TABLE 15.2
Modified DSM-IV Criteria for Dementia Syndrome

Multiple cognitive deficit, including memory impairment and at least one of the following:
  Aphasia: Abnormality in the production or comprehension of language
  Apraxia: Incapacity to execute purposeful movements even when there is no motor or sensory impairment
  Agnosia: Lack of ability to perceive or recognize, especially people
  Disturbed executive functioning: Impaired planning, sequential organization, and attention span problems
Cognitive deficits that are severe enough to interfere with working and/or social life
Cognitive deficits that represent a decline from previous levels
Deficits that do not occur exclusively during the course of delirium

Source: Based on American Psychiatric Association.[9]

The ICD-10 defines dementia as a disorder in which the deterioration of both memory and thinking are severe enough to affect the patient's activities of daily living. Memory impairment is typically found to affect the registering, storing, and retrieval of new information. One of the definition requirements is that, apart from memory impairment, the patient must also suffer a cognitive decline and problems with reasoning.

Dementia is defined by the ICD-10 as a syndrome that is caused by a brain disease, has a chronic or progressive nature, and affects multiple cognitive domains such as memory, thinking capacity, orientation, comprehension, learning, calculation, and language abilities. However, the patient's level of consciousness remains unaltered.

The condition is associated with emotional lability, abnormalities in the patient's social behavior, lack of motivation, and a considerable cognitive decline, which have a negative impact on daily necessities such as washing, eating, and excreting functions.

The criteria given by ICD-10 show some discrepancies with those established by DSM-IV. These are the following:

1. Mild, moderate, or severe verbal and nonverbal memory deficit (essential requirement)
2. Mild, moderate, or severe cognitive deficit characterized by thinking problems and difficulty processing information

3. Lack of effect on the level of consciousness
4. Emotional lability, lack of motivation, and behavioral changes
5. Elements 1 and 2 must have appeared at least 6 months earlier

15.5 DIFFERENTIAL DIAGNOSIS: IS DEMENTIA PRESENT?

Determining whether a patient suffers dementia can be a difficult diagnostic task. Retrospective studies have indicated error rates of 30 to 50% in this determination in the past; however, with a new and better definition of the clinical syndrome, much greater accuracy is now possible. The diagnostic difficulties are threefold: differentiating early dementia from mild memory changes that are a normal age-related condition; differentiating dementia from primary psychiatric syndromes, particularly depression; and determining the presence of decline limited to just one cognitive domain.[11]

15.5.1 AGE-RELATED COGNITIVE IMPAIRMENTS

The age-related worsening of the memory is a frequent cause of concern for patients. Memory deficits in elderly people can be caused by a variety of reasons other than dementia.[12–14] In this respect, the following should be distinguished:

1. **Age-related memory impairment:** This is considered a more severe alteration, but its progression toward dementia is not accepted by many authors. It is a short-term memory deficit that affects people over 50 years of age but is not associated with other systemic, neurological, or psychiatric diseases, and does not imply a cognitive impairment (Table 15.3).
2. **Age-related cognitive deterioration:** This cognitive deficit, which is suffered by elderly people, can affect other cognitive domains apart from memory. There are mild alterations, which have little or no effect on the individual's abilities and are reversible within 6 months.

TABLE 15.3
Criteria for AAMI (Age-Associated Memory Impairment)

50 years old or older

Patient complains of gradual memory deficit that has a negative impact on daily life activities

Difference in the memory tests of at least one standard deviation below the average obtained by young adults in a secondary standardized memory test with data according to specifications

Cognitive function obtaining at least a 9 score in the vocabulary subtest of Wechsler's intelligence test

Lack of dementia determined by a 24 or higher score in the MMSE

Ruling out criteria of medical conditions, risk factors of vascular dementia, cranial trauma, drug abuse, or psychotropic medication, which can affect cognitive functions

15.5.2 Delirium

Delirium is also known as acute confusional syndrome. The main characteristics of this acute or semiacute alteration of various etiologies are alterations in the level of consciousness and difficulty in sustaining concentration. It can last from days to several weeks, with the patient's swinging from a hallucinatory and agitated state (mainly nocturnal) to a quiet and sleepy mood (Table 15.4).[15]

Although delirium can coexist with dementia or be one of its early manifestations, it can also have a completely independent nature.

TABLE 15.4
Delirium

Sudden and rapid onset with identifiable date
Acute illness, generally lasting days to weeks, but rarely for longer than 1 month
Usually reversible, often completely
Early disorientation
Variability from moment to moment, hour to hour, throughout the day
Striking physiological changes
Clouded, altered, and changeable level of consciousness
Strikingly short attention span
Disturbed sleep–waking cycle with hour-to-hour variation
Marked psychomotor changes (hyperactive or hypoactive)

Source: Modified from Reference 15.

15.5.3 Focal Cerebral Syndromes

Certain focal cerebral syndromes cause selective deficits in cognitive functions such as aphasias or amnesias. The concept of global cognitive deterioration, which is used as one of the definitions of dementia, can help in the differentiation of these syndromes from dementia.[16]

However, some patients with dementia have a focal onset, which, together with progressive aphasia, hinders the diagnosis. In these cases, clinical features alone will not be sufficient to attain an accurate diagnosis.

15.5.4 Depression

It is estimated that around 27% of the studied patients with cognitive impairment have in fact a depressive syndrome.[17] The progression of both depression and dementia can be associated or can be completely independent. Therefore, distinguishing a depressive pseudodementia from a real dementia is a very difficult task as it requires a comprehensive follow-up of the patient, involving on some occasions an assessment carried out by more than one specialist and the support of psychiatrists.

The following should be distinguished:

1. **Depressive pseudodementia.** This impairment has an essentially emotional nature with some neurological symptoms that are hardly detectable during the course of the patient's examination. The basic clinical features include attention span problems, anhedonia, frequent complaints about memory problems, apathy, pessimism, and sleeping and eating disorders. Response to antidepressive treatment is generally good.
2. **Depression associated with dementia.** As many as 50% of the patients with dementia can develop a depressive syndrome while suffering from the condition. This is more common in the early stages of dementia. The possibility that dementia and the depressive syndrome may have the same underlying cause has been suggested (Table 15.5).

TABLE 15.5
Distinctions between Depressive Dysfunction and Alzheimer's Disease

Depressive Dementia	Alzheimer´s Disease
Clinical Course	
Onset can be dated with some precision	Onset dated only within broad limits
History of previous psychiatric illness of similar kind common	Previous psychiatric history of similar kind unusual
Family usually very aware of the dysfunction and its severity	Family usually very unaware of the dysfunction and its severity
Clinical Features	
Patients complain considerably of cognitive loss	Patients complain little of cognitive loss
Patients emphasize failure	Patients conceal disability
Patients make little effort to perform even the simplest of tasks	Patients delight in accomplishments
Patients usually communicate strong sense of distress	Patients often appear unconcerned
Nocturnal accentuation of dysfunction uncommon	Nocturnal accentuation common
Features of Cognitive Dysfunction	
Memory gaps for specific events common	Memory gaps for specific events unusual
Marked variability in performing tasks of similar difficulty	Consistently poor performance on tasks of similar difficulty

Source: Modified from Reference 1.

15.6 CLINICAL ASSESSMENT

Examination of both the patient's history and mental status are the most critical aspects concerning the evaluation of a patient with dementia. However, the diagnosis of dementia continues to be predominantly clinical. As physicians do not normally have the patient's biological and analytical data available for the diagnosis, the clinical history becomes our most basic and essential working tool. This must be as complete and detailed as possible and should include all the information provided by family and carergivers about the most recent changes in the patient's life.[18,19]

15.6.1 CLINICAL HISTORY

A detailed and comprehensive clinical history and a careful examination of the patient's cognitive functions are essential for clinical evaluation.

The *clinical history* is a crucial element for the diagnosis of dementia. Because of the mental deterioration, much of the information about the patient's condition will have to be provided by a family informant. Therefore, confirmation by a reliable source of the patient's cognitive decline is an instrument of paramount diagnostic importance (this information must include a detailed account of the activities that the patient was able to perform in the past but is no longer able to do). It is important to analyze:

- Characteristics of the mental deterioration
- Early symptoms (memory deficit, behavioral changes, reasoning difficulties, depression)
- Time profile: type of onset, progression period, and type of progression
- Presence of symptoms denoting focal neurological deficits
- Patient or family record of previous systemic, neurological, or psychiatric disease associated with dementia or depression
- Intake of toxic substances or medicine

Chronic substance abuse can induce persistent dementias. The most common substances include alcohol, inhalants, sedatives, hypnotics, anxiolytics, anticonvulsants, antineoplasic drugs, and other toxic products such as lead, mercury, carbon monoxide, insecticides, organophosphorated chemicals and industrial solvents. However, there are many other commonly used chemicals that can also induce cognitive impairments. These include metals (aluminium, bismute, or lithium) and drugs such as antiparkinson and cardiovascular medication (antihypertensive, antiarrhythmic, or vasodilator drugs), corticoids, interferon-α, aciclovir, opioids, or simply aspirin.

The clinical history should always include an evaluation of the patient's functional abilities in his or her activities of daily living (ADL), such as whether the individual is able to shop, carry out financial operations, or have a normal social and working life. Quantifying functional decline is essential as it can serve as an indicator of the progression of the disease. The instrumental activities of daily living, or IADL, are affected in the early stages; however, when the extent of dementia becomes moderate or severe, the most basic ADL are affected (these include getting dressed and washing and excreting functions). Determining the level of functional decline is also a useful way of quantifying the response to different therapies.

15.6.2 Examination

Another aspect that is important in the diagnostic assessment of dementia is *neurological exploration*, which mainly aims at the following:

- Finding focal neurological signs denoting a localized cerebral pathology (tumor, vascular lesion)
- Finding signs that allow the determination of a particular subtype: myoclonias, extrapyramidal signs (subcortical dementia)
- Studying characteristic signs of dementia that can provide information about the extent and severity of the neurological condition: glabellar reflexes, sucking movement, conjugate gaze alteration, irritability, paratonia, and other signs of diffuse neurological dysfunction (such as nuzzling, grasping, palmomental reflex)
- Identifying associated behavioral and emotional disorder.; other abnormalities such as hallucinations, agitation crises, depression, or delirious ideas, which are frequent problems, are basically conditioned by both the etiology and the extent of the dementia and by the patient's social and familial environment

The neurological examination confirms whether the patient suffers an isolated dementia (which is usually caused by primary degenerative dementias such as AD or Pick's disease); or a "plus" dementia, which is usually secondary to focal or multifocal deficits of the nervous system (tumors, vascular lesions); or extensive abiotrophic processes, which are different from the degenerative primary dementias (such as Parkinson's, progressive supranuclear paralysis, olivopontocerebellar atrophy, and various other similar conditions that are usually associated with extrapyramidal, cerebellar, or bilateral dysfunction symptoms or signs).

A general examination allows the detection of atherosclerosis, arterial hypertension, carotid murmur, palpation of peripheral pulse, evidence of cardiac pathology, etc.

15.6.3 Mental Status Examination

The mental status examination is a direct way of determining the presence and nature of the cognitive deficit. The examination can be carried out with different degrees of specialization that range from the simplest and smallest scales (which are easy to use and provide a global estimation of the cognitive decline) to the most detailed and comprehensive neuropsychological battery tests (which provide a detailed classification of the various cognitive deficits and are helpful for subsequent follow-ups).[20]

In primary care, universal psychometric tools are used, which are easy to learn and do not require interpretation by a specialist. Each examination should include at least a test evaluating concentration span, recent memory, past memory, language and visuospatial abilities, praxis, and ability to respond to commands.[21]

The Mini-Mental State Examination developed by Folstein includes most of these elements and is currently widely used. This test takes 5 to 10 min to complete and provides an evaluation of time and spatial awareness, fixation and recent memory, calculation and language abilities, and constructive apraxia. The scale uses scores of 0 to 30. A score ranging between 24 and 30 is considered normal; a score below 23 denotes the presence of cognitive decline. Despite having some disadvantages (low sensitivity in the detection of mild deficits, sensory deficits, influence of previous intelligence and socioeducational level, etc.), this scale is a universal and easy-to-use instrument.

15.6.4 ADDITIONAL TESTS

Since the primary aim of additional tests is to rule out dementia induced by curable and treatable causes, the choice of a particular additional test will depend on the nature of the etiology of the setting. Although the diagnosis of a dementia syndrome is essentially a clinical assessment, additional tests can be useful for the differential diagnosis of the various subtypes.[22,23]

15.6.4.1 Additional Analysis and Tests

The following additional tests should always be performed:

- Hematology: detailed hemogram, erythrocyte sedimentation rate
- Serumal biochemical test: glycemia, urea, creatinine, uric acid, cholesterol, transaminases, bilirubin, alkaline phosphatase, ionogram, calcium, sideremia, total proteins, thyroid hormones, vitamin B_{12}
- Luetic serology
- Electrocardiogram
- Thoracic X-ray

15.6.4.2 Lumbar Puncture

There is much controversy concerning the indication of lumbar puncture. This procedure allows the examination of cerebrospinal fluid (CSF) and diagnosis of chronic meningitis, which may manifest as dementia. It is important to perform a lumbar puncture if there are suspicions of cancer, CNS infections, positive serology of syphilis, hydrocephaly, dementia in a patient younger than age 55, inmunosuppression, signs of potential vasculitis in diseases affecting the connective tissues, and in cases of dementias with unusual clinical features or rapid progression.

15.6.4.3 Electroencephalogram

The electroencephalogram (EEG) is a useful ally in differential diagnosis. It is critical for identifying a patient's cognitive deficit that is secondary to electrical seizure activity in the brain that has failed to produce overt behavioral seizures.[24] The EEG is indicated during the progression of dementia when it is necessary to:

- Suggest the organic nature of the disorder (diffuse slowing of AD)
- Study EEG characteristic findings: complex periodic waves (Creutzfeldt–Jakob), three-phase waves (hepatic disease), etc.
- Detect the signs of a focal abnormality that can denote the presence of a tumor, cerebral infarctions, etc.

15.6.4.4 Brain Imaging

Brain imaging using computed tomography (CT) or magnetic resonance imaging (MRI) is useful in most cases for ruling out structural brain lesions (tumors, hydrocephalus, and stroke). These scans can also show evidence of the extent of brain atrophy in AD (which is often asymmetric and mainly involves the temporal lobes).[25]

15.6.4.5 Positron Emission Tomography

Positron emission tomography (PET) provides a method for determining regional changes in glucose and oxygen metabolism; it is very sensitive to functional changes, including the presence of dementia, but the measurements obtained are also sensitive to ongoing sensory input, the performance of tasks, and even thinking. In AD, there is a decrease in parietal metabolism. The lower the level of the activity, the greater the severity of the dementia. The most advanced cases present a frontal lesion.[26]

15.6.4.2 Brain Biopsy

The performance of a brain biopsy in the patient with a dementia is only indicated if needed for:

- Diagnosing a curable process: e.g., Whipple
- Diagnosing transmissible dementia: e.g., Creutzfeldt–Jakob
- Studying a disease that is difficult to diagnose: e.g., ceroid lipofuscinosis

15.6.4.7 Other Additional Tests

Some tests performed in patients with dementia have a questionable diagnostic value.

- VIH serology is usually requested when there are risk factors
- Transcranial Doppler scans: Changes in arterial pulse constitute an additional and noninvasive criterion for the differential diagnosis of AD and vascular dementia[27]
- Evoked potentials
- Genetic markers[28]
- Biologic markers: Tau protein, amyloid protein[29,30]

However, the additional explorations recommended in primary care are hematological battery, biochemical and hormonal tests, electrocardiogram, thoracic X-ray studies, and CT. The findings can be used for confirming or ruling out "treatable" dementia (Table 15.6), many of which are related to general medical or extraneuro-logical diseases. The remainder of the tests should only be used in specialized care.[31]

TABLE 15.6
Dementias That Are Secondary
to Potentially Treatable Processes

Depression
    Metabolic alterations
    Hypothyroidism
    Hypophysial insufficiency
    Cushing's disease
    Chronic hypoglycemia
    Hepatic or kidney failure
    Vitamin B_{12} deficiency, pellagra
    Hereditary metabolic diseases
    Deposit diseases
Toxic
    Carbon monoxide intoxication
    Postanoxic encephalopathy
    Alcoholism
    Heavy metals
Infections
    Prion diseases (Creutzfeldt–Jakob)
    HIV infection
    Chronic meningitis (tuberculosis, brucellosis, luetic disease)
    Abscesses
    Progressive multifocal leukoencephalopathy
    Subacute sclerosing panencephalitis
    Herpetic encephalitis
Neurosurgical processes
    Cranial trauma
    Cerebral tumors
    Hydrocephaly
    Subdural hematoma

REFERENCES

1. Wells, C. E., Diagnostic evaluation and treatment in dementia, in *Dementia*, Wells, C. E., Ed., F. A. Davis, Philadelphia, 1977.
2. Erkinjuntti, T., Ostbye, T., Steennhuis, R., and Hachinski, V., The effect of different diagnostic criteria on the prevalence of dementia, *N. Engl. J. Med.*, 337, 667–674, 1997.
3. Sandson, T. A. and Price, B. H., Diagnostic testing and dementia, *Neurol. Clin.*, 14(1), 45–59, 1996.
4. Grupo de estudio de la demencia, Sociedad Española de Neurología, *DECLAMEO: Definición, Clasificación y Estudio del Paciente Demente*, J.R. Prous, Barcelona, 1989.

5. Adams, R. D., Victor M., and Ropper A. H. Degenerative disease of the nervous system, in *Principles of Neurology*, 6th ed., Adams, R. D., Victor, M., and Ropper A. H., Eds., McGraw-Hill, New York, 1997, 1046–1107.

6. Fleming, K. C. and Evans, J. M., Dementia: diagnosis and evaluation, *Mayo Clin. Proc.*, 70, 1093–1107, 1995.

7. Cummings, J. L. and Benson, D. F., Cortical dementias: Alzheimer disease and other cortical degenerations, in *The Dementias. A Clinical Approach*, 2nd ed., Cummings, J. L. and Benson, D. F., Eds., Butterworth-Heinemann, Boston, 1992, 45–93.

8. Albert, M. L., Feldman, R. G., and Willis, A. L., The subcortical dementia of progressive supranuclear palsy, *J. Neurol., Neurosurg. Psychiatr.*, 37, 121–130, 1974.

9. American Psychiatric Association, *Diagnostic and Statistical Manual of Mental Disorders*, 4th ed., APA, Washington, D.C., 1994.

10. CIE-10, Trastornos mentales y del comportamiento, 10th Reunión de la Clasificación Internacional de las Enfermedades, O.M.S., 1993.

11. Consensus Conference, Differential diagnosis of dementing diseases, *JAMA*, 258, 3411–3416, 1987.

12. Petersen, R. C., Smith, S. C., Waring, S. C., Ivnik, R. J., Kokmen, E., Tangelos, E. G., and Kokmen, E., Mild cognitive impairment. Clinical characterization and outcome, *Arch. Neurol.*, 56, 303–308, 1999.

13. Brayne, C. and Calloway, P., Normal ageing, impaired cognitive function, and senile dementia of the Alzheimer's type: a continuum? *Lancet*, 1, 1265–1267, 1988.

14. Levy, R., Working party of International Psychogeriatric Association, Report: Aging-associated cognitive decline, *Int. Psychogeriatr.*, 6, 63–68, 1994.

15. Ham, R. J., Confusion, dementia and delirium, in *Primary Care Geriatrics, A Care Based Approach*, 3rd ed., Ham, R. J. and Sloane, P. D., Eds., C. V. Mosby, St. Louis, 1997, 217–259.

16. Cummings, J. L. and Benson, D. F., *Dementia: A Clinical Approach*, Butterworths, Stoneham, MA, 1983.

17. Reding, M., Haycox, J., and Blass, J., Depression in patients referred to a dementia clinic: a three-year prospective study, *Arch. Neurol.*, 42, 894–896, 1985.

18. Corey-Bloom, J., Thal, L. J., Galasko, D. et al., Diagnosis and evaluation of dementia, *Neurology*, 45, 211–218, 1995.

19. Report of the Quality Standards Subcommittee of the American Academy of Neurology, Practice parameter for diagnosis and evaluation of dementia (summary statement), *Neurology*, 44, 2203–2206, 1994.

20. U.S. Preventive Services Task Force. Screening for dementia, in *Guide to Clinical Intervention*, Williams & Wilkins, Baltimore, 1989, 251–255.

21. Folstein, M. F., Folstein, S. E., and McHugh, P. R., Mini-Mental State, a practical method for grading the cognitive state of patients for the clinician, *J. Psychiatr. Res.*, 12, 189–198, 1975.

22. American Academy of Neurology, Quality Standards Subcommittee. Practice parameter for diagnosis and evaluation of dementia, *Neurology*, 44, 2203–2206, 1994.

23. McCormick, W. C. and Larson, E. B., Pragmatismo y probabilidades diagnósticas en la demencia, *Hosp. Pract.* (ed. Española), 6(5), 21–31, 1991.

24. Petit, D., Montplaisir, J., Riekkinen, P., Soninen, H., and Riekkinen, P., Electrophysiological tests, in *Alzheimer's Disease. Clinical Diagnosis and Management*, Gauthier, S., Ed., Martin Dunitz, London, 1996, 107–126.

25. Kidron, D., Black, S. E., and Stanchev, P. et al., Quantitative MR volumetry in Alzheimer's disease. Typographic markers and the effects of sex and education, *Neurology*, 49, 1504–1512, 1997.

26. Brooks, D. J., PET: its clinical role in neurology, *J. Neurol. Neurosurg. Psychiatr.*, 54, 1–5, 1991.
27. Alayón Fumero, A., Role of transcranial Doppler sonography in the differentiation of multi-infarct and Alzheimer-type dementia, *Stroke*, 25, 2505–2506, 1994.
28. Sadovnick, D. and Lovestone, S., Genetic counseling, in *Clinical Diagnosis and Management of Alzheimer's Disease*, Martin Dunitz, London, 1996, 343–358.
29. Galasko, D., Clark, C., Chang, L. et al., Assessment of CSF levels of tau protein in mildly demented patients with Alzheimer's disease, *Neurology*, 48, 632–635, 1997.
30. Hulstaert, F., Blennow, K., and Ivanoin, A., Improved discrimination of AD patients using B-amyloid (1-42) and tau levels in CSF, *Neurology*, 52, 1555–1562, 1999.
31. Downs, M. G., The role of general practice and the primary care team in dementia diagnosis and management, *Int. J. Geriatr. Psychiatr.*, 11, 937–942, 1996.

16 Neurobehavioral Syndromes in Patients with Cerebrovascular Pathology

María Dolores Jiménez, Eva Cuartero, and Jorge Moreno

CONTENTS

16.1 Introduction 337
16.2 Basic Concepts of Acute Cerebrovascular Pathology
with Neuropsychological Implications 338
16.3 Neuropsychiatric Syndromes in Patients
with Cerebrovascular Pathology 342
    16.3.1 Aggressive Behavior 342
    16.3.2 Emotional Incontinence 344
    16.3.3 Apathy 345
    16.3.4 Fatigue 347
    16.3.5 Depression...347
16.4 Vascular Dementia 351
References..360

16.1 INTRODUCTION

This chapter discusses the behavioral, emotional and cognitive alterations resulting from a pathology with a great prevalence in the elderly population: cerebrovascular disease (CVD). This population includes patients with chronic multiple medical and psychiatric impairments. Their mental deterioration clearly limits therapy and subsequent rehabilitation after a cerebrovascular accident (CVA). This deterioration, although it is treatable, poses a very serious problem that requires early and precise evaluation and management by various medical specialists who can each contribute to patient management.

This chapter not only gives a detailed account of the psychiatric syndromes that are associated with the clinical signs of CVD, but also analyzes the repercussions that this often overlooked condition have on the management of the cerebrovascular pathology.

16.2 BASIC CONCEPTS OF ACUTE CEREBROVASCULAR PATHOLOGY WITH NEUROPSYCHOLOGICAL IMPLICATIONS

In 1976, the World Health Organization defined CVA as "the sudden appearance of clinical signs of a focal (sometimes global) alteration in the working of the brain which lasts longer than 24 hours or results in a death apparently caused by none other than a vascular condition."

Unfortunately, the various official definitions and classifications of CVD are essentially based on neuropathology and tend to overlook the nonphysical symptoms in the acute stage such as behavioral, cognitive, and emotional alterations.

In 1990, The National Institute of Neurological and Communicative Disorders and Stroke (NINCDS)[1] provided one of the most widely accepted classifications of the past few years. The aim of the classification was to provide a precise definition of the different types of CVD and their various diagnostic and etiopathogenetic aspects. According to this classification, the clinical presentations can be divided into four categories: (1) asymptomatic cerebrovascular disease, (2) cerebral focal dysfunction, (3) vascular dementia, (4) hypertensive encephalopathy.

Asymptomatic cerebrovascular disease is a condition that, although it displays no apparent previous neurological symptoms, has already caused vascular damage. This is typical of asymptomatic carotid stenosis. This classification also includes patients suffering from leukoaraiosis, a term used to describe the periventricular or subcortical rarefaction of the cerebral white matter, which can be detected by neuroimaging techniques. These areas, which are more frequently seen in older patients with vascular risk factors, have been found responsible for many late-developing psychiatric disorders. For some authors[2] the meaning of leukoaraiosis differs according to whether the areas of rarefaction are detected by computed tomography (CT) or solely by magnetic resonance imaging (MRI). They conclude that when the areas are also shown on the CT it is likely that the rarefaction is associated with dementia. Association with dementia has also been linked with a higher tendency for the periventricular areas to be affected;[3] however, subcortical leukoaraiosis seems to be the disorder with a clearer ischemic origin. The most widely accepted conclusion is that leukoaraiosis in patients with vascular risk factors is more prevalent in those who develop vascular dementia (VaD).

The term silent cerebral infarction[4] refers to the incidental finding in neuroimaging tests of ischemic lesions in patients who have never had any signs or evident clinical symptoms. These CVAs are not always so silent. They can produce a recurrent or very subtle clinical condition, which, although the patient may have failed to notice it, can be detected by careful exploration performed by a specialist.

In a large series of studies on the epidemiology of CVD in Massachusetts, such as that by Kase et al.[5] in 1989, it was observed that as many as 10% of patients with a clinical diagnosis of CVD show radiological evidence of having suffered a previous silent CVA. However, the ultimate relationship between a previous silent infarction and a high incidence of dementia or short-term impairment has not been proved.[6]

In 1986, Dunne et al. used the term *nonobvious* CVD to refer to patients with clinical signs exclusively of behavioral alterations without symptoms or physical evidence of focal neurological abnormality. These authors found that 3% of hospitalized patients with CVD confirmed by CT or autopsy showed only behavioral alterations. From this study, it can be inferred that a proportion of the cerebral infarctions are considered silent present symptoms that do not suggest the initial diagnosis of a cerebrovascular pathology. As a consequence, diagnostic tests that would reveal the disorder are not performed.

The second group included in the classification given by the NINCDS is "symptomatic CVD." This includes focal cerebral dysfunction with transient ischemic attack (TIA), ictus, VaD, and hypertensive encephalopathy (HE).

Focal cerebral dysfunction includes, depending on whether the neurological deficit reverts in the first 24 h or not, TIA and ischemic or hemorrhagic cerebral infarction. In TIA and cerebral infarction, there is a partial or focal decrease in the blood supply to the brain. However, in other cases these conditions can lead to global deficit affecting the whole of the encephalon in a synchronic way that results in a global cerebral ischemia. This tends to occur in situations in which the pressure of cerebral perfusion is affected, such as when there is a fall in cardiac output or there has been a condition of prolonged shock. This global ischemia can lead to conditions of extremely varied prognosis, which can range from a slight cognitive deficit, affecting mainly memory and attention, to a persistent vegetative condition or death caused by brain stem lesion.

TIAs are defined as focal episodes of cerebral ischemia that last less than 24 h. The deficit they cause is reversible, and they usually have a multiple or recurrent presentation. Because of their reversible nature, there should be no evidence of infarction in neuroimages, although it is not rare to find such evidence. The TIA tends to last between 2 and 15 min. Because they last less than an hour and because when the patient is evaluated the deficit has usually disappeared, information obtained by detailed anamnesis is crucial.

Transient ischemia has the same etiopathogenic mechanisms as that of cerebral infarction: extra- or intracranial atherothrombosis; embolic arterioarterial, cardiac, pulmonary, or paradoxical; and hemodynamic, which may also be exacerbated by the coexistence of significant stenosis or arterial occlusion. According to the vascular region involved, TIAs can be divided into carotid, vertebrobasilar, or of uncertain territory. They can also affect the retinal area (causing amaurosis fugax) or the encephalon, with symptoms including motor, sensory, and language impairment.

Accurate diagnosis is important because the TIA may be the first or only manifestation of an occlusion or an important carotid stenosis. Another objective, which is also of paramount importance, is to rule out other pathologies of various origins such as syncope, hypoglycemia, partial epileptic seizure, migraine, and anxiety crisis. In this respect, anxiety crises and agoraphobia are devastating experiences that can cause confusion and extreme alarm in both the patient and the medical staff. Because of the great intensity of the symptoms they present, such as dizziness, tremor, sweating, tachycardia, precordial pain, dyspnea, and paresthesias in feet and hands, these attacks manifest themselves in the form of a convincing mock organic pathology.

On some occasions, these patients suffer an uncontrollable fear of having a myocardial infarction or a CVA. This fear can exacerbate such symptoms as dizziness and paresthesia, which can hinder the differential diagnosis. Simple phobias can, in some cases, lead to syncope of a vasovagal origin, which must be differentiated from epileptic seizures and, more easily, from TIA. Witnessing these seizures or becoming familiar with precipitating factors can contribute to definitive information for their diagnosis. A problem arises when the anxiety crises are caused by fear of suffering a new stroke, as in these instances the possibility of a TIA or a new cerebral infarction must be ruled out. This anxiety usually affects patients with a good functional recovery rate who are independent, have very little family support, and few social contacts.[7]

Ictus is included in the second division of focal cerebral dysfunction established by the NINCDS. This group includes ictus with an ischemic origin (parenchymatous or intraventricular) cerebral hemorrhage, subarachnoid cerebral hemorrhage, and arteriovenous-associated malformation. Ischemic ictus or cerebral infarction occurs when blood flow deficiency is sufficiently prolonged that it produces an area of anatomopathological necrosis. According to the pathogenic mechanism, these clinical categories or etiological subtypes can be thrombotic, embolic, and hemodynamic; the various clinical categories or etiological groups are atherothrombotic, cardioembolic, and lacunar. Other types are related to the vascular area affected.

The clinical symptoms are determined by the size and localization of the ischemic lesion. Thus, there is a lesion topography related to each arterial area. This distribution was given by the classification proposed in 1991 by the Oxfordshire Community Stroke Project[8] (Table 16.1).

Localizing the functional areas of the brain is beginning to be possible thanks to detailed and careful clinical observation, studies carried out after postmortems, and, in the last few decades, information gained from neuroimaging and neuropsychological tests. Although initially neuropsychological tests were initially designed for the diagnosis of lesions in specific cerebral areas, the latest advances in neuroimaging (CT and MRI) and functional techniques (transcranial Doppler ultrasonography and regional cerebral blood flow, Xe-CT, SPECT, and PET) have centered mainly on the ability to evaluate the impairment of a determined function rather than on the localizing potential. In neuropsychological practice, the abovementioned tests are usually grouped into batteries that evaluate the functions of the frontal, parietal, temporal, and occipital lobe.

Because of its high prevalence, cerebral vascular pathology has contributed very important data for localization of functional areas in the brain. A factor that works against this is that, in contrast to experimental lesions in animals, in practice one can find multiple, simultaneous, or stepwise lesions that hinder determination

TABLE 16.1
Subgroups of Cerebral Infarction (CI) from the Oxfordshire Community Stroke Project (OCSP)

CI Subtypes	Symptoms and Signs	Anatomical Basis	Pathological Mechanism
1. Lacunar infarcts (LACI)	Pure motor stroke Pure sensitive stroke Sensory-motor stroke Ataxic hemiparesis Disarthria — clumsy hand syndrome	Perforating artery	Lipohyalinosis Microatheroma
2. Total anterior circulation infarcts (TACI)	New higher cerebral dysfunction (e.g., dysphasia, dyscalculia, visuospatial disorder) Homonymous visual field defect Ipsilateral motor and /or sensory deficit of at least two areas	Deep and superficial territories of the middle cerebral artery (MCA) and anterior cerebral artery (ACA)	Cardioembolic Spread of thrombus from a more proximal occlusion
3. Partial anterior circulation infarcts (PACI)	Only two of the three components of the TACI syndrome Higher cerebral dysfunction Motor or sensory deficit confined to one limb, or to face and hand	Upper or lower division of the MCA	Embolic (cardiogenic, artery-to-artery) Spread of thrombus
4. Posterior circulation infarcts (POCI)	Ipsilateral cranial nerve palsy with contralateral motor and/or sensory deficit Bilateral motor and/or sensory deficit Disorder of conjugate eye movement Cerebellar dysfunction Isolated homonymous visual field defect	Vertebrobasilar arteries	*In situ* thrombosis Cardioembolic

of the anatomofunctional relationship. On the other hand, each function is the result of the integration of a determined system and its multiple connections with other cerebral areas. This principle rules out the traditionally held simplistic theory which maintained that each specific function was related to a single area of the cerebral cortex. Today, thanks to the study of neurotransmitters and the localization of their receptors through ligands bound by isotopes, the trajectories of the above-mentioned neurotransmitters are beginning to be defined and, with this, the functional anatomy of the integrator systems.

Apart from specific localizations, it seems that mental alteration is more characteristic of lesions located in the right than in the left hemisphere. The right hemisphere has been found responsible for creativity, will power, metaphorical and humorous use of language, as well as visuospatial, perceptive, and constructive tasks, abstract reasoning, and the ability to identify commonly used objects and to express or comprehend the emotional components of language. Some studies have linked the higher rate of behavioral disorders caused by right hemispheric lesions with the lower amount of residual physical impairments, including language, and therefore with a higher tendency to be able to express feelings or to be influenced by negative feelings.

In contrast to this, there are patients who are anosognosic and systematically deny their impairment, which can also be caused by a right hemispheric lesion. These patients can either act recklessly and be at risk of having accidents or show indifference toward their limitations. This denial or anosognosia greatly hinders rehabilitation therapy and leads to a poor prognosis, especially if it is also associated with visuospatial negligence and visual field deficits.[9]

16.3 NEUROPSYCHIATRIC SYNDROMES IN PATIENTS WITH CEREBROVASCULAR PATHOLOGY

The following sections describe the main neuropsychological syndromes that accompany the acute phase of a CVA or are secondary to it. These syndromes include behavioral, mood, and cognitive disorders.

16.3.1 AGGRESSIVE BEHAVIOR

Rage and violence after a CVA are extremely troubling problems because they cause management difficulties in the patient's family and social environment. The World Health Organization (WHO), in its ICD-10, defines this as an organic personality disorder characterized by irritability and angry outbursts. This aggressiveness is usually manifested in the form of verbal and even physical assaults against patients' caregivers and, more frequently, their partners. These patients are incapable of fully appreciating or describing their aggressive feelings.

In 1952, Goldstein described cerebral lesions in patients with extreme and exaggerated anger reactions attributed to their frustration about tasks that present some degree of difficulty. He called this Goldstein's catastrophic reaction. Later, this problem was also studied in relation to localization of an ischemic cerebral lesion[10] that manifests itself by rage, crying, and giving up on a task (in left hemispheric lesions) and by indifference (in right lesions).

Aggressive conduct has been associated with various neurotransmitters (decrease of γ-aminobutyric acid and 5-hydroxindolacetic acid; increase of acetylcholine and the catecholamines) and with specific localizations of the ischemic lesion. These areas include the tonsil, the cingulum, the hypothalamus, and the temporal and frontal lobes. On the other hand, violent behavior can also be part of the acute confusional status or delirium in the acute phase of an ictus, especially in patients with a history of previous cognitive deterioration. Their aggressiveness is usually manifested against fictitious attackers and is a response to delirious and hallucinatory episodes that usually lead to an exacerbation of motor activity in a disorganized way.

Some toxic agents pathogenically related to the CVD, such as alcohol, cocaine, or drugs that are frequently used by these patients, could be responsible for their aggressive behavior. The authors believe that it is important to draw attention to the possibility that hospitalized affected patients can develop delirium tremens a few hours later or display cocaine withdrawal syndromes or paradoxical reactions to anxiolytics, conditions that are particularly striking in elderly patients.

Antipsychotic medication is frequently administered to treat aggressive behavior, although it is always necessary to be careful with its extrapyramidal, anticholinergic and cardiovascular effects, which can have very significant clinical repercussions in this type of patient. It is preferable to use atypical neuroleptics such as risperidone as it has fewer extrapyramidal effects and is easy to use clinically. Furthermore, its sedative effects are lighter than those of the typical neuroleptics, a factor that is extremely advantageous for the patient's intellectual and social performance. However, if the patient shows psychomotor agitation, this medication may be inadequate. Clozapine is another atypical neuroleptic that was tried as an alternative to classical neuroleptics. Its main disadvantages are high risk of causing orthostatic hypotension, difficult management with cerebrovascular and elderly patients, and potential cause of severe blood dyscrasia.

Because of their serotoninergic properties, other non-neuroleptic drugs such as carbamazepine, buspirone, selective serotonin reuptake inhibitors (SSRIs) and trazodone have been used. Carbamazepine has a primary neural action over the voltage-dependent sodium channels and seems to be extremely useful in cases of violence with partial and complex crises and in patients with dementia. Other indications in this group of patients are acute manic episodes, emotional lability, and alcohol withdrawal. Its side effects are dose dependent and appear at the initial stage of treatment. Therefore, this drug must be introduced gradually. Another aspect that must be taken into account is that both the dosage and the therapeutic levels are always lower than those used in the treatment of epilepsy. Its main side effect in elderly patients is sleepiness. Buspirone is a nonbenzodiazepinic anxiolitic whose main drawback is that it has a latent action (a minimum of 2 weeks) and this makes it mandatory to use an additional drug with a faster action in that latent period. Trazodone has been widely used for treating agitation because it has powerful sedative effects and hardly any significant side effects, except perhaps orthostatic hypotension, which can be caused by the α1-adrenergic block.

In those cases in which immediate sedation becomes necessary, it is common to use intravenous (IV) or intramuscular (IM) administered short-acting benzodiazepines (BZD) such as lorazepam, phenothiazines, or haloperidol. These require constant monitoring as they can cause cardiorespiratory depression. In addition to the therapeutic measures, a patient with violent reactions after a CVA requires multidisciplinary management in which neurologists, psychiatrists, neuropsychologists, and caregivers play an essential role. After examination of records, the kinds of behavior, and the consequences of each aggression, one would also need to evaluate whether it is necessary to apply behavior-modifying techniques, whenever people surrounding the patient are available to collaborate. However, it is desirable for caregivers to avoid conduct that the patient could interpret as threatening.

16.3.2 EMOTIONAL INCONTINENCE

An apparent mood alteration that is frequently observed in patients with CVA is emotional incontinence or emotional lability. This is not exclusive to the CVD, as it can also be linked to various other central nervous system (CNS) pathologies such as multiple sclerosis (MS) and amyotrophic lateral sclerosis (ALS).

Emotional incontinence is defined as a lack of ability to control emotions in response to minor stimuli. As a result, a person can laugh, or cry, or be extremely angry for no apparent reason. Some patients try to apologize constantly as they find that their reactions are unjustifiable and uncontrollable, but the majority of them find it difficult to express how they are feeling.

Emotional incontinence can be part of so-called supranuclear bulbar or pseudobulbar paralysis. This name relates to that fact that the condition, although in a less severe form, presents similar symptomatology as that of bulbar lesions (dysarthria, dysphagia, bilateral facial paralysis, motor deficit in extremities), with the lesion level located in the geniculate bodies of the corticobulboprotuberantial tract. With a lesion at this level, the motor troncoencephalic nuclei become disconnected from cortical control. Emotional incontinence is often the key to differentiating bulbar from pseudobulbar paralysis, as the disorder is present only in the latter.

Voice impairments in pseudobulbar paralysis are very easily identifiable: speech is used with the wrong intonation and, as the subject talks, the voice becomes fainter than usual (hypophonesis). Patients with this disorder can also suffer palilalia, or involuntary repetition of words at the end of a sentence, and, in advanced stages, they can also suffer anarthria, or loss of the power to articulate speech.

Emotional incontinence reaches its maximum expression with crying and laughter crises of a spasmodic nature. These are caused by peribuccal muscles contracting in response to a minor emotional situation. On some occasions these crises include expiratory and suffocation shaking, which are caused by the contraction of the expiratory muscles.

Despite their similarity, pseudobulbar paralysis and the lacunar state must not be considered synonymous conditions. The lacunar status is a histological concept that was described by French classical authors (*etat lacunar*) as multiple lacunar infarctions. It can manifest itself as a pseudobulbar syndrome associated with motor disorders in lower extremities and with multi-infarction dementia. Although both conditions often coexist, in pseudobulbar paralysis the lacunae must be found on the geniculate bodies. On the other hand, not all infarctions causing pseudobulbar conditions are lacunae; they can be larger infarctions.

No links have been found between emotional incontinence, particularly pathological crying, in patients with CVA and a higher prevalence of depression. The WHO in its ICD-10 defines the "right hemispheric emotional impairment" as a condition in which patients present emotional incontinence and seem to be depressed, although no evidence of this depression is shown in the corresponding scales.

Finally, it is necessary to add that there is evidence suggesting that the physio-pathogenic basis of emotional incontinence is a serotoninergic disorder of neu-rotransmission. In a study carried out by Andersen et al. in 1994,[11] pathological crying was more intense in pontine bilateral lesions that affected the nuclei of the serotonin-producing raphe nuclei. Following this line of research, trials with SSRIs such as fluoxetine, sertraline, and paroxetine have produced spectacular results.[12]

16.3.3 APATHY

Patients' motivation plays a fundamental role in rehabilitation after a CVA. Apathy or lack of motivation should not always be regarded as intentional or secondary to social factors that can induce dependence. In most cases, apathy is the result of a series of factors that are often associated with CVA. These include neurological deficits that go unnoticed in the first explorations, confusion, fatigue, depression, dementia, appearance of concurrent medical diseases, and the use of psychotropic medication. In patients who have suffered a CVA, concurrent mental disorders such as depression, dementia, or personality alterations can cause and simulate apathy. Depression, a symptom that is similar to apathy, is one of the main factors involved in rehabilitation failure. Depression is discussed in Section 16.3.5.

In the advanced stages of dementia, patients suffer difficulties expressing their feelings and show a true emotional apathy. Such a severe degree of dementia is not usually the effect of a CVA; rather, the deterioration of a previous dementia increases with a later CVA. Negativism is one of the characteristics of schizophrenia, which can cause the patient to appear apathetic. Patients with some personality disorders and evasive, passive–aggressive, and dependent patients tend to benefit less from rehabilitation therapy. Apathy can also be secondary to extensively used medication in patients with vascular disorders: neuroleptics, hypnotics, anxiolitics, antiepilep-tics, and β-blockers. The diagnosis and treatment of apathy requires multidisciplinary management, ruling out of iatrogeny and finding a potentially treatable cause.

Several degrees of apathy are included in various psychomotor syndromes. These can range from aboulia to akinetic mutism. According to Fisher, aboulia includes medium to moderate apathy, lack of spontaneity and poor language and movement. Akinetic mutism was described by Cairus in 1941 as a state of alertness with profound apathy, indifference to nociceptive stimuli (thirst and hunger), and absolute lack of psychic, verbal, or motor initiative. This is manifested by lack of spontaneous movement or response to questions or orders.

Some researchers have tried to relate some localizations of CVA with apathy. In these studies, the frontal lobes, the thalamus, the nucleus caudatus, and the posterior arm of the internal capsule[13] have been found to be the most affected areas. The anterior-most positions of the frontal lobes are very well developed in humans. They have been related to the initiation of a planned action, although they also seem to enable the patient to take the effect of the completed action into account and to verify whether or not such action has been performed following a suitable program. Evidence of anterior akinetic mutism has been found in ischemic lesions affecting both anterior cerebral arteries with bilateral damage of the gyrus cinguli, and in the unilateral occlusion with transient akinetic mutism. In contrast to this, other cases can show completely different symptoms, such as euforia, moria, and loss of self-control, which can also hinder the progress of rehabilitation and, especially, of family and social reintegration.

Apart from these mood and attention alterations, the frontal syndrome also includes memory alterations, as the condition leads to failures in the process necessary for retaining and associating new ideas, as well as to incapacity for persevering with ideas or learned motor actions and therefore difficulty switching from one requested task to another. All these problems greatly hinder rehabilitation programs.

The thalamus is another of the areas that has been usually related to apathy. Its arterial contribution comes from terminal branches without functional anastomosis that are made up of four pedicles: polar or tubero-thalamic, posterior thalamo-subthalamic; thalamo-geniculate; and posterior choroidal arteries. The first two are often the most involved in the condition discussed in this chapter. '

Polar artery infarction causes sleepiness, apathy, loss of initiative and spontaneity, bradypsychia, judgment impairment, amnesic deficit, and perseverance. The condition mainly affects the dorsomedial nucleus and its connections with the ipsilateral frontal lobe and the mammillary bodies.

Infarctions in the posterior thalamo-subthalamic artery are usually bilateral (butterfly wing infarctions) when both arteries stem from a single pedicle coming from the basilar communicating arteries. In these cases, the lesion reaches the rostral mesencephalon causing akinetic mutism episodes that are due to the destruction of the dopaminergic pathways and the partial lesion of the ascending reticular activating system.

Some authors have described apathy episodes in relation to caudal nuclei infarctions, including the "*syndrome athymhormique*" described by Habib et al. in 1991. This syndrome produces sudden mental changes that involve loss of interest in work or leisure, inactivity, and complete lack of sensitivity. However, there is no evidence of depression or dementia.

Apathy must be differentiated at an early stage from other subtle neurological deficits that could interfere with active collaboration in the patient's rehabilitation: sensory deficits and extrapyramidal and cerebellar disorders.

Sensory deficits include language impairments such as aphasia; sensory disorders, such as loss of self-awareness and inability to discriminate between two points; and loss of visual field, such as hemianopsias contralateral to the lesion. These deficits can isolate the patient as they cause lack of insight, and therefore can hinder the physiotherapist's or rehabilitator's task, especially when these deficits remain silent. To avoid these types of difficulties at the time of designing the rehabilitation program, as much information as possible should be gathered including data from the detailed neurological examination, and the neuroimaging and neuropsychological tests (especially those evaluating parietal functions).

Extrapyramidal symptomatology can be found secondary to strategic infarctions located in the basal ganglia. However, most of the extrapyramidal pathology in patients with ischemia is caused by a previous degenerative pathology in the same system or by side effects caused by medication. It is important to keep in mind that errors are possible if one mistakes the hypokinesia that is typical of parkinsonism, for apathy, depression, or catatonia. Among the abnormalities found in movement, hemiballism (involuntary violent twitching and jerking affecting one part of the body) can be secondary to an ischemic lesion on the Luys subthalamic nucleus, which loses its inhibitor effect over the globus pallidus. When this anomalous movement affects both parts of the body, the condition is referred to as ballism, and, in this case, it is usually a psychogenic disorder.

16.3.4 FATIGUE

Fatigue associated with CVA is a widely recognized condition that contributes to the failure of rehabilitation and to functional deterioration at least during the first year after the infarction.

In 1999, Ingles et al.[14] published the results of a 13-month follow-up study of 88 patients who had suffered a CVA. They used the Fatigue Impact Scale (measuring the presence and severity of fatigue and its impact on psychological, physical, and cognitive functions) and the Geriatric Depression Scale. The study found that 68% of the patients and only 36% of the controls suffered from fatigue. The study found no relationship with the severity or the localization of the infarction and also suggested that fatigue was independent of the presence of depression, although the negative impact of fatigue on functional abilities increased very significantly when coexisting with depression. It is important to point out that in this study up to 40% of the patients considered fatigue the worst or one of the worst residual symptoms of CVA. They also found that fatigue had great relevance to patients' functional limitations. The authors believe that these data justify the need to detect and treat fatigue at an early stage to achieve the maximum possible functional recovery.

16.3.5 DEPRESSION

Depression, with an estimated global frequency of 40%,[15] is perhaps the most frequent emotional disorder following a cerebral infarction. Depression can manifest itself as major depression (26% of cases), minor depression (14% of cases), or bipolar disorder. Thus, because of its high levels of prevalence, and its role as a condition that affects the patient's mood and cognitive system, depression should not be overlooked. Depression not only has a negative impact on functional recovery but also a high rate of mortality.[16]

In 1982, Feibel and Springer[17] suggested that depression is the cause rather than the consequence of patients' reducing their everyday life activities after a CVA. This theory contradicts the generally accepted assumption that loss of dignity and self-esteem or giving up everyday life activities can cause depression after a CVA that has produced some degree of physical impairment.

As for the risk of suffering postinfarction depression, no differences have been found in relation to sex, age, level of education, type of infarction, or history of previous CVA. However, evidence of higher incidence has been found in patients with a depressive history before a CVA, and in patients with early impairments during the acute stage of the CVA. These early impairments, considered predictors of a later development of depression, mania, or anxiety, include disinhibition, indifference, and aggressivity (the accuracy of these findings has not yet been established in studies carried out in large population cohorts).

When classifying postinfarction depression as a reactive depression, the psychiatric nomenclature uses the terms "adaptative impairment with depressive mood" (as defined in the DSM-IV by the American Psychiatric Association) and "depressive reaction" (as defined by WHO in its ICD-10).

There are no specific scales for postinfarction or vascular depression. The commonly used scales require that the patients be able to express themselves. Logically, this is a limitation for patients with aphasia or vascular dementia. Several authors had carried out various trials to design evaluating scales for aphasic patients that are based on objective estimation and eliminate self-report, thus allowing items related to physical symptoms and self-care ability to become less relevant. However, no consensus on this matter has yet been reached, and neither of the currently used scales, the Geriatric Depression Scale[18] and the Hamilton Rating Scale for Depression,[19] contribute any accuracy to the clinical diagnosis reached by a specialist.

Attempts have been made to define a relationship between the localization of the infarction and the presence or severity of postinfarction depression. Lishman,[20] in his classic study on the frontal lobe in soldiers with traumatic cerebral lesions, found a clear link between right frontal lesions and severe and persistent depression. Later on, several authors supported the association of infarctions located in anterior regions of the left hemisphere and in the posterior regions of the right hemisphere. However, this suggestion has not yet been confirmed by meta-analysis.

Other long-term follow-up studies, Äström et al.[21] in 1993 and Shimoda and Robinson[22] in 1999, showed that the correlation between postinfarction depression and the location of the lesion varies as time passes after the infarction. They were able to reconcile the differences between the various studies. In 1999, Shimoda and Robinson published the results of a follow-up study of 60 patients who had suffered a CVA. The study revealed that there was a significant association between depression and anterior left hemispheric lesions only in those patients whose depression had already manifested itself during the acute stage of the CVA. Most of these patients developed major depression. In subsequent controls, 3 to 6 months later, they found a correlation with a higher lesion volume and with lesions located near both the left and right frontal poles. At 1 and 2 years after the CVA, they found an association with the lesion volume and right hemispheric lesions as well as lesions located near the occipital pole.

There are some objections to the hypothesis that left anterior lesions cause depression. These are based on the fact that it is possible to reach a wrong diagnosis if one considers only autonomous or vegetative symptoms since an ischemic lesion in the above-mentioned location could cause these by itself, without the need for the patient to show other additional signs of depression. In contrast, Fedoroff et al.[23] found that vegetative symptoms (anxiety, foreboding, weight loss, asthenia, loss of libido, sleeping difficulties, early awakening, and morning depression) were closely linked to depressive mood in patients with acute CVA.

On the other hand, in the low-dose dexamethasone suppression test (DEX), endocrine alterations were found associated with mood changes after a CVA, especially when these abnormalities persist after the acute stage of the infarction.[24] Other authors link these endocrine changes with extensive infarctions rather than with the presence or absence of depression.

The depletion of some neurotransmitters seems to play an essential physiopathogenic role in the development of depression. The neurotransmitters most involved are serotonin and the catecholamines dopamine, noradrenaline, and adrenaline. Thus, infarctions localized in places where these neurotransmitters are synthesized, such as the locus coeruleus and the substantia nigra, or those damaging their cortical afferent pathways, would cause the development of major depression after a CVA. On the other hand, ictus-posterior dysthymic impairments could be related to previous personality abnormalities and other psychosocial factors.

The depressive condition tends to revert a year after the CVA. However, old age and the incidence of other concurrent medical diseases can worsen the prognosis. It seems that depression in late stages has a clear reactive origin (the patient loses hope that important impairments will disappear).

Stenager et al.[25] published in Denmark in 1999 an epidemiological study of the risk of suicide after suffering a CVA. The incidence in the general population was higher than expected, with women's figures being higher. These authors did not find any relationship with the number of years passed since a CVA.

Mania is another mood disorder often associated with depression in a bipolar affective illness. According to the DSM-IV (American Psychiatric Association, 1994) mania is a period of abnormally and persistently elevated, expansive, or irritable mood, sufficiently severe to cause marked impairment in occupational functioning or in usual social activities, not due to effects of a sustance (e.g., a drug of abuse or a medication) or a general medical condition.

Several neurological conditions have been correlated with secondary mania. In patients with poststroke mania, the strongest associations are with lesions of the right hemisphere, above all the orbitofrontal cortex, thalamus, or perithalamic regions, caudate nuclei, and the basotemporal area.

Early detection and treatment of postinfarction depression are clearly advantageous for the patient's physical and cognitive recovery. Both psychotherapeutic and pharmacological treatments are indicated. However, patients with this kind of depression can suffer difficulties with oral communication, which greatly hinders the application of psychotherapy and assessment of the efficacy of the treatment.

When prescribing antidepressants, it is important to take into account that, in general, sufferers of CVA tend to be elderly patients who usually have other concurrent medical pathologies and who, therefore, can be taking a large amount of drugs with consequent risk for development of adverse effects and drug interactions. Whatever the treatment chosen, it must be monitored carefully and plasmatic level controls must be performed as often as possible.

The trials performed so far have yielded ambiguous results. In general, it is widely accepted that both nonselective amine reuptake inhibitors (tricyclic antidepressants, or TADs, such as nortriptyline[26] and imipramine, and others such as trazodone and mianserin) and selective serotinin reuptake inhibitors (SSRIs) (such as citalopram and fluoxetine)[27] are effective.

Apart from their widely recognized peripheral anticholinergic effects (dry mouth, constipation, blurred vision, urinary retention, sexual impotency, worsening of closed-angle glaucoma, etc.), the TADs can produce confusion, anticholinergic delirium, and orthostatic hypotension in this type of patient. Regarding cardiovascular effects, therapeutic doses of TADs behave as type Ia antiarrhythmics. In high doses, they can cause a decrease in cardiac contractility, hypotension, tachycardia, and electrocardiographic alterations (such as flattening of T waves, prolonged QT intervals, and depressed ST segments). Other TADs such as clomipramine and maprotiline lower the convulsive threshold and therefore must be avoided in patients who develop post-CVA vascular epilepsy.

These side effects are worsened in elderly patients with cardiac pathology (a group with a high prevalence in the cerebrovascular pathology). Therefore, TADs must be reserved for patients who show no response to SSRIs or have a history of previous depression and have had a good or exclusive response to TADs.

SSRIs are used nowadays as first-choice drugs. In contrast to TADs, they have better tolerance, produce a less profound sedative effect, and are safer in case of overdose. Their most frequent side effects are of a gastrointestinal nature (anorexia, nausea, and diarrhea) and disappear within a few days. Other effects that have also been described in relation to these drugs include agitation, insomnia, cephalea, and sexual dysfunction.

The SSRIs increase the effect of drugs commonly used in patients with cerebrovascular pathology. These include, among others, warfarin (especially paroxetine and sertraline), antiepileptic drugs (fluoxetine and fluvoxamine), and haloperidol (fluoxetine).

These drugs must never be administered in combination with monoamine oxidase inhibitors (MAOI). Because of the risk of producing a serotoninergic syndrome (hyperpirexia, hypertension, profuse sweating, myoclonus, epileptic seizures, and coma) it is advisable to delay the introduction of SSRI medication until 2 weeks after the MAOI has been withdrawn. This syndrome can also be caused by the association of various SSRIs, and therefore it is advisable always to use this type of medication in monotherapy.

In general, the treatment of major depression must last between 6 and 9 months although 40% of the elderly patients present residual symptoms that require prolonged treatment. Dosage must be adjusted according to age and concurrent pathology. However, it is always advisable to use the smallest effective dose, and the agents must be introduced and withdrawn gradually. Before deciding that a treatment is not effective, one must always make sure that it has been followed properly. As compliance is usually irregular and side effects are frequent, a great number of patients decide to suspend antidepressive treatment themselves after a short period.

The presence of delirious ideas, vegetative signs of endogenous depression, and low response to the pharmacological treatment are widely accepted indications in the scientific community for the use of electroconvulsive therapy (ECT). For the patient with CVA, the need to apply anesthetics is more of a risk than the ECT itself. The increase in arterial pressure (over 20 mmHg) that occurs during ECT has not been found to be dangerous even in cases of intracerebral aneurysm. No cases of subcranial hemorrhages caused by ECT have been described. A study by Murray et al.[28] revealed that there was no neurological worsening induced by the ECT. However, it is advisable to bear in mind that it is important to perform cognitive function controls before and after the ECT. The most frequent undesirable effects of ECT (post-treatment confusion and agitation, cephalea, and memory impairments) are generally reversible.

16.4 VASCULAR DEMENTIA

Vascular dementia (VaD) is a frequent cause of cognitive deterioration in elderly people. In Western industrialized countries, it is the second most frequent cause of dementia after Alzheimer's disease (AD), and it is the origin of 20% of the dementias in the population older than 65. In Russia, Japan, and other Eastern countries, VaD is the most frequent cause of dementia.[29]

However, postmortem studies reveal a lower incidence of VaD than is clinically suspected. It is clear that vascular disorders contribute significantly to the development of other types of dementias, which are called mixed dementias. This discordance between classical epidemiological and postmortem studies seems to be due to the difficulty in establishing precise differential criteria between VaD and primary degenerative dementias.

In 1955, Roth[30] defined the main characteristics of vascular dementia. He described the sudden onset, the presence of neurological focal symptoms or signs that point to cerebrovascular pathology (pyramidalism, urinary incontinence, emotional lability, pseudobulbar paralysis, etc.), and the evidence of vascular-associated risk factors (old age, hypertension, diabetes mellitus, cardiopathy, hyperlipidemia, polyglobulia, heavy smoking habit, alcoholism, and history of previous ictus).

Patients with VaD usually present a subcortical profile, which includes walking with small steps, early alterations in sphincter control, evidence of parkinsonian syndrome, and pseudobulbar syndrome in final stages. The psychopathological features classically considered to be specific to the condition include relative preservation of insight, emotional lability, incontinence, nocturnal confusion, and depression.

In 1974, Hachinski et al.[31] proposed a scale for ischemia (Table 16.2), with an empirical basis that has been extensively used for clinical and epidemiological research. Several neuropathological studies have validated this scale, although they also prove its limitations when trying to differentiate mixed forms of dementia. Furthermore, low specificity of the scale means that a significant number of degenerative dementias are included as vascular dementias.[32] On the other hand, a strict use of Hachinski's criteria has the risk of excluding an important number of patients with VaD who do not have a history of previous cerebrovascular episodes and can present a non-stepwise, but progressive deterioration.

The current criteria used for diagnosing VaD were established between the end of the 1980s and the beginning of the 1990s. In general, these criteria parallel those established for the diagnosis of AD, but require the existence of a cognitive impairment within the context of underlying cerebrovascular disease. This cognitive impairment must always include the deterioration of memory to the detriment of other more clinically relevant early disorders (such as aphasia, agnosia, apraxia, and alteration of the executive functions) caused by this type of dementia, which could allow a more efficient diagnosis and treatment.

The most widely accepted and better-known diagnostic criteria are those established by the DSM-IV,[33] the ICD-10,[34] the NINDS-AIREN,[35] and the CAMDEX.[36] Of all of them, the criteria given by the NINDS-AIREN (Table 16.3) seem most useful both for clinical practice and for epidemiological research, because they do not exclude hemorrhagic causes and have a proven interobserver reliability. These criteria, which are also based on the ICD-10, provide a more-restricted definition and detailed exclusion criteria. They also propose that the term *mixed dementia* be avoided, and they establish four different degrees of diagnostic probability for vascular dementia (uncertain, probable, possible and definite dementia). The cerebrovascular disease must be proved by clinical (focal neurological signs or history of ictus) and neuroimaging data. One of the most controversial aspects of the NINDS-AIREN criteria is provision of a maximum limit of 3 months between the cerebrovascular episode and the development of dementia. This would exclude patients with MRI evidence of diffuse white matter alterations, as they can develop dementia several years later.

TABLE 16.2
Ischemia Scale of Hachinski

Features	Score
Abrupt onset	2
Stepwise deterioration	1
Fluctuating course	2
Nocturnal confusion	1
Relative preservation of personality	1
Depression	1
Somatic complaints	1
Emotional incontinence	1
History or presence of hypertension	1
History of strokes	2
Evidence of associated atherosclerosis	1
Focal neurological symptoms	2
Focal neurological signs	2

Note: A score of 4 or more suggests that the patient does not have pure Alzheimer's disease, and that a vascular component is a cause of or contributes to the clinical syndrome. A score of 7 or more suggests vascular dementia.

TABLE 16.3
Criteria for the Diagnosis of Vascular Dementia

I. CRITERIA FOR THE CLINICAL DIAGNOSIS OF *PROBABLE VaD*:

1. *Dementia* defined by:
    - Cognitive decline severe enough to INTERFERE with activities of daily living not due to physical effects of stroke alone.
    - Excludes preexisting mental impairment.
    - Loss of memory and deficits in at least two or more cognitive domains (orientation, attention, language-verbal skills, visuospatial abilities, calculations, executive functions, motor control, judgment, and praxis).
    - Established by clinical examination and documented by judicious neuropsychological testing.
    - *Exclusion criteria of dementia*: disturbance of consciousness, delirium (not delusions), psychosis, severe aphasia or major sensorimotor impairment. Systemic disorders or other brain diseases (AD) that could account for deficits in memory and cognition.

2. *Cerebrovascular disease* defined by:
    - Presence of focal neurologic signs consistent with stroke (with or without a history of stroke).
    - Evidence by brain imaging (CT or MRI) of radiologic lesions associated with dementia (multiple large-vessel infarcts, single strategically placed infarct, multiple basal ganglia and white matter lacunes, or extensive periventricular white matter lesions or combinations thereof).

3. These two disorders must be reasonably related by:
    a. Temporal association (onset of dementia within 3 months following a recognized stroke).
    b. Abrupt or stepwise deterioration in cognitive functions.

4. Clinical features consistent with the diagnosis of *probable VaD*:
    a. Early presence of a gait disturbance;
    b. History of unsteadiness and frequent, unprovoked falls;
    c. Early urinary frequency, urgency, and other urinary symptoms;
    d. Pseudobulbar palsy;
    e. Personality and mood changes.

II. CLINICAL DIAGNOSIS OF *POSSIBLE VaD*:
    - May be made in the presence of *dementia* with focal neurological signs when:
      a. Brain imaging studies to confirm definitive CVD are missing;
      b. Absence of clear temporal relationships between dementia and stroke;
      c. Subtle onset and variable course of cognitive deficits and evidence of relevant CVD.

III. CRITERIA FOR THE DIAGNOSIS OF *DEFINITIVE VaD*:
    - Clinical criteria for *probable* vascular dementia;
    - Histopathological evidence of CVD;
    - Absence of neurofibrillary tangles and neuritic plaques exceeding those expected for age;
    - Absence of other clinical or pathological disorder capable of producing dementia.

To classify VaD, efforts have been made to unify etiopathogenic aspects of the cerebrovascular disease with other anatomic and physiopathological concepts. In daily practice, this condition is usually classified following neuropathological criteria with the data obtained from the clinical exploration and the neuroimaging tests. In this way, the classification would include dementia caused by multi-infarction; strategic infarction; disease in small vessels, subcortical and/or cortical; ischemic–hypoxic and hemorrhagic dementia; and a combination of them all.

A more schematic classification would include two essential kinds of VaD: cortical and subcortical VaD. Etiopathogenically cortical VaD is often associated with atherothrombotic, cardioembolic CVAs and infarctions in bordering areas, whereas subcortical VaD is usually linked with a deep white matter alteration and lacunar infarctions. Clinically, VaD has a rapid onset of the cognitive deficit and shows a predominance of aphasic-apraxic-agnosic manifestations and signs of focal hemispheric deficit. The characteristics of VaD with cortical appearance usually include pure motor hemiparesia and other lacunar syndromes, dysartria, depression, early alterations in sphincter control, gait impairment, evidence of parkinsonian syndrome, and pseudobulbar syndrome in late stages.

A subject of discussion is whether cortical and subcortical VaD reflect the existence of other diseases or are different manifestations of a condition that shares the same causes but presents lesions in different localizations. In clinical practice, most patients show an overlapping of both cortical and subcortical profiles, although in early cases one type of VaD or the other is predominant.

Clinically, two theories arose to explain the physiopathology of cognitive deterioration and vascular dementia. The volumetric hypothesis[37] emphasizes the importance of the total volume of cerebral tissue affected by the infarction. This theory establishes a critical threshold beyond which any amount of tissue affected would exceed the compensatory functional reserve of the brain and lead to dementia. This theory has lost credibility over the last decade. In the 1970s, the minimum volume threshold of damaged tissue was set at 100 ml. Later on, evidence suggested that a volume lower than 40 ml could cause VaD. Today, it is widely accepted that VaD can exist even when there has been no cerebral infarction.

Although it seems logical that the higher the number of lesions, the higher the probability of developing VaD, this is not a determining factor in itself. Evidence suggests that a low number of lesions or even one single lesion in a strategic location can lead to the development of VaD. This is the basis of the localizationist theory. Strategic cerebral areas are zones where lesions produce an important cognitive deficit. In some cases, such damage is out of proportion to the size of the lesion. These strategic areas are both cortical and subcortical and produce characteristic focal syndromes. The localizations that have been described as strategic include the medial side of the frontal and temporal lobe in the dominant hemisphere, the hippocampus, the limbic system, and the thalamus.

Several studies have pointed out the relevance of lesions located in the dominant hemisphere, whereas others insist that the lesions must be bilateral. Neuropathological studies have found evidence suggesting that up to 96% of patients with VaD have suffered bilateral infarctions (91% are temporal, 65% parietal, 61% occipital, 56% frontal and 48% are located in the hippocampus)

As for cortical areas, the occlusion of the posterior division of the left middle cerebral artery (MCA) produces one of the most representative cortical VaD syndromes caused by a strategic infarction: the gyrus angularis syndrome. A lesion in this area interrupts the integration of language, mathematical, and constructive praxis functions. When the lesion is complete, it causes fluent aphasia, anomia, and verbal paraphasias, and because the patient is aware of these impairments, this causes great frustration. Other disorders related to this lesion include alexia with agraphia, acalculia, left and right disorientation, digital agnosia, and constructive alterations without visuospatial impairments. If the infarction is located in the angular convolution of the nondominant hemisphere, it can cause agitation and confusion associated with visuospatial deficits.

As for the subcortical areas, the thalamic infarction (anterior left or right thalamus and medial left thalamus) causes the disconnection of the frontal–subcortical circuits, an episode that causes VaD and is extensively found in the literature.[38] Other subcortical localizations are the caudal nucleus (left or right), the knee of the internal capsule (left), the anterior hippocampus, and the tonsil (left).

The main characteristics of thalamic dementia are apathy, slow thought processing, and amnesic deficits. This disorder can be caused by infarctions of the polar artery or the posterior thalamo-subthalamic arteries, syndromes, like those caused by infarction of the caudatus and of the knee of the internal capsule, that have already been described in the section on apathy and akinetic mutism.

The ictal amnesic syndrome in bilateral infarctions or only in left infarctions of the posterior cerebral artery (PCA) affects the temporal branches (hippocampus) and the perforans pedicle (thalamus). In extensive bilateral lesions of the PCA, apart from severe amnesia, other disorders can include cortical blindness, color anomia, visual agnosia for objects, and difficulty in recognizing already known faces.

In 1990, Mesulam[39] proposed a model unifying both the volumetric and the localizationist theories. In this model, cognitive functions have an anatomofunctional basis: complex neurocognitive networks that include cortical areas, subcortical nuclei, and connecting pathways crossing the white matter. According to this model, one area can be the seat of several functions, and one function can have anatomic components in different areas.

Apart from the cerebral infarction, cerebral or subcortical atrophy is a constant neuroradiological finding in patients with VaD, with the widening of the lateral ventricules the most consistent feature. This aspect is not the cause of the volume vs. localization controversy that we discussed earlier in this chapter. Most of the published research establishes a significant association between cerebral atrophy and dementia. The atrophy in the corpus callosum has also been linked with the cognitive deterioration of patients with cerebrovascular disease.

Most of the current classifications of VaD identify subcortical deterioration with the cerebral small vessel pathology (arteriosclerosis). They distinguish three different entities with no clearly established boundaries since they all share the same clinical–radiological manifestations and risk factors: ischemic leukoencephalopathy, lacunar state, and Binswanger's disease (BD). On the other hand, microangiopathy or small vessel disease is not limited only to subcortical regions. Conditions such as hypertensive angiopathy, amyloid angiopathy, and caliginous vasculopathy with dementia also affect the cortico-subcortical regions.

The rarefaction of white matter in patients with "arteriosclerotic" dementia had already been described by Alzheimer and Binswanger at the turn of the century. With the introduction of CT and, later, MRI, it was possible to detect an unusually high frequency of rarefactions in the white matter, which are known as leukoaraiosis (or rare white matter). These lesions are located in the periventricular areas and in the semioval centers and are arranged in a symmetrical and bilateral way. They have a higher prevalence in older patients and in those with cerebrovascular pathology; these findings are associated with the presence of arterial hypertension (AHT) and with obtaining worse scores in the cognitive scales. Thus, small areas of leukoaraiosis have been found in up to 25% of the CT of patients with long-term hypertension, in 40% of patients with AD, and, due to the high sensitivity of this technique, in 80% of normal MRI controls.

These signal changes in the white matter can be due to normal structures such as the subcallosal facicullus, areas of granular ependymitis, and augmentation of the Virchow–Robin spaces. They can even be due to demyelinization areas in multiple sclerosis. Therefore, these images are not necessarily due to arteriosclerosis or changes of an ischemic nature. In patients with VaD, areas with leukoaraiosis that suggest ischemic leukoencephalopathy are typically big, patchy, bilateral, with diffuse confluent edges and are either separated from the ventricle or joined to it but spread toward the subcortical white matter.

Many patients with leukoaraiosis caused by ischemic leukoencephalopathy have no previous record of ictus or neuroradiological findings of lacunar infarctions. This is the reason some authors maintain that both entities have different etiopathogenic mechanisms even though their vascular nature is the same.

The cognitive deterioration associated with isolated leukoaraiosis is more restricted than that caused by the lesion of the base gray nuclei, with memory, abstract thinking, and visuoconstructive abilities and language remaining unimpaired.[40] The ischemic leukoencephalopathy is associated with the slowing of mental tasks and the speed of processing of information, as well as attention impairments and low performance in frontal functions tests.

The lacunar state is the result of a series of small-sized subcortical multiple infarctions (lacunae) caused by the arteriosclerosis occlusion of the basal and medullar long perforans vessels. The affected areas are the internal capsule, the basal ganglia, the thalamus, the protuberance, the cerebellum, and the semioval center. The lacunar state does not necessarily have to be connected to dementia. The degree of cognitive deterioration and dementia depend more on the localization and number of lacunae rather than on their size (the localization of these subcortical strategic infarctions has already been described).

Clinically, the lacunar state manifests itself in the form of cognitive disorders of the frontal area, apathy, alteration of attention and memory, perseverative tendency, and marked psychomotor slowness. In the exploration, hypertonia in the lower extremities, gait impairment, and evidence of parkinsonian syndrome are the striking features.

BD was described in 1894 as a clinicopathological entity. Its onset has been established at between 50 and 65 years of age, and its main characteristics are slow and progressive mental deterioration, ictus clinical manifestations, epileptic seizures, and agitation episodes. The anatomopathological profile is that of atrophy of the white matter with little cortical incidence.

Caplan's criteria are the most commonly used in the diagnosis of this disease.[41] They include the main clinical and neuroradiological findings, the associated conditions, and the neuropathological characteristics of BD. Among the clinical findings, emphasis is placed on a 5- to 10-year period of stepwise progression of motor, cognitive, and behavioral deficits. During this period, there are stabilization and even improvement phases. As for the motor abnormalities, gait impairment, similar to that of a Parkinson's disease sufferer, is one of the distinctive features of the disease. In the early stages, although memory remains usually unimpaired, it is possible to find deterioration of constructive functions. Later on, language, memory, and visuospatial functions are severely affected. From the onset of the disease, apathy and aboulia mix with irritability and agitation, as well as impairment of judgment and sensitivity and loss of insight.

The diagnosis is essentially clinical and is supported by various neuroimaging findings. Thus, lacunar infarctions are found in the white matter and in basal ganglia, predominant leukoaraiosis in the frontal horn and in the parietal-occipital region, and moderate ventricular dilatation caused by subcortical atrophy and, in some cases, cortical atrophy. BD has been associated with arterial hypertension, amyloid angiopathy, elasticum pseudoxantoma, antiphospholipid antibody syndromes and another small vessel disease known since 1993 as cerebral autosomic dominant angiopathy with subcortical infarctions and leukoencelopathy (CADASIL).

CADASIL affects young people of either sex with lacunar infarctions and a history of previous migraine with aura and depression. The lacunar infarctions are multiple and affect basal ganglia, the thalamus, and the white matter. It is thought that they are caused by the hyaline and fibrinoid degeneration of long perforans small arteries. These changes have also been detected in the skin vessels and in the muscle. This disease can be inherited with an autosomal dominant pattern bound to chromosome 19, and Notch-3 gen are found in the 19q12 locus.

There is no specific neuroradiological pattern for the CADASIL. There are combinations of multiple subcortical infarctions (associated cortical infarctions have not been described) with diffuse leukoaraiosis of the periventricular and subcortical white matter. The main characteristics of dementia in the CADASIL are slow and progressive frontal cognitive deterioration, memory deficit, and neuropsychiatric manifestations (such as emotional lability, apathy, lack of interest, and depression), which can be quite acute. As with the lacunar state, this condition presents gait impairment (with rigidity and general spasticity), corticospinal signs, and other focal findings.

Its diagnosis is easy since patients are young and do not present with vascular risk factors. They have a family history of migraine, subcortical vascular dementia, depression, or leukoencephalopathy. Apart from the neuroimaging studies, skin or muscle biopsy can prove to be useful to find evidence of the characteristic angiopathy.

Among the localizations of corticosubcortical microangiopathies, attention should be drawn to the amyloid angiopathy that is caused by a deposit of amyloid protein in the middle and adventitia layers of cerebral arteries with small to medium caliber. This anatomopathological alteration has been observed in up to 80% of patients with AD, but is not exclusive to it. The condition known as amyloid angiopathy is particularly developed by older female patients, both sporadically and as a consequence of family history. The involvement of arteries typically produces spontaneous lobar hematomas. In addition to this, recurrent ischemic infarctions and leukoencephalopathy can be found.

As hemorrhagic events occur, the patient develops within weeks or months a dementia with a rapidly progressive course. The family history is inherited in an autosomal dominant manner and clinical presentation is usually cerebral hemorrhage in adults who are younger than 50. However, this condition can also manifest itself in the form of slowly progressive dementia.

Other vascular causes of dementia are ischemic–hypoxic and hemorrhagic dementia. Ischemic–hypoxic dementia is the result of a permanent neuronal loss caused by a prolonged hypoxic episode. Among the most frequent causes of this condition are global cerebral ischemia, pulmonary hypoventilation, and alterations in the transportation of oxygen. The most areas affected during a prolonged hypoxia are located in the big artery territories, in the boundaries between the medial cerebral artery, in the posterior and anterior cerebral arteries, in the basal ganglia, and in the hippocampus. Dementia secondary to intracranial hemorrhage is a consequence of lesions that are residual to bleeding and develop in combination with various clinical syndromes depending on the region of the bleeding. The origin of the hemorrhage can be spontaneous or can be related to arterial hypertension, congenital or mycotic aneurysm, arteriovenous malformations, coagulopathies, vasculitis, hemorrhagic encephalitis, or toxic encelopathies. Post-traumatic hemorrhage can manifest itself in the forms of epidural, subdural, or parenchymatous hematoma, acute subarachnoid hemorrhage, or intraventricular hemorrhage.

Epidural and subdural hematomas can manifest themselves exclusively as a confusional syndrome, with no patent signs of any neurological focality. The chronic subdural hematoma develops in old age after a trauma that can be of no significance and has even been forgotten. Cerebral atrophy, diminishing of intracranial pressure, alcoholism, or other coagulation disorders seem to favor its development. Clinical features tend to be unspecific and can be labeled as ictus, senile dementia, or normotensive hydrocephaly. Generally, its manifestations include continuous cephalea, gait impairment, loss of sphincter control, and dementia with subacute course. The diagnosis is reached by means of CT exploration (with iso-, hypo- or hyperdense signal).

Post-traumatic parenchymatous hematomas tend to be more frequent in the frontal and temporal lobes and are caused by a blow and countercoup in the cranial skullcap. These cause various focal cognitive impairments, which will depend on their localization. An intraventricular hemorrhage can damage the limbic system in an irreversible way causing character impairments and severe amnesic failures.

Accurate diagnosis of VaD requires clinical neurology expertise and judicious use of a specific neuropsychological test battery that demonstrates cortical and subcortical deficits. The test selected should have sensitivity in evaluating language and motor functions and in detecting subcortical deterioration, which are more commonly defective in VaD than in AD. The Mini-Mental State Examination (MMSE)[42] has disadvantages in VaD screening because this test emphasizes language and memory, is relatively insensitive to mild deficits, is influenced by education, and appears to be more sensitive to cortical than to subcortical dysfunctions. Other tests that could be useful for VaD are the Wechsler Adult Intelligence Scale–Revised (WAIS-R),[43] the Wechsler Memory Scale–Revised (WMS-R),[44] the Rey Complex Figure Test,[45] the Boston Diagnostic Aphasia Examination,[46] and the Western Aphasia Battery.[47]

The treatment of VaD has an essential preventive nature as treatment can prevent CVA by means of strict control of the vascular risk factors from both a primary and a secondary approach. The treatment includes platelet antiaggregation medication (acetylsalicylic acid, dipyridamole, triflusal, ticlopidine, clopidogrel).[48] Depending on the origin of the ischemic condition and the patient's state, anticoagulation treatments or interventionist therapies to prevent symptomatic carotid stenosis can also be considered. To date, the benefits of endarterectomy on symptomatic carotid stenoses when the VaD has already developed have not been reported. However, some authors suggest that it has some preventive effect on the development of VaD.

In this sense, it is possible that once the VaD has fully developed, controlling risk factors will contribute to slow its progression as this would prevent new ischemic lesions or improve the blood supply to hypoperfused areas.

Another research line tries to find drugs whose hemorrheologic action can improve the cerebral blood flow (by reducing blood viscosity and increasing erythrocytic deformability), thus preventing the progression of the VaD. This approach includes drugs such as pentoxifylline, cyclandelate, and vinpocetine. However, results concerning the efficacy of these drugs have been inconsistent.

As with an Alzheimer-type dementia, there are various groups of drugs used to try to stop the course of VaD by modifying the oxidative stress (MAOI such as seligiline, vitamin E), by reducing free intraneuronal calcium (with calcium antagonists such as nimodipine), or by easing the general cerebral metabolism (nootropic agents such as pirazetam, nebrazetam, and other GABA derivatives). These drugs produced significant improvements in some studies.

Another important aspect of the treatment of VaD is the control of dementia symptoms such as behavior changes, anxiety, agitation, emotional lability, and depression. An antidepressive treatment based on clinical suspicions can help in the differential diagnosis of a true VaD from a pseudodementia, since striking cognitive improvements occur after treatment of the latter condition.

Psychotic symptoms (delirious ideas and hallucinations) have a high incidence in BD (they are present in 40% of the patients). The most frequent delirious contents are suspiciousness, oversensitivity to the environment, belief that there are strangers in the house, abandonment, grandeur, and infidelity. These symptoms increase the emotional burden of the caregivers, which usually leads to institutionalization of the patients. Other behavioral symptoms that hinder patient management even more include restlessness, agitation, hostility, urinary incontinence, and insomnia. Furthermore, the appearance of psychotic symptoms is related to a more rapid cognitive deterioration. Therefore, controlling all the above-mentioned problems is crucial for managing a patient with VaD. Neuroleptics can reduce aggressivity and agitation, which improves the patient's standard of living and care. The minimum effective dosage should always be used to prevent the frequent undesirable effects (extrapyramidal alterations, somnolence, cognitive deterioration, and anticholinergic and paradoxical effects). There is no evidence that one neuroleptic drug is better than another. However, the efficacy of haloperidol, thioridazine, thiothixene, and loxapine has been demonstrated. More recently, low doses of modified neuroleptic drugs such as clozapine, olanzapine, and risperidone have allowed the control of psychotic symptoms with hardly any extrapyramidal or anticholinergic adverse effects.

Cognitive therapy uses compensatory strategies after identifying by means of neuropsychological tests the most affected areas in each patient. With these techniques, improvements can be achieved that, although modest, have been shown to have a positive impact on the patient's ability to carry out everyday life activities and to be integrated into the family environment. That VaD is not necessarily progressive can contribute to achieving more encouraging results than those obtained for other types of dementias, such as AD.

REFERENCES

1. National Institute of Neurological Diseases and Stroke, Classification of cerebrovascular disease, III, *Stroke*, 21, 637, 1990.
2. Kobari, M., Meyer, J. S., and Ichigo, M., Leuko-areiosis, cerebral atrophy and cerebral perfusion in normal aging, *Arch. Neurol.*, 47, 161, 1990.
3. Matsubayashi, K. et al., Incidental brain lesions on magnetic resonance imaging and neurobehavioral functions in the apparently healthy elderly, *Stroke*, 23, 175, 1992.
4. Kempster, P. A., Gerraty, R. P., and Gates, P. C., Asymptomatic cerebral infarction in patients with chronic atrial fibrillation, *Stroke,* 19, 955, 1988.
5. Kase, C. S. et al., Prevalence of silent stroke in patients presenting with initial stroke: the Framingham study, *Stroke*, 20, 850, 1989.
6. Ricci, S. et al., Silent brain infarctions in patients with first-ever stroke, *Stroke,* 24, 647, 1993.
7. Äström, M., Generalized anxiety disorder in stroke patients, *Stroke*, 27, 270, 1996.
8. Bamford, J. et al., Classification and natural history of clinically identifiable subtypes of cerebral infarction, *Lancet,* 337, 1521, 1991.
9. Cassidy, T. P. et al., The association of visual field deficits and visuospatial neglect in acute right-hemisphere stroke patients, *Age-Ageing*, 28(3), 257, 1999.
10. Gainotti, G., Il comportimento emozionale dei cerebrolesi destri e sinistri in situazione di test neurolopsicologico, *Arch. Psicol. Neurol. Psichiatr.,* 31, 457, 1970.
11. Andersen, G. et al., Pathoanatomic correlation between poststroke pathological crying and damage to brain areas involved in serotonergic neurotransmission, *Stroke*, 25, 1050, 1994.
12. Nahas, Z. et al., Rapid response of emotional incontinence to selective serotonin reuptake inhibitors, *J. Neuropsychiatr. Clin. Neurosci.*, 10(4), 453, 1998.
13. Starkstein, S. E. et al., Apathy following cerebrovascular lesions, *Stroke*, 24, 1625, 1993.
14. Ingles, J. L. et al., Fatigue after stroke, *Arch. Phys. Med. Rehabil.*, 80(2), 173, 1999.

15. Pohjasvaara, T. et al., Frequency and clinical determinants of poststroke depression, *Stroke,* 29(11), 2311, 1998.
16. Robinson, R. G., Neuropsychiatric consequences of stroke, *Annu. Rev. Med.,* 48, 217, 1997.
17. Feibel, J. H. and Springer, C. J., Depression and failure to resume social activities after stroke, *Arch. Phys. Med. Rehabil.,* 63, 276, 1982.
18. Brink, T. L., Yesavage, J. A., and Lum, O., Screening test for geriatric depression, *Clin. Gerontol.,* 1, 37, 1982.
19. Hamilton, M. A., A rating scale for depression, *J. Neurol. Neurosurg. Psychiatr.,* 23, 56, 1960.
20. Lishman, W. A., Brain damage in relation to psychiatric disability after head injury, *Br. J. Psychiatr.,* 114, 373, 1968.
21. Äström, M., Adolfsson, R., and Asplund, K., Major depression in stroke patients: a 3-year longitudinal study, *Stroke,* 24, 976, 1993.
22. Shimoda, K. and Robinson, R. G., The relationship between poststroke depression and lesion location in long-term follow-up, *Biol. Psychiatr.,* 45(2), 187, 1999.
23. Fedoroff, J. P. et al., Are depressive symptoms non-specific in patients with acute stroke? *Am. J. Psychiatr.,* 148, 1172, 1991.
24. Ästrom, M., Olsen, T., and Asplund, K., Different linkage of depression to hypercorticolism early versus late after stroke, *Stroke,* 24, 52, 1993.
25. Stenager, E. N. et al., Suicide among patients with apoplexy. An epidemiological study, *Ugeskr Laeg.,* 161(21), 3099, 1999.
26. Lipsey, J. R. et al., Nortriptyline treatment of post-stroke depression: a double blind study, *Lancet,* 1, 297, 1984.
27. Reding, M. J. et al., Antidepressant therapy after stroke: a double blind trial, *Arch. Neurol.,* 43, 763, 1986.
28. Murray, G. B., Shea, V., and Conn, D. K., Electroconvulsive therapy for post-stroke depression, *J. Clin. Psychiatr.,* 47, 258, 1986.
29. Jorm, A. F., Korten, A. E., and Henderson, A. S., The prevalence of dementia: a quantitative integration of the literature, *Acta Psychiatr. Scand.,* 76, 465, 1987.
30. Roth, M., The natural history of mental disorders arising in senium, *J. Ment. Sci.,* 101, 281, 1955.
31. Hachinski, V. C., Lassen, N. A., and Marshall, J., Multi-infarct dementia. A cause of mental deterioration in the elderly, *Lancet,* 2, 207, 1974.
32. Fischer, P. et al., Prospective neuropathological validation of Hachinski's ischemic score in dementias, *J. Neurol. Neurosurg. Psychiatr.,* 54, 580, 1991.
33. American Psychiatric Association, *Diagnostic and Statistical Manual of Mental Disorders,* 4th ed., American Psychiatric Association, Washington, D.C., 1994.
34. World Health Organization, *The ICD-10 Classification of Mental and Behavioural Disorders. Diagnostic Criteria for Research,* World Health Organization, Geneva, 1993.
35. Román, G. C. et al., Vascular dementia: diagnostic criteria for research studies. Report of the NINDS-AIREN International Work Group, *Neurology,* 43, 250, 1993.
36. Roth, M. et al., CAMDEX: a standardized instrument for the diagnosis of mental disorders in the elderly with special reference to the early detection of dementia, *Br. J. Psychiatr.,* 149, 698, 1986.
37. Tatemichi, Y. K., Sacktor, N., and Mayeux, R., Dementia associated with cerebrovascular disease, other degenerative diseases, and metabolic disorders, in *Alzheimer's Disease,* Terry, R. D., Katzman, R., and Bick, K. L., Eds., Raven Press, New York, 1994, 123.

38. McPherson, S. E. and Cummings, J. L., Neuropsychological aspects of vascular dementia, *Brain Cogn.,* 31, 269, 1996.
39. Mesulam, M. M., Large-scale neurocognitive networks and distributed processing for attention, language and memory, *Ann. Neurol.,* 28, 597, 1990.
40. Schmidt, R. et al., Neuropsychologic correlates of MRI white matter hyperintensities: a study of 150 normal volunteers, *Neurology,* 43, 2490, 1993.
41. Caplan, L. R., Binswanger's disease revisited, *Neurology,* 45, 626, 1995.
42. Folstein, M., Folstein, S., and McHugh, P. R., Mini-Mental State: a practical method for grading the cognitive state of patients for the clinician, *J. Psychiatr. Res.,* 12, 189, 1975.
43. Wechsler, D., *The Wechsler Adult Intelligence Scale–Revised,* The Psychological Corporation, New York, 1981.
44. Wechsler, D., *Wechsler Memory Scale–Revised Manual,* The Psychological Corporation, San Antonio, TX, 1987.
45. Osterreich, P. A., Le test de copie d'une figure complexe, *Arch. Psychol.,* 30, 206, 1944.
46. Goodglass, H. and Kaplan, E., *Boston Diagnostic Aphasia Examination,* Lea & Febiger, Philadelphia, 1973.
47. Kerstesz, A., *The Western Aphasia Battery Test Manual,* Grune & Stratton, Orlando, FL, 1982.
48. Lindsay, J., Hèbert, R., and Rockwood, K., The Canadian study of health and aging. Risk factors for vascular dementia, *Stroke,* 28, 526, 1997.

17 Treating Depression in Elderly People

José M. González Infantes,
José I. Ramírez Benítez,
and Pilar Moya Corral

CONTENTS

17.1 Introduction 363
17.2 Pharmacological Treatment...364
    17.2.1 Cyclical and Heterocyclical Antidepressants.................................365
    17.2.2 Monoamine Oxidase Inhibitors 366
    17.2.3 Selective Serotonin Reuptake Inhibitors..366
    17.2.4 Novel Antidepressants: Venlafaxine, Mirtazapine, Nefazodone,
            and Reboxetine 367
17.3 Electroconvulsive Therapy 368
17.4 Psychotherapy and Depression in Elderly People......................................369
    17.4.1 Support Psychotherapy..370
    17.4.2 Psychodynamic Psychotherapy 370
    17.4.3 Behavioral Treatment 372
    17.4.4 Cognitive–Behavioral Intervention 372
    17.4.5 Psychoeducational Intervention 374
            17.4.5.1 Program for Confronting Depression 374
            17.4.5.2 Life Satisfaction Course 375
    17.4.6 Interpersonal Psychotherapy 375
References...376

17.1 INTRODUCTION

When working within the frame of reference of the "medical model," the thera-peutic ideal is to carry out an etiological treatment. The problem with applying this ideal to disturbances of a psychological nature is that the etiology is so polymorphic that an etiological treatment, as such, is difficult to attempt. In the case of depressive syndromes, clear lines cannot be drawn between successive etiological and pathogenetic moments. Because of this, etiopathogeny is generally considered a set of co-causes and motivations that culminate in the onset of affective disorder. One should always try to treat psychopathological symptoms from this etiopathogenetic standpoint.

Another doctrinal aspect that determines a treatment program is working from a holistic conception of a person and his or her illness. This helps establish an integrated therapy and avoid treating depressive symptoms unilaterally. Working from this perspective somatic therapies (psychopharmacological medication and electroconvulsive therapy, or ECT), psychological techniques (psychotherapy) can be integrated with social-therapeutic measures (social therapy).

This approach is fundamental when dealing with elderly people, as patients who suffer depression for the first time at an advanced age have little or no family history of affective disorders (in other words, a lower genetic predisposition) and a greater number of individual and social factors triggering the depressive symptoms (especially bereavement and somatic disturbances).

This chapter focuses primarily on the biological and psychological treatments for depressed elderly people, without losing sight of the importance of social and rehabilitative measures.

17.2 PHARMACOLOGICAL TREATMENT

What is known about the effectiveness and safety of antidepressants with regard to the elderly population is based on research conducted on otherwise healthy patients 60 years of age. These drugs should therefore be used with caution in elderly patients who are weakened or have other coexisting illnesses. Antidepressants in the context of controlled clinical trials appear to be effective in 50 to 60% of depressed elderly patients.

At present, there exists a wide arsenal of antidepressants, including cyclic and heterocyclic antidepressants, monoamine oxidase (MAO) inhibitors, selective serotonin reuptake inhibitors (SSRI), noradrenaline, and novel antidepressants, such as mirtazapine and nefazodone.

In addition to the effectiveness of a drug, other aspects such as tolerance, safety, and potential drug interactions take on particular importance when treating elderly people. As regards tolerance, it is known that elderly people are more susceptible to side effects from psychiatric drugs as a result of the physiological changes produced with aging. This can affect the patient's quality of life and may cause the patient to abandon treatment, which in turn aggravates the preexisting illness. The following recommendations, together with a thorough knowledge of the patient's pathology, can be followed to palliate this problem.

1. Begin treatment with one third the recommended adult dosage.
2. Increase the administered dosage of medication gradually, aiming for the minimum effective dosage.
3. To prevent reinforcing toxic effects, avoid the simultaneous use of several medications.
4. Choose the most appropriate time of day for taking the medication.

Given the high risk of suicide in depressed older people, safety measures must be taken with medications to avoid overdose.

It also must be taken into account that elderly patients are often under pharmacological treatment for other illnesses. It is very important to be aware of the possible interactions of the antidepressant treatment with other medications that are being administered. Special precaution should be taken with anticoagulants, antiarrhythmic drugs, antiepileptic seizure medications, β-blockers, cardiotonics, oral hypoglucemiants, new antihistamines, opiates, and psychopharmacological drugs.

Other aspects to consider when choosing an antidepressant are as follows:

1. The symptomatic profile of the depression
2. Previous reactions to a medication in a past depressive episode, or the effectiveness the same treatment had on a family member
3. Convenience and ease of the dosage (single as opposed to multiple doses)

The following is a brief review of different categories of antidepressants, emphasizing the particular characteristics of their use in elderly people.

17.2.1 CYCLICAL AND HETEROCYCLICAL ANTIDEPRESSANTS

Potent antidepressants, the tricyclic and tetracyclic antidepressants, for many years were virtually the only pharmacological option, and therefore there has been a great deal of experience with their use. The side effects of the tricyclic drugs (Table 17.1) and numerous pharmacological interactions limit their use in elderly people. Currently, these drugs are reserved for treatment of major depressions with melancholy and for patients who do not respond to other antidepressants.

TABLE 17.1
Main Side Effects of Tricyclic Antidepressants and Their Clinical Consequences

	Side Effects		Consequence
CNS	Confusion		↑Cognitive deficits especially
	Memory alterations		in dementias
	Sedation		Falls → fractures
Peripheral	Cardiovascular alterations	Orthostatic hypotension	Falls → fractures
		Cardiac arrythmia Heart block	↑Previous cardiovascular pathology
		Cardiac toxicity of amitryptiline	↑Previous cardiovascular pathology
	Urinary retention		Acute retention in prostate hypertrophy
	Constipation		Fecalomas in previously constipated patients (intestinal obstruction)

In general, the secondary amines (nortriptyline, desipramine, and protryptiline) seem to be better tolerated in old age than the tertiary amines (imipramine, amitryptiline, chlorimipramine, and doxepine). Trazodone stands out among the tricyclic antidepressants with the fewest anticholinergic effects. With regard to choice of medication according to the symptomological profile, clomipramine tends to be used for inhibited depressions and obsessive–compulsive symptoms. Amitryptiline is used in anxious agitated depressions, and trazodone is particularly useful in treating depressed patients who cannot sleep.

The tetracyclic antidepressants used are mianserin and maprotyline. Mianserin is widely used in older adults. It is characterized by a lack of anticholinergic and sedative effects and is used to treat depressed elderly people suffering from cardiovascular disease. Maprotyline is a noradrenaline reuptake inhibitor and is characterized by its sedative action. It is used in cases of anxious–agitated depressions when anticholinergic drugs are not tolerated. Arterial hypotension and the appearance of some cases of agranulocytosis are noteworthy among the described adverse reactions from mianserin. The most notable adverse reaction in the case of maprotyline is the production of epileptic crises with greater frequency than with other antidepressants.

17.2.2 MONOAMINE OXIDASE INHIBITORS

The irreversible MAO inhibitors have a very limited use in the older adult. The difficulties caused by the need to avoid certain food and drug combinations are practical arguments for avoiding their use. Rarely are these drugs used as a first choice, only in atypical and refractory depressions. In the cases when they are used, tranylcipromine is preferable to fenelzine given that the effects of the former disappear in 24 h whereas in the latter the effects persist for a week. The most frequent side effect is hypotension. Other important side effects are nervousness, insomnia, hypertensive crisis, and weight gain.

The reversible and selective inhibitors of MAO-A (RIMA) are used in mature adults with inconsistent results. In a review, Gareri et al.[13] pointed out that moclobemide is not very effective in elderly patients, whereas other investigators observed good results, especially with patients with Alzheimer's dementia or Parkinson's disease. These authors found improvements both in the depression and in some of the symptoms of the underlying illness (improvement in cognition and in tremors, respectively). Gibert Rahola and Micó[14] observe the effectiveness in depression following a stroke and in the association of tricyclic–RIMA for the treatment of resistant and recurring depression. The side effects of the RIMA drugs are dry mouth, headaches (cephalea), dizziness, insomnia, tremors, sweating, and constipation.

17.2.3 SELECTIVE SEROTONIN REUPTAKE INHIBITORS

The pharmacological action of these drugs is the selective inhibition of the reuptake of serotonin, thus increasing the concentration of this neurotransmitter at the receptor site. Binding to any of the other presynaptic or postsynaptic receptors is minimal. Thus, the sedative, cardiovascular, or anticholinergic effects that limit the use of tricyclics are not produced by SSRIs. Thus, they are considered by many clinicians to be the first choice for the elderly patient. There seems to be a general consensus on using SSRIs as the treatment of choice in medium to moderately intense depressions. This is in spite of the fact that it has not been proved that the antidepressive action of the SSRIs is as effective as that of the tricyclics in every type of affective disorder.

The available inhibitors are fluvoxamine, fluoxetine, paroxetine, sertraline, and citalopram. The differences among them are basically pharmacokinetic (short/long half-life) and in relation to pharmacological interactions. Fluoxetine has a longer half-life than aroxetine and sertraline. As well, norfluoxetine (an active metabolite of fluoxetine) has a half-life of 4 to 16 days, which has clinical consequences in elderly people, as the plasma levels of norfluoxetine persist long after the interruption of the treatment with fluoxetine. When treatment is interrupted because of adverse side effects or drug interactions, it is important to keep this plasma level persistence in mind. A benefit is that discontinuation of treatment syndrome appears less frequently if patients forget to take their medicine. During prolonged treatments with fluoxetine or paroxetine, it should be taken into account that both present nonlinear pharmokinetics and danger of accumulation of the drugs and their active metabolites. The high potential of union between sertraline and the plasmatic proteins can induce important plasmatic modifications in other coadministered drugs, thereby causing serious side effects. Therefore, extreme caution must be taken in administering the drug to an older adult. In the case of the polymedicated elderly patient, citalopram appears to be the SSRI of choice.

In reference to comorbidity, in patients with Parkinson's disease SSRIs can produce an increase in the motor symptoms. There are studies that note good results with citalopram in depressions following a cerebrovascular accident and in patients with depression with dementia.

There are some differences in the clinical profile of different SSRIs. Paroxetine and fluvoxamine show a better action on anxiety and could be preferred in anxious depressions. Paroxetine and sertraline may show a better effect on atypical depression than other SSRIs. Citalopram may be used in aged patients taking other medications. SSRIs should not be prescribed with MAO inhibitors. Lithium levels should be strictly monitored when used with SSRI but this association is not recommended. Combination of tricyclic antidepressants with SSRI should be restricted to refractory depression.

17.2.4 NOVEL ANTIDEPRESSANTS: VENLAFAXINE, MIRTAZAPINE, NEFAZODONE, AND REBOXETINE

Venlafaxine inhibits the reuptake of noradrenaline and serotonin but, unlike the tricyclics, does so without accentuated action on postsynaptic receptors; thus, it possesses an effectiveness similar to that of the tricyclics but without the negative reactions and with a more rapid initial action. It is useful in the case of resistant depression. At high dosages, an increase in arterial pressure has been described. This is information that must be kept in mind when prescribing this medicine to elderly people.

Mirtazapine works as an antagonist at the α-2 noradrenergic receptors. Thus, it produces an indirect increase of the liberation of serotonin, at the same time that it is an antagonist at the 5-HT$_2$ and 5-HT$_3$ receptors. Thus it is effective in treating depression as well as anxiety, although it has a marked sedative action. The therapeutic profile for this drug is for use in patients with depression who also suffer anxiety and insomnia. It is also an alternative treatment for depressions that, after having improved with SSRIs, become worse, or when there is intolerance for SSRIs because of sexual dysfunction, nausea, or gastrointestinal disorders.

Nefazodone possesses a weak action as a 5-HT reuptake inhibitor and as a potent 5-HT$_2$ antagonist. In addition to its antidepressant properties, it acts as a sedative and a sleep regulator, and possibly as an analgesic, as well. Its use could therefore be indicated in depressed patients who suffer illnesses that provoke pain. The therapeutic profile is similar to that of mirtazapine.

Reboxetine is an selective reuptake inhibitor of noradrenaline. Montgomery,[24] found a similar effectiveness when comparing this drug with imipramine in elderly patients suffering from major depression. Findings also showed a lower incidence of hypotension and other related symptoms than with imipramine.

To conclude, another group of drugs used to treat depression in elderly people should be mentioned: stimulants and lithium. Stimulants are used in secondary depressions associated with chronic illnesses; the most popular is methylfenidate. Among its advantages, the most notable is the rapidity with which patients respond to the treatment. There is noticeable improvement in 24 to 48 h. If in 72 h there is no response, treatment should be suspended. Among the disadvantages of this drug is the phenomenon of tolerance and dependence.

Lithium is used in patients with bipolar type 1 depressions and as a stimulator of antidepressive action in resistant depressions. On these occasions, extreme caution should be exercised to avoid neurotoxic effects, even with low doses. The response to lithium is individual; lithemias of 0.4 to 0.6 are sufficient. On the other hand, and above all when dealing with the elderly population, interactions must be kept in mind. The most important interactions to consider are those with diuretics, non-steroidal anti-inflammatories, neuroleptics, and antiarrhythmic drugs.

17.3 ELECTROCONVULSIVE THERAPY

Today, electroconvulsive therapy (ECT) is considered a safe and effective technique for the elderly population. The effectiveness oscillates between 70 and 80% of total recuperations or very important improvements for this age group. Steck et al.,[36] after reviewing 18 studies on effectiveness, found a percentage between 50 and 100% for significant clinical improvements. In addition, in general, ECT is tolerated better than psychiatric drugs and there are no clear data on cognitive decline in the long term associated with this therapy, although as a precaution, the initial use of non-dominant unilateral ECT is recommended. Additionally, it is necessary to modify the dosage of the drugs normally used and to increase the intensity of the convulsive stimulus (with age, the threshold increases). In practice, while the patients receive ECT treatment they should continue taking antidepressants as well, maintaining the dose for at least 6 months, because ECT does not prevent relapses.

The more endogenous symptoms a patient's depression presents, the better the patient responds to ECT. This type of treatment is resorted to in the following circumstances:

1. Depression with psychotic symptoms
2. Inhibited and/or rapidly progressive depressions (due to its rapid action)
3. Cases of elevated risk of suicide
4. Cases of impossibility of antidepressant treatment (intolerance of the side effects)
5. Resistant depressions
6. Cases of serious somatic repercussions of the depression (alarming weight loss, dehydration)
7. Depressive pseudodementia (ECT usually proves to be more effective than psychiatric drugs)

Comorbidity is an important issue to keep in mind. The coexistence of dementia does not constitute a counterindication of any kind for the application of ECT, as additional deterioration has not been observed. The coexistence of endogenous depression and Parkinson's disease is considered an indication for ECT, given the simultaneous improvement of both disorders (improvement of the motor symptoms in Parkinson's disease). It is recommended that the dose of L-dopa be reduced to one half and that the the rest of the medication be suspended. The presence of vascular cerebral accidents is a relative counter indication.

A similar situation occurs in patients with cardiovascular problems, especially if it is kept in mind that mortality attributed to ECT results in great part from cardiovascular accidents during treatment or immediately afterward. These accidents appear to be associated with two factors: the previous cardiovascular condition of the patient and the physiological changes induced by the treatment. Patients with cardiac illnesses have a significantly higher rate of these types of adverse effects and, in fact, some prefer to abstain from applying ECT in the cases of patients who have suffered a recent heart attack. However, Agelink et al.[1] found that ECT was well tolerated by cardiovascular patients. The risk of cardiac failure can be reduced with preoxygenation and prior treatment with nitroglycerin and adrenergic block.

In patients with broncopulmonary disorders the risks are hypoxia and laryngospasm. Mortality in ECT has been associated with treatment with theophyline.

17.4 PSYCHOTHERAPY AND DEPRESSION IN ELDERLY PEOPLE

Currently, it seems that no one doubts that the depressed elderly patient can benefit from certain types of psychotherapeutic interventions,[7,18,22,33] especially if these are combined with drug therapy.[5,15,26,27,30] However, this opinion, which today is supported by multiple investigations, was not always viewed this way. The authors recall the pessimism of Freud in regard to the utility of psychoanalysis of mature patients (those over 40)[2] because of the lack of sufficient elasticity in the mental process, the rigidity of character and the defenses, and the length of duration of accumulated material.[8] Subsequently, this pessimism originating from Freud in reference to the use of psychotherapy softened within the school of psychoanalysis.[31]

With regard to the effectiveness of different psychotherapeutic modalities for the treatment of depression in the elderly patient, there seem to be data in favor of the behavioral[29] and cognitive–behavioral approaches,[19] as well as the somewhat more recent applications in elderly people of the so-called interpersonal psychotherapies.[38]

This section, without intending to be exhaustive, describes the most popular psychotherapeutic modalities for treatment of depression of the elderly person, beginning with the so-called support psychotherapy, continuing with psychodynamic psychotherapies, behavioral therapies, cognitive–behavioral, and psychoeducative interventions. The section ends with interpersonal psychotherapy.

17.4.1 Support Psychotherapy

This type of psychotherapy has the aim of attenuating or suppressing anxiety so that patients can return to their previous situation before the crisis, as well as attempt to try out new behaviors during the psychotherapeutic period. The role of the therapist is educative-directive. It is expected that the real link with the therapist also exerts a corrective influence.

The specific objectives of this psychotherapeutic modality are to support the evaluation of reality, to obtain support for the ego, and to maintain or reestablish the level of normal functioning. Its duration can be limited or according to the necessities of the case. The techniques employed are usually accessibility of the therapist in a predictable way; utilization of interpretation to fortify the defenses; the therapist maintaining a professional relationship, based on reality, support, concern, and problem solving; suggestion, reinforcement, advice, evaluation of reality, cognitive reconstruction, and reaffirmation; and vital psychodynamic narration.

This type of therapy has been applied to elderly patients with depression;[8] the therapist takes a much more active role in identifying and clarifying the problem of the patient and in trying to mobilize the patient toward a greater commitment to his or her own life and problems.

17.4.2 Psychodynamic Psychotherapy

Previously, the difficulties of the application, according to Freud, of this type modality of intervention in the elderly patient were mentioned. Nevertheless, subsequent psychoanalytic authors clarified this perspective. For example, Abraham contemplated this difficulty but put greater emphasis on the "age" of the neurosis rather than on the age of the patient. On the other hand, Jung saw the age of 40 as a good moment for carrying out important changes in the personality (recall that Freud considered people "old" after the age of 40).

One of the first authors to publish an analysis of a mature patient was H. Segal,[31] in 1958, in his article entitled "Fear of Dying. Notes on the Analysis of an Elderly Man." Segal emphasizes and considers the cause of psychotic depression that his patient suffered from at the age of 73 as the unconscious fear of dying.[31]

Hinze[17] centers his psychotherapeutic work on the analysis of the transference and countertransference of the aged patient. He attempts to show that prejudices in relation to growing old and countertransference problems have been at the core of the lack of previous interest for treating this type of patient. These issues of counter-transference in reference to aging could be summed up in four points:[4]

1. The elderly patient stimulates therapists' own fears about their own old age.
2. Elderly patients arouse conflicts in therapists about their relationships with parental figures.
3. Therapists often consider that they do not have anything useful to offer because the elderly person cannot change.
4. Therapists think that their psychotherapeutic abilities are wasted in work with elderly people.

From the point of view of psychoanalysis and psychoanalytically oriented psy-chotherapy, according to Beá Montagut,[2] some of the characteristics of depressive states in old age are as follows:

1. Mourning as a consequence of changes in the type of objectal relationship that constitutes the foundation of personal identity, which is transformed and enriched in these processes.
2. In old age the amount of bereavement is very intense. In the corporal sphere (illnesses, reactionary factors, etc.), in the social aspect (decline in activity, family modifications, etc.), and in the mental arena (awareness of these facts, continuous remembrance of the reality of death, etc.).

The elaboration of these conflicts does not always go hand in hand with maturation growth or development of the *Mental Id*, but it can easily reactivate unresolved primitive conflicts, returning to points of fixation, that are at the base of different psychopathological disturbances, among them depressive states.

Therefore, in accordance with Simón Brainsky,[32] a fundamental aspect of psy-chotherapeutic work with older adults maintains a relationship with the elaboration of grief and the resonance that the recent losses evoke in the elderly patient, running the risk that such losses are replaced by a greater narcissistic charge of the body itself with resulting hypochondria. Continuing in this line, just as Pollock[25] considers, when discharging the energy linked to lost people and/or situations, a liberation of feelings, emotions, thoughts, and potential actions is originated, which will be free to adjust to new situations and recognize new significant objects. Therefore, a psychotherapeutic activity is to channel these energies toward transactions that are personally and socially acceptable.

17.4.3 Behavioral Treatment

The behavioral therapies emphasize carrying out activities and learning-determined skills, trying to produce or provoke in this way a modification in the target behavior of the intervention.

One type of behavioral treatment that has been demonstrated to be successful in treating depression in elderly people is the program developed by Lewinsohn et al.,[21] applied to and investigated in this population by Gallagher[12] with certain modifications that affect the form of presentation of the material, in "time" with and to the rhythm imposed by the therapist.[11] This program, based on the theory of the same author, is founded on the manifest relationship between the positive consequences derived from carrying out activities of a pleasant (or unpleasant) nature and mood. Succinctly, the treatment tries to increase the pleasant activities and augment the satisfaction that these produce in the subject. The program, which is extremely structured, comprises the following phases:

1. Initial sessions: Explanation to the patient about the nature of the therapy. In this phase self-reports are usually used to collect information about positive and negative events (pleasant events scale, PES; unpleasant events scale, UES).
2. Intermediate sessions: The objective in this phase is to show patients the relationship between activities and depression by means of the completion of a diary of self-registry of moods and activities. As a result of this, a plan for increasing pleasant activities and reducing unpleasant ones will be developed. In this phase, it is sometimes necessary to teach certain skills of self-management, for example, relaxation training, social skills, etc.
3. Final sessions: Reviewing what has been learned, making explicit the maintenance plan for change that is going to be put into practice after the termination of the therapy.

The authors recommend having "brush-up" sessions at 6 and 12 weeks with the objective of reinforcing the continuity in the use of learned behavioral skills.

17.4.4 Cognitive–Behavioral Intervention

The cognitive theory considers that feelings of depression are determined by thoughts and especially by errors in logic. The investigation of depression among elderly people has established that this can be defined, in good measure, by the high number of negative cognitions maintained in relationship with themselves, the world, and their future. So, as well, the logical errors of depression determine the erroneous beliefs that predispose the subject to feeling unhappy and worried, and generating thoughts of failure and indefensiveness.

The cognitive intervention consists of the identification of logical errors that are associated with the depressed state, as well as the elimination of the negative cognitions, learning to substitute them with others that are more adaptive and logical about themselves and others. One type of cognitive therapy such as that of Beck,[3] published in 1976, was adapted for use with elderly people by Emery.[9] It is a structured therapy organized as follows:

1. First sessions: The therapy begins with a systematic register of daily activities and the level of pleasure and expertise of execution that is associated with each of them. Beginning this way is only a modification of the therapy for elderly people, since it is found that this group has the greatest difficulties in the utilization of cognitive strategies that demonstrate that thought affects mood. Besides, terminating with behavioral changes alleviates some of the symptoms of subjects and motivates them to continue with the therapy. An intervention is planned and applied to increase the activities that are pleasant, or that are carried out with skill, by means of planning daily activities. At this time, the therapist introduces the explanation of the relationship between thoughts and feelings.
2. Intermediate sessions: When the relationship between thought and fluctuations of mood is understood by the subject, the identification of the specific cognitive distortions implicated in the negative thoughts of the subject takes place. It is convenient that patients recognize the logical errors that they commit to focus the therapy on their correction. The most frequent logical errors and negative thoughts in elderly people with depression are listed here.
   - *Arbitrary Interference*: Establishing conclusions that are specific to situations and realities without the necessary evidence for doing so.
   - *Selective Abstraction*: Producing judgments and thoughts based on isolated details while ignoring other important characteristics of the situation.
   - *Overgeneralization*: Making general conclusions based on isolated facts and applying them to situations related and unrelated to them.
   - *Magnification and Minimization*: Minimizing their skills and overvaluing the difficulties of the events.
   - *Personalization*: Relating certain external facts to themselves, even when there is no evidence for doing so.
   - *Dichotomous Thinking*: Classifying experiences in opposite categories and classifying themselves in the negative extreme.

   Older patients with major depression refer a series of negative thoughts, such as physical worries, negative thoughts about the past, disappointment with their sons and daughters, death of relatives and friends, changes in physical appearance, loss of social roles, caretaking of disabled relatives, fear of being victims of unlikely accidents or criminal offenses, or decline of their sexual life (Gallagher, 1981).

   The identification of negative thoughts is done via a self-register in which primarily the situations in which the patient feels depressed are identified, and, if possible, what the patient was thinking in these moments. In mature adults, difficulties can appear at this point in the therapy, although it is a central element of the same issue and the therapist should try by way of questions to discover the before-mentioned negative thoughts.

3. Final sessions: After identifying the negative thoughts, it is necessary to help the subject recognize what specific distortions underlie such thoughts. It is a question of the patients, in everyday life, identifying their thoughts and recognizing cognitive distortions that they make and later to generate rational alternatives and responses to these erroneous thoughts. The therapist, therefore, should show the subject by way of cognitive strategies, such as reattribution, evaluating the evidence, listing the pros and cons of maintaining an idea, and examining the consequences that follow this idea, to evaluate their thoughts and generate alternatives. These techniques help patients develop greater perceptual and cognitive flexibility. Often older people need more time and to be motivated in greater measure to reach this objective, since they are more resistant to modifying their ideas and beliefs.

17.4.5 PSYCHOEDUCATIONAL INTERVENTION

The term *psychoeducative* is associated more directly with the conceptualization of Bandura's social learning. Psychoeducative intervention is based on vicarious learning. It is symbolic, and in the processes of self-regulation, assigns the individual an important role in the modification of his or her own environment. The following describes two types of psychoeducative programs for depression amply applied to older people.

17.4.5.1 Program for Confronting Depression

Lewinsohn et al.[21] designed this program, which represents a reorganization of some of the traditional strategies of behavioral treatment of depression. It is a course that can be imparted in small groups with an educative format. This course is composed of six sessions focused on education of the techniques of self-control relevant to thoughts, pleasant activities, relaxation, and personal interaction.

This program was adapted in 1983 by Thompson et al.[37] for older people with the following modifications: increasing the time of each skill that the elderly person should learn, reduction of the number of skills to teach, maintaining the basic skills to increase the pleasant events and reduce the negative events, and elimination of advanced skills (assertiveness and relaxation training).

The sessions are conducted once a week, with groups of six to eight people with two instructors for 2 hours for a total of 6 weeks. The sessions are very structured, with the following content:

1. First session: Centered on "mood control."
2. Second session: Identification of daily pleasant events.
3. Third session: Identification of negative events that influence mood, the relationship between level of activity and mood. Manipulation of activity.

4. Fourth session: Identification of the specific problem, object of change for each person. Teaching self-reinforcement. Promotion of choice of specific attainable objectives.
5. Fifth session: The program of change is amplified in each subject with a second objective.
6. Sixth session: Work on the "maintenance of progress." In 2 months the group is brought together again for a review session.

This program has been used successfully with elderly patients with moderate symptoms of depression (by the same authors). Hedlund and Thompson[16] also had successful results with older people diagnosed with major depression. Despite its effectiveness, the authors have modified certain aspects that they considered deficient, thus creating another program: Life Satisfaction Course.[37]

17.4.5.2 Life Satisfaction Course

This is designed for mature adults who reside in communities. Those who suffer from major depression may not participate in this program; however, those who have mild depression or frequent mood swings may. The course consists of nine sessions of 2 hours each over the period of 9 weeks. In each group six to ten participants take part with two instructors.

The sessions are quite structured, always following the same format: revision and discussion of the "homework," reinforcing the progress of the participants and resolving whatever doubts may come up; presentation of the new information by means of a brief reading; and, last, a seminar in which the participants apply the new material with the supervision of the instructors. In the fifth and sixth sessions "skills for self-change" are taught. The last two sessions are focused on the revision of the plan for change, elaborating a new plan for the systematic increase of positive and satisfactory activities and generalizing the skills to other problematic areas. Follow-up sessions are conducted at the end of 1 and 6 months.

The effectiveness of this course has been tested by Fernández-Ballesteros et al.,[10] who obtained ambiguous results.

17.4.6 INTERPERSONAL PSYCHOTHERAPY

This is a type of psychotherapy in the short term developed by Klerman et al.[20] It is brief psychotherapy that lasts from 12 to 16 weeks focused on current interpersonal problems. It was developed primarily for unipolar depressed patients who are non-psychotic ambulatory patients, but subsequently its use has been extended to other clinical symptoms, as well as to different population groups, including elderly patients.[23,34,35]

Interpersonal psychotherapy (IPT) is derived from the interpersonal psychiatric school founded by Adolf Meyer and Harry Steck Sullivan. Most of this psychotherapy is based on the psychodynamic theory.

The first stage of therapy is begun by taking a detailed history (inventory) of the symptoms, generally utilizing a structured interview. The symptoms are reviewed with the patient who is explicitly informed of the natural course of the depression. The fact of legitimizing to the patient the role of being ill is highlighted. As well, at this stage an evaluation of the interpersonal problems is done, attempting to identify one or more of the following four problematic areas: reaction to grief, interpersonal disputes, role transitions, and interpersonal deficits.

At the middle stage of the treatment, efforts are directed toward resolving the problematic areas. The basic techniques for managing each problematic area consist of the clarification of the positive and negative emotional states, identification of past models of relationships, and guidance and stimulation of the patient in examination and choice of alternative behaviors. Emphasis is maintained on current problems and not on previous interpersonal problems. The focus of this therapy is directed more toward interpersonal events than toward intrapsychotic or cognitive events.

Studies on the effectiveness of this type of intervention show that good results are obtained in maintenance of the improvement of social functioning, in recuperation from depression and reduction of symptoms, and in improvement of functioning during the acute stage of an episode of depression. These effects are not made apparent until after 6 or 8 months. The results improve when this type of intervention is combined with pharmacological treatments,[28] including as well as one of the factors associated with a lesser rate of recurrence of the depressive symptoms in elderly patients when IPT is maintained.[6] Thus, the combination of pharmacological treatment and this type of psychotherapy is efficacious in the long term.[28]

REFERENCES

1. Agelink, M. W. et al., Benefits and risks of electroconvulsive therapy in elderly patients with cardiovascular risk factors, *Nervenarzt*, 69(1), 70, 1998.
2. Beá Montagut, J., Aspectos psicodinámicos de la depresión en la tercera edad, *Inf. Psiquiátr.*, 142, 481, 1995.
3. Beck, A. T. et al., Terapia cognitiva de la depresión, Desclée de Brower, Bilbao, 1983.
4. Butler, R. N., Psiquiatría geriátrica, in *Tratado de Psiquiatría*, Vol. 2, Kaplan, H. I. and Sadock, B. J., Eds., Salvat, Barcelona, 1989.
5. Butler, R. N. et al., Late-life depression: treatment strategies for primary care practice, *Geriatrics*, 52, 51–52, 58–60, 63–64, 1997.
6. Buysse, D. J. et al., Longitudinal effects of nortriptyline on EEG sleep and the likelihood of recurrence in elderly depressed patients, *Neuropsychopharmacology*, 14(4), 243, 1996.
7. Collins, E., Katona, C., and Orrell, M. W., Management of depression in the elderly by general practitioners: referral for psychological treatments, *Br. J. Clin. Psychol.*, 36, 445, 1997.
8. De La Serna, I.. *Psicogeriatría*, Jarpyo Editores, Madrid, 1996).
9. Emery, G., Cognitive therapy with the elderly, in *New Directions in Cognitive Therapy*, Emery, G., Hollon, S., and Bedrosian, R., Eds., Guilford, New York, 1981.
10. Fernández-Ballesteros, R. et al., Satisfacción de la vida y vejez: evaluación de un programa, in *Cong. Interamericano de Psicología*, Cuba, 1987.
11. Fernández-Ballesteros, R. et al., *Evaluación e Intervención Psicológica en la Vejez*, Martínez Roca, Barcelona, 1992.

12. Gallagher, D., Behavioral group therapy with elderly depressives: an experimental study, in *Behavioral Group Therapy*, Vol. 3, Upeer, D. and Ross, S., Eds., Research Press, Champaign, IL, 1981.

13. Gareri, P. et al., Antidepressant drugs in the elderly, *Gen. Pharmacol.*, 30, 465, 1998.

14. Gibert Rahola, J. and Micó, J. A., Tratamiento farmacológico de la depresión en el anciano, in *Grandes Síndromes Psiquiátricos*, 3ª Unidad Didáctica: Síndrome depresivo. Ferrer Internacional S.A., 1997.

15. González Infante, J. M. et al., Integración de la farmacoterapia y la socioterapia en el tratamiento de ciertas entidades específicas, *Psicopatología*, 4(2), 135, 1984.

16. Hedlund, B. and Thompson, L. W., Teaching the Elderly to Control Depression Using an Educational Format, American Psychological Association, Montreal, 1980.

17. Hinze, E., La transferencia y contratransferencia en el tratamiento psicoanalítico de pacientes de edad avanzada, *Libro Anual de Psicoanálisis,* Vol. 3, 1987.

18. Jorgensen, M. B., Dam, H., and Bolwig, T. G., The efficacy of psychotherapy in nonbipolar depression — a review, *Acta Psychiatr. Scand.*, 98, 13, 1998.

19. Katon, W. et al., A multifaceted intervention to improve treatment of depression in primary care, *Arch. Gen. Psychiatr.*, 53, 924, 1996.

20. Klerman, G. L. et al., *Interpersonal Psychotherapy of Depression,* Basic Books, New York, 1984.

21. Lewinsohn, P. M. et al., A behavioral group therapy approach to the treatment of depression, in *Handbook of Behavioral Group Therapy*, Upeer, D. and Ross, S., Eds., Plenum Press, New York, 1982.

22. McCusker, J. et al., Effectiveness of treatments of depression in older ambulatory patients, *Arch. Intern. Med.*, 158, 705, 1998.

23. Miller, M. D. et al., Interpersonal psychotherapy (IPT) in a combined psychotherapy/medication research protocol with depressed elders. A descriptive report with case vignettes, *J. Psychother. Pract. Res.*, 7, 47, 1997.

24. Montgomery, S. A., El lugar de la reboxetina en el tratamiento antidepresivo, *J. Clin. Psychiatr.*, 59(14), 1998.

25. Pollock, G., On aging and psychopathology, *Int. J. Psychoanal.*, 63, 27, 1982.

26. Reynolds, C. F. et al., Treatment outcome in recurrent major depression: A post hoc comparison of elderly ("young old") and midlife patients, *Am. J. of Psychiatr.*, 153(10), 1288, 1996.

27. Reynolds, C. F. et al., Nortriptyline and interpersonal psychotherapy as maintenance therapies for recurrent major depression. A randomized controlled trial in patients older than 59 years, *JAMA*, 281(1), 39, 1999.

28. Reynolds, C. F. et al., Treatment of 79(+)-year-olds with recurrent major depression. Excellent short-term but brittle long-term response, *Am. J. Geriatr. Psychiatr.*, 7, 64, 1999.

29. Rokke, P. D., Tomhave, J. A., and Jocic, Z., The role of client choice and target selection in self-management therapy for depression in older adults, *Psychol. Aging*, 14, 155, 1999.

30. Schukberg, H. C. et al., Treating major depression in primary care practice. Eight-month clinical outcomes, *Arch. Gen. Psychiatr.*, 53, 913, 1996.

31. Segal, H., *El Temor a la Muerte: Notas sobre el Análisis de un Anciano*, Paidós, Argentina, 1989.

32. Simón Brainsky, L., Psicoterapia en la tercera edad, *Psiquis*, 44, 1986.

33. Small, G. W. et al., Recognizing and treating anxiety in the elderly, *J. Clin. Psychiatr.*, 58, 41, 1997.

34. Sole Puig, J., Psicoterapia interpersonal (I), *Rev. Psiquiatr. Univ. Med. Barcelona*, 22(4), 91, 1995.
35. Sole Puig, J., Psicoterapia interpersonal (II), *Rev. Psiquiatr. Univ. Med. Barcelona*, 22(5), 120, 1995.
36. Steck, M. L., Beekman, A. T., and Verwey, B., Electroconvulsive therapy in late life depression: a review, *Tijdschr. Gerontol. Geriatr.*, 28 (3), 106, 1997.
37. Thompson, L. et al., Evaluation of the effectiveness of professionals and nonprofessionals as instructors of "coping with depression" classes for elders, *Gerontologist*, 23, 390, 1983.
38. Weissman, M. M., Interpersonal psychotherapy: current status, *Keio J. Med.*, 46, 105, 1997.

18 Advances in the Prevention and Treatment of Age-Related Organic Memory Disorders

José León-Carrión,
María Rosario Domínguez-Morales,
and Juan Manuel Barroso y Martín

CONTENTS

18.1 Introduction 379
18.2 Memory Terminology 381
18.3 Age-Related Memory Changes.. 382
18.4 Principles and Goals of Age-Related Memory Neurorehabilitation 386
18.5 Advances in the Prevention of Age-Related Memory Problems 388
18.6 Behavioral Training for Age-Related Memory Disorders......................... 391
18.7 Neuropharmachological Advances in the Treatment
     of the Age-Related Memory Deficits... 393
18.8 Concluding Remarks.. 397
References.. 397

18.1 INTRODUCTION

Aging can be approached from at least three different perspectives: physiological, cultural, and political. It seems clear that there are biological systems that age quickly and later are regenerated (blood cells). However, the nervous system seems to be one of the most stable and, in general, can be well conserved even after 80 years of life, although there are problems with reparation and regeneration. Other systems can be particularly active during certain ages and not in others (motor system). According to Flannigan et al.,[1] the effects of aging on skeletal muscle can be recognized in three ways. First, muscle mass and strength both undergo a general decline. Second, alterations in muscle histopathy, mainly mitochondrial abnormalities, reflect underlying physiological changes that occur with aging. Third, and perhaps reflecting the influence of the two previous points, susceptibility to certain neuromuscular diseases is age related.

From a cultural point of view, "old age" is a concept that depends on the relative age of individuals. To a 15-year-old, someone who is 30 is "old," whereas for a 40-year-old, someone of 65 is "young-old." From a political point of view, "old age" depends on legislation that sets the age of a "senior citizen" to coincide with the age at which one receives a pension.[2] The concept of normality for old age changes according to how habits, customs, and lifestyles also change for the general population. Normality is usually understood as what is normal according to the statistics for a certain age group.

From a neuropathological point of view, Odenheimer[2] (p. 563) finds that aging is associated with a decline in functional abilities normally as a result of neurological conditions. With advanced age, complex or instrumental activities of daily living, such as managing finances, preparing meals, grocery shopping, or driving a car, are often impaired. Of people between the ages of 65 and 69, about 10% will require assistance in activities of daily living, while this type of assistance will be required for more than 50% of those aged 85 or more. However, the simplest activities of daily life (bathing, going to the toilet, grooming, eating, and walking) are fairly resistant and tend to remain intact in at least 80% of people over 85 years of age. The weight of the brain also seems to change with age, the greatest change occurring between the second and third decades, beginning to diminish in the middle of the fifth decade with losses of cerebral volume of 2 to 3% in the following decades,[3,4] with gyral atrophy and ventricular dilation. The areas most affected by gyral atrophy are the parasagittal region, median limbic areas, and the poles of the frontal and temporal lobes.

The effect of advanced age on the neuron content of the cerebral cortex shows that the loss of gray and white matter is not uniform throughout life. During the second and fifth decades the decrease in volume is greater in gray matter; thereafter, the loss of white matter is greater.[5] Frontopolar, premotor, and temporal association areas lose between 12 and 15%; hippocampus and parts of the amygdala lose 20 to 25% of cells; locus ceruleus loses 20 to 40%; and the substantia nigra loses 50% of cells by the ninth decade. All these changes lead to losses of synaptic densities, especially in the association cortices.[6]

The ratio between intracranial and cerebral volume remains relatively constant until the 60s after which it falls by nearly 20% between the seventh and tenth decades of life. In addition, some authors have found progressive neural loss in the hippocampus (one third of individuals from 55 to 88 years was found to demonstrate hippocampal atrophy) and an age-related decline in neural population of the putamen and thalamus (see Schochet).

Different authors have proposed that there is a fall in cerebral blood flow and oxygen metabolism from childhood to adolescence, followed by a more gradual reduction throughout the remaining age span. An interesting study was done by Hagstadius and Risberg,[8] measuring the regional cerebral blood flow (rCBF) of 97 normal subjects aged 19 to 68 years old while resting. Results showed that the mean

CBF level decreased progressively with age. The decrease was more pronounced in frontotemporal and inferior Rolandic areas bilaterally. Frontal areas showed the highest values in all age groups. This hyperfrontality weakened somewhat with age. Mean CBF in the right hemisphere was significantly higher than in the left, as was flow in superior frontal, inferior frontal, and parietal areas. These asymmetries were age invariant. The age-related decrease of rCBF is interpreted by the author as reflecting aging of the brain per se, although the influence of asymptomatic brain disease cannot be ruled out. The flow asymmetries are interpreted as related to functional lateralization of some aspects of attentional activation.

Interestingly, the functional effectiveness of the nervous system at age 50 can be much better than at age 20 due to functional changes that have occurred from experience, although it is probable that cerebral energetic consumption is different in a young person than in an adult. However, one should not forget that cerebral self-regulation can deteriorate with age. According to Choi et al.,[9] the normal cerebralvascular bed responds to blood pressure, O_2 tension, CO_2 tension, and cerebral metabolism, and these responses decrease with age. Other factors with long-term adverse effects on self-regulation include uncontrolled hypertension, cardiac dysfunction, and smoking. According to these authors, these conditions and aging may have a compounding impact on the cerebrovascular system. Three of the most common neurological diagnoses found in elderly people are Alzheimer's disease, Parkinson's disease, and stroke.

18.2 MEMORY TERMINOLOGY

The following briefly presents the most common terminology used in the field of neuropsychology of memory.

Amnesia. A general term used to refer to any form of temporary or permanent global memory loss. Permanent stable amnesia is normally known as the amnesic syndrome.

Anterograde amnesia. Produced when a patient has difficulty or is unable to store, evoke, or retain new information.

Confabulation. A tendency to produce false memories. These are implausible memories the patient has no doubt are true. It is associated with frontal damage.

Explicit memory. All those memories that can be evoked or recognized consciously. They can be explicit or declarative.

Focal retrograde amnesia. A memory impairment in which the primary deficit is a loss of remote memory with no low scores in the performance of anterograde tests.

Implicit memory. All those memories that cannot be declared. They are memories that are implicit in procedures and in activities.

Post-traumatic amnesia. The loss of memory produced once a person has regained consciousness after suffering a brain injury or recover from coma. It can last minutes, hours, and days.

Primary memory. A memory that requires only brief retention and retrieval
of information. It is limited in terms of the quantity of information that can
be retained at a certain time. Also called short-term memory.

Psychogenic memory deficits. Those memory problems where the existence
of a neurological illness or brain injury has been discarded.

Retrograde amnesia. The incapacity to remember facts, events, or information
learned prior to the neurological disorder.

Transient global amnesia. Condition normally originates from a temporary
neurological condition. When resolved the patient recovers normal memory.
It tends to be more common in elderly people and those suffering migraines.

18.3 AGE-RELATED MEMORY CHANGES

All the data seem to indicate that age-related memory changes do exist. However,
the originating causes are not clear. Much data indicate that these memory problems
in elderly people are caused by physiological aging affecting certain areas of the
brain involved in different memory processes. It is also true that, probably because
of genetic factors and lifestyles, not all people age biologically the same way. Aging
does not affect all cognitive functions uniformly. The study carried out by Ritchie
et al.[10] shows that intellectual ability factors decline principally in persons with low
education and that a high initial IQ level provides a protective effect over age 75.
Persons with higher levels of education show relative stability over time on language
and secondary memory tasks but deteriorate as rapidly as persons with low education
on visuospatial tasks.

One also must consider that psychological and environmental factors play an
important role in memory processes. For example, depressive moods affect the
content of personal memories as well as the way of thinking. Negative moods can
block the storage of new information, and stressful conditions significantly decrease
(declarative) memory performance, as well.[11] Because of motivational aspects, there
are no topics that interest the person and therefore the individual does not pay enough
attention for the information to be stored. When depression in an elderly person is
very severe, as with a young person, biological factors also play a role (for example,
alteration of rapid eye movement, or REM sleep) in the capacity of information
storage and recovery. Memory disorders may seriously affect activities of daily living
and can be incapacitating.

There exist, however, what can be called "normal" memory problems that one
not pathological in old age but rather associated with normal aging; pathological
memory disorders directly derived from some neurological illness; and functional
memory problems related to depression and situational aspects. It can be said that
people feel old more because of the illnesses they suffer at those ages than because
of other factors.

Research on age-related memory changes has been conducted to find out the
concerns older adults have about their subjective decline in the ability to remember.[12–15] But memory is not a unitary construction; it is more multimodal and mul-
tisystemic (Table 17.1). In addition, different lesions and malfunctions in the central
nervous system can lead to different types of memory deficits. *Memory problem* is

TABLE 18.1
Different Concepts of Memory Type and Divisions

Memory Type	Divisions	
Short-term	Working Memory	
	Multiple Working Memory	
Long-term	Declarative (explicit)	Episodic
		Semantic
	Procedural (implicit)	Skills
		"Priming"
		Simple classic conditioning, etc.

a general term that should be avoided; rather, the type of memory deficit presented by the person, as well as its known or presumed origin, should be specified.

Studies on *sensorial memory* have found that as age increases perceptive difficulties appear that cause elderly people to need more time to identify complex visual stimuli, indicating that with age a certain deterioration of visual sensorial memory is produced. However, this impairment may be due to typical loss of visual discrimination in elderly people. Lehrner et al.[16] conducted a study to investigate olfactory threshold, odor identification, and their relationship to odor memory across the human life span, concluding that in the elderly population olfactory functions gradually decline. The most significant decline is in odor memory and odor identification, which indicates mayor alterations of olfactory processing in advanced age. These findings correlate with the work of Geisler et al.[17] These authors used cognitive olfactory event–related potentials and found a decline in speed of cognitive processing with age. Other authors have found that the decline in sensory memory with age is minimal.[18]

Working memory is understood as the volume of information people have available on their mental screen to process the information that simultaneously reaches the senses. If the volume available is low, all the other cognitive processes can be slowed or altered. The storage of processed information is carried out simultaneously with ongoing acquisition of even newer data. It is a process where temporal storage, recovery, and information manipulation occur at the same time. Following Fuster,[19] working memory and long-term memory share in part the same neural substrate in the cerebral cortex, which consists of a system of widespread, partly overlapping, interconnected, and hierarchically organized networks of cortical neurons. This system works because any neuron or group of neurons can be part of many networks; thus, working memory is the temporary activation of one such network of long-term memory for any purpose.

Poor performance in different cognitive tasks has been associated with a reduction in working memory in aging people.[15] For some authors, visual memory shows few if any losses with age. In primary memory, most studies have found nonsignificant age-related differences in digit span forward and in word span, and have found moderate differences in letter span. Older subjects show as much of a recency effect as younger ones. Others have found that the latency of response within working memory is increased.[20] Small et al.[21] developed a study to evaluate annually a sample of 212 healthy people of different ages with a neuropsychological battery testing memory and other cognitive domains. They found that the old age group displayed a relative decline in memory performance with time; in contrast, no decline was observed in tests of language, visuospatial ability, and abstract reasoning. Furthermore, age-related decline was restricted to a specific aspect of memory, such as acquisition and early retrieval of new information, and not in a measure of memory retention.

According to Albert,[20] contrary to what occurs with primary memory, there are substantial changes in secondary memory. According to Albert, the degree of loss is related to the type of material to be remembered and the method of assessment. Free recall seems to be very sensitive at relatively early ages and decrements are greater in recall than in recognition tasks.

Different studies have been conducted on age-related impairment in *prospective memory*. Prospective memory abilities seem to decline with age, and these memory problems are exacerbated by an increase of memory load of both the actual tasks and the context in which the tasks are to be performed. Prospective memory takes place within the context of ongoing activities, and the level of engagement required by an activity is important in determining whether an event will be remembered. There exists an overall deterioration of prospective memory performance with age. These age-related differences in prospective memory were observed even when differences in the selected background variables were taken into consideration.

Different authors have proposed that age-related impairment in memory is associated with executive functioning and the frontal lobe. Rapp et al.[22] suggested that memory decline in human aging partly reflects a compromise of executive memory processes supported by frontal lobe regions of the brain, combined with a deterioration of explicit memory capacities supported by the hippocampal system. Nolde et al.[23] suggested that the left prefrontal cortex is activated during remembering, depending on the reflective demands of the task. As more complex, reflective processes are required, left prefrontal cortex activity is more likely to occur. Other studies using functional neuroimaging techniques have indicated that the right prefrontal cortex is activated while people remember events. The work of Desgranges et al.[24] reviewing the structures implicated in the encoding and retrieval of episodic information shows the involvement of the prefrontal cortex. They also observed a hemispheric encoding/retrieval asymmetry: the left side is preferentially involved in encoding and the right in retrieval. McDaniels et al.,[25] using measures of prospective memory in older adults, compared the scores of frontal and temporal lobe functions and found than high-functioning frontal subjects showed better prospective remembering that low-functioning frontal subjects. There were no significant differences in prospective memory performance attributable to medial temporal functioning. The results clearly suggest that the frontal lobe play a key role in prospective memory. Reduction in information processing speed is a fundamental contributor to normal age-related memory loss. Nonetheless, there are circumstances where other mechanisms, such as working memory, executive function, and sensory processes, are important.

Regarding *implicit memory*, researchers seem to agree that it is more resistant to decline with normal aging. Thomas-Antérion et al.[26] found that implicit learning abilities appear before explicit memory and within the adult life span there appears to be little significant deterioration in implicit memory abilities. In the same way, Jelicic[27] found that older subjects perform normally on perceptual implicit tasks, but show somewhat reduced priming in conceptual implicit tasks. For Russo and Parkin[28] all differences in implicit memory were more apparent than real; and for Maki et al.[29] age has a small but reliable influence on implicit memory. *Knowing how, memory without awareness, procedural knowledge*, and *habits* are synonyms of implicit memory. Implicit memories are those in which conscious recollection does not occur, for example, riding a bicycle. Old age is characterized by increases in both retrieval and acquisition (encoding) difficulties. Regarding acquisition, the related deficit appears to be limited to the formation of new associations, perhaps because such formation is capacity demanding.

Memory for continuous performances of various tasks (e.g., solving anagrams), or *activity memory,* in elderly people has also been studied. The age deficit in recall of activities is clearly greater for some activities than for others. There is evidence to indicate that activities demanding a high degree of mental effort to be performed are especially recallable for elderly subjects. However, the age deficit in recall appears to be as pronounced for tasks requiring primarily motor activity as for tasks requiring primarily cognitive activity. Russo and Parkin[28] found that age reduced skill learning.

Some authors have taken care to relate physical activity, age, and cognitive/motor performance to find ways to prevent, postpone, or compensate for the possible decline in cognitive performance with age. Stones and Kozma[30] focused their work on regular physical activity as one such intervention, that is, on the impact of physical activity on the functional capability of aging humans. According to them, physical activity is associated with both tonic and overpractice effects. The tonic effect of chronic aerobic exercise is generalized across interrelated physical and psychological domains of function. Overpractice effects result in resistance to age-related deterioration in the performance of highly overpracticed tasks.

A number of degenerative illnesses exist, especially the demential processes they follow, and generally begin with memory deficits, showing different types of amnesia that often worsen as time goes by. Gabrieli[31] analyzed the effects on memory of normal aging and two age-related neurodegenerative diseases, Alzheimer's disease (AD) and Parkinson's disease. These analyses found an occipital memory system that may mediate implicit visuoperceptual memory and appears to be unaffected by aging or AD. A frontal system that may mediate conceptual memory is affected by AD but not by normal aging. Another frontal system that mediates aspects of working and strategic memory is affected by Parkinson's disease and, to a lesser extent, by aging. The aging effect appears to occur during all ages of the adult life span. Finally, a medial-temporal system that mediates declarative memory is affected by the late onset of AD. Studies of intact and impaired memory in age-related diseases suggest that normal aging has markedly different effects upon different memory systems.

18.4 PRINCIPLES AND GOALS OF AGE-RELATED MEMORY NEUROREHABILITATION

The rehabilitation process for memory deficits in elderly people is complex and should be structured and designed in relation primarily to five factors: (1) the characteristics of the memory deficits to be treated; (2) the characteristics of the neuropathological processes that serve as a basis for the memory disorder; (3) the objectives being pursued; (4) the idiosyncratic characteristics of the patient; and (4) the means available.

The *characteristics of the memory deficits* the patient presents should be considered. In the first place, the patient may have specific memory deficits or deficits derived from or associated with other cognitive deterioration or disorder. Specific memory deficits refer to, for example, difficulties in evocation of past events, as occurs in retrograde amnesia. Desired deficits refer to a problem of evocation due to an organization problem of mnesic material derived from a lesion or deterioration in the prefrontal area that makes subjects unable to organize their memories and therefore unable to evoke them correctly. The first will need specific rehabilitation programs and pharmacological treatment for memory (see León-Carrión[32]), whereas the second will have to begin with programs of frontal lobe training (see Mateer[33]).

Second, one must consider the *characteristics of the neuropathological process* from which memory the disorders presented by the patient are derived. It is fundamental to know the nature of the disorder, especially whether it is static or degenerative. Static disorders are those in which memory deficits are established, are not concurrent with other neurocognitive deficits, and may remain at the same level of signs — they do not worsen and have possibilities of treatment with certain levels of effectiveness. When memory disorders are due to degenerative illnesses such as dementing processes already established in a patient, the possibilities of treatment with minimum effectiveness are limited if not impossible.

Third, one must be very clear about what is wanted, *the objective of the treatment* that is to be applied. There are normally three objectives: recover, compensate, or maintain memory. The majority of the patients and their families ask for *recovery* even in degenerative cases. Recovery is understood in the case of patients with retrograde amnesia as the ability of patients again to make use of their memories and voluntarily to evoke past events and knowledge acquired previously; or, as the ability of patients to retain new memories, all at the same levels of efficiency as before the appearance of the memory disorder. The recovery of the mnesic functions is one of the most difficult objectives to achieve; however, it is possible with some patients. Injured neurons can recover via a number of mechanisms, for example, resolution of edema, restitution of flow, recovery from diaschisis, unmasking of phylogenetically older pathways, and new dendritic sprouting and synaptogenesis. It must be noted that much neuroplasticity in the adult human brain may be due to structural and neurophysiological cortical reorganization and subcortical connections.[34]

Compensation is the most common strategy for memory disorders, but not the best. It is a type of cognitive prothesis, in that it helps the patient to remember using exterior help: for example, the use of a day planner for patients to remember what they must do during the day or the use of a programmed watch to remind patients to do something at a certain moment. Almost all compensation methods are oriented toward the deficits of prospective memory, for which the patients remember a time they must do a certain activity (see Sgaramella et al.[35]). Compensation as a method to treat memory disorders should only be used when the deficit presented by the patient has been demonstrated as resistant to any other method of treatment. This recommendation is based on the fact that when a patient uses compensation other methods that can be used naturally by the patient or in therapy are impeded.

Memory maintenance is another strategy. This is only used when patients have severe cognitive deterioration and, since it is improbable the patients will experience any cognitive improvement, the objective is that, at least, they not worsen. One tries to maintain patients at their present memory levels.

The fourth factor to consider when designing a memory rehabilitation program for patients with age-related memory disorders is the *idiosyncratic characteristics of the patient*. It is very important to know patient's previous personality characteristics, their prior intellectual level, their lifestyle, the role memory played in their life, what they used memory for aside from survival aspects, etc. Here one should apply a fundamental principle of rehabilitation: nothing is built in a void.[32] Rehabilitation of memory processes should be done by building on what remains of the cognitive system. It is not the same to reconstruct as to create new. During the rehabilitation process, patients may have two options. First, they may have reconstructed memories from what had remained or, second, they may have created new memories about previous personal events. This occurs when patients who do not recognize their prior personal memories are obliged or induced to believe in them. These new memories are not based on the rest of their memories, and this does not imply their truly remembering. For example, patients can accept the fact that they are married because they see a photograph and a video of their wedding, but although they accept it they cannot remember it. What then occurs is that the patient creates a new induced memory that, in a way, is false.

Obviously treatment of organic memory problems will be carried out with greater or lesser effectiveness in accordance with the *rehabilitation methods applied*. Maximum effectiveness will be found when there is a coordinated interdisciplinary team with all members fulfilling their role in the structure designed to carry out the treatment. Three options are the most common when facing cognitive decline, especially memory in adult age. The first is prevention, which centers its methodology on the lifestyles and on dietary or pharmacological supplements that delay or avoid the appearance of mnesic deficits. The second option, once the memory deficits have appeared, applies techniques of neuropsychological rehabilitation, either alone or accompanied with administration of a chemical substance able to act on the cerebral areas used for memory. The third option is pharmacological. The following sections describe each of these options.

18.5 ADVANCES IN THE PREVENTION OF AGE-RELATED MEMORY PROBLEMS

Stroke is one of the most common age-related disorders producing important motor, behavioral, and cognitive impairments.[36-39] An interesting study was conducted to understand cognitive decline after stroke.[40] Data clearly showed that strokes have a massive effect on many cognitive processes. More than 70% of patients were notably slow with information processing, whereas at least 40% of all patients had difficulty with memory, visuospatial and constructive tasks, language skills, and arithmetic. Other studies have shown that the presence of vascular risk factors (such as diabetes mellitus and hypercholesterolemia) in a stroke-free group of elderly persons may lead to cognitive decline.[37]

Older patients not only are at risk of dementia processes of vascular or nonvascular origin, but also are exposed to a serious increase in their vulnerability to cognitive deterioration due to the side effects of medication, overmedication, other systemic diseases, etc. According to Gray et al.[39] nearly any drug can cause cognitive impairment in a susceptible individual; however, certain classes are more commonly implicated (see Chapter 14 on neuropharmacology). Benzodiazepines, opioids, anticholinergics, and tricyclic antidepressants are probably the worst offenders. Older hypertensive agents (reserpine, clonidine) have negative effects on cognition; however, large clinical trials in elderly subjects indicate that commonly used agents, e.g., thiazide diuretics, calcium antagonists, ACE inhibitors (captopril, enalapril), and β-blockers (atenolol), have minimal effects on cognition. Newer antidepressants such as selective serotonin reuptake inhibitors (SSRIs) and reversible inhibitors of monoamine oxidase (MAO) seem to have lesser negative effects on cognition. Although some drugs have shown low risk for causing cognition disorders in research studies, risk may be increased in frail older adults taking several medications, and each case should be reviewed carefully. These authors conclude that identification of drug-induced cognitive impairment is crucial to early detection and resolution of symptoms. Preventive strategies directed at avoiding high-risk medications when possible, appropriately adjusting doses based on age-related changes, and close follow-up may prevent these conditions.

The older the patient and the higher the blood pressure, the greater the hypotensive effect of salt restriction. For example, the average difference in systolic blood pressure associated with a 100 mmol/24 h difference in sodium intake was 5 mmHg for the 20- to 29-year-old age group but 10 mmHg for the 60- to 69-year-old age group. This calculated hypotensive effect, especially in elderly and hypertensive people, is comparable with that of antihypertensive medication.

Therefore, prevention of cognitive decline related to aging must be one of the first goals, especially in at-risk patients. Prevention of age-related memory disorders should begin by avoiding stroke risk factors. Lifestyle regulation is very important, especially when referring to physical activity, diet, and control of biological systems, especially uncontrolled hypertension, cardiac dysfunction, and smoking.

Moderate and controlled *physical activity* is a factor that contributes to reducing the risk of stroke or heart attack and can contribute to lowering blood pressure and improving glucose tolerance, among other beneficial aspects. *Diet* influences the risk of stroke by affecting blood pressure and arteriosclerosis development. While a diet rich in potassium seems to protect health, salt and animal fats are detrimental.

Also, obesity itself is an independent risk factor, generally associated with cerebral atherothrombotic infarct. *Hypertension* (>160/95) is one of the main risk factors for stroke, and risk factors increase directly with the increase of arterial pressure, which undoubtedly, should be controlled. People with *cardiac disorders* are at high risk of suffering a stroke since several types of heart disease can clearly produce an ischemic stroke of embolic cardiac origin. The risk in *smokers* is twice that of nonsmokers.

Avoiding stress is also recommended in elderly people. McEwen and Sapolski[40] found that stress affects cognition in a number of ways, acting rapidly via catecholamines and more slowly via glucocorticoids. Catecholamine actions involve β-adrenergic receptors and the availability of glucose, whereas glococorticoids biphasically modulate synaptic plasticity over hours and also produce longer-term changes in dendritic structure that last for weeks. Prolonged exposure to stress leads to loss of neurons, particularly in the hippocampus. Recent evidence suggests that the glucocorticoid and stress-related cognitive impairments involving declarative memory are probably related to the changes they effect in the hippocampus, whereas the stress-related effects on emotional memories are postulated to involve such structures as the amygdala.

The treatment of neuropsychological memory disorder is very complex to describe in just a few pages. The organic ethiology of such disorders is diverse, as are the various memory systems that can be affected. Also, different treatment systems have been practiced with differing responses. There are those who believe treatment of organic memory disorders is an impossible objective and those who think improvement is possible and is only a question of methodology and design. What cannot be disputed is that treatment should be specifically designed for each patient. All data seem to indicate that all patients should undergo exploration and neuropsychological assessment before beginning a treatment program for memory problems, and the design for this program should be based on these results. Only expert neuropsychologists who know a lot about both neuropsychology of memory and rehabilitation should design this type of proper personalized treatment.

Neuropsychological rehabilitation should begin with a complete neuropsychological assessment (Table 18.2) that shows not only memory problems, but also the patient's neurocognitive profile. A systematic study of neuropsychological treatment of organic memory problems can be found in León-Carrión.[32]

It also seems important as a preventive activity that elderly people not abandon intellectual activity. Being intellectually active reading, participating with friends or groups in activities of cultural or political discussions, taking an interest in things occurring around one and in other parts of the world, having projects and dreams are all factors that, in the authors' experience, can contribute greatly to help prevent cerebrovascular disorders. This is especially true when combined with control of the risk factors described above, and it also contributes to improving the deficits and sequelae in cases where there has already been a stroke. As with avoiding excess stress, it is also recommended to avoid depression and social isolation.

TABLE 18.2
Neuropsychological Assessment Tests and Batteries for Older Adults

Cognitive Areas	Tests	
Intellectual functioning	Wechsler Adult Intelligence Scale (WAIS) Raven's Progressive Matrices	Verbal and performance IQ General intelligence
Attentional mechanism	BNS Letter Cancellation Tests (BNS Attention Subtests)	Tonic alertness (simple attention) Phasic alertness (vigilance)
Memory process	Luria Memory Curve Functional Organic Questionnaire (FOM) Wechsler Memory Scales (WMS)	Memory and learning processes Functional organic memory problems Memory
Language	COWAT/FAS Boston Naming Test	Verbal fluency measure Expressive speech, accuracy, and vocabulary level
Executive functioning	The Stroop Test The Tower of Hanoi-Seville The Trail Making Test Serial Seven Digit Backward	Neurocognitive interference (activation/inhibition responses) Problem solving; planning, monitoring, prospective, and control Attention mediated by frontal lobe, mental flexibility, shifting of an ongoing activity Mental tracking, complex mental operations
Visuoperceptive and visuoconstructive	BNS Tachistoscopic Task	Inattention, negligence, hemi-inattention, anopsia, quadrantaopsia in visual field
Sensory and motor skills	Tactual Performance Test (TPT) Seashore Rhythm Test Speech Sound Perception Test The Finger Tapping Test The Senso-Perceptive Examination Grooved Pegboard The Lateral Dominance Examination Luria Motor Function Examination	Motor accuracy, coordination, nonverbal auditory perception Motor skills, psychomotor coordination Finger agnosia, dominant/nondominant hand Manual dexterity Motor abilities
Personality, affective, and emotional problems	Neurologically Related Changes in Personality Inventory (NECHAPI)	Emotional changes
Dementing processes	Aphasia test Agnosia test Apraxia test Barthel Index IQCODE Blessed Deteriorating Scale CAMDEX ADAS Beck Depression Scale Hamilton Depression Scale Yesavage Scale	Language problems Recognition Sequences of movements Functional dysfunctions Depression

It is also advisable to use compound substances, normally through dietary supplements, that help prevent stroke and cognitive decline related to age. Recently, a substance, vinpocetine (Intelectol), has been proposed as a powerful memory enhancer to use as a dietary supplement because it increases the concentration of some neurotransmitters involved in memory functioning.

Vinpocetine is a synthetic derivative of vincamine, the natural alkaloid of *Vinca minor*;[41] it is a vasoactive and neuroprotective agent that has been used for nearly 20 years as a substance with cerebral blood flow–enhancing, antihypoxic, and anti-ischemic properties, that also increases cerebral metabolism. The neuroprotective action of vinpocetine is related to the inhibition of the operation of voltage-dependent neuronal NA^+ channels, indirect inhibition of some molecular cascades initiated by the rise of intracellular CA^{2+} levels and, to a lesser extent, inhibition of adenosine reuptake. Vinpocetine has been shown to be a selective inhibitor of Ca^{2+} calmodulin-dependent cGMDP-PDE. It seems that this inhibition enhances intracellular GPM levels in the vascular smooth muscle leading to a reduced resistance of cerebral vessels and an increase of cerebral flow. This effect might also beneficially contribute to the neuroprotective action.

Various authors have shown the effects of vinpocetine on memory. Nootropic effects of vinpocetine and its effects on memory were studied by DeNoble et al.[42] They evaluated the abilities of vinpocetine, vincamine, aniracetan, and hydergine to prevent scopolamine-induced and hypoxia-induced impairment of passive avoidance retention (24 h) in rats. Results showed that vinpocetine, aniracetam, vincamine, and hydergine prevented memory disruption by scopolamine. Data support the view that vinpocetine has cognitive-activating ability as defined in models of both sco-polamine-induced and hypoxia-induced memory impairment in rats. In another study, DeNoble[43] found that vinpocetine has cognition-activating abilities as defined by an animal model of memory retrieval. Human studies are still needed to replicate results obtained with animals.

The use of dietary and/or pharmacological complements to prevent cognitive decline in elderly people is much more effective when accompanied by the healthy lifestyles pointed out at the beginning of this section and when risk factors that can increase the possibilities of suffering a stroke or any other neurological illness are avoided.

18.6 BEHAVIORAL TRAINING FOR AGE-RELATED MEMORY DISORDERS

Cognitive techniques have achieved the best results in neuropsychological training in age-related memory disorders. In one group, *associated pairs* are used. These pairs can either be read or listened to and, through repetition, storage and correct retrieval of the information is exercised. This technique can become progressively more complicated, thereby requiring the patient to define the content more sharply, thus refining these memory mechanisms. An example of this kind of task is the use of lists of words of different lengths, which must be remembered in both direct and reverse order. Similarly, pictures, geometric forms, musical tones, even odors, can be used. This can be done using the individual groups or by relating the different groups (e.g., picture–musical tone; odor–geometric form).

Another method to minimize the effects of aging on memory performance is the use of strategies that assist the older adult in encoding (organizing information) and then retrieving this information on demand. This technique, known as *mnemonics* or the use of memory aids, attempts to provide meaning to the information, to organize it, and to form meaningful associational networks.[18] The technique uses what is called the chain system,[45] which consists of making a meaningful sequential association between the first and second items, then between this and item three, continuing in like manner to the last item. A variation of this technique uses the imagery mnemonic method, in which the information to be recalled is first visualized. The main drawback of the chain system, because of the sequential nature of the chain, is that when one word is forgotten, retrieval of the rest of the list is impossible.

The *Loci system,* attributed to Cicero in 500 B.C., is another method used in age-related memory disorders. This technique requires the subject to visualize the location or logical order in which items are placed. To retrieve these items, the subject has only to take a *mental walk* through the location. This method seems to present fewer complications than the chain system.

The peg-word or book system is a similar method and is used for the retrieval of discrete information. The first item is associated with the number 1, the second with number 2, and so on. Subjects can then recall any item by its associated number. Much more complex techniques have also been developed, using such things as syllables, nursery rhymes, or phonetic systems, but the underlying mnemonic principle is the same.

These methods can be used for long-term memory training by introducing a longer period of time between training and retrieval. However, a different kind of content, which requires subjects to elaborate at a higher level, is generally used for long-term memory. Content matter such as short texts from books or advertisements from newspapers, television programs, or short television news announcements, radio announcements, and so forth are being successfully used with this method. The same mechanism as previously described is used, i.e., breakdown into smaller chunks of information and storage of these "smaller chunks" through continued repetition. In addition, in the context of a rehabilitation program, patients are encouraged to recount the details of the content of the exercises done during the day, or previous days, as painstakingly as possible. The use of cues in this type of task will aid the subject in retrieval of the information.

Another group of techniques is based on a theoretical hierarchical model that presents the conceptualization of memory in dichotomies. In other words, the model presents procedural vs. declarative and semantic vs. episodic memory.

In the first of these techniques, procedural memory refers to the ability to learn rule-based or automatic behavioral sequences, such as motor skills, conditioned responses, or the ability to carry out sequences for operating things. The following is an example of the use of this model with patients who are incapable of remembering if they have performed an activity, or where it was performed. The patient is trained, through repetition, to perform a given motor activity, such as turning a crank in a certain way to start a fan. After several sessions, patients able to initiate the activity correctly on their own, and even improve performance in doing so, all the while denying that they have ever performed the activity before. This helps to increase the quality and quantity of the information that is remembered..

In the semantic vs. episodic memory model, the first concept, semantic memory, refers to knowledge of word meaning, ideas, information that is independent of the context in which it has been learned — information that we know, but that we do not know when or where we learned. The best way to train semantic memory is by repetition — names of therapists, new friends, meals, and so forth.

Problems with episodic memory, information about the place in time and space events were experienced, information linked with context, can be addressed by using preserved semantic or procedural memory. This helps elderly adults compensate for the lack of episodic memory.

Techniques taking advantage of the priming effect may also be used. These techniques[46] use the method of *vanishing cues*. Using a fragment from a textbook or something similar, the authors create a systematic reduction of letter fragments to be relearned words across trials. This relearning depends on first-letter cues and patients acquire vocabulary to produce target words in the absence of fragment cues.

Another group of techniques compensates for memory deficits by using external aids. The most often used aids are memory books (in which items to be remembered are written down) and beeping watches or electronic daily planners, which give an acoustic signal when it is time to carry out an activity (take medication, make a phone call, etc.).

18.7 NEUROPHARMACHOLOGICAL ADVANCES IN THE TREATMENT OF THE AGE-RELATED MEMORY DEFICITS

People over 65 years old in United States take at least one medication, normally three, and medication use increases with age, women consuming more than men. Average medication use in this age group is 5 to 12 drugs per day, and less than 5% of the elderly population uses no medication. This widespread use of medication is not only due to the higher prevalence of chronic illnesses in this population, but also to inappropriate prescriptions and misuse of prescribed and over-the-counter drugs. Medication presents special problems in elderly people because of their altered drug disposition and responses as a consequence of important physiological changes that occur with normal aging, which are independent of the multiple illnesses that are so often present in elderly patients.[47]

The most common therapeutic agents used in elderly people are antihypertensives, non-narcotic analgesics, antirheumatics, and vitamins. Medication use increases with age. Other studies indicate that the average number of drugs prescribed for elderly people is around three. Studies in the United Kingdom and Scandinavia indicate that the average number of drugs per elderly inpatient ranges from 2.5 to 6.3, with the oldest patients receiving 5 medications. The most widely prescribed drugs are cardiovascular (54.7%), central nervous system agents (11.4%), and analgesics (9.4%). The most often used over-the-counter medications were analgesics (39.6%), vitamins and nutritional supplements (32.9%), and gastrointestinal agents including laxatives (21.6%). Psychoactive drugs are used by one third of people over 65 with little medical supervision or understanding by staff members of their possible side effects.[48] Drug reactions seem to be directly responsible for about 10% of the hospital admissions of older people.

In the 1970s certain laboratory groups and researchers began to offer data on the theory of a deficit of acetylcholine activity in patients showing severe memory problems, especially in patients with AD. The research activity on therapy of organic memory disorders focused on the administration of choline, which is capable of haltering the processes of mnesic deterioration and, at times, restoring function..

The following describes the discoveries obtained with a drug that, in the authors' clinical and research experience, offers the best results for improvements in mnesic deficits presented by patients with severe organic memory disorders. The use of this drug, CDP-choline, is an important step in the treatment of these disorders.

Cytidinediphosphocholine (CDPc) is a mononucleotoid made up of ribose, citosine, pyrofosphate, and choline and the chemical structure corresponds to 2-oxi-4-aminopirimidine. CDPc acts as an essential intermediary in the synthesis of phospholipids of the neuron membrane.[49–53] Different studies have shown that CDPc inhibits phospholipase A2, impeding the destruction of phospholipids in the membrane.[54–56] The increase of dopamine synthesis in the striatum was observed by Agut et al.[57] and an increase of the adrenergic activity by Lopez et al.[58] CDPc is a hydrophile and adminitrade taken orally and is easily absorbed with a high bioavailability. It has been shown that when orally administered it promotes several favorable physiological actions with CDPc endogen. Its administration increases metabolic renovation of inositol phospholipids as a result of an increase of acetylcholine availability that acts on muscarinic receptors. It is well tolerated and has few side effects (less than 2% of patients).[59]

CDPc has proved to be effective in the treatment of cerebrovascular disorders. According to Weiss,[61] when administered through oxygen, it prevents, reduces, or reverses the effects of ischemia or hypoxia in a large percentage of the animal or cellular models studied. In the brain injury models studied, CDPc reduced and limited the lesions of the neuronal membrane, reestablished sensibility and function of regulatory intracellular enzymes, and limited edema. So, the therapeutic uses of CDPc have been indicated for cerebrovascular illnesses, brain injury, Parkinson's disease, cardiovascular diseases, aging, AD, learning, and cholinergic stimulation memory disorders.

One of the hypotheses on cognitive decline in elderly people is the lack of availability of the necessary quantities of choline for the brain to carry out certain cognitive functions easily. A study done by Cohen et al.[62] showed that cerebral captation of choline decreases with age. After choline administration, the proportion of cerebral choline-creatine increased noticeably (60%) in young people, while in elderly people the average increase was only 16% and, therefore, significantly inferior to the increase observed in the young people. According to these authors this fact may contribute to easing the appearance of degenerative diseases, especially dementia, at an advanced age as a consequence of the existing limitation of choline availability for the cholinergic neurons. Babb et al.[63] reached similar results. Their results seemed to confirm the decrease of cerebral choline reuptake as age increases. If plasmatic concentrations increased in all cases after CDPc administration, relative concentrations of cerebral choline after treatment application corresponded to a decrease of 5.8% in the oldest group and an increase of 18% in the younger people. The observations also suggest that in elderly people the administration of CDPc can increase the synthesis of phosphotydilcholine in the cellular membrane of the brain through the incorporation of choline.

Morra and Marchi[64] have also studied the effects of CDPc on cerebral senile deterioration. They studied 197 outpatient and hospitalized patients between age 65 and over 80 with senile mental deterioration at low ($n = 85$) and moderate ($n = 112$) levels. They were administered two cycles of treatment lasting 21 days each, with 1 week of pharmacological wash between. The treatment consisted of 1000 mg of CDPc a day with intramuscular administration. The results showed that treatment for 21 days produced a statistically significant improvement of mental, physical, and social symptomatology that increased during the second treatment cycle. During the period of pharmacological wash between the two cycles persistence of the therapeutic effect from the first cycle was observed. The treatment produced statistically significant improvements in cognitive and behavioral parameters of independence/autonomy, life relation/social life, behavior, and interest/attention. According to these authors, the results obtained show that CDPc treatment is therapeutically effective for clinical, functional, and social recovery in patients with cerebral senescence as a consequence of its effects on cognitive and behavioral capacity of these patients.

The study of choline transportation and biotransformation in the human brain can be important in several neuropsychiatric disorders. In the study done by Nitsch et al.[65] a decrease of 40 to 50% appeared in cerebral concentrations of choline in the frontal and parietal cortex of patients with AD as compared with control patients.

In an experimental study done with rats to determine histological cerebral changes and the behavioral clinical effect of treatment with CDPc in an ischemic cerebral focal model, the results indicated that a threshold of biological cerebral membrane lesions may exist, under which CDPc is able to reestablish the content and disposal of phospholipids and to preserve the integrity of the membrane with the achieved therapeutic effect.[66] According to Schäbitz et al.,[67] prolonged treatment with CDPc at high doses reduced the volume of cerebral infarct in an ischemic temporal focal model, in which they observed a tendency for cerebral edema and mortality to be reduced. According to these authors these effects may be related to the stabilization of the membrane and inhibition of liberating free fatty acids.

In another study by Önal et al.[68] effects of synergetic neuroprotectors of CDPc and an NMDA antagonist in the transitory focal experimental ischemia were found. This synergy is reached with lower than optimal doses of one or both products, although it is necessary to determine the complete effectiveness of a treatment with complete doses. According to the authors, their results suggest that CDPc can allow a reduction of the NMDA antagonist doses, and therefore the side effects, maintaining the neuroprotection.

A multicenter clinical report by Clark et al.[69] indicated that treatment with CDPc taken orally can be used safely with minimum side effect in acute ictus. CDPc seems to improve the functional results and reduce the neurological deficit. A dose of 500 mg seems ideal for this end.

The results obtained by Bruhwyler et al.[70] in a study of 127 patients hospitalized for acute brain infarct appearing at most 48 h before the study, showed that consciousness level, orientation, speech and motor functions improved significantly with time. Of the patients, 79% improved their score in the scale measuring these functions. According to Bruhwyler et al., the results showed that CDPc is an effective and well-tolerated treatment in patients presenting with acute cerebral infarct. Equally, the results obtained by Warach et al.[71] suggest a reduction in the volume of ischemic cerebral infarct lesions with the administration of CDPc. A significant reduction in the size of cerebral infarcts in a cerebral ischemia model in animals was also found by Andersen et al. [72] For Clark et al.,[73] CDPc is a safe drug that can produce favorable effects in a subgroup of patients presenting with moderate or large-sized ictus.

CDPc has been widely used in the treatment of memory disorders. In a study done by León-Carrión et al.[60] with patients with traumatic brain injury with hypoperfused left temporobasal brain areas, CDPc was found to induce a normalization of the blood flow in the temporobasal hypoperfused zones. These authors suggest that CDPc is a procognitive drug that acts only in the cerebral areas related to memory. As the authors' experience shows, to be effective, neuropsychological treatment of organic memory problems should simultaneously include memory training and a drug (CDPc) that is able to restore and maintain blood flow in the damaged sites associated with memory, usually the left inferoposterior temporal area. CDPc and memory training are the best combination to improve organic-related memory disorders, together enhancing the power of the treatment. Treatment with only the drug or with only the training has very modest results.

Dixon et al.,[74] in a study with microdialysis in rats with CDPc administration, observed a rapid increase in production of CDPc regarding its basal value after only one intraperitoneal administration of this substance. Also, it remained higher for a period of up to 3 h in the dorsal hippocampusand the neocortex, compared with control animals. These discoveries suggest that this type of treatment could be useful in the chronic postlesion phase of memory deficit treatment for people with cerebral lesions.

The effects of CDPc in a subcortical dementia associated with Parkinson's disease assessed by qualitative electroencephalography have been studied by Garcia-Mas et al.[75] After the administration of CDPc they observed an important increase in the slow rhythms, theta and especially delta, that led to an increase in the total potentials and a tendency to a slight reduction of the alpha/theta index. According to these authors, CDPc seems to reestablish the normal values of the potentials related to cognitive functions, especially in alpha waves.

Eberhard and Dehrr[76] studied 11 patients aged between 57 and 85 with clinical diagnosis of senile cerebral insufficiency compatible with a degenerative type of dementia who were treated with CDPc (200 mg three times a day) and placebo for 5 weeks. The results showed marked differences in favor of CDPc in the cognitive tests and geriatric scales. Antón-Alvarez et al.[77] reached similar conclusions, finding that CDPc improved memory performance in elderly subjects, mainly in free recall tasks, at doses ranging from 300 to 1000 mg/day.

The results obtained by Spiers et al.[78] showed that CDPc therapy improved verbal memory functioning in older individuals with relatively inefficient memories. According to these authors, CDPc may prove effective in treating age-related cognitive decline that may be a precursor of dementia.

In a multicenter report by Serra et al.,[79] the clinical data obtained demonstrated that treatment with CDPc is able to determine an improvement of symptomology from the first cycle of therapy and a further improvement in the second cycle. The treatment with CDPc 1000 mg/day for two 21-day cycles in patients suffering from brain aging determined a significant improvement of independence/autonomy, social life, attention, interest, and individual behavior.

Fioravanti and Yanagi[80] reached the conclusion in a Cochrane review that there is some evidence that CDPc has a positive effect, at least in the short term, on memory and behavior. The evidence of benefit from global impression is stronger, but is still limited by the duration of the studies. There is evidence that the effect of treatment is more homogeneous for patients with cognitive impairment secondary to cerebrovascular disorders. In the authors' experience, CDPc is the best option to treat organic memory disorders, and the best results are obtained when CDPc is used simultaneously with neuropsychological memory training.

18.8 CONCLUDING REMARKS

Normal aging is characterized by a series of slow and continual changes in different cognitive areas that affect the global functioning of the individual. These changes are especially patent and well documented in the domain of memory and, due to the subjective complaints of individuals, are a frequent source of constant worry, both to the individual and to those around him or her. Research has found that not all types of memory decline, nor are the same alterations found to the same degree in all elderly people. In fact, many memories remain intact. This makes it all the more necessary to study the characteristics and treatment methods of memory deficits, with the aim of forestalling their devastating consequences and reducing their impact on elderly people.

It is hoped this chapter will extend a message of optimism with regard to this problem. There are memory problems that inexorably accompany the aging process. Fortunately, progress has been made in preventing these problems and with neuropsychological training and advances in neuropharmacological treatment a way has been found to cushion the blow of the effects of memory loss on elderly people.

REFERENCES

1. Flanigan, K. M. et al., Age-related biology and diseases of muscle and nerve, *Neurol. Clin.*, 16, 659, 1998.
2. Odenheimer, G. L., Geriatric neurology, *Neurol. Clin.*, 16, 561, 1998.

3. Terry, R. D., DeTeresa, R., and Hansen, L. A., Neocortical cell counts in normal human adult aging, *Annu. Neurol.*, 21, 530, 1987.

4. Esri, M. H. et al., Aging and the dementias, in *Grensfield's Neuropathology,* Vol. 1, Graham, D. I. and Lantos, P. L., Eds., Oxford University Press, New York, 1997, 153.

5. Anderson, J. M. et al., The effect of advanced age on the neurone content of the cerebral cortex: observations with an automated image analyser point counting method, *J. Neurol. Sci.,* 58, 235, 1983.

6. Hovarth, T. B. and Davis, K. L., Central nervous system disorders in aging, in *Handbook of the Biology of Aging,* Schneider, E. L. and Rowe, J. W., Eds., Academic Press, New York, 1990, 306.

7. Schochet, S. S., Neuropathology of aging, *Neurol. Clin.,* 16, 569, 1998.

8. Hagstadius, S. and Risberg, J., The effects of normal aging during resting and functional activation, *rCBF Bull.,* 6, 1160, 1983.

9. Choi, J., Morris, J. C., and Hsu, C. Y., Aging and cerebrovascular disease, *Neurol. Clin.,* 16, 687, 1998.

10. Ritchie, K. et al., Establishing the limits and characteristics of normal age-related cognitive decline, *Rev. Epidemiol. Sante Publ.,* 45(5), 373, 1997.

11. Lupien, S. J. et al., Stress-induced declarative memory impairment in healthy elderly subjects: relationship to cortisol reactivity, *J. Clin. Endocrinol.,* 82(7), 2070, 1997.

12. Smith, A., Memory, in *Handbook of the Psychology of Aging,* Birren, I. and Schaine, K., Eds., Academic Press, San Diego, CA, 1996.

13. Kauser, D., *Learning and Memory in Normal Aging,* Academic Press, New York, 1994.

14. Salthouse, I., *Theoretical Perspectives on Cognitive Aging,* Lawrence Erlbaum Associates, Hillsdale, NJ, 1991.

15. Light, L., Memory and aging: four hypotheses in search of data, *Annu. Rev. Psychol.,* 42, 333, 1991.

16. Lehrner, J. P., Glück, J., and Laska, M., Odor identification, consistency of label use, olfactory threshold and their relationships to odor memory over the human lifespan, *Chem. Senses,* 24(3), 337, 1999.

17. Geisler, M. W. et al., Neuropsychological performance and cognitive olfactory event-related brain potentials in young and elderly adults, *J. Clin. Exp. Neuropsychol.,* 21(1), 108, 1999.

18. Poon, L., Memory training for older adults, in *Geriatric Mental Health,* Abrahams, J. P. and Crooks, V., Eds., Grune & Stratton, Orlando, FL, 1984.

19. Fuster, J. M., Cellular dynamics of network memory, *Z. Naturforsch.,* 53(7), 670, 1998.

20. Albert, M. S., General issues in geriatric neuropsychology, in *Geriatric Neuropsychology,* Albert, M. S. and Moss, M. B., Eds., Guilford Press, New York, 1988.

21. Small, S., Stern, Y., and Mayeux, R., Selective decline in memory function among healthy elderly, *Neurology,* 52(7), 1392, 1999.

22. Rapp, P. R., William, C., and Heindel, C., Memory system in normal and pathological aging (review article), *Curr. Opin. Neurol.,* 7, 294, 1994.

23. Nolde, S. F., Johnson, M. K., and Raye, C. L., The role of prefrontal cortex during test of episodic memory, *Trends Cogn. Sci.,* 2, 399, 1998.

24. Desgranges, B., Baron, J. C., and Eustache, F., The functional neuroanatomy of episodic memory: the role of the frontal lobes, the hippocampal formation and other areas, *Neuroimage,* 8(2), 198, 1998.

25. McDaniels, M. A. et al., Prospective memory: a neuropsychological study, *Neuropsychology,* 13(1), 103, 1999.

26. Thomas-Antérion, C. et al., Aging and procedural memory. Study of a series of test on microcomputers, *Rev. Med. Intern.,* 15(9), 581, 1994.

27. Jelicic, M., Aging and performance on implicit memory tasks: a brief review, *Int. J. Neurosci.*, 82(3–4), 155, 1995.

28. Russo, R. and Parkin, A. J., Age differences in implicit memory: more apparent than real, *Mamoria Cogn.*, 21(1), 73, 1993.

29. Maki, P. M., Zonderman, A. B., and Weingartner, H., Age differences in implicit memory: fragmented object identification and category exemplar generation, *Psychol. Aging*, 14(2), 284, 1999.

30. Stones, M. J. and Kozma, A., Physical activity, age, and cognitive motor performance, in *Cognitive Development in Adulthood*, Howe, M. L. and Brainerd, J., Eds., Springer-Verlag, New York, 1988, 273.

31. Gabrieli, J. D., Memory systems analyses of nemonic disorders in aging and age-related diseases, *Proc. Natl. Acad. Sci.*, 93(24), 1353, 1996.

32. León-Carrión, J., Ed., *Neuropsychological Rehabilitation. Fundamentals, Innovations and Directions*, St. Lucie Press, Delray Beach, FL, 1997.

33. Mateer, C., Rehabilitation of individuals with frontal lobe impairment, in *Nuove Frontiere in Neurorehabilitazione*, Mazzucchi, A., Ed., Realizacione Editorial, Bologna, 1991.

34. Alexander, D. N., Geriatric neurorehabilitation, *Neurol. Clin.*, 16, 713, 1998.

35. Sgaramella, T., Bisiacchi, P., and Zettin, P., For a componential analysis to a cognitive of everyday planning, in *Neuropsychological Rehabilitation. Fundamentals, Innovations and Directions*, León-Carrión, J., Ed., St. Lucie Press, Delray Beach, FL, 1997.

36. Babikian, V. et al., Cognitive changes in patients with multiple cerebral infarcts, *Stroke*, 21, 1013, 1990.

37. Desmond, D. et al., Risk factor for cerebralvascular disease as correlates of cognitive function in a stroke free cohort, *Arch. Neurol.*, 50(20), 162, 1993.

38. Ogden, J., Mee, E. W., and Henning, M., A prospective study of cognition and memory and recovery after subarachnoid haemorrhage, *Neurosurgery*, 333(4), 572, 1993.

39. Gray, S. L., Lay, K. V., and Larson, E. B., Drug-induced cognition disorders in the elderly: incidence, prevention and management, *Drug Saf.*, 21, 101, 1999.

40. McEwen, B. C. and Sapolski, S. B., Stress and cognitive function (review article), *Curr. Opin. Neurobiol.*, 5, 205, 1995.

41. Lörinc, C., Szász, K., and Kisfaludy, L., The synthesis of apovincaminate, *Arzten-mittelforschung*, 26, 1907, 1977.

42. DeNoble, V. et al., Vimpocetine: nootropic effects on scopolamine-induced and hypoxia-induced retrieval deficit of a step-through passive avoidance response in rats, *Pharmacol. Biochem. Behav.*, 24, 1123, 1986.

43. DeNoble, V., Vinprocetine enhances retrieval of a step-through passive avoidance response in rat, *Pharmacol. Biochem. Behav.*, 26, 183, 1987.

44. Smith, A., Age differences in encoding, storage and retrieval, in *New Directions in Memory and Aging*, Poon, W. C., Fozard, J. L., Cermak, L. et al., Eds., Proceedings of the George Tallad Memorial Conference, Lawrence Erlbaum Associates, Hillsdale, NJ, 1980.

45. Higbec, H., *Your Memory. How It Works and How to Improve It*, Prentice-Hall, Englewood Cliffs, NJ, 1977.

46. Glisky, E., Schachter, D., and Tulving, E., Learning and retention of computer-related vocabulary in memory-impaired patients: method of vanishing cues, *J. Clin. Exp. Neuropsychol.*, 8, 292, 1989.

47. Kompoliti, K. and Goetz, C., Neuropharmacology in the elderly, *Neurol. Clin.*, 16, 599, 1998.

48. Vestal, R. and Cusack, B., Pharmacology of aging, in *Handbook of the Biology of Aging*, Schneider, E. L. and Rowe, J. W., Eds., Academic Press, New York, 1990, 343.

49. De la Morena, E., Goldberg, D.M., and Werner, M., Citidindifosfato de colina y biosíntesis de fosfolípidos, in *Citicolina: Bioquímica, Neurofarmacología y Clínica*, De la Morena, E., Ed., Salvat, Barcelona, 1985, 25.

50. Giuffrida, A. M. et al., Biochemical changes of lipids, nucleic acid and protein metabolism in brain regions during hypoxia: effects of CDP-choline, in *Novel Biochemical. Pharmacological and Clinical Aspects of Cytidinediphosphocoline*, Zappia, V. et al., Eds., Elsevier Science Publishers, New York, 1985, 105.

51. Jane, F., Algunos aspectos de la farmacología de la citicolina, in *Citicolina: Bioquímica, Neurofarmacología y Clínica*, De la Morena, E., Ed., Salvat, Barcelona, 1985.

52. Jiménez-Collado, J., Distribución de los fosfolípidos colinodependientes. Acción de la CDP-colina, in *Citicolina: Bioquímica, Neurofarmacología y Clínica*, De la Morena, E., Ed., Salvat, Barcelona, 1985, 39.

53. Kennedy, E. P., The function of cytidine coenzymes in the biosynthesis of membrane lipids, in *Novel Biochemical Pharmacological and Clinical Aspects of Cytidinediphosphocoline*, Zappia, V. et al., Eds., Elsevier Science Publishers, New York, 1998, 53.

54. Freysz, L. et al., Metabolism of neuronal cell cultures: modifications induced by CDP-choline, in *Novel Biochemical, Pharmacological and Clinical Aspects of Cytidinediphosphocholine*, Elsevier, New York, 1985.

55. Agut, J. and Ortiz, J., Effect of oral cytidine-(5′)-diphosphocholone (CDP-choline) administration on the metabolism of phospholipids in the rat brain during normobaric hypoxia, *Alzheimer's Dis. Adv. Basic Res. Ther.*, 18, 327, 1987.

56. Arrigoni, E., Averet, N., and Cohandon, F., Effects of CDP-choline on phospholipase A2 and cholinephosphotranspherase activities following a cryogenic brain injury in the rat, *Biochem. Pharmacol.*, 36, 3697, 1987.

57. Agut, J., Coviella, I., and Wurtman, R., Cytidine (5′) diphosphocholine enhances the ability of haloperidol to increase dopamine metabolites in the striatum of the rat and to diminish stereotyped behavior induced by apomorphine, *Neuropharmacology*, 23, 1403, 1984.

58. López, I. et al., Effects of cytidine (5′) diphosphocholine (CDP-choline) on the total urinary excretion of 3-metoxy-4-hydroxyphenylglycol (MHPG) by rats and humans, *J. Neural Transm.*, 66, 129, 1986.

59. Dórlando, K. J. and Sandage, B. W., Citicholine (CDP-choline): mechanisms of action and effects in ischemic brain injury, *Neurol. Res.*, 17, 281, 1995.

60. León-Carrión, J. et al., The role of citicholine in neuropsychological training after traumatic brain injury, *Neurorehabilitation*, 14, 33, 2000.

61. Weiss, G. B., Metabolism and actions of CDP-choline as an endogenous compound and administered exogenously as citicoline, *Life Sci.*, 56, 637, 1995.

62. Cohen, B. M., Renshaw, P. F., Stoll, A. L., Wurtman, R. J., Yurgelun-Todd, D., and Babb, S. M., Decreased brain choline uptake in older adults: an *in vivo* proton magnetic resonance spectroscopy study, *JAMA*, 274, 902, 1995.

63. Babb, S. M. and Appelmans, K. E., Differential effect of CDP-choline on brain cystolic choline levels in younger and older subjects as measured by proton magnetic resonance spectroscopy, *Psychopharmacology*, 127, 88, 1996.

64. Morra, G. and Marchi, E., CDP-colina y deterioro mental senil, *Ressegna Geriátr.*, 26, 489, 1990.

65. Nitsch, R. M., Blusztajn, J. K., Pittas, A. G., Slack, B. E., Growdon, J. G. and Wurtman, R. J., Evidence of a membrane deficit in Alzheimer's disease brain, *Proc. Natl. Acad. Science U.S.A.*, 89, 1671, 1992.

66. Aronowski, J., Strong, R., and Grotta, J., Citicholine for treatment of experimental focal ischemia: histolofic and behavioral outcome, *Neurol. Res.*, 18, 570, 1996.

67. Schäbitz, W. et al., The effects of prolonged treatment with citicholine in temporary experimental focal ischemia, *J. Neurol. Sci.*, 138, 21, 1996.

68. Önal, M. Z. et al., Synergistic effects of citicoline and MK-801 in temporary experimental focal ischemia, *Stroke,* 28, 1060, 1997.

69. Clark, W. et al., A randomized dose–response trial of citicholine in acute ischemic stroke patients, Citicholine Stroke Study Group, *Neurology,* 49, 671, 1997.

70. Bruhwyler, J., van Dorpe, J., and Géczy, J., Multicentric open-label study of the efficacy and tolerability of citicholine in the treatment of acute cerebral infarction, *Curr. Ther. Res.,* 58, 309, 1997.

71. Warach, S. et al., Reduction of lesion volume in human stroke by citicholine detected by diffusion-weighted magnetic resonance imaging: a pilot study, *Ann. Neurol.*, 40, 527, 1996.

72. Andersen, M., Overgaard, K., Meden, P., Boysen, G., and Choi, S. C., Effects of citicholine combined with thrombolytic therapy in a rat embolic stroke model, *Stroke,* 30, 1464, 1999.

73. Clark, W. M., Williams, B. J., Selzer, K. A., Zweifler, R. M., Sabounijian, L. A., and Gammans, R. E., A randomized efficacy trial of citicholine in patients with acute ischemic stroke, *Stroke,* 30, 2592, 1999.

74. Dixon, C.E., Ma, X., and Marion, D., Effects of CDP-choline treatment on neurobehavioral deficits after TBI and hippocampal and neocortical acetylcholine release, *J. Neurotrauma,* 14, 161, 1997.

75. García-Mas, A., Rossinol, A., Roca, M., Lozano, R., Rossello, J., and Llinas, J., Effects of citicholine in subcorticl dementia associated with Parkinson's disease assessed by quantified electroencephalography, *Clin. Ther.,* 14, 718, 1992.

76. Eberhard, R. and Dehrr, I., Eficacia y tolerancia de CDP-colina en pacientes geriátricos con insuficiencia cerebral senil. Estudio doble ciego cruzado, *Rev. Esp. Geriatr. Gerontol.,* 24, 73, 1989.

77. Anton-Alvarez, X. et al., Coticoline improves memory performance in elderly subjects, *Met. Find. Exp. Clin. Pharmacol.,* 19, 201, 1997.

78. Spiers, P. et al., Citicoline improves verbal memory in aging, *Arch. Neurol.,* 53, 441, 1996.

79. Serra, F. et al., CDP-choline effects on brain aging. Multicenter experience on 237 patients, *Minerva Med.,* 81, 465, 1990.

80. Fioravanti, M. and Yanagi, M., Cytidinediphosphocholine for cognitive and behavioural disturbances associated with chronic cerebral disorders in the elderly, The Cochrane Library, 1989.

19 Anticonvulsvant Drugs and Cognitive Functions in Elderly Patients with Epilepsy

Francesco Monaco and Cristoforo Comi

CONTENTS

19.1 Introduction 403
19.2 Effects of AEDs 406
References...408

19.1 INTRODUCTION

The special management problems of elderly people with epilepsy are receiving increasing attention, and because populations are aging in the developed countries, the problem of the occurrrence of new cases of epilepsy in the elderly population is quite relevant. In the United States about 13% of the total population is aged 65 years or older, with a constantly growing rate. The incidence of seizures in elderly people is at least as high as in the first decade of life,[1] and detailed reports obtained from a primary care database[2] indicate the following numbers: a prevalence of 1090, 1200, and 1310 per 100,000 adults for those aged 60 through 69, 70 through 75, and 80 years or older, respectively, with an overall rate of 1180 per 100,000 adults in those older than 60 years. The overall prevalence of active epilepsy in one study including 5559 persons aged 55 to 95 years was 0.9%.[3] The prevalence increased with age from 0.7% for those aged 55 to 64 years to 1.2% for those aged 85 to 94 years, with the increase detected both for men and women. More recent studies have shown that seizures in elderly people are cryptogenic in 11 to 50%; secondary to stroke in 22 to 39%; and secondary to tumor in 2 to 22%.[4] Other disorders associated with seizures in this specific age group are Alzheimer's disease, cerebral amyloid angiopathy, toxic-metabolic syndromes such as nonketotic hyperglycemia, and postcardiac arrest. Some seizures may also be caused by drugs. Recognition of seizures is often complicated by their clinical presentation and differential diagnosis with similar disturbances of consciousness. Nonconvulsive status epilepticus may present as recurrent episodes of confusion.

Adults with epilepsy are often confronted with a complex array of psychological and psychosocial challenges. Among the most significant challenges are the cognitive deficits frequently seen in persons with epilepsy. The extent of cognitive weakness varies markedly among patients, with some patients with epilepsy reporting no significant problems.[5]

The cognitive difficulties noted in individuals with epilepsy may occur in one or several domains, including attention,[6] speeed of mental processing,[7] memory and learning,[8] executive function (i.e., shifting of cognitive set),[9] and school achievement.[10] No consensus has been reached regarding what specific neuropsychological tests are most useful in each form of epilepsy. Here are report Tables 19.1 through 19.4, the main types of psychological testing.

TABLE 19.1
Summary of Tests Used to Evaluate Attention Area of Cognition

Arithmetic scale of Lurija-Nebraska Battery
Computation test, arithmetic task
Corsi block span alternating S test
Cross-out cancellation test
Dot cancellation test
H barrage test, Bell barrage test, Tolouse Pieron test
Italian attention matrix (modified digit cancellation)
Letter cancellation test
PASAT (paced additive serial additive)
Stroop test

TABLE 19.2
Assessment of Intellectual Function

CIA adult intelligence scale (Brazil)
Coding task
Intellectual function scale of Lurija-Nebraska Battery
National Adult Reading Test
Object naming test (recognition test)
Pauli test
Raven
Reaction time tests
Uchida–Kraepelin test
Verbal fluency test: Wechsler Adult Intelligence Scale–Revised
Wonderlic personnel test

TABLE 19.3
Tests of Short-Term Memory Function

Number scanning tests
Verbal learning tests
Visual memory tests

TABLE 19.4
Tests of Psychomotor Function

Bilateral hand movements
Motor function scale, rhythm function scale, tactile and visual
  function scale of Lurija-Nebraska Battery
Pegboard tests
Tapping test
Tracking tests
Trailmaking test/digit symbol

The possibility that the epileptic activity per se may worsen the age related cognitive impairment in elderly people is important. In fact, uncontrolled seizure activity has been associated with a decline in cognitive functioning, and transitory cognitive impairment with disruption of function in the area of seizure origin has been described in 50% of patients showing frequent subclinical epileptiform discharges.[11] Partial seizures are more common in elderly people than generalized ones, so that psychiatric manifestations of temporal lobe epilepsy in older adults may be represented by changes in behavior or cognition, mistakenly ascribed to "normal aging."[12] Furthermore, depression is the most frequent mood disorder associated with epilepsy, and it is not rare in elderly people following a stroke, especially in the left hemisphere.[13]

The main factors that may influence cognitive impairment are the disease type, the site of epileptogenic focus, and the effect of antiepileptic drugs (AEDs).

The type of disease is a determining factor in the form of cognitive impairment a patient might experience. Patients with generalized seizures usually have attention impairment caused by the dysfunction of the activating thalamic system.[14] Memory disturbances are more common in patients who have complex partial seizures that are sometimes caused by lesions of the amygdaloid and hippocampal neuronal circuits. Patients with idiopathic disease generally experience no cognitive impairment because no lesions occur in the brain to cause such a disturbance.

Cognitive impairment is more evident in patients with complex partial seizures who have recurrent prolonged seizures. Cognitive deficits also might correlate with subclinical epileptic activity, frequently associated with interictal electroencephalographic (EEG) abnormalities. This is the so-called transient cognitive impairment described by Stores.[15]

The site of the epileptogenic focus influences the form of cognitive impairment.[16] In patients with temporal lobe lesions, memory impairment primarily involves learning abilities, as has been confirmed by electrophysiological and cerebral blood flow studies.[17] Frontal lesions, on the other hand, cause both memory and attention disturbances.[14] Left hemisphere involvement has been correlated with impaired verbal learning, verbal memory, and denomination; right hemisphere involvement might cause affective disturbances, nonverbal memory impairment, and visuospatial analysis impairment.

Additional factors to consider in determining the cause of cognitive impairment are age at disease onset, duration and frequency of seizures, the presence of other neurological abnormalities, and the patient's educational and psychosocial background.

19.2 EFFECTS OF AEDs

AEDs may cause adverse cognitive effects, and thus further worsen a critical situation already at risk for behavioral and cognitive dysfunction. It must also be remembered that cognitive side effects of AEDs may develop slowly and insidiously, and may easily be confounded by, or mistaken for, the gradual and progressive mental decay associated with aging. Last but not least, the memory and intellectual deficits, associated with motor impairment or altered special sensory function, may also have an adverse effect on compliance.

Age-related changes in pharmacokinetcs and pharmacodynamics demand special alertness when prescribing drugs for an elderly patient. Neuronal loss and/or neural sensitivities play an important role in altering the kinetics and the uptake of drugs by brain tissue. Because decreased albumin and decreased protein binding are associated with aging, free drug concentrations of AED may be higher than normal and should be assessed in the elderly patients, Treating these patients with epilepsy therefore involves many challenges, including the presence of concomitant disease and hence the frequent polytherapy.

As the recurrence risk following a first unprovoked seizure after age 65 is unknown, but probably higher than in young adults, immediate AED treatment in this case may be reasonable, but, because treatment may be associated with an even greater risk for side effects, deferral of treatment should also be considered.[18] Once the decision to initiate treatment has been made, therapy should be tailored to the individual patient, with an initial low dosage and a slow, progressive increase. Whenever possible, AED blood levels (including free levels) should be determined on a routine basis at fixed intervals.

To date, there is no drug of first choice for the treatment of epilepsy in elderly people. Therefore, the choice must be made on the basis of knowledge of the mechanism of action, the efficacy, and the side effects of available old and new AEDs in younger people.

The sedative action of some AEDs, such as phenobarbital, primidone, and the benzodiazepines, can contribute to impaired cognitive function. In particular, phenobarbital and primidone have been found to induce memory impairment, especially in the areas of short-term memory and attention. The effects of phenytoin on cognitive function have been under investigation for some time, and a "Dilantin dementia" was described by Rosen in 1966,[19] but it appears that the syndrome is associated with higher plasma drug concentrations.[20] In a single blind, randomized study designed to compare the impact of phenytoin and valproic acid on cognitive function in elderly people,[21] the authors were able to show only slight effects of the AEDs and only very trivial differences between the two drugs. Other anticonvulsants, such as ethosuximide, clobazam, and carbamazepine, appear to cause insignificant neuropsychological side effects. In a placebo-controlled study in elderly patients taking carbamazepine, valproate, or phenytoin as monotherapy, no cognitive impairment developed when the dose was modestly increased within the target range for each drug.[22]

Of the newer drugs, gabapentin, lamotrigine, and vigabatrin caused minimal or no effects on cognitive functioning in young healthy adults or patients with epilepsy, whereas topiramate demonstrated potential acute and steady-state adverse cognitive effects. No deterioration in cognitive performance was observed in patients on long-term treatment with oxcarbazepine and tiagabine[23,24] (Table 19.5).

TABLE 19.5
Risk for Adverse Effects of AEDs
on Cognitive Function

Benzodiazepines[a]	++
Phenobarbital	++
Primidone	+
Phenytoin	±
Ethosuximide	0
Carbamazepine	0
Valproic Acid	0
Oxcarbazepine	0
Vigabatrin	0
Lamotrigine	0
Gabapentin	0
Tiagabine	0
Topiramate	+

[a] Not clobazam, which shows no detrimental effect on cognition.

In conclusion, the choice of the AED in the treatment of late-onset seizures needs particular skill and competence.[25,26] Optimizing the pharmacological management of epilepsy in elderly people requires a particular proneness to detect the subtlest signs of mental deterioration and even a sensitivity to the psychological and social problems that occur in this population. The preservation of cognitive function is therefore mandatory, and the antiepileptic drug must be chosen considering this aspect of the problem as one of major concern.

REFERENCES

1. Thomas, R. J., Seizures and epilepsy in the elderly, *Arch. Intern. Med.*, 157, 605–617, 1997.
2. De la Court, A., Breteler, M., Meinardi, H. et al., Prevalence of epilepsy in the elderly: the Rotterdam study, *Epilepsia*, 37, 141–147, 1996.
3. Hauser, W. A., Annegers, J. F., and Kurland, L. T., Incidence of epilepsy and unprovoked seizures in Rochester, Minnesota: 1935–1984, *Epilepsia*, 34, 453–468, 1993.
4. Holt-Seitz, A., Wirrell, E. C., and Sundaram, M. B., Seizures in the elderly: etiology and prognosis, *Can. J. Neurol. Sci.*, 26, 110–114, 1999.
5. Rausch, R., Le, M. T., and Langfitt, J. T., Neuropsychological evaluation — adults, in *Epilepsy A Comprehensive Textbook*, Engel, J. and Pedley, T. A., Eds., Lippincott-Raven, Philadelphia, 1998, 978.
6. Mitchell, W. G., Zhou, Y., Chavez, J. M., and Guzman, B. L., Reaction time, attention, and impulsivity in epilepsy, *Pediatr. Neurol.*, 8, 19–24, 1992.
7. Rugland, A. L., Neuropsychological assessment of cognitive functioning in children with epilepsy, *Epilepsia*, 31(Suppl. 4), S41–S44, 1990.
8. Dodrill, C. B., Correlates of generalized tonic-clonic seizures with intellectual neuropsychological, emotional, and social function in patients with epilepsy, *Epilepsia*, 27, 399–411, 1986.
9. Strauss, E., Hunter, M., and Wada, J., Wisconsin card sorting performance: effects of age of onset of damage and laterality of dysfunction, *J. Clin. Exp. Neuropsychol.*, 15, 896–902, 1993.
10. Seidenberg, M., Beck, N., Geisser, M. et al., Academic achievement of children with epilepsy, *Epilepsia*, 27, 753–759, 1986.
11. Stores, G., Effects on learning on subclinical seizure discharge, in *Education and Epilepsy*, Aldenkamp, A. P., Alpherts, W. C. J., and Meinardi, H., Eds., Swets & Zeitlinger, Amsterdam, 1987, 14–21.
12. Robertson, M., Mood disorders associated with epilepsy, in *Psychiatric Comorbidity in Epilepsy. Basic Mechanisms, Diagnosis, and Treatment*, McConnell, H. W. and Snyder, P. J., Eds., American Psychiatric Press, Washington, D.C., 1998, 133–168.
13. Puryear, L. J., Kunik, M., Molinari, V. et al., Psychiatric manifestations of temporal lobe epilepsy in older adults, *J. Neuropsychiat. Clin. Neurosci.*, 7, 235–237, 1995.
14. Trimble, M. R. and Reynolds, E. H., *Epilepsy, Behaviour, and Cognitive Functioning*, John Wiley & Sons, Chichester, U.K., 1988.
15. Stores, G., Effects of learning on "subclinical" seizure discharge, in *Education and Epilepsy*, Aldenkamp, A. P., Alpherts, W. C. J., and Meinardi, H., Eds., Swets & Zeitlinger, Amsterdam, the Netherlands, 1987, 14–21.
16. Piccirilli, M., D'Alessandro, P., Sciarma, T. et al., Attention problems in epilepsy: possible significance of the epileptogenic focus, *Epilepsia*, 35, 1091–1096, 1994.
17. Aldenkamp, A. P., Alpherts, W. C. J., Dekker, M. J. A. et al., Neuropsychological aspects of learning disabilities in epilepsy, *Epilepsia*, 31, 9–20, 1990.
18. Scheuer, M. L., Drug treatment in the elderly, in Engel, J., Jr. and Pedley, T. A., Eds., *Epilepsy: A Comprehensive Textbook*, Lippincott-Raven, Philadelphia, 1998, 1211–1219.
19. Rosen, J. A., Dilantin dementia, *Trans. Am. Neurol. Assoc.*, 93, 276, 1966.
20. Reynolds, E. H., Mental effects of antiepileptic medication: a review, *Epilepsia*, 24(8 Suppl. 2), S85–S95, 1983.

21. Craig, I. and Tallis, R., Impact of valproate and phenytoin on cognitive function in elderly patients: results of a single-blind randomized comparative study, *Epilepsia*, 35, 381–390, 1994.
22. Read, C. L., Stephen, L. J., Stolarek, I. H. et al., Cognitive effects of anticonvulsant monotherapy in elderly patients: a placebo-controlled study, *Seizure*, 7, 159–162, 1998.
23. Monaco, F., Cognitive effects of Vigabatrin: a review, *Neurology*, 47(Suppl. 1), S6–S11, 1996.
24. Martin, R., Kuzniecky, R., Ho, S. et al., Cognitive effects of topuiramate, gabapentin and lamotrigine in healthy young adults, *Neurology*, 52, 321–327, 1999.
25. Scheuer, M. L., Seizures and epilepsy in the elderly, in *Recent Advances in Epilepsy*, Vol. 6, Pedley, T. A. and Meldrum, B. S., Eds., Churchill Livingstone, Edinburgh, 1995, 247–270.
26. Willmore, L. J., Management of epilepsy in the elderly, *Epilepsia*, 37(8 Suppl. 6), S23–S33, 1996.

20 Multiple Sclerosis: Impact on Elderly People

Jack Burks, G. Kim Bigley, and Haydon Hill

CONTENTS

20.1 Introduction 412
20.2 Pathogenesis 412
20.3 Clinical Patterns of Multiple Sclerosis...413
20.4 Risk Factors..415
20.5 Clinical Manifestations of Multiple Sclerosis..416
20.6 Diagnosis..416
20.7 Treatment..417
    20.7.1 Disease Course Therapy...417
    20.7.2 Symptom Management 418
        20.7.2.1 Fatigue 419
        20.7.2.2 Spasticity 419
        20.7.2.3 Weakness 419
        20.7.2.4 Dizziness..419
        20.7.2.5 Depression 419
        20.7.2.6 Paroxysmal Disorders...420
        20.7.2.7 Dysarthria 420
        20.7.2.8 Cognitive Problems 420
        20.7.2.9 Pain 420
        20.7.2.10 Bladder Dysfunction...420
        20.7.2.11 Bowel Dysfunction 421
        20.7.2.12 Sexual Dysfunction 421
        20.7.2.13 Autonomic Dysfunction 421
        20.7.2.14 Dysphagia 421
20.8 The Impact of Multiple Sclerosis in Elderly People...422
20.9 Summary 422
Acknowledgment 422
References..423

20.1 INTRODUCTION

In 1868, the famous French neurologist Jean Marie Charcot described the clinical and pathological features of an illness that is now called multiple sclerosis. Multiple Sclerosis (MS) is likely to have existed for centuries before, but it was not described in detail until the 19th century.[1] In the past, MS has been described as an uncommon, relapsing–remitting, demyelinating disease of young Caucasian adult women.

These early perceptions have changed somewhat. Although most patients begin with relapsing–remitting disease, most transition to a chronic progressive disease after several years. While demyelination is prominent, axonal loss can also be significant, especially in acute lesions.[2] MS is not rare. In fact, MS is the most common neurological disease diagnosed between the ages of 20 and 50 in the United States. Over 1 million people worldwide are diagnosed with MS. Although MS usually begins before the age of 50, many MS patients live well into their senior years. With the discovery of new MS treatments in the past 8 years, the percentage of patients with MS who are active in the elderly population will continue to rise.

20.2 PATHOGENESIS

MS is believed to be an autoimmune inflammatory disease initiated by T cells activated by specific (unknown) antigen(s) (Table 20.1). The antigen(s) may be related to myelin components and/or to an environmental exposure such as a virus during adolescence in a genetically susceptible person. Macrophages destroy myelin. Cytokines help regulate the process.[3] The disease also has a B-cell or antibody-mediated component as well as a degenerative component.[4-7] As people with MS reach their 50s and 60s, the inflammatory changes in the central nervous system (CNS) are reduced and the progressive degenerative process is more prominent. While new immunomodulating therapies have a robust therapeutic effect on the inflammatory changes in MS, they may have less effect on the progressive degenerative process.

TABLE 20.1
Mechanisms of MS Damage

Types	Primary Processes Involved
I	Activated T lymphocyte, macrophages, cytokines
II	Type I with an antibody- and complement-mediated components
III	Ischemic-type changes with diffuse inflammation
IV	Myelin-producing, oligodendroglial cell apoptosis

The magnetic resonance imaging (MRI) scan has added significant new insights into the pathogenesis of the disease. The MRI scan shows a dynamic process with myelin destruction and repair, even when patients remain asymptomatic. Axonal loss, evidenced by brain atrophy and "black holes" on MRI, can occur early with only minimal clinical signs.[8] Also, the MRI helps in predicting the future disease course.[9] Based on clinical and MRI data, the National Multiple Sclerosis Society (NMSS) has recommended the treatment of all patients with MS who are relapsing.

Recently emphasized cognitive deficits may be partially attributable to axonal loss. Axonal loss is thought to be less reversible than myelin loss. Lucchinetti[6] and Lassman[7] and colleagues have further challenged the understanding of MS by identifying four separate pathological patterns in MS.[6,7] The first is the activated T-cell-mediated immunological damage. The second adds an element of antibody-mediated CNS tissue destruction. The third pattern is a diffuse inflammatory process such as seen in ischemia. The fourth is progressive destruction of oligodendroglia, the cells that make myelin.

These new concepts have significant implications for future treatment. For example, the current anti-inflammatory treatments may need to be combined with neuroprotective agents and specific B-cell treatments to have maximum therapeutic benefit.

Myelin and axonal damage may not be necessarily permanent. Remyelination, at least in part, does occur in the CNS. Damaged axons can undergo a reparative process. Immunomodulating therapy may enhance both of these repair mechanisms.

20.3 CLINICAL PATTERNS OF MULTIPLE SCLEROSIS

The classification of various forms of MS is currently undergoing review, and will likely be reclassified in the near future (Table 20.2). This reclassification will better reflect patients' response to certain treatments. For example, since patients with a clinically isolated syndrome (CIS) and multiple MRI lesions are likely to develop MS, a new, early MS classification has been suggested.

TABLE 20.2
Types of MS

Type	Features
Clinically isolated syndrome (CIS)	Pre-MS demyelinating event with MRI lesions
Relapsing–remitting multiple sclerosis (RRMS)	Exacerbations separated by clinical stability
Secondary progressive multiple sclerosis (SPMS)	Follows RRMS, progressive with or without exacerbations Inflammatory lesions early; degenerative lesions later
Primary progressive multiple sclerosis (PPMS)	Older age, progression from onset, less inflammation, more degeneration
Malignant multiple sclerosis (Marberg)	Rare, rapidly progressive plus exacerbations, may be fatal
Benign MS	10% of patients, few attacks, good recovery, mostly sensory symptoms, no progression

Nearly 80% of MS begins as relapsing–remitting MS (RRMS).[10] However, most patients develop a progressive form of the disease after several years (secondary progressive MS, or SPMS). Since all axons in the brain and spinal cord have myelin sheaths, the destruction of myelin in RRMS can cause a host of neurological signs and symptoms. These signs and symptoms can appear rapidly and last from a few days to several months. Recovery may be incomplete with the remaining signs and symptoms lasting a lifetime. Between exacerbations in RRMS, neurological symptoms are stable. However, patients may have good days and bad days where symptoms may wax and wane. Also, patients are likely to feel worse in the late afternoon, after exercise, or after exposure to extreme heat based on body temperature elevation.

SPMS may be divided into two types. Patients with progression who still have relapses and MRI evidence of inflammation may be classified as early SPMS or late RRMS. These patients may benefit from immunomodulating therapy more than those patients with a progressive course and little inflammation on MRI.

The severity of the disease course varies dramatically for each patient. Even identical twins with MS may have markedly different disease courses. A greater number MRI lesions, especially gadolinium-enhancing lesions, are generally associated with more disability in the future.

Approximately 10% of patients with MS have primary progressive MS (PPMS), which is a relentlessly progressive form of the disease without exacerbations. PPMS affects older patients, and spinal cord involvement prevails. Their symptoms often begin with progressive weakness and spasticity in the lower extremities as well as parethesias and bladder, bowel, and sexual dysfunction. Possibly, PPMS and SPMS are two distinct illnesses with two separate pathogeneses.

A "malignant" form of MS is rare. Malignant MS (Marberg variant) can result in a relentless progression coupled with severe exacerbations. Death may ensue within a matter of months or a few years.

Benign MS occurs in about 10% of patients, but it is usually a retrospective diagnosis after 15 years. These patients have only a few exacerbations, which are usually sensory, followed by recovery. The time between attacks is prolonged and patients do not transition to SPMS. Patients who are considered to have benign MS should have regular medical examinations and MRIs to ascertain subclinical damage in the brain in these asymptomatic patients.

MS usually has an onset between the ages of 20 and 50. However, since MS is only rarely fatal, most patients have a nearly normal life expectancy. Therefore, MS has a significant impact on the lives of those affected throughout their adult lives. Even as patients with MS become elderly, the tendency is to relate all their symptoms to MS. This often leads to misdiagnosis and inappropriate treatment.

Most patients with RRMS transition to a progressive illness in later life (SPMS). The mechanism of neurological tissue destruction likely changes as patients get older. Early in adulthood, the disease is likely to be characterized by relapses and remissions with intense inflammation in the brain. Later in life, the lesions assume a more degenerative characteristic as the patients have fewer attacks and a steadier progression.

PPMS, with spinal cord involvement and no relapses in an older MS population, occurs in 10 to 20% of patients. Treatment trials for PPMS have lagged behind the treatment trials for young adults with the relapsing–remitting form of the disease. However, PPMS clinical trials are currently under way.

The elderly patient with MS with progressive disease often presents a confusing medical picture to the clinician. What symptoms are related to aging vs. MS? For example, a sudden neurological deterioration may result from MS exacerbation or a stroke.

20.4 RISK FACTORS

The risk for developing MS is reduced dramatically after age 50 (Table 20.3). Nonetheless, MS is common in later life because of its chronic, nonfatal course. Women are affected two to three times more frequently than men. Caucasians are affected more than other races. A predilection for people in higher socioeconomic status is seen in some countries. Northern Europe, Canada, and the Northern United States are high-risk areas for MS. Temperate climates in the Southern Hemisphere also have more MS than tropical climates. However, an increasing risk for MS has been identified in southern Europe. The explanation remains a mystery.

TABLE 20.3
Risk Factors for MS

Factor	Ages 20–50 at Onset
Race	Mostly Caucasian
Gender	Females 3:1 more than males
Genetics	Increased in first-degree relatives and even higher in monozygotic twins
Environmental exposure	? Virus, other agent(s)

Genetics also plays a role in the pathogenesis of MS.[4] Although a specific MS gene is unlikely, certain histocompatibility antigens are more common in MS.[11,12] HLA DRW2 is overrepresented in most populations of patients with MS. However, since MS may not be a uniform disease, the genetic factors may differ. For example, HLA DR4 is observed in Sardinian and Mexican patients with MS and HLA DR6 is observed in Jordanian Arab patients with MS.[13]

Twin studies have shown that dizygotic twins have a concordance rate for MS of 5%, whereas monozygotic twins have a concordance rate of about 30%.[14] People with close family members with MS have a 10 to 20 times increased risk for getting the disease, although the overall risk remains at less than 5%, except for monozygotic twins.

Specific environmental factors (virus) have yet to be confirmed, but clusters of MS have been reported. In addition, people who migrate from a high-risk MS area in the world to a low-risk area carry the high risk of the disease if they move after adolescence, but not if they move before adolescence.[15] Children adopted into families with MS do not have an increased risk of the disease. Also, spouses of patients with MS are not at higher risk. Therefore, it seems unlikely that MS is directly transmissible.

Risk factors for attacks of MS have also been defined. For example, viral infections increase the risk of attacks of MS.[16] However, vaccinations for influenza do not increase the risk of an MS attack. Although patients with MS may have attacks after vaccination, the risk does not appear to be greater than those patients who did not have the vaccinations.[17]

The risk for MS attacks is decreased during pregnancy and increased dramatically in the postpartum period.[18] Therefore, hormonal influences are likely to be a risk factor for MS attacks. However, breastfeeding does not appear to have an affect on the risk for an attack.

Trauma, especially to the nervous system, has been postulated to increase the risk for attacks of MS. However, a thorough review has not substantiated this risk.[19]

Stress precipitating exacerbations has been emphasized by some patients who identify stress before an attack. However, recall bias is obviously present. Studies on the influence of stress on exacerbations have revealed differing results.[19] One problem is defining stress. Possibly the perception of stress may be more important than the actual stress itself.

20.5 CLINICAL MANIFESTATIONS OF MULTIPLE SCLEROSIS

MS is known for its diverse clinical presentation. Sensory symptoms often predominate early in the disease course. However, ensuing motor symptoms usually result in the disability seen later in the course of the disease.

Decreased vision associated with optic neuritis may be the first symptom of the disease. Numbness and tingling in the extremities are also early signs. Eventually, weakness, spasticity, ataxia, dysarthria, dysphagia, pain, cognitive problems, and bowel, bladder, and sexual dysfunction may be evident.

20.6 DIAGNOSIS

The diagnosis of MS is primarily made based on a neurological history and physical examination. The diagnosis is suspected when multiple episodes of neurological dysfunction are recognized that involve multiple areas of the CNS. Once a diagnosis is suspected, the MRI and spinal fluid evaluations provide additional support for the diagnosis.

The diagnostic MRI is likely to show multiple white matter lesions, especially periventricularly. Lesions can also involve the corpus callosum, cerebellum, brain stem, and spinal cord. The lesions may or may not enhance with gadolinium. As many as 95% of patients with MS will have an abnormal MRI within 3 years of the onset of symptoms. Multiple MRI lesions that are ovoid, greater than 6 mm, located periventricularly, and located in the brain stem and/or corpus collosum are strong indications of MS in a patient with multiple clinical episodes.

The cerebral spinal fluid shows evidence of immunological dysfunction with the production of oligoclonal bands and intrathecal immunoglobin-G. These findings may not be specific for MS, since other inflammatory and infectious agents of the

CNS may produce similar results. However, once those conditions have been ruled out, MS rises to the top of the diagnostic list.

Other diseases may mimic MS, but blood work, neuroimaging, cerebral spinal fluid evaluation, and ancillary tests usually make the diagnosis clear.

The MRI can also be helpful in determining prognosis. A patient with a clinically isolated (CNS) syndrome (CIS) with multiple MRI lesions is very likely to have more clinical episodes and a diagnosis of MS. On the other hand, a patient with a CIS with a normal MRI is unlikely to develop MS within 5 years. Patients with gadolinium-enhanced lesions at onset are likely to develop significant disability if not treated early.

20.7 TREATMENT

20.7.1 DISEASE COURSE THERAPY

Immunomodulating therapy has emerged as first line therapy for MS (Table 20.4). Before 1993, the treatment for MS was primarily high-dose intravenous methylprednisolone for exacerbations. In 1993, interferon-ß-1b (Betaseron) was approved by the Food and Drug Administration (FDA) for the treatment of RRMS.[20] Interferon-ß-1b reduced relapses and dramatically reduced disease burden and gadolinium-enhanced lesions on the MRI. The higher dose was more effective than a lower dose. Limited 5-year data support continued long-term efficacy.[21]

TABLE 20.4
Immunomodulation Therapies

Name	Dosage	Delivery	Approved for
Interferon-ß-1b (Betaseron)	28 MIU/week	Subcutaneous, every other day	RRMS (World) and SPMS (Europe)
Interferon-ß-1a (Avonex)	6 MIU/week	Intramuscular, once a week	RRMS (World)
Interferon-ß-1a (Rebif)	36 or 18 MIU/week	Subcutaneous, three times a week	RRMS (Europe and Canada)
Glatiramer acetate (Copaxone)	20 mg/day	Subcutaneous, daily	RRMS (World)
Mitoxantrone (Novantrone)	12 mg/m^2	Intravenous, every 3 months	Progressive MS

In 1996, an interferon-ß-1a (Avonex) was also approved by the FDA in a once-a-week, intramuscular injection. In addition to effects on relapses, Interferon-ß-1a was shown to have an affect on progression of disability in RRMS patients.[22] More recently, interferon-ß-1a has shown efficacy in extending the time between a CIS and the diagnosis of MS.[23]

Glatiramer acetate (Copaxone), a non-interferon treatment, was added to the list of treatments for MS shortly after interferon-ß-1a was introduced.[24,25] Glatiramer acetate has fewer side effects than the interferons, but requires a subcutaneous injection daily. Limited 6-year data indicate long-term positive effects.[25]

Outside the United States, another interferon-ß-1a (Rebif) is also approved and widely used.[26] The 4-year data continue to show efficacy. It is given subcutaneously three times per week. The higher dose showed better results than the lower dose in many parameters.

In SPMS, interferon-ß-1b (Betaseron) was markedly effective in reducing disease progression in a large European trial, leading to approval for treatment.[27] A similar, but not identical North American trial had mixed results with no effect on progression.[28] The patients in the North American trial had suffered from MS longer and their lesions were less active than those of patients in the European trial. A degenerative process may have played a more prominent role in progression in the North American trial.

In 2000, the FDA approved Mitoxantrone (Novantrone), a chemotherapeutic agent for neoplastic disease, for progressive MS.[29,30] While effective, it has the potential to produce a dose-related irreversible cardiotoxicity. Therefore, it is only given for a limited time (2 to 3 years). As with other chemotherapeutic agents, the rare risk of future leukemia is also of some concern.

Investigational treatments include stem cell transplantation, intravenous immunoglobin-G, anti-T-cell antibodies, α-interferon, antibodies against adhesion molecules associated with the blood–brain barrier, antimetalloproteinases, and T-cell vaccinations. Experimental therapies for remyelination such as insulin-like growth factor 1 and nerve growth factor are also being tested.

20.7.2 SYMPTOM MANAGEMENT

Almost any CNS symptom may occur with MS. These symptoms may last for a few days or a lifetime. One goal of treatment is to increase the functional status of the patient by alleviating the symptoms.[31] This is best accomplished by a health-care team, which may consist of the following: neurologist, physiatrist, ophthalmologist, physical therapist, occupational therapist, speech and language pathologist, recreational therapist, rehabilitation nurse, dietician, psychologist, social worker, vocational rehabilitation counselor, driver education specialist, and chaplain or minister.[32] In addition to specific symptom management, general health screening is also important to counteract the tendency to attribute all symptoms to MS. MS symptoms, especially in elderly people, may actually represent other medical or neurological conditions.

Since MS symptom management can be overwhelming to the individual practitioner and patient, a disease management team approach to MS has been adopted by many of the major comprehensive MS centers in the world. In some centers, the MS specialist may be responsible for the ongoing general medical care of people with MS. A nurse care coordinator is often the patient's point person for care. The disease management process includes prevention, diagnosis, acute management, rehabilitation, long-term medical and neurological follow-up, community integration, and end-of life-management.

20.7.2.1 Fatigue

Fatigue is the most common symptom in MS. MS fatigue is often worse in the late afternoon and with temperature elevation. Cognitive decline and an increase in other MS symptoms may be present during periods of fatigue. The treatment of fatigue is multidisciplinary. Exercise and modification of work activity are used initially along with treatment of depression, sleep deprivation, and pain, if present. Cooling via cool baths, ice chips, and/or cooling vests may provide some relief.

Medications for fatigue are only partially effective. Amantadine (Symmetrel) is often the first-line treatment. CNS-stimulating drugs such as pemoline (Cylert), methylphenidate (Ritalin), and dexedrine sulfate (Dexedrine) are helpful but are fraught with potential problems. Selective serotoninergic reuptake inhibitors (SSRIs) may also be helpful. More recently, modafinil (Provigil) has been shown to be very effective in the treatment in MS fatigue and has become the first-line treatment for a growing number of physicians.[33] Last, 4-aminopyridine is being studied for the treatment of fatigue. However, 4-aminopyridine may precipitate seizures.

20.7.2.2 Spasticity

Spasticity is also common in MS. Physical therapy and cooling are the first lines of treatment. Pharmacological intervention with baclofen (Lioresal) and/or tizanidine (Zanaflex) may dramatically reduce spasticity, although side effects of these medications need close scrutiny. For severe spasticity, which does not respond to oral medications, intrathecal baclofen via a pump has proved to be very effective.

20.7.2.3 Weakness

Weakness in MS is difficult to treat specifically. Muscles that have lost their CNS connections do not respond to the usual strengthening exercise programs. However, exercising complementary muscles may allow for increased strength in an extremity. Disuse is a treatable cause of muscle weakness. As muscle weakness increases, adaptation through ambulatory aids and/or a wheelchair may be necessary to increase mobility and decrease fatigue.

20.7.2.4 Dizziness

Dizziness and vertigo in MS can be vexing problems. Antihistamines such as meclizine (Antivert), diphenhydramine (Benadryl), and dimenhydrinate (Dramamine) may be helpful. A transdermal scopolamine patch may be used temporarily for dizziness and vertigo in MS. The benzodiazapines may have some limited use in the patients suffering from dizziness as well.

20.7.2.5 Depression

Depression in MS is common. A combination of psychotherapy and medications is ideal. The tricyclic antidepressants can be helpful, but they cause significant anti-cholinergic side effects. Therefore, the SSRIs are usually the first line of medical

treatment. Other medications such as trazodone, nefacodone (Serzone), and bupro-
pion HCl (Wellbutrin) are also helpful in depression associated with MS.

20.7.2.6 Paroxysmal Disorders

Paroxysmal disorders are intermittent symptoms that occur suddenly and last a few
minutes before disappearing. They occur in approximately 10% of patients with MS.
Paroxysmal pain, spasms, sensory symptoms, including trigeminal neuralgia, dysarthria, ataxia, and diplopia, as well as Lhermitte's sign are all examples of paroxysmal symptoms in MS. A clinical challenge is recognizing paroxysmal disorders
as part of MS symptomatology. Once recognized, gabapentin (Neurontin) often
eliminates these symptoms. Carbamazepine (Tegretol), and phenytoin (Dilantin)
have also been shown to have some positive benefits in paroxysmal disorders.

20.7.2.7 Dysarthria

Dysarthria in MS usually represents a combination of problems including weakness,
spasticity, and ataxia of the muscles in the lips, tongue, mandible, soft pallet, vocal
cords, and diaphragm. A speech and language pathologist can provide considerable
symptomatic help for these patients.

20.7.2.8 Cognitive Problems

Cognitive problems have recently been recognized to occur early in MS in some
patients. This can be a major contributor to a lower quality of life and employability.
Cognitive retraining techniques have benefit in helping the patient recognize the
problems and adapt strategies to function better. Medications for Alzheimer's disease
have been studied in a few patients with MS with mixed results. Cognitive problems
may also be precipitated by medications for other symptoms.

20.7.2.9 Pain

Pain was once thought to be uncommon in MS. However, recent studies have shown
that up to 65% of patients with MS suffer from pain. Pain can be divided into two
groups. The first group is neurogenic pain, which is usually characterized as light-
ning-like, burning, or dysesthetic in nature. This pain is best treated with gabapentin
(Neurontin) and other anticonvulsants.

   The second type of pain in MS is related to musculoskeletal stressors from
weakness, incoordination, and spasticity. Rehabilitation programs with stretching
and exercise can help these patients.

20.7.2.10 Bladder Dysfunction

Bladder dysfunction in MS is a leading cause of social isolation. Patients fear going
out of the house because of frequency, urgency, and incontinence. Bladder problems
are divided into three groups. The first group consists of a small spastic bladder

(failure to store urine). Anticholinergic medications such as tolterodine tartrate (Detrol), and oxybutynin (Ditropan) are mainstays of treatment. Intrathecal baclofen pump may also be helpful in severe cases. The second type of bladder dysfunction is a large flaccid bladder (failure to empty urine). No medication is very helpful. These patients require intermittent catheterization for relief of their symptoms.

The third type of bladder dysfunction is dyssynergia, with incoordination between bladder wall contraction and external sphincter contraction. When both contract at the same time, urine flow is disturbed and reflux may occur toward the kidneys. Treatment is aimed at relaxing the bladder wall contractions and coordinating sphincter and bladder wall musculature. α-Blockers such as terazosin (Hytrin) or dibenzyline as well as baclofen (Lioresal) may be helpful in the treatment of the dyssynergic bladder. Intermittent catheterization is often necessary.

20.7.2.11 Bowel Dysfunction

Bowel dysfunction is equally disturbing to patients with MS. Constipation is the most common problem, but diarrhea and incontinence may occur. Medications used to treat other MS symptoms may be an additional aggravating factor in constipation. Bowel training, high-fiber diet, bulk-forming agents, and stool softeners combined with adequate fluid intake are the mainstays of therapy. Suppositories and laxatives should be used sparingly.

20.7.2.12 Sexual Dysfunction

Sexual dysfunction is much more common than previously discerned, especially in women. Sexual dysfunction therapy involves extensive education and understanding. Psychological and other medical factors (including medication side effects) may contribute to sexual dysfunction and can be addressed. Sildenafil citrate (Viagra) has shown remarkable positive benefits in some men with sexual dysfunction. In addition to medical management, reframing the concept of sexuality can make a significant difference in intimacy issues within a couple's relationship.

20.7.2.13 Autonomic Dysfunction

Autonomic dysfunction can also be part of MS. Obviously bladder, bowel, and sexual function are controlled by the autonomic nervous system. In addition, problems with vasomotor control may result in cold extremities, which may be swollen and blue or pale. Orthostatic hypotension is an uncommon, but difficult-to-treat problem in MS.

20.7.2.14 Dysphagia

Dysphagia or problems with swallowing can lead to regurgitation of food and even aspiration pneumonia. Fatigue is often a major contributing factor in dysphagia. Therefore, smaller, more frequent meals are recommended so patients do not become fatigued eating a large meal. Swallowing training is often useful.

20.8 THE IMPACT OF MULTIPLE SCLEROSIS IN ELDERLY PEOPLE

In elderly people, MS is often a progressive illness. Managing progressive symptoms is a significant challenge. For example, fragile skin can more easily lead to decubitous ulcers. Failure to empty urine from the bladder may lead to bladder infections and sepsis, which can be life-threatening. Mobility issues in MS are compounded by mobility problems due to arthritis and other conditions.

One of the most common problems in elderly patients with MS is attributing all of their symptoms to MS. This may lead to delayed diagnosis and treatment for important medical conditions. The clinician should remain hypervigilant for medical problems, especially as patients get older.

Many patients with MS are on multiple medications for several MS symptoms. These medications can have a profound deleterious effect in elderly people. For example, cognition may be dramatically worsened with some of the medications for MS symptoms. The judicious use of medications and the careful adjustment of their dosage are imperative to maximizing function in elderly people.

The use of ambulatory aids and wheelchairs for mobility is especially important in the elderly patient with MS. For example, a wheelchair to transport the patient may reduce fatigue and preserve the person's ability to function at a much higher level once the destination is reached. Pulmonary and cardiac problems are compounded in patients with MS.

20.9 SUMMARY

Although MS can present an overwhelming challenge to the patient and the healthcare provider, a systematic, disease management, team approach allows for maximum function. The results are fewer symptoms and a higher quality of life. The disease-modifying agents such as interferons, glatiramer acetate, and mitoxantrone may not be as effective in elderly patients with advanced progressive MS. However, their use is not contraindicated. Occasionally, MS in the elderly patient stops progressing spontaneously ("burned out MS").

Fortunately, most elderly patients with MS have discovered that their quality of life is much more related to interpersonal relationships and creativity than to mobility. And mobility is still possible with adaptive equipment. Therefore, many elderly patients with properly treated MS have a high quality of life, in spite of significant disabilities.

ACKNOWLEDGMENT

The authors thank Brandi Dupont for her assistance with the manuscript.

REFERENCES

1. Burks, J. S. and Johnson, K. P., Eds., *Multiple Sclerosis: Diagnosis, Medical Management, and Rehabilitation*, Demos, New York, 2000, chap. 1.
2. Trapp, B. D. et al., Axonal transection in the lesions of multiple sclerosis, *N. Engl. J. Med.*, 338, 278, 1998.
3. Steinman, L., Multiple sclerosis: a coordinated immunological attack against myelin in the central nervous system, *Cell*, 85, 299, 1996.
4. Noseworthy, J. H. et al., Multiple sclerosis, *N. Engl. J. Med.*, 343, 938, 2000.
5. Storch, M. K. et al., Multiple sclerosis: in situ evidence for antibody- and complement-mediated demyelination, *Ann. Neurol.*, 43, 465, 1998.
6. Lucchinetti, C., Heterogeneity of multiple sclerosis lesions: implications for the pathogenesis of demyelination, *Ann. Neurol.*, 47, 707, 2000.
7. Lassman, H., The new pathology of MS, *ACTRIMS*, 2000.
8. Simon, J. H. et al., A longitudinal study of T1 hypointense lesions in relapsing MS: MSCRG trial of interferon ß-1a, *Neurology*, 55, 185, 2000.
9. Burks, J. S. and Johnson, K. P., Eds., *Multiple Sclerosis: Diagnosis, Medical Management, and Rehabilitation*, Demos, New York, 2000, chap. 6.
10. Poser, C. M. et al., New diagnostic criteria for multiple sclerosis: guidelines for research protocols, *Ann. Neurol.*, 13, 227, 1983.
11. Haines, J. L. et al., A complete genomic screen for multiple sclerosis underscores a role for the major histocompatibility complex, *Nat. Genet.*, 13, 472, 1996.
12. Weinshenker, B. G. et al., Major histocompatibility complex class II alleles and the course and outcome of MS: a population-based study, *Neurology*, 51, 742, 1998.
13. Rosati, G. et al., Epidemiology of multiple sclerosis in northwestern Sardinia: further evidence for higher frequency in Sardinians compared to other Italians, *Neuroepidemiology*, 15, 10, 1996.
14. Sadovnick, A. D. et al., A population-based study of multiple sclerosis in twins: update, *Ann. Neurol.*, 33, 281, 1993.
15. Dean G., Annual incidence, prevalence, and mortality of multiple sclerosis in white South-African-born and in white immigrants to South Africa, *Br. Med. J.*, 2, 724, 1967.
16. Sibley, W. A., Bamford, C. R., and Clark, K., Clinical viral infections and multiple sclerosis, *Lancet*, 1, 1313, 1985.
17. Miller, A. E. et al., A multicenter, randomized, double-blind, placebo-controlled trial of influenza immunization in multiple sclerosis, *Neurology*, 48, 312, 1997.
18. Confavreux, C., Pregnancy in multiple sclerosis group. Rate of pregnancy-related relapse in multiple sclerosis, *N. Engl. J. Med.*, 339, 285, 1998.
19. Goodin, D. S. et al., The relationship of MS to physical trauma and psychological stress: report of the Therapeutics and Technology Assessment Subcommittee of the American Academy of Neurology, *Neurology*, 52, 1737, 1999.
20. The IFNB Multiple Sclerosis Study Group, Interferon beta-1b is effective in relapsing-remitting multiple sclerosis. I. Clinical results of a multicenter, randomized, double-blind, placebo-controlled trial, *Neurology*, 43, 655, 1993.
21. The IFNB Multiple Sclerosis Study Group, University of British Columbia MS/MRI Analysis Group, Interferon ß-1b in the treatment of multiple sclerosis: final outcome of the randomized controlled trial, *Neurology*, 45, 1277, 1995.

22. Jacobs, L. D. et al., Intramuscular interferon beta-1a for disease progression in relapsing multiple sclerosis, *Ann. Neurol.*, 39, 285, 1996.

23. Jacobs, L. D. et al., Intramuscular interferon beta-1a therapy initiated during a first demyelinating event in multiple sclerosis, *N. Engl. J. Med.*, 343, 898, 2000.

24. Johnson, K. P. et al., Copolymer 1 reduces relapse rate and improves disability in relapsing-remitting multiple sclerosis: results of a phase III multicenter, double-blind, placebo-controlled trial, *Neurology*, 45, 1268, 1995.

25. Johnson, K. P. et al., Extended use of glatiramer acetate (Copaxone) is well tolerated and maintains its clinical effect on multiple sclerosis relapse rate and degree of disability, *Neurology*, 50, 701, 1998.

26. PRISMS (Prevention of Relapses and Disability by Interferon ß-1a Subcutaneously in Multiple Sclerosis) Study Group, randomised double-blind placebo-controlled study of interferon ß-1a in relapsing/remitting multiple sclerosis, *Lancet*, 352, 1498, 1998.

27. European Study Group on Interferon ß-1b in Secondary Progressive MS, Placebo-controlled multicentre randomised trial of interferon ß-1b in treatment of secondary progressive multiple sclerosis, *Lancet*, 352, 1491, 1998.

28. Goodkin, D. E., North American Study Group on Interferon beta-1b in Secondary Prevention MS, Interferon beta-1b in secondary progressive MS: clinical and MRI results of a 3-year randomized controlled trial, *Neurology*, 54, Suppl., 2352, 2000.

29. Edan, G. et al., Therapeutic effect of mitoxantrone combined with methylprednisolone in multiple sclerosis: a randomised multicentre study of active disease using MRI and clinical criteria, *J. Neurol. Neurosurg. Psychiatr.*, 62, 112, 1997.

30. Kita, M. et al., A phase II trial of mitoxantrone in patients with primary progressive multiple sclerosis, *Neurology*, 54(Suppl. 3), A22, 2000.

31. Schapiro, R. T., *Symptom Management in Multiple Sclerosis,* 3rd ed., Demos, New York, 1998.

32. Maloney, F. P., Burks, J. S., Ringel, S. P., *Interdisciplinary Rehabilitation of Multiple Sclerosis and Neuromuscular Disorders*, J.B. Lippincott, Philadelphia, 1985, chap. 2.

33. Rammohan, K. W. et al., Modafinil — efficacy and safety for the treatment of fatigue in patients with multiple sclerosis, *Neurology*, 54(Suppl. 3), A24, 2000.

21 Vitamin, Mineral, Antioxidant, and Herbal Supplements: Facts and Fictions

Victor Herbert

CONTENTS

21.1   Introduction 425
21.2   Free Radicals 426
21.3   Antioxidants 426
21.4   Vitamin Supplements 427
21.5   Vitamin E 427
21.6   β-Carotene and Vitamin A 428
21.7   Vitamin D 428
21.8   Vitamin C 429
21.9   Calcium 429
21.10 Chromium 430
21.11 Selenium 430
21.12 Multivitamin Preparations 430
21.13 Diet 431
21.14 PGA and Crystalline Vitamin B_{12} 431
21.15 Herbs as Supplements 433
References 435

21.1 INTRODUCTION

The history of dietary supplements (vitamins, minerals, antioxidant, herbs, etc.) is the history of science (facts: evidence-based delineation of ratios efficacy to safety) vs. snake oil (fictions: deceptions by omission of adverse facts).[5,6,29,53] The first snake oil nutrition salesman was the snake in the Garden of Eden, who convinced Eve to get Adam to eat that apple, promising it would give him wisdom, but deceiving her by omitting the adverse fact that eating it would result in Adam and Eve being expelled forever from the Garden of Eden.

0-8493-2066-/01/$0.00+$1.50
© 2001 by CRC Press LLC

Deception by omission of adverse facts, and the use of deceptive and misleading "buzz words" has remained the hallmark of snake oil salesmen down through the ages. They remain today the basis for the sale to the public of billions of dollars annually of unneeded, unnecessary, and often worthless to harmful dietary supplements.

A table summarizing then-known harms from supplements of fiber, omega-3 fatty acids, vitamin A, β-carotene, vitamin C, vitamin E, iron, lecithin, niacin, and selenium was published by Herbert and Kasdan.[56] Today's leading deceptive, misleading, and often just plain false "buzz words" such as " dietary supplement" (to describe a product that adds a nutrient to a diet that already has it in adequate quantity) "natural" (when used to describe factory-produced synthetics), "vitamin" (when used to characterize nonvitamins such as coenzyme Q10, laetrile, and and "vitamin B_{15}"[30]), "antioxidant" (used to benignly characterize redox agents), "nutraceutical" (to describe a food supplement), "functional food" (to describe a food to which a nutraceutical has been added),[66] "potent" (a benign description for a high dose), "potentize" (the homeopath's descriptor for "diluted"), "succussed" (the homeopath's descriptor for "shaken"). By using these delusional descriptors, sellers can charge more for a homeopathic remedy 100-fold diluted 30 times and shaken each of those 30 times ($30\times$) than for one that has been diluted and shaken only 10 times ($10\times$). Both the $10\times$ and the $30\times$ are essentially water containing no active agent. A 100-fold dilution, 30 times repeated, yields a product diluted so far past Avogadro's number that there would be about a molecule of active agent in a container more than 30 billion times the size of the Earth (see chapter on "The Ultimate Fake" in Reference 5).

21.2 FREE RADICALS

Free radicals are the price we pay for breathing. We breathe in oxygen and urinate out water, which requires the generation of free radicals along the way. Moderate amounts of free radicals are essential for normal cell metabolism. Excesses are harmful. Slight excesses are prevented from doing harm by various body proteins and enzymes, such as superoxide dismutase. Superoxide dismutase pills are a fraud; as proteins, they are destroyed by gastric and pancreatic proteases and are not absorbed.

21.3 ANTIOXIDANTS

Most Americans, including physicians, have been gulled by an avalanche of media promotions and supplement-industry-funded peer-reviewed papers[5] into believing that if a supplement is labeled "antioxidant," it is good for you. Nothing could be farther from the truth.[40]

"Antioxidant" is a shorthand "buzz word" for "redox agent." All "antioxidant" supplements are in fact redox agents, antioxidant in some circumstances (mainly in dietary reference intake, or DRI,[20,21] and in lower amounts).[34] As naturally present in any fruit, fruit juice, vegetable, or grain, they are balanced by over 150 other phyto (plant) chemicals, at least a dozen of which are also redox agents. Thus, one absorbs over 150 phytochemicals, which balance each other out to produce a redox potential close to zero, preventing prooxidant harm. No such protective balance exists in "antioxidant" supplements.

21.4 VITAMIN SUPPLEMENTS

With the exception of vitamin B_{12}, which is factory biosynthesized, vitamin supplements currently produced in the United States are factory chemically synthesized, whereas some of those produced in Europe are biosynthesized.[71] Chemical synthesis produces racemic (D,L) product (i.e., two mirror-image molecules, facing each other), one of which is natural (i.e., the form found in bacteria and plants, and the nutrient in humans), and the other of which is synthetic, not found in nature, and may have harmful properties.[34,34a,71] Representing racemic vitamins, amino acids, and sugars as "natural" is false advertising. Biosynthesis is carried out by fermentation, using live microorganisms or their enzymes, and produces only the natural form, which is the D-form for vitamins and sugars, and the L-form for amino acids.

21.5 VITAMIN E

Vitamin E supplements are promoted as antioxidant and immune enhancing. This ignores the fact that immune enhancement may do more harm than good.[41] It also ignores that the vitamin E in plants is 80% γ-tocopherol and only 20% α-tocopherol. The only form in nearly all supplements is α-tocopherol. It blocks cell uptake of γ-tocopherol, thereby promoting rather than retarding NO_x free-radical damage, such as in the substantia nigra in parkinsonism, and in Alzheimer's disease, where NO_x free radicals are generated from NO (nitric oxide).[41] The experimental use of vitamin E supplements to retard progression of Alzheimer's disease has so far not shown value in a New York City group,[7] but has been associated with hemorrhagic strokes in two patients with Alzheimer's disease in a Syracuse (New York) group.[86] As Ames's group[12] published, γ-tocopherol binds and thereby inactivates both NO_x and oxygen free radicals, whereas α-tocopherol only acts against oxygen free radicals. To make matters worse, α-tocopherol supplements prevent cell uptake of food γ-tocopherol, with the result that the cells take up no γ-tocopherol and therefore have no protection against NO_x free radicals. Christen et al.[12] suggest that the solution to the problem is to add γ-tocopherol to α-tocopherol supplements. Herbert[41] suggests that the solution to a harmful pill is not taking it in the first place, rather than adding its antidote. The primary food source for vitamin E is liquid oil from grains; the usual diet provides about 15 IU/day. Stephens et al.[87] found that in patients with angioscopically proven coronary atherosclerosis, taking 400 or 800 IU of α-tocopherol daily for a median of 510 days (range 3 to 981) led to a statistically significant reduction in the incidence of nonfatal myocardial infarction. However, the incidence of cardiovascular death and all-cause mortality was slightly higher in the patients who took α-tocopherol than in those who took placebo. In a placebo-controlled, prospective study of 27,271 Finnish male smokers aged 50 to 69, Virtamo et al.[91] found that supplementation with 50 mg daily of α-tocopherol had only marginal effect on the incidence of fatal coronary heart disease and no influence on nonfatal myocardial infarction. Steiner[85] had found that, *in vivo*, as little as 50 mg daily of supplement α-tocopherol effectively inhibits platelet adhesion, which would be protective against vascular occlusions (such as heart attacks), but promotional of vascular hemorrhages (such as fatal hemorrhagic strokes). Indeed, this proved to be the case in the Finnish study.[91] α-Tocopherol may be a more potent platelet adhesion inhibitor (and general cell adhesion inhibitor) than "γ-tocopherol." Additionally, supplements of vitamin E higher than 800 IU can also cause severe bleeding via antagonizing the action of vitamin K.

Of the two vitamin E over-the-counter compounds most commonly purchased, the biological potency of RRR-α-topherol (the natural form) is twice that of all-rac-α-tocopherol (the synthetic racemic [D,L] form).[61] Horwitt, the world's leading authority on, and proponent of, vitamin E has stated, "Very high levels of antioxidants in blood and tissue may make them prooxidants. A number of reports have shown that the tocopherols can inhibit platelet adhesion and aggregation... My position on health claims on labels is that they should be absent or stated very conservatively" (cited in Reference 56).

21.6 β-CAROTENE AND VITAMIN A

Primary food sources for carotenoids are dark-colored fruits and vegetables. Primary foods sources for preformed vitamin A are meats, fish oil, and vitamin A–fortified dairy products.

The Virtamo et al. study,[91] of 27,271 Finnish men, randomly assigned the men to receive vitamin E (50 mg), β-carotene (20 mg), both agents, or placebo daily for 5 to 8 years (median 6.1 years). It found that supplementation with β-carotene has no primary preventive effect on major coronary events.

β-Carotene and other carotenoids in the vitamin A family are all redox agents, and epidemiological studies have found that higher levels of carotenoids in the diet and higher serum levels of carotenoids are associated with a lower incidence of cardiovascular disease and cancer. High serum β-carotene against disease.[37,40,43] In fact, the latest research[1,2] suggests that the reason above-DRI (Daily Reference Intake) supplements of β-carotene increase lung cancer rates among smokers is that smoke (and the high oxygen levels in lung cells) converts the supplemental β-carotene stored in the lungs to oxidized metabolites, which destroy retinoic acid, a tumor suppressor, and increase a protein that activates cell division, thereby promoting precancerous lesions.

It is now generally agreed among non-supplement-industry-funded health scientists, such as those at Harvard, Mount Sinai, the University of Helsinki, the National Cancer Institute, and the FDA, that no one should take β-carotene supplements.[37,40-44,91]

The carotenoids protective against macular degeneration appear to be lutein and its isomer, both normally present in high concentrations in the macula. It was recently discovered[2] that proteins associated with 3-carotenoids are light-harvesting complexes (LHCs), which capture light for photosynthesis in higher plants. One wonders if there is a similar carotenoid-dependent LHC in the human retina, which needs lycopene and zeaxanthin.

21.7 VITAMIN D

This vitamin is made in human skin adequately exposed to sunlight.[20] A recent unpublished study in the nursing home of the Bronx VA Medical Center indicates vitamin D deficiency in elderly people not exposed to sunlight is prevented by having them sit every day for 30 min at a round table playing cards with their sleeves rolled up to the elbow and an ultraviolet lamp above the middle of the table. In that 30 min daily, they make enough vitamin D in their exposed skin to sustain normal blood vitamin D levels around the clock.

21.8 VITAMIN C

Higher intakes of fruits and vegetables, each of which contains over 150 phytochemicals, of which vitamin C is just one, result in high phytochemical levels in the serum, including a high serum vitamin C level. This has been repeatedly associated with less cataract, cancer, coronary artery disease, and a higher high-density lipoprotein (HDL) cholesterol concentration. In fact, the lower incidence results from the total of all the phytochemicals absorbed from food, which cancel out any harmful effects from vitamin C alone. No long-term intervention studies showing a definite value of supplement vitamin C alone have been published. However, Podmore et al.[78] reported that, in a study of 30 healthy adult male volunteers, half given 500 mg daily of a vitamin C supplement and half given a placebo, for 6 weeks, those given the vitamin C developed oxidative damage in one part of the DNA of their peripheral blood lymphocytes. Their levels of 8-oxoadenine increased by a factor of four, from a norm of 0.05 nmol/mg, reflecting severe prooxidative damage. This DNA harm would probably occur with only 100 mg daily, because a 100-mg vitamin C supplement daily completely saturates all human cells,[69] and, as Herbert[38] pointed out, saturating normal human macrophages with synthetic vitamin C kills them prematurely by releasing too many free radicals all at once from their ingested heme. Levine et al.[69] found that 200 mg of vitamin C daily saturated not only all the cells, but also all the serum. Noting that 200 mg synthetic vitamin C daily could cause excessive menstrual blood loss, they excluded all females from their study. As Herbert pointed out in critiquing their study,[38] they also excluded from their study the more than one third of all Americans who, for genetic reasons,[84] can be harmed by 200 mg synthetic vitamin C per day, namely, the approximately 30% of African Americans and 12% of non–African Americans who are heterozygous for hemochromatosis; the approximately 1% of Americans who are homozygous for hemochromatosis (for whom vitamin C supplements will sharply accelerate irreversible organ damage and death); the one sixth of Americans who are stone-formers because they are genetically unable to catabolize ascorbate past oxalate; the millions of Americans with diabetes mellitus; and the Americans with hereditary hemolytic animas (i.e., sickle cell anemia, G6PD deficiency, or paroxysmal nocturnal hemoglobinuria), etc.

21.9 CALCIUM

Women are constantly not only remodeling bone daily, but also laying down new bone until approximately age 35, after which there is a holding action of remodeling and very slow, genetically predisposed, loss of bone, accelerated by menopause loss of estrogen, to eventual osteoporosis (for genetic reasons, earlier in whites than in blacks). This process is retarded by adequate calcium, which makes calcium supplements desirable starting at age 35 in women and age 50 in men (menopause in men starts about 15 years later than in women).[20]

21.10 CHROMIUM

Chromium is an essential nutrient in trace amounts. Grains are a major food source.[75] A glass of beer a day supplies all the chromium one needs, and its alcohol content raises HDL cholesterol (the "good cholesterol").

21.11 SELENIUM

Clark et al.[13] agreed in essence with the debunking by Herbert[45] of their suggestion that selenium supplements (as high-selenium yeast) should be taken to protect against cancer. Herbert[45] pointed out that the Clark study found no reduction by selenium of all-cause morbidity and mortality. Clark et al. disagreed with Kuller,[67] who presented evidence from the Surveillance, Epidemiology, and End Results (SEER) program that what Clark et al. had actually found was not a reduced incidence of cancer in those taking the selenium supplements, but rather an increased incidence of cancer in the placebo group. However, both the placebo and the yeast-selenium were coated with titanium, to prevent the study subjects from being able to detect a yeast aroma. Titanium is listed as a carcinogen. This author would speculate that yeast-selenium may prevent the absorption of titanium. Should this prove true, it would explain why those taking the placebo, with no yeast selenium in it to block titanium absorption, would develop more cancer.

21.12 MULTIVITAMIN PREPARATIONS

Chandra[11a] reported (1992), in a study of 96 elderly Newfoundland patients, that those who took multivitamin preparations for 12 months showed signs of better immune function and had fewer sick days, which would be expected in Newfoundland, where sick days are usually due to infectious disorders (which immune enhancement fights). However, immune enhancement brings out and maintains latent autoimmune disorders, such as autoimmune hemolytic anemia, rheumatoid arthritis, lupus erythematosis and multiple sclerosis, and a multitude of neoplasms, such as malignant lymphoma and thyroid and epithelial cell cancers.[41] In a CDC (Centers for Disease Control) study of a large cohort of Americans, Kim et al.[65] found that those who took vitamin and mineral supplements fared no better in overall morbidity and mortality than those who did not take supplements. At the Symposium on Prooxidant Effects of Antioxidant Vitamins[38] (cited in Kim et al.,[65] p. 1199S), Kim confirmed and extended this finding indicating that supplements help some, harm others, and have no effect on most; so the bottom line is a wash.

21.13 DIET

Many substances found in foods may reduce the occurrence of heart disease and malignancy; few are vitamins. Supplementing the diet with vitamins is a totally inadequate substitute for the beneficial effects of a balanced diet rich in grains, fruits, and vegetables, and moderate in milk and milk products, which are the main American source of absorbable calcium, and meat and meat products, which are the main American source of absorbable iron (five times as absorbable as plant iron) and of vitamin B_{12}).

21.14 PGA AND CRYSTALLINE VITAMIN B_{12}

For the health and safety of elderly people, folate (PGA—pteroylglutamic acid) food fortification or supplements must always be accompanied by crystalline vitamin B_{12}.

Holotranscobalamin II* (holo TCII) is a surrogate Schilling test, in that it becomes low within a week after cessation of absorption of food vitamin B_{12} usually because of gastric atrophy sufficient to stop production of gastric acid and enzymes.[35,58] Flynn et al.[18] found in 171 (139 men, 32 women) healthy elderly Missouri Caucasians (mean age 65) that 49% had low (below 60 pg/ml serum) holo TCII, meaning they were no longer able to absorb food vitamin B_{12}; 52 (60%) also had vasculotoxically high serum homocysteine (Hcy) (>17.5 nmol/ml). Of these 52, only 7 also had low total serum vitamin B_{12} (<200 pg/ml). The remaining 31 who had reduced food B_{12} absorption, as measured by holoTC < 60 pg/ml, did not yet have high Hcy. All 171 had normal red cell folate (>136 ng/ml) and serum folate >1.6 ng/ml. Flynn et al. are conducting a follow-up study with Green and colleagues at University of California, Davis[24,50] to determine how much of this gastric atrophy is of the genetically predisposed variety, how much is due to *Helicobacter pylori*, and how much to both. The data support that, starting at age 50, older people should take a daily oral supplement of not less than 25 or more than 100 µg of crystalline B_{12}. This recommendation, and the reasons for it, are embodied in a petition to the FDA by Herbert and Bigaouette.[54] White the vitamin B_{12} DRI[21] of 2.4 µg/day will suffice in elderly people for the years that the gastric atrophy has not yet proceeded to loss of gastric intrinsic factor (IF), once IF is finally lost, physiological absorption of vitamin B_{12} ceases and the only mechanism remaining for absorption of oral vitamin B_{12} is pharmacologic mass action diffusion, which produces absorption of 1% of any oral dose.[16,27,35]

As first suggested by Hibbard and Smithells,[59] confirmed by many others since,[74] and reviewed by Eskes,[17] about half of newborns with neural tube defects (NTD) can have their NTDs prevented if their mothers take folic acid supplements starting a few months before becoming pregnant. The neural tube forms so early in pregnancy that it may be deformed before a woman knows she is pregnant.[15,76]

Folate-preventable NTDs (and some other birth defects)[17] are related to a defect in the genes for 5, 6, 7, 8-tetrahydrofolate reductase, a defect that makes the reductase

---

* As of 1998, the Roman numeral II is no longer used.

thermolabile.[63] The genetic defect is homozygous in 5% of Americans,[63] including, of course, elderly people, and is overcome by supplying daily above-physiological amounts of folate.[73] This, plus other considerations[55,81] makes folate supplements in elderly people appropriate. The physiological minimum amount of folate (as synthetic pteroylglutamic acid, PGA) needed orally daily to prevent folate deficiency in healthy nonpregnant adult females with no known genetic defect is only 50 pg.[45] PGA (a synthetic oxidized monoglutamate) is about twice as stable and well absorbed as food folates (reduced folate PGA).[64,83]

Spearheaded by the CDC's Godfrey Oakley (1997), folate (PGA) fortification of all fortified grains (breads, cereals, and pastas) to prevent NTDs became U.S. FDA law in January 1998.[19] Supplements containing 400 pg PGA daily were (and are) also heavily promoted (Oakley 1997). PGA, the synthetic oxidized folate monoglutamate, is used because of its shelf-stability,[47] a property that Colman et al.[14] has successfully used to fortify grain with PGA in a large study in South Africa more than two decades ago. Synthetic PGA is a racemic, and it is possible the human-active isomer given alone would be safer.

A caveat is that when 400 µg of PGA is ingested, it is a little too much to be polyglutamated and reduced to natural forms in the process of absorption, resulting in absorption of some unaltered synthetic PGA, which may act as an antifol.[50,63]

If folate fortification (and supplementation) does not also include adding crystalline vitamin B_{12}, millions of elderly people (as well as fertile females of black heritage) will be harmed. Fortification with B_{12} is necessarily not only because it is cost-effective,[35] but also because current screening tests for total serum vitamin B_{12} have poor positive and negative predictive value,[24] and assays for homocysteine and methionine are confounded by a number of variables.[24] As Green et al.[24] state, "Some clinical evidence supports the concept that measurements of holo-TCII levels may provide a better index of cobalamin status, but reliable commercial screening assays for holo-TCII have just become available."*

Fertile females of black African descent rarely have the gene defect for folate-preventable NTD babies, but do have a different gene defect: one for early pernicious anemia (PA), as described in fertile South African Black females,[60,70] and fertile U.S. Afro-American females[11]) reviewed in References 35 and 49). In such women, PGA will mask the hematological damage of their vitamin B_{12} deficiency, slowing the diagnosis of B_{12} deficiency until well after they develop B_{12} deficiency neurological damage, some of it irreversible. One such woman[8] diagnosed at age 33 with PA (with combined system disease) and only sporadically treated, who had serum antibody to intrinsic factor, gave birth at age 40 to a child with temporary vitamin B_{12} deficiency associated with transplacentally acquired antibody to intrinsic factor.

Ever since Combe in the 1820s and Addison in the 1850s first described PA, it has been generally recognized that PA is intimately associated with gastric atrophy and is a disease primarily of elderly people. Partly on a genetically predisposed basis and partly due to acquired gastric insults (such as iron deficiency,

---

* HoloTC commercial assays are available in Europe from Axis-Shield ASA of Oslo, Norway, and in the United States from ICN Diagnostics at www.icndiagnostics.com.

H. pylori, etc.), gastric atrophy begins in nearly all Americans sometime between age 50 and 90, and gradually progresses, first with loss of gastric acid and pepsin, causing inability to split B_{12} from its peptide bonds in food, and then, after a number of years, loss of gastric intrinsic factor, producing inability to absorb crystalline B_{12} by the efficient physiological mechanism, but still able to absorb about 1% of any oral dose of crystalline B_{12} by simple mass action diffusion (see Reference 30 for citations).

To care for those elderly people who have lost only gastric acid and pepsin, the DRI[21] for vitamin B_{12} states: "The RDA [Recommended Dietary Allowance) for adults is 2.4 μg of B_{12}/day. Since 10 to 30 percent of older people [i.e., those over age 50] may be unable to absorb naturally occurring B_{12} normally, it is advisable for those older than 50 years to meet their RDA mainly by taking foods fortified with [crystalline] B_{12} or a [crystalline] B_{12} containing supplement." Intake of 100 μg of vitamin B_{12} orally daily is able to reduce their hyperhomocysteinemia.[20,52] This was easily predictable, since patients with PA absorb by mass action about 1% of any oral dose of crystalline vitamin B_{12},[39] and only 0.1 μg of cobalamin must be absorbed daily to sustain normality.[88]

In those elderly people who have lost intrinsic factor secretion, eating 25 μg vitamin B_{12} will result in absorption of about 0.25 μg and eating 100 μg will result in absorption of about 1 μg. Although the MDR (minimum daily absorbed requirement) to sustain normality is only 0.1μg,[35] when a multivitamin pill containing the RDA for iron, 200 mg of vitamin C, and the RDA for B_{12} and folate dissolves in the stomach, within 30 min (the gastric half-emptying time) the vitamin C and iron destroy about half the B_{12} and 20% of the folate[36] because of "vitamin C–driven free radical generation from iron."[36] Worse, the vitamin C and iron convert the B_{12} to anti-B_{12} molecules, which are absorbed with the undestroyed B_{12} and prevent call uptake of the undestroyed B_{12}.[36] For these reasons, supplements of vitamin B_{12} should be taken alone, and taken either on wakening or between meals (so as not to attach to the protein in meals and thus become unabsorbable).[36a-c]

Kuzminski et al.[68] reported that 1 mg oral B_{12} daily was better than 1 mg injections monthly for treating B_{12} deficiency. This is because daily oral B_{12} produces a sustained normal serum vitamin B_{12} level, rather than the roller-coaster serum up-and-down level produced by monthly injections.[28] Daily to weekly intranasal B_{12} is also an option, especially for those with disorders producing generalized intestinal malabsorption. Data suggest that 0.1 mg (100 μg) of oral vitamin B_{12} daily will adequately sustain normal serum levels and in fact will prevent gastric atrophy–associated vitamin B_{12} deficiency from occurring in the first place.[24,35,36a-c,63]

21.15 HERBS AS SUPPLEMENTS

The science of herbs as medicines from natural sources is pharmacognosy, a branch of pharmacology.[4,5,77,89] Herbology is a melange of observation with no controls, anecdote, and misperception of nonspecific coincidence, suggestion, and placebo effect as specific medicinal effect. Herbology is to pharmacognosy what astrology is to astronomy.

To quote Barrett:[4]

> Herbal or other botanical ingredients include processed or unprocessed plant parts (barks, leaves, flowers, fruits, and stems) as well as extracts and essential oils. They are available as teas, powders, tablets, capsules, and elixirs, and may be marketed as single substances or combined with other herbs, vitamins, minerals, amino acids, or non-nutrient ingredients. The fact that an herb is known to be toxic does not ensure its removal from the marketplace ... most published information about herbs is unreliable ... with safe and affective medicine available, treatment with herbs rarely makes sense.

Barrett[4] quotes Tyler[39] as observing:

> More misinformation about safety and efficacy of herbs is reaching the public currently than at any previous time.... The literature promoting herbs includes pamphlets, magazine articles, and books ranging in quality from cheaply printed flyers to elaborately produced studies in fine bindings with attractive illustrations. Practically all these writings recommend large numbers of herbs for treatment based on hearsay, folklore, and tradition. The only criterion that seems to be avoided in these publications is scientific evidence. Some writings are so comprehensive and indiscriminate that they seem to recommend everything for anything. Even deadly poisonous herbs are sometimes touted as remedies, based on some outdated report or a misunderstanding of the facts. Particularly insidious is the myth that there is something almost magical about herbal drugs that prevents them, in their natural state from harming people.

Hemlock is natural. It has been known at least since Socrates that hemlock is a lethal poison. U.S. Senator Hatch's Dietary Supplement and Health Education Act (DSHEA) (characterized in the title of a *New York Times* 1993 editorial as "The Snake Oil Supplement Act"), which became law in 1994, decrees that herbs are foods and not drugs.[5] DSHEA forbids the FDA from protecting the public against the direct marketing of lethal doses of hemlock as a supplement! Brody[9,10] recently reviewed some of the harms from a wide variety of over-the-counter herbs unleashed on the American public by the DSHEA,[9,10] as did Grady.[22] At the other end of the scale, one study of 64 "pure" ginseng products found that 60% of them were so diluted with cheaper herbs as to be worthless.[10]

The bottom line is that definitive studies have yet to be done in the United States to show that popular herbs sold in the United States, none of which have any federal controls on content, such as St. John's wort, ginseng, gingko biloba, kava, saw palmetto, valerian, echinacea, and feverfew, are effective, safe, and do more good than harm. In fact, studies in the United States have shown that almost every brand of any herb sold as a supplement in the United States differs in content, from too little to too much of each active ingredient, from each competing brand. For dietary supplements, the United States is still in the age of the Wild West.[3-5,22,36a]

REFERENCES

1. Anonymous, Why Megadoses of Beta Carotene May Promote Lung Cancer, Food & Nutrition Research Briefs, Agricultural Research Service, U.S. Department of Agriculture, Beltsville, MD, January 1999.
2. Anonymous, A different light trap, *Chem. Eng. News*, 77(6), 1999.
3. Barrett, S., Fad diagnosis: an epidemic of nonsense in nutrition and "fringe" medicine, *Nutr. For.*, 15(6), 41, 42, 44, 1999. (Comprehensive update coverage of harms from dietary supplements and herbs can be accessed on Dr. Barrett's Web site, available at http://www.quackwatch.com.)
4. Barrett, S., The herbal minefield; what we don't know is scary, *Nutr. For.*, 16(1), 5, 1998.
5. Barrett, S. and Herbert V., *The Vitamin Pushers: How the "Health Food" Industry Is Selling America a Bill of Goods*, Prometheus Books, Amherst, NY, 1994.
6. Barrett, S. and Herbert, V., Fads, frauds, and quackery, in *Modern Nutrition in Health and Disease*, Shils, M. E., Olson, J. A., Shike, M., and Ross, A. C., Eds., Williams & Wilkins, Baltimore, MD, 1999, chap. 109.
7. Brin, M., personal comunication, 1999.
8. Bar-Shany, S. and Herbert, V., Transplacentally antibody to intrinsic factor with vitamin B_{12} deficiency, *Blood*, 30, 777, 1967.
9. Brody, J., Americans gamble on herbs as medicine: with few regulations, no guarantee of quality, *New York Times*, 9 February, F1, F7, 1999.
10. Brody, J., Natural, "drug-free" herb may have risks of its own, *New York Times*, 9 February, F6, 1999.
11. Carmel, R. and Johnson, C. S., Racial patterns in pernicious anemia: early age at onset and increased frequency of intrinsic-factor antibody in black women, *N. Engl. J. Med.*, 298, 647, 1978.
11a. Chandra, R. K. Taking multivitamins may reduce sick days, *Lancet*, 340, 1124, 1992.
12. Christen, S., Woodall, A. A., Shigenaga, M. K., Southwell-Keely, P. T., Duncan, N. W., and Ames, B. N., γ-Tocopherol traps mutagenic electrophiles such as NO_x and complements α-tocopherol: physiological implications, *Proc. Natl. Acad. Sci. U.S.A.*, 94, 3217, 1997.
13. Clark, L. C., Combs, G. F., Turnbull B. W., and State, E. H., Selenium supplementation and cancer rates, *JAMA*, 277, 881, 1997.
14. Colman, N., Larson, J. V., Barker, M. et al, Prevention of folate deficiency by food fortification. III. Effect in pregnant subjects of varying amounts of added folic acid, *Am. J. Clin. Nutr.*, 28, 465, 1975.
15. Czeizel, A. E. and Dudas, I., Prevention of the first occurrence of neural tube defects by periconceptional vitamin supplementation, *N. Engl. J. Med.*, 327, 1832, 1992.
16. Ellenbogen, L., Herbert, V., and Williams, W. L., Effect of D-sorbitol on absorption of vitamin B_{12} by pernicious anemia patients, *Proc. Soc. Exp. Biol. Med.*, 99, 257, 1958.
17. Eskes, T. K. A. B., Genetic defects, hyperhomocysteinemia, and neural tube defects, *Nutr. Rev.*, 56, 236, 1998.
18. Flynn, M. A., Herbert, V., Nolph, G. B., and Krause, G., Atherogenesis and the homocysteine-folate-cobalamin triad: do we need standardized analysis? *J. Am. Coll. Nutr.*, 16, 258, 1997.
19. Food and Drug Administration, Food standards: amendment of standards of identity for enriched grain products to require addition of folic acid, *Fed. Regis.*, 61, 878, 1996.

20. Food and Nutrition Board, Dietary Reference Intakes for Calcium, Phosphorus, Magnesium, Vitamin D, and Fluoride, National Academy Press, Washington, D.C., 1997.

21. Food and Nutrition Board, Dietary Reference Intakes for Thiamin, Riboflavin, Niacin, Vitamin B_6 Folate, Vitamin B_{12} Pantothenic Acid, Biotin, and Choline, National Academy Press, Washington, D.C., 1998.

22. Grady, D., Articles question safety of dietary supplements: use can endanger lives of ailing people, *New York Times*, 17 September, A23, 1998.

23. Green, R., Screening for vitamin B_{12} deficiency: caveat emptor, *Ann. Intern. Med.*, 124, 509, 1996.

24. Green, R., Miller, J. W., Herbert, V., and Flynn, M. A., Oral vitamin B_{12} supplementation decreases homocysteine in healthy elderly people with suboptimal vitamin B_{12} status, *FASEB J.*, February, 1999.

25. Guzik, H. J., Tommasulo, B. C., Mandel, F. S., Kasdan, T. S., and Herbert, V., Prevalence of negative vitamin B_{12} balance in well- and malnourished frail elderly, *J. Am. Geriatr. Soc.*, 41(10), SA27, 1993.

26. Herbert, V., Cuneen, N., Jaskiel, L., and Kapff, C., Minimal daily adult folate requirements, *Arch. Intern. Med.*, 110, 649, 1962.

27. Herbert, V. et al., Oral treatments of pernicious anemia, *Lancet*, 2, 801, 1958.

28. Herbert, V., *The Megaloblastic Anemias,* Grune & Stratton, New York, 1959.

29. Herbert, V., *Nutrition Cultism; Facts and Fictions,* George Stickly, Philadelphia, 1980.

30. Herbert, V., Pseudovitamins, in *Modem Nutrition in Health and Disease*, 7th ed., Shils, M. E. and Young, V. R., Eds., Lea & Febiger, Philadelphia, 1988.

31. Herbert, V., Folate and neural tube defects, *Nutr. Today*, 27(6), 30, 1992.

32. Herbert, V., Folate deficiency to protect against malaria, *N. Engl. J. Med.*, 328, 1127, 1993.

33. Herbert, V., Vitamin C supplements and disease-counterpoint, *J. Am. Coll. Nutr.*, 14, 2112, 1995.

34. Herbert, V., Chair, Symposium: Prooxidant Effects of Antioxidant Vitamins, *J. Nutr.*, 126 (Suppl.), 1197S, 1996.

34a. Herbert, V., Underreporting of dietary supplements to health care providers does great harm, *Mayo Clinic Proc.*, 74, 531, 1999.

35. Herbert, V., Vitamin B_{12}, in *Present Knowledge in Nutrition*, 7th ed., Ziegler, E. E. and Filer, L. J., Eds., International Life Sciences Institute (ILSI) Press, Washington, D.C., 1996, chap. 20.

36. Herbert, V., Anti-hyperhomocysteinemic supplemental folic acid and vitamin B_{12} are significantly destroyed in gastric juice if co-ingested with supplemental vitamin C and iron, *Blood*, 88 (10 Suppl. 1), 492a (Abstr. 1957), 1996.

36a. Herbert, V., Vitamin B_{12}: an overview, in *Vitamin B_{12} Deficiency,* Herbert, V., Ed., Round Table Series No. 66, Royal Society of Medicine Press, Lohdon, 1999.

36b. Herbert, V., Preventing early morbidity and mortality in millions of elderly, and saving $ billions: new evidence that 100μg free vitamin B_{12} (cobalamin) orally daily from age 50 will prevent gastric atrophy of the elderly from producing subtly progressive B_{12}-deficiency neuropsychiatric dementia and stumbling and later anemia, *FASEB J.*, 14(4), A754, 2000.

36c. Herbert, V., Loss of recent memory (Where in the parking lot is my car? etc.) in persons age >50 is often unrecognized subtle vitamin B_{12} deficiency, producing inadequate synthesis of new brain cells, but no anemia, *FASEB J.*, 15(5), A59, 2001.

37. Herbert, V., Shaw, S., and Jayatilleke, E., Vitamin C-driven free radical generation from iron, *J. Nutr.*, 126 (Suppl. 4), 1213S, 1996. (*Note:* Figure 3 as printed is incorrect; see Errata containing the correct Figure 3 and correct citation to Ames, 1983, published in *J. Nutr.*, 126, 1746, 1996 and Errata adding Herbert, V. to the Ran et al. reference and correcting units of ferritin iron to ng fe/ml of serum, published in *J. Nutr.*, 126, 1902, 1996.)

38. Herbert, V., Introduction. American Institute of Nutrition (AIN) Symposium on Prooxidant Effects of Antioxidant Vitamins, *J. Nutr.*, 126 (Suppl. 4), 1197S, 1996.

39. Herbert V., Anti-hyperhomocysteinemic supplemental folio acid and vitamin B_{12} are significantly destroyed in gastric juice if co-ingested with supplemental vitamin C and iron, *Blood*, 88(10 Suppl. 1), 492a, 1996.

40. Herbert, V., The value of antioxidant supplements vs. their natural counterparts, *J. Am. Diet. Assoc.*, 97, 375, 1997.

41. Herbert, V., Destroying immune homeostasis in normal adults with antioxidant supplements, *Am. J. Clin. Nutr.*, 65, 1901, 1997.

42. Herbert, V., Nutrition status misassessment maims and kills millions, *FASEB J.*, 11(3), A185, 1997.

43. Herbert, V., Genetics determines which supplements are safe (Ex: folate + B_{12} but not folate alone) and which are unsafe (Ex: antioxidants; minerals), in *Proc. 16th International Congress of Nutrition*, (Abstr.), July 27–August 1, 1997, Montreal, Canada. Poster presentation.

43a. Herbert, V., Gene mutations can produce polymorphisms which alter minimal daily micronutrient requirements, *Clin. Invest. Med.*, 24(1), 54–55, 2001.

44. Herbert, V., Fraudulent "alternatives" and scam "supplements" scam millions and steal $ billions, *J. Invest. Med.*, 45, 301S, 1997.

45. Herbert, V., Selenium supplements and cancer rates, *JAMA*, 277, 880, 1997.

46. Herbert, V., The elderly need oral vitamin B_{12}, *Am. J. Clin. Nutr.*, 67, 39, 1998.

47. Herbert, V., A triple hematologic nightmare: grossly underdiagnosing and not treating the most common U.S. genetic disorder (hemochromatosis) and garbaging each year so many tons of good hemochromatosis donor blood as to create donor blood shortages in each of the past 30 years, *Am. J. Hematol.*, 59, 261, 1998.

48. Herbert, V., Relationship of dietary folate and vitamin B_6 with coronary heart disease in women: without vitamin B_{12} supplements, extra folic acid and vitamin B_6 will do elderly women more harm than good, *JAMA*, 280, 418, 1998.

49. Herbert, V., Vitamin E supplementation and immune response in elderly patients, *JAMA*, 279, 505, 1998.

50. Herbert, V., Folic acid, in *Modern Nutrition in Health & Disease*, 9th ed., Shils, M. E., Olson, J. A., Shike M., and Ross, A. C., Eds., Lea & Febiger, Philadelphia, 1999, chap. 26.

51. Herbert, V. and Spivack, M. FDA now approves hemochromatosis blood as normal donor blood. Measuring serum iron status as part of routine blood testing will: 1. prevent phenotypic disease in millions; 2. save healthcare $ billions; 3. end U.S. biannual blood shortages, *J. Invest. Med.*, 49(2), 241A, 2001; *FASEB J.*, 15(5), A973, 2001.

52. Herbert, V., To prevent vasculotoxicity from hyperhomocysteinemia, give children vitamin B_6, give fertile females folate, and give all >50 daily oral 25 to 100 µg vitamin B_{12}, *FASEB J.*, 13(4), A227, 1999.

53. Herbert, V. and Barrett, S., Alternative nutritional therapy claims, in *Modern Nutrition in Health and Disease*, 9th ed., Shils, M. E., Olson, J. A., Shike, M., and Ross, A. C., Eds., Williams & Wilkins, Baltimore, MD, 1999, chap. 110.

54. Herbert, V. and Bigaouette, J., Call for endorsement of a petition to the Food and Drug Administration to always add vitamin B_{12} to any folate fortification supplement, *Am. J. Clin. Nutr.*, 65, 572, 1997.

55. Herbert, V. and Das, K. S., Folic acid and vitamin B_{12}, in *Modern Nutrition in Health and Disease*, 8th ed., Lea & Febiger, Philadelphia, 1994, 402–425.

56. Herbert, V. and Kasdan, T. S., Misleading nutrition claims and their gurus, *Nutr. Today*, 2 (3), 28, 1994.

57. Herbert, V., Flynn, M. A., Nolph, G. A., and Krause, G., 50% of healthy American elderly have low serum transcobalamin, diagnosing reduced vitamin B_{12} absorption; 60% also have high serum homocysteine; none have low red cell folate; all elderly should get 25 to 100 µg oral free crystalline vitamin B_{12} daily as food fortificant or supplement, *Neth. J. Med. Sci.*, 52 (Suppl.), S8, 1998.

58. Herzlich, B. and Herbert, V., Depletion of serum holotranscobalamin II. An early sign of negative vitamin B_{12} balance, *Lab. Invest.*, 58, 332, 1988.

59. Hibbard, E. D. and Smithells, R. W., Folic acid metabolism and human embryopathy, *Lancet*, 1, 1254, 1965.

60. Hift, W., Moshal, M. G., and Pillay, K., Pernicious anaemia-like syndromes in the nonwhite population of Natal, *S. Afr. Med. J.*, 21, 915, 1963.

61. Horwitt, M. K., My valedictory on the differences in biological potency between RRR-α-tocopherol and all-rac-α-tocopherlol acetate, *Am. J. Clin. Nutr.*, 69, 2, 341, 1999.

62. Institute of Medicine, Panel on Folate, Other B Vitamins, and Choline, Dietary Reference Intakes: Thiamin, Riboflavin, Vitamin B_6 Folate, Vitamin B_{12} Pantothemic Acid, Biotin, and Choline, National Academy Press, Washington, D.C., 1998.

63. Kang, S. S., Wong, P. W. K., and Malinow, M. R., Homocysteinemia as a risk factor for occlusive vascular disease, *Annu. Rev. Nutr.*, 12, 279, 1992.

64. Kelly, P., McPartlin, J., Goggins, M., Weir, D. G., and Scott, J. M., Unmetabolized folic acid in serum: acute studies in subjects consuming fortified food and supplements, *Am. J. Clin. Nutr.*, 65, 1790, 1997.

65. Kim, I., Williamson, D. F., Byers, T., and Koplan, J. P., Vitamin and mineral supplement use and mortality in a U.S. cohort, *Am. J. Publ. Health*, 83, 546, 1993.

66. Kolata, G., Drug or food? Patients stumble into gray area, *The New York Times*, 9 February, F6, 1999.

67. Kuller, L. H., Selenium supplementation and cancer rates, *JAMA*, 277, 880, 1997.

68. Kuzminski, A. M., Del Giacco, E. J., Allen, R. H. et al., Effective treatment of cobalamin deficiency with oral cobalamin, *Blood*, 92, 1191, 1998.

69. Levine, M., Conry-Cantilena, C., Wang, Y., Welch, R. W., Wanshko, P. W., Dhariwal, K. R., Park, J. B., Lararev, A., Graumlich, J. F., King, J., and Cantilena, L. R., Vitamin C pharmokinetics in healthy volunteers: evidence for a recommended dietary allowance, *Proc. Natl. Acad. Sci. U.S.A.*, 93(8), 3704, 1996.

70. Metz, J., Randall, T. W., and Kniep, C. H., Addisonian pernicious anemia in young Bantu females, *Br. Med. J.*, 1, 178, 1961.

71. McCoy, M., Chemical makers try biotech paths, *Chem. Eng. News*, 22 June, 13, 1998.

72. McCully, K. S., Relationship of dietary folate and vitamin B_6 with coronary heart disease in women, *JAMA*, 280, 419, 1998.

73. Molloy, A. M., Daly, S., Mills, J. L. et al., Thermolabile variant of 5-10 MTHFR associated with low red cell folate: implications for folate intake recommendations, *Lancet*, 349, 1591, 1997.

74. MRC Vitamin Study Research Group, Prevention of neural tube defects: results of the Medical Research Council Vitamin Study, *Lancet*, 338, 131, 1991.

75. Nielsen, F. H., Chromium, in *Modern Nutrition in Health and Disease*, 9th ed., Shils, E., Olson, J. A., and Shike, M., Eds., Lea & Febiger, Philadelphia, 1999.

76. Oakley, G. P., Jr., Let's increase folio acid fortification and include vitamin B_{12}, *Am. J. Clin. Nutr.*, 65, 1889, 1997.

77. PDR, *PDR (Physicians' Desk Reference) for Herbal Medicines*, Gruenwald, J., Ed., Medical Economics Company, Montvale, NJ, 1998, medical director of a German phytomedicine company. On page iv, it is stated that "The publisher has performed no independent verification of the data reported herein...." The book updates the German Commission E reports, and adds hundreds of other products sold in the United States, listing alleged effects and side effects, and some contraindications.

78. Podmore, I., Griffiths, H., Herbert, K., Mistry, N., Mistry, P., and Lunec, J., Vitamin C exhibits pro-oxidant properties, *Nature*, 392, 559, 1998.

79. Ran, J. Y., Dou, P., Wang, L. Y., Qin, Y., Jin, S. Y., Li, X. F., and Herbert, V., Correlation of low serum folate and total B_{12} with high incidence of esophageal carcinoma (EC) in Shanxi, China, *Blood*, 82 (Suppl. 1), 532a, 1993.

80. Ran, J. Y., Dou, P., Wang, L. Y., Yuan, R. X., Hao, J. M., Zhang, H., Jin, S. Y., Li, P., Qin, Y., and Herbert, V., In a high-frequency esophageal carcinoma (EC) area, folate and B_{12} deficient subjects with esophageal dysplasia (ED) improve with added folate and B_{12}, *Blood*, 82 (Suppl. 1), 532a, 1993.

81. Rimm, E. B., Willet, W. X., Hu, F. B., Colditz, G. A., Sampson, L., Manson, J. E., Hennekens, C. H., and Stampfer, M., Relationship of dietary folate and vitamin B_6 with coronary heart disease in women, *JAMA*, 280, 418, 1998.

82. Russell, R., Mild cobalamin deficiency in older Dutch subjects., *Am. J. Clin. Nutr.*, 68, 222, 1998.

83. Seyoum, E. and Selhub, J., Properties of food folates determined by stability and susceptibility to intestinal pteroylpolyglutamate hydrolase action, *J. Nutr.*, 12B, 1956, 1998.

84. Simopoulos, A., Herbert, V., and Jacobson, B., *Genetic Nutrition: Designing a Diet Based on Your Family Medical History*, Macmillan, New York, 1993. (Reprinted in 1995 as a text-unchanged softcover with a new title *The Healing Diet: How to Reduce Your Risks and Live a Healthier Life If You Have a Family History of Cancer, Heart Disease Hypertension, Diabetes, Alcoholism, Obesity, Food Allergies*.)

85. Steiner, M., Vitamin E inhibits blood coagulation, *J. Am. Coll. Nutr.*, 10, 466, 1991.

86. Steiner, J., personal comunication, 1999.

87. Stephens, N. G. et al., Vitamin E and mortality, *Lancet*, 347, 781, 1996.

88. Sullivan, L. W. and Herbert, V., Studies on the minimum daily requirement for vitamin B_{12} hematopoietic responses to 0.1 microgram of cyanocobalamin or coenzyme B_{12} and comparison of their relative potency, *N. Engl. J. Med.*, 272, 340, 1965.

89. Foster, S. and Tyler, V., *Tyler's Honest Herbal*, 4th ed., Haworth Press, Binghamton, NY, 1999.

90. Van Asselt, D. Z. B., De Groot, L. C. P. G. M., Van Stavere, W. A., Blom, H. J., Wevers, R. A., Biemond, I., and Hoefnagels, W. H. L., Role of cobalamin intake and atrophic gastritis in mild cobalamin deficiency in older Dutch subjects, *Am. J. Clin. Nutr.*, 68, 328, 1998.

91. Virtamo, J., Rapola, J. M., Ripatti, S., Heinonen, O., Taylor, P. R., Albanes, D., and Huttunen, J K., Effect of vitamin E and beta carotene on the incidence of primary nonfatal myocardial infarction and fatal coronary heart disease, *Arch. Intern. Med.*, 158, 668, 1998.

Index

A

ABAB statistical design, 301
Aboulia, 345
Acoustical normalization, 155
Activities of daily living (ADL), 330
    instrumental, 330
Adler, Alfred (1870–1937), 16
Administration, modes of drug, 311–312
Adolescents, frontalization of motor
        functions in, 139–140
Adrenocortical system, early work on, 26
ADS Test, 270–271
Affective anosognosia (unawareness of
        deficit), 246
Affective disorders, *see also* specific
        disorders
    in narcolepsy–cataplexy syndrome, 229
    in sleep apnea syndrome, 228–229
    sleep disorders and, 231–233
Affective, emotional, and personality
        assessment, 245–246, 265–267
Age-associated memory impairment
        (AAMI), 279–286, 327, 382–385,
        see also Mild cognitive impairment
Aggressive behavior
    in cerebrovascular disease, 342–344
    as co-morbid condition, 186, 187
Aging
    analytic perspective, 15–18, *see also*
        Analytic perspective
    cognitive changes with normal, 85–108,
        111–112–114, *see also under*
        Cognitive dysfunction
    contemporary views, 20–21
    decremental theory of, 134
    development concept of, 126
    historical perspective on, 3–15, *see also*
        Historical perspective
    modern developments related to, 18–20
    pharmacokinetics in, 27–28
    as related to disease, 29–30
    sleep changes in normal, 204–206,
        see also Sleep disorders

    sociocultural attitudes toward, 133–134,
        172, 187–188, 197, 380
Aging Associated Cognitive Decline
        (AACD), 217–218
Agitation, 119, 194
    nocturnal, 214
    vs. mania, 186
Agnosia, 246
    DSM-IV criteria, 326
Agoraphobia vs. cerebrovascular disease,
        340
Akinetic mutism, 345
Alcohol/alcohol abuse, 189, 195, *see also*
        Substance abuse
    frontal lobe atrophy in, 77–78
    history, 246–247
    sleep-related side effects, 209
α-tocopherol vs. γ-tocopherol, 428
Alprazolam, 314, *see also*
        Benzodiazepines
Alzheimer's disease (AD), 29, *see also*
        Dementia
    aggression in, 187
    Biondi ring tangles in, 71
    cerebral atrophy in, 68
    corpus callosum atrophy in, 75–76
    depression in, 185–186, 189, 192–193
    diagnostic criteria for, 138, 267–268
    diagnostic language deficits in, 246
    differential diagnosis, 29
    economic impact of early diagnosis, 283
    epidemiology, 43–46
    executive dysfunction in, 219
    family response to, 194–196
    frontal variant of, 78
    language deterioration in, 159, 166,
        173–175
    limb apraxia studies in, 142, 143–145
    manual-skills decline as diagnostic, 138
    memory dysfunction in, 112–113, 385
    mild cognitive impairment (MCI) and,
        279–286, *see also* Mild cognitive
        impairment

neuropsychiatric symptoms in, 119
sleep disorders in, 214–215
vs. depressive dysfunction, 329
Amantadine
in multiple sclerosis, 419
in Parkinson's disease, 314
American Geriatrics Society, 24
American Psychological Association, 20
4-Aminopyridine, in multiple sclerosis, 419
Amnesia, 380
anterograde, 380
focal retrograde, 380
post-traumatic, 380
retrograde, 381
sleep medications and, 226
transient global, 381
Amyloid plaques, 282–283, 358
Analytic perspective, 15–18
Charlotte Bühler's "Course of Life,"
16–17
Erikson's views, 17–18
Anesthetics, cognitive side effects of topical,
319
Angiopathy, amyloid, 282–283, 358
Anisotropy, diffusional, 73–74
Anopsia, 272
Anosognosia, affective (unawareness of
deficit), 246
Anterograde amnesia, 380
Antiaging medicines, 31–32
Antibiotics, drug interactions of, 319
Anticholinergics
aging and pharmacokinetics of, 42
sleep-related side effects, 209
Anticoagulants, in cerebrovascular disease,
359
Anticonvulsants
cognitive effects of, 248
in epilepsy, 406–409
in multiple sclerosis, 420
Antidepressants, 315–317, 364–368
cyclical and heterocyclical, 365–366
dosage considerations, 349
MAO inhibitors, 314, 350, 359, 366
memory impairment and, 388
novel, 367–368
mirtazepine, 367–368
nefazodone, 368
rebazetine, 368
stimulants and lithium, 368

venlafaxine, 367
selective serotonin reuptake inhibitors
(SSRIs), 349–350, 366–367
tricyclic, 349–350, 365–366
Antihistamines, in multiple sclerosis, 419
Antihypertensives
memory impairment and, 388
side effects, 248
cognitive, 318–319
sleep-related, 209
Antineoplastics, sleep-related side effects,
209
Antioxidants, dietary, 426, see also Dietary
supplements
Antiparkinsonian drugs, 42, 313–314
sleep-related side effects, 209
Antipsychotics, see Neuroleptics
Anxiety
as co-morbid condition, 186–187
vs. cerebrovascular disease, 340
Anxiolytics, 314–315
adverse effects of, 42
in insomnia, 226
Apathy
in cerebrovascular disease, 345–347
vs. depression, 345
Aphasia, 173–175, 271
in Alzheimer's disease (AD), 246
in cerebrovascular disease, 346
DSM-IV criteria, 326
Apolipoprotein A, 46
Apolipoprotein E, white matter
hyperintensity and, 70
Approximation to validity, 292
Apraxia, 140–141, 246, see also Motor
functions
conceptual, 141
DSM-IV criteria, 326
gait, 141
limb, 141–143
melokinetic, 140
Aristotle (Greek philosopher), 5, 187
Arizona Long-Term Care System (ALCS),
289
Arteriosclerosis, vascular dementia and,
353–356, see also Vascular
dementia
Assessment, 243–277
affective, emotional, and personality
problems, 265–267

attentional processes, 253–254
baseline, 244–251
  premorbid intellectual functioning,
    248–249
  psychological and health biography,
    245–248
  social and work history, 249–250
in cerebrovascular disorders, 271–272
for dementia, 329–334
  clinical history, 330
  examination (neurological
    exploration), 332
  tests and modalities, 332–334, *see also*
    specific methods
of dementing processes, 267–271
  cognitive symptoms, 268
  functional alterations, 269–271
  psychiatric and behavioral symptoms,
    268–269
for depression, 348
of emotional disturbance, 184, 186
of executive functioning, 259–262
  digits backward test, 262
  frontal lobe functions (Tower of
    Hanoi/Seville), 260–261
  neurocognitive interference (Stroop
    effect), 259–260
  Trail Making Test, 261
of intellectual functioning, 251–253
  Raven's Progressive Matrices,
    77, 253
  Wechsler Adult Intelligence Scale
    (WAIS), 89–90, 157–158,
    216–217, 251–253
of intervention programs, 287–307,
    see also Statistical issues; Validity
  conceptual foundations of validity,
    290–294
  concluding remarks, 303–304
  design issues for improving, 294–302
  importance of, 289–290
  methodological implications,
    302–303
  overview, 288–289
of language, 257–258
  Boston Naming Test, 258
  verbal fluency, 257–258
of memory processes, 254–256, 390
  Functional Organic Memory
    Questionnaire (FOM), 255–256

  verbal memory and learning,
    254–255
  Wechsler Memory Scales–Revised,
    256
MicroCog software for, 90–91
of mild cognitive impairment (MCI),
    279–286, *see also* Mild cognitive
    impairment
for multiple sclerosis, 416–417
reliability and validity issues in, 251
of sensory and motor skills, 283–285
of sleep disorders, 227
in traumatic brain injury, 272
for vascular dementia, 358–359
of visuoperceptive and visuoconstructive
    processes, 262–263
Assisted living, 197, 232
Associated pairs task, 391–392
Asthma medications, sleep-related side
    effects, 209
Asymptomatic carotid stenosis, 338
Atrophy
  cerebral, 67–79, 68–69, 380
  gastric, 431, 432–433
Attention, 102, 215
  changes in normal aging, 102, 103
  disengagement deficit, 102
  divided, 102
  language and, 155, 156
  in patients with epilepsy, 404
  selective, 102
  transient visual, 100, 101
Attentional processes assessment, 253–254
Auditory changes, in normal aging, 87–88
Auditory impairment, language and,
    154–155
Auditory stimulation, therapeutic reduction
    of, 119
Automatic vs. effortful processing, 98
Autonomic dysfunction, in multiple
    sclerosis, 421

B

Baclofen, in multiple sclerosis, 419
Bacon, Sir Francis (1561–1626), 8–10
Baltimore Longitudinal Study on Aging
    (BLSA), 24, 25
Barona Estimation of Premorbid IQ,
    248–249

Barthel Index for Daily Living Activity, 269
Basal ganglia
    aging and, 78–80
    in motor function, 129
Baseline assessment, 244–251
    premorbid intellectual functioning,
        248–249
    psychological and health biography,
        245–248
    social and work history, 249–250
β-blockers, sleep-related side effects, 209
Beck Depression Inventory (BDI),
    269–270
Behavioral side effects, of pharmacologic
    treatment, 318–319
Behavioral therapy, 372
Behavioral training, in memory disorders,
    391–393
Behaviorism, 19
Benign multiple sclerosis, 414
Benign senescent forgetfulness, *see* Mild
    cognitive impairment
Benton's Visual Retention test, 158
Benzodiazepines, 313, 314–315
    aging and pharmacology of, 42
    in insomnia, 226
β-carotene, 428
Bias
    cultural, *see* Cultural bias
    medical against case studies, 191
Binswanger's disease, 355, 357
Biological markers, 284, 333
Biondi ring tangles, in Alzheimer's disease
    (AD) vs. normal aging, 71
Biopsy, brain, in dementia evaluation,
    333
Biosynthesized vs. chemically synthesized
    dietary supplements, 427
Bipolar disorder, 368, *see also* Affective
    disorders
    in cerebrovascular disease, 347, 349
Birren, James E., 24
Bladder dysfunction, in multiple sclerosis,
    420–421
Blessed Scale of Deterioration, 269
Blindness, cortical, 272
Body deterioration theory of aging, 9
Body-part-as-object (BPO) response,
    143–145
Boston Naming Test, 158, 166, 258

Bowel dysfunction, in multiple sclerosis,
    421
Brain, neuroanatomy of functional aging,
    67–81
    basal ganglia and cerebellum, 78–80
    cerebral atrophy in elderly persons,
        68–69, 380
    cerebral ventricles, 71–74
    corpus callosum, 74–76
    frontal lobe, 77–78
    limbic structures, 76
    other structures, 80
    white and gray matter, 69, 70, 72, 338
Brain biopsy, in dementia evaluation,
    333
Brain imaging, in dementia, 333
Brain injury, traumatic, *see* Traumatic brain
    injury
Broca's aphasia, 271
Bromocriptine, in Parkinson's disease,
    314
Buffon, Comte de (Georges Leclerc,
    1707–1788), 10–11
Bühler, Charlotte (1883–1974), 16–17
Buspirone, in aggressive conduct, 343
Busse, Ewald, 24
Butterfly-wing infarctions, 346
Butters, Dr. Nelson, 191

C

Cabanis, Pierre Jean (1757–1808), 11–12
CADASIL (cerebral autosomic dominant
        angiopathy with subcortical
        infarctions and leukoencelopathy),
        357–358
Caffeine, sleep-related side effects, 209
Calcium-channel blockers
    drug interactions, 319
    in vascular dementia, 359
Calcium supplements, 429–430
CAMDEX criteria for vascular dementia,
    270, 351
Caplan's criteria, for leukoaraiosis, 357
Carbamazepine, *see also* Anticonvulsants
    in aggressive conduct, 343
    cognitive effects of, 407
Cardiac medications
    cognitive side effects, 319
    side effects, 248

Cardiovascular disease
  cognitive performance and, 220
  as risk factor, 389
Carotid stenosis, asymptomatic, 338
Case studies, lack of in scientific literature,
    191
Caudate nuclei infarctions, 346
Cerami, Anthony, 25
Cerebellum, aging and, 78–80
Cerebral atrophy, 67–79, 380, *see also*
    Brain, neuroanatomy of functional
    aging
Cerebral blood flow
  age-related changes in, 380–381
  medications increasing, 359
Cerebral cortex, *see* Cortex; Cortical entries
Cerebral ventricles, aging and, 71–74
Cerebrolysin, 318
Cerebrovascular disease, 337–362
  assessment of, 271–272
  classification of, 338–342
  neuropsychiatric syndromes in, 342–350,
    see also Vascular dementia
    aggressive behavior, 342–344
    apathy, 345–347
    depression, 347–350
    emotional incontinence, 344–345
    fatigue, 347
    nonobvious, 339
    suicide risk and, 349
    TIAs and, 339–340
    vascular dementia in, 43–46, 351–360,
      see also Vascular dementia
    vitamin E and risk of stroke, 427
    white matter hyperintensity
      (leukoaraiosis) and, 69, 70, 72, 338
Charcot, Jean Marie, 29
Chemotherapy-related encephalopathy, 319
Choline, as mechanism in memory
    disorders, 394–395
Choroid plexus, Biondi ring tangles in, 71
Chromium supplements, 430
Circadian sleep–wake rhythms, 205–206,
    211
Circumlocution, 164
Citalopram, 366–367, *see also*
    Antidepressants; Selective
    serotonin reuptake inhibitors
Clobazam, cognitive effects of, 407
Clozapine, in aggressive conduct, 343

Cocaine, 247, *see also* Substance abuse
Cognition-enhancing (nootropic) drugs,
    318, 391
Cognitive and behavioral side effects, of
    pharmacologic treatment, 318–319
Cognitive–behavioral psychotherapy,
    372–374
Cognitive function
  limbic structure and, 76
  sleep disorders and, 223–233
  ventricular size and, 72–73
Cognitive impairment
  in depression, 232–233
  in epilepsy, aging and, 405–406
  executive dysfunction
    assessment of, 259–262, *see also under*
      Assessment
    effect on family of, 118
    in frontal lobe dementia and Pick's
      disease, 114
    interventions for, 118–119
    neuropsychology of, 113–116
    in normal aging, 100–101, 113–114,
      218–219
    in Parkinson's disease, 114–115
    prefrontal zone atrophy and, 78
    in traumatic brain injury, 115–116
  frontal lobe atrophy and, 77
  language and, 154–161
    attention and memory, 155–157
    contextual aspects of, 157–161
    motor deficiencies, 157
    visual and auditory perceptual
      impairments, 154–155
  memory dysfunction, *see also* Memory
    entries
    in Alzheimer's disease (AD), 112–113
    interventions for, 116–117
    neuropsychology of, 111–113
    in normal aging, 111–112
  in multiple sclerosis, 420
  neuropsychology of, 111–116, *see also*
    Executive functioning; Memory
    dysfunction
  of normal aging (mild cognitive
    impairment), 215–223
    in attention, 102, 103
    cognitive performance pattern,
      215–218
    general cognitive changes, 99–92

general processing resources, 92–96
general sensory changes, 86–88, 103
in memory, 96–99, 103, 219
neural basis of, 220–223
reasoning and frontal aging hypothesis,
100–102, 103
sleep disorders and, 223–231, *see also
under* Sleep disorders
summary and conclusions, 102–104
in visuospatial processing, 99–100, 103
of normal aging (mild cognitive
impairment), 85–108, 215–223,
279–286, 327
transient, 405
Cognitively Impaired, Not Demented
(CIND) classification, 218
Cognitive therapy, *see* Psychotherapy
Cohort defined, 300
Color vision, 86
Communication
importance of, 28
language as aspect of, 152–153
Comorbidity
depression and dementia, 48–49
emotional disorders and, 184–187
manic syndromes and dementia, 48
Comparison (recognition) cycle, 93–94
Compensation
for language deficits, 170–173
in memory disorders, 117, 386–387
Computed tomography (CT scan)
in cerebrovascular disease, 338, 340
in dementia evaluation, 333
Conceptual apraxia, 141
Confabulation, 380
Confrontation naming, 98
Constructive praxias, 268
Construct validity, 291
Consultations and referrals history, 245
Continuous positive airway pressure (nasal
CPAP), in sleep apnea, 228
Controlled Oral Word Association Test/FAS
(COWAT/FAS), 257–258
Corpus callosum, aging and, 74–76
Cortex, motor, 127–129, *see also* Motor
cortex
Cortical blindness, 272
Cortical dementia of Alzheimer's type, *see*
Alzheimer's disease (AD)
Cotman, Carol W., 26

Cross modal priming studies, 162
Crying, pathological, 344
Crystal vs. fluid intelligence, 217
Cultural bias, 133–134, 172, 187–188, 197,
380
intellectual in Western medicine, 187–188
toward aging and elderly, 133–134, 172,
187–188, 197
toward mental illness, 189
Current Contents database, 295–297
Cyclandelate, 359
Cytidinediphosphocholine (CDPc), in
memory disorders, 394–397

D

Darwin, Charles (1809–1822), 3–4, 13
Databases, for evaluation of interventions,
295–297
Death, causes of, 30
de Beauvoir, Simone, 7
Declarative (explicit) memory, 383
Decremental theory of aging, 134
Degenerative diseases, dementia in, 325
Delirious ideas, in vascular dementia,
359–360
Delirium (acute confusional syndrome), 327
Delirium tremens, 247
Delusions/hallucinations, 119
Dementia, *see also* Executive functioning;
specific disorders
assessment of processes, 267–271
cognitive symptoms, 268
functional alterations, 269–271
psychiatric and behavioral symptoms,
268–269
clinical assessment, 329–334
clinical history, 330
examination (neurological
exploration), 332
tests and modalities, 332–334, *see also*
specific methods
as comorbidity
in depression, 48–49
with manic syndromes, 48
cortical of Alzheimer's type, see
Alzheimer's disease (AD)
definition and severity, 42–43, 324
with depression, 368
depressive pseudodementia, 233, 329

diagnostic criteria, 326–327
differential diagnosis, 327–329
  age-related cognitive deterioration, 327
  age-related memory impairment, 327
  delirium (acute confusional syndrome),
    328
  depression, 328–329
  focal cerebral syndromes, 328
  vs. medication effects, 42, *see also*
    Medication side effects
epidemiologic studies 1995-2000, 56–65
epidemiology
  incidence, 43
  prevalence, 44–45
  risk factors, 45–46
etiology, 324–325
executive dysfunction in, 114
family response to, 194–196
groups affected by, 50
impairments falling short of, 217–218
limited, *see* Mild cognitive impairment
mild, *see* Mild cognitive impairment
minimal, *see* Mild cognitive impairment
mixed, 351
multi-infarction, 344, *see also*
    Cerebrovascular disease; Vascular
    dementia
neuropsychiatric symptoms of,
    interventions for, 119
phenytoin-related, 407
in primary care, 323–336
questionable, *see* Mild cognitive
    impairment
secondary to potentially treatable
    processes, 334
sleep disorders in, 213, 214–215
vascular, *see* Vascular dementia
Demographics, 37–41, *see also*
    Epidemiology
Demyelinating disease, 70, *see also* specific
    diseases
Dentures, as related to oral praxis skills, 137
Dependency, *see also* Substance abuse
  on benzodiazepines, 315
Deprenyl, 314
Depression, 189
  anxiety coexisting with, 186
  assessment instruments for, 269–270
  bipolar, 347, 349, 368
  in cerebrovascular disease, 347–350

characteristics particular to elderly, 47
as co-morbid condition, 48–49, 185–186,
    368
electroconvulsive therapy (ECT) in, 350,
    368–369
emotional incontinence (emotional
    lability) and, 344
epidemiology, 46–48
in family members, 195
fatigue and, 347
mortality and, 47–48
in multiple sclerosis, 419–420
in narcolepsy–cataplexy syndrome, 229
in obsessive–compulsive disorder,
    190–191
postinfarction, 347–348
sleep apnea syndrome and, 228
sleep disorders and, 231–232
subsyndromal, 231
in traumatic brain injury, 116
treatment of, 363–378
  electroconvulsive therapy (ECT), 350,
    368–369
  pharmacological, 315–317, 364–368,
    see also Antidepressants
  psychotherapy, 369–376, *see also*
    Psychotherapy
vs. apathy, 345
Depressive pseudodementia, 233, 329
Deterioration theory of aging, 9
Development concept of aging, 126
Dexamethasone suppression test, in mood
    disorders, 348–349
Diazepam, 28
Diet, 431
  preventive value of, 388–389
Dietary Supplement and Health Education
    Act, 434
Dietary supplements, 425–437, see also
    specific vitamins and minerals
  antioxidants, 426
  biosynthesized vs. chemically
    synthesized, 427
  free radicals and, 426
  herbs as, 433–434
  mineral supplements, 429–430
  vitamin supplements, 427–429, 430,
    431–433
Diffusional anisotropy, 73–74
Digit-number matching test, 99

Digits backward test, 262
Digoxin, cognitive side effects, 319
Dilantin dementia, 407
Disconnection symdrome, 272
Discourse comprehension and elderspeak, 169–170
Disease prevention, 28–29
Disengagement deficit, 102
Disinhibition vs. mania, 186
Disopyramide, cognitive side effects, 319
Divided attention, 102
Dizziness, in multiple sclerosis, 419
DNA glycosylation, early work on, 25
Dopamine depletion, 134
Dopaminergic agonists, 313–314
  sleep-related side effects, 209
Drug abuse, 247
Drug interactions, *see* Medication side effects
DSM-IV criteria
  for dementia, 326–327
  for postinfarction depression, 348
  for vascular dementia, 351
Duke University study, 25
Dysarthria, 246
  in multiple sclerosis, 420
Dyskinesia, tardive, 313
Dysphagia, 137
  in multiple sclerosis, 421

E

Economic costs, of Alzheimer's disease (AD), 283
Educational level, cognitive changes and, 90–92, 245
Educational Resources Information Center (ERIC) database, 295–297
Elderly persons, medical practice considerations for, 26–27
"Elderspeak," 153, 169–170, 171
Electroconvulsive therapy (ECT), 350, 368–369
Electroencephalography (EEG), in dementia evaluation, 332–333
Emotional disorders, 183–201, *see also* Sleep disorders and specific entities
  assessment considerations in, 184
  conclusions, 197

organic etiology: co-morbid conditions, 184–187
  aggression, 187
  anxiety, 186–187
  depression, 185–186
  mania, 186
psychosocial etiology, 187–197
  cultural bias and, 133–134, 172, 187–188, 197
  preexisting conditions, 189–191
    exacerbation of symptoms, 189
    expression of psychopathology, 190–191
  reactive conditions, 191–197
    awareness of deterioration, 191–193
    breakdown of social support, 194–196
    lifestyle changes, 196–197
    social isolation, 193–194
Emotional incontinence, 344–345
Emotional lability, 344–345
Encephalopathy
  chemotherapy-related, 319
  toxic, 250
Endartarectomy, 359
Epidemiology, 35–65
  behavioral and affective, 46–48
  comorbidity, 48–49
  concluding remarks, 49–51
  dementia studies 1995–2000, 56–65
  internet addresses, 55
  neurological, 42–46
  neuropharmacologic issues, 41–42
  summary, 51–52
  world demography of aging, 37–40
  world epidemiology of aging, 40–41
Epilepsy, 314
  cognitive function/dysfunction in, 403–406, *see also* Anticonvulsants
Episodic memory, 393
Epworth Sleepiness Scale, 227
Erikson, Erik (1902–1994), 17–18
Erikson's life stages, 17–18
Ethanol, *see* Alcohol/alcohol abuse
Ethosuximide, cognitive effects of, 407
Etymologiae (St. Isidore), 7
European Community Concerted Action on Epidemiology and Prevention of Dementia, 44
Evaluation, *see* Assessment

Evolutionary theory, 3–4, 13
Executive dysfunction, *see also* Executive
    functioning
  effect on family of, 118
  interventions for, 118–119
  neuropsychology of, 113–116
    in frontal lobe dementia and Pick's
      disease, 114
    in normal aging, 113–114, 218–219
    in Parkinson's disease, 114–115
    in traumatic brain injury, 115–116
  in normal aging, 100–101
  prefrontal zone atrophy and, 78
Executive functioning, *see also* Executive
    dysfunction
  assessment, 259–262
    digits backward test, 262
    frontal lobe functions (Tower of
      Hanoi/Seville), 260–261
    neurocognitive interference (Stroop
      effect), 259–260
    Trail Making Test, 261
  disturbed (DSM-IV criteria), 326
  memory decline and, 384–385
Exercise, 8, 28–29
  mental and cognitive performance, 223
  in multiple sclerosis, 419
  preventive value of, 388–389
Explicit (declarative) memory, 380, 383
Extended Complex Figure Test recall, 98
External validity, 291–293

F

Family
  executive dysfunction and, 118
  toll of neurological deterioration on,
    194–196
Family history, 245
Fan effect, 98
Fatigue
  in cerebrovascular disease, 347
  depression and, 347
  in multiple sclerosis, 419
Fatigue Impact Scale, 347
Feedback, 139
Feeding skills, 137
Finger Oscillation (Finger Tapping) test,
  264
Florida [apraxia] Battery, 142

Fluency problems, 164–166, *see also*
    Language; Lexical retrieval
Fluid vs. crystal intelligence, 217
Fluoxetine, 366–367, *see also*
    Antidepressants; Selective
    serotonin reuptake inhibitors
Focal cerebral dysfunction, 339, *see also*
    Cerebrovascular disease
Focal retrograde amnesia, 380
Folate supplementation, 431–432
Free radicals, 31–32, 426, 429
Frontal aging hypothesis, 77–80, 100–102
Frontalization of motor functions, 139–140
Frontal lobe dementias
  apathy and, 345–347
  executive dysfunction in, 114
Frontal lobe functions, assessment (Tower
    of Hanoi/Seville), 260–261
Frontal lobes
  hyper- and hypofrontality, 110
  in memory and executive dysfunction,
    109–123, 384–385, *see also*
    Executive dysfunction; Memory
    dysfunction
FSTA Current database, 295–297
Functional Organic Memory Questionnaire
    (FOM), 255–256
Functional system theory, of motor
    programs, 131–132
  perceptual and motor integration, 131
  sequencing, 132
  variability, 131–132

G

Gabapentin (neurontin)
  cognitive effects of, 407
  in multiple sclerosis, 420
Gait
  age-related functional changes, 136
  changes as adaptive vs. pathological, 136
Gait apraxia, 141
Galton, Sir Francis, 13
γ-aminobutyric acid (GABA), in aggressive
    conduct, 342
Gastric atrophy, 431, 432–433
Gender differences, *see* Sex differences
General slowing model, 160
Genetic factors, in multiple sclerosis, 415
Geriatric Assessment, 26–27

Geriatric Depression Scale, 347, 348
Geriatrics
  antiaging interventions, 31–32
  caring for older patients, 29–30
  health promotion and disease prevention
    in, 27–29
  history of, 24–26
  holistic approach in, 27–28
  origin of term, 24
  physician attitudes toward, 30–31
  specialty training in, 25
  studies comprising field of, 26–27
Gerontological Society of America, 24
Gerontology, 23–33, *see also* Geriatrics
Gerstman's syndrome, 271
Gestures, transitive vs. intransitive,
    142–143
Ginkgo biloba leaf extract, 318
Glatiramer acetate, in multiple sclerosis,
    417–418
Global amnesia, transient, 381
Global validity, 293–294
Goddard-Segin Board, 263
Goldstein's catastrophic region, 342
Gray matter, aging in, *see also*
    Leukoaraiosis
Grayness-of-hair analogy, 95
Grecian views on aging, 4–5
Grooved Pegboard test, 264

H

Hachinski scale for ischemia, 351–352
Hall, Granville Stanley, 13, 14–15
Hallucinations, 119
  in vascular dementia, 359–360
Halperidol, *see* Neuroleptics
Hamilton Rating Scale for Depression, 348
Hamilton's depression test (HAMD), 270
Handbooks, evolution of specialized,
    20–21
Hastead–Reintan test battery, 264
Hayflick limit, 26
Headache, hypnotic, 213
Health promotion, 28–29
Hearing
  changes in normal aging, 87–88
  language and, 154–155
Heart attack, as risk factor, 45–46
Heavy metal poisoning, dementia in, 330

Hematoma
  clinical presentation, 358
  post-traumatic parenchymatous, 358
Hematoma-related dementia, 358
Hemianopsia, 272
Hemochromatosis, vitamin C and, 429
Herbal supplements, 433–444
Hippocampal formation atrophy, 76
Historical perspective, 3–15
  Greece, 4–5
  Middle Ages, 6–7
  modern age, 7–15
    Hall's *Senescence* (1922), 14–15
    19th century, 11–13
  Rome, 5–6
History (patient's)
  importance of, 26
  psychological and health biography,
    245–248
  social and work, 249–250
(The) History of Life and Death (Bacon),
    8–10
Holistic approach, 27–28
Humanities Index, 295–297
Huntingdon's disease, 187, 192
Hydrocephalus, idiopathic normal-pressure,
    71
5-Hydroxyindolacetic acid, in aggressive
    conduct, 342
Hyperarousal, insomnia and, 225–226
Hyperfrontality, 110
Hypersomnia (excessive daytime sleepiness,
    EDS), 226–227, *see also* Sleep
    disorders
Hypertension, as risk factor, 389
Hypnotic headache, 213
Hypnotics, in sleep disturbance, 208–209,
    226
Hypofrontality, 110
Hypokinesia, 346
Hypoxemia, sleep apnea and, 227

I

Ictal amnesiac syndrome, 355
Ictus, ischemic, 340, *see also*
    Cerebrovascular disease;
    Infarction
Ideational praxias, 141, 141.141
Ideomotor praxias, 141, 268

Idiopathic normal pressure hydrocephalus, 71
Immune enhancement, adverse effects of, 428, 430
Immune suppression, drug interactions in, 319
Immunomodulating therapy, in multiple sclerosis, 417–418
Implicit (procedural) memory, 383, 385
Incidence, see Epidemiology
Infarction, see also Vascular dementia
　butterfly-wing, 346
　caudate nuclei, 346
　silent cerebral, 338–339
　thalamic, 355
　thalamo-subthalamic artery, 346
Infectious diseases, dementia in, 325
Information processing, changes with normal aging, 92–96
Inhalation, administration by, 311
Inhibition deficit hypothesis of language, 171
Inhibition theory, of attention, 156
Inhibitory control, 101–102
Insomnias, 224–226, see also Sleep disorders
　hyperarousal and, 225–226
　psychophysiological, 207–208
　"restless legs" syndrome and, 210–211
Institutionalization, sleep disorders and, 232
Instrumental Activities of Daily Living (IADL), 330
Intellectual functioning assessment, 251–253
　Raven's Progressive Matrices, 77, 253
　Wechsler Adult Intelligence Scale (WAIS), 89–90, 157–158, 216–217, 251–253
Intelligence, fluid vs. crystal, 217
Interferon-β variants, in multiple sclerosis, 417, 418
Internal validity, 291
Internet resources, epidemiological, 55
Interpersonal psychotherapy, 376–377
Intervention programs, see also Treatment
　improvement of evaluation, 296–302
　state-of-the-art evaluation, 295–296
　statistical assessment, 287–307, see also Statistical issues; Validity

　conceptual foundations of validity, 290–294
　concluding remarks, 303–304
　design issues for improving, 294–302
　importance of, 289–290
　methodological implications, 302–303
　overview, 288–289
Intracranial hemorrhage, dementia secondary to, 358
Intravenous injection, 311
Intraventricular CSF pulsation artifact, 71–72
Involuntary vs. voluntary movement, 126
Iowan Elderly Outreach Program, 289
IQ, see also Intelligence; Wechsler entries
　Barona Estimation of Premorbid, 248–249
　changes with normal aging, 89–90
　language and, 157–158
IQ CODE (informant interview), 269
Iregren (solvent), 250
Ischemia, Hachinski scale for, 351–352
Ischemic–hypoxic vascular dementia, 358
Ischemic ictus, 340, see also Cerebrovascular disease; Infarction
Ischemic leukoencephalopathy, 355–356

J

James, William, 3
Journal of Gerontology, 20
Jung, Carl G. (1875–1961), 16

K

Korsakoff's disease, 247
Kral criteria, for normal vs. pathological aging, 217–218

L

Lability, emotional, 344–345
Lacunar state, 355–356, see also Vascular dementia
Lamotrigine, cognitive effects of, 407
Language, 151–181
　aspects preserved during aging, 161–163
　prosody, 163
　semantic memory, 161–162

syntax, 162–163
cognitive impairments and, 154–161
   attention and memory, 155–157
   contextual aspects of, 157–161
   motor deficiencies, 157
   visual and auditory perceptual
      impairments, 154–155
communication and, 152–153
discourse comprehension and elderspeak,
   169–170
discourse production and compensation
   mechanisms, 170–173
lexical retrieval as core issue, 163–168
   orthographic representations,
      167–169
   phonological representations,
      163–167
      naming/verbal fluency problems,
         164–166
      tip-of-the-tongue phenomenon,
         166–167
pathological evolution in Alzheimer's
   disease (AD), 173–175
social isolation in response to
   inappropriate, 193–194
summary, 175–177
Language assessment, 257–258
   Boston Naming Test, 258
   verbal fluency, 257–258
Lateral Dominance Examination, 264
Laying on of hands, 28
Learning, 215–218
   of motor tasks, 139
Leclerc, Georges (Comte de Buffon,
   1707–1788), 10–11
Leukoaraiosis (white matter hyperintensity),
   69, 70, 72, 338
Leukoencephalopathy, ischemic, 355–356
Levo-dopa (L-dopa), 313–314
Lexical retrieval, 163–168
   orthographic representations, 167–169
   phonological representations, 163–167
      naming/verbal fluency problems,
         164–166
      tip-of-the-tongue phenomenon,
         166–167
Libre de Bon Amor (Ruiz), 7
Life expectancy, 20–21
Lifespan, 30
Lifestyle, historical views of, 10, 15

Lifestyle change, emotional response to,
   196–197
Limb apraxia, 141–143
Limbic structures, aging and, 76
Limb praxis
   functional changes, 135
   in healthy elderly, 140–145
      qualitative analysis, 143–145
      quantitative analysis, 140–143
Lithium, 367, 368
Loci system, in memory disorders, 117, 392
Lorazepam, 315, *see also* Benzodiazepines
Lumbar puncture, in dementia evaluation,
   332
Luria/Cristensen test battery, 264
Luria's Memory Curve, 254–255

M

Magnetic resonance imaging (MRI)
   in cerebrovascular disease, 338, 340
   in dementia evaluation, 333
   in mild cognitive impairment, 283, 284
   in multiple sclerosis, 416–417
Magnetization transfer ratio, 74
Maimonides, Moses (1135–1204), 28
Malignant multiple sclerosis, 413, 414
Mania
   in cerebrovascular disease, 349
   as co-morbid condition, 48, 186
   misdiagnosis of, 186
Manual skills, 137–139
   age-related functional changes, 137–139
Manual/visual integration, 157
MAO inhibitors, 350
   in Parkinson's disease, 314
   reversible and selective MAO-A (RIMA),
      366
   in vascular dementia, 359
Marijuana, 247
Maslow, Abraham (1908–1970), 18
Maze-learning task, 99
Medical education, neglect of geriatrics in,
   30–31
Medication compliance, 117
Medication side effects, 134, 247–248,
   318–319, 393–394, *see also*
      specific agents
   of 4-aminopyridine, 419
   of antidepressants, 364–365

apathy as, 345
memory impairment and, 388
of multiple medications, 365
of neuroleptics, 350
of selective serotonin reuptake inhibitors
    (SSRIs), 350
sleep-related, 208
Medieval views on aging, 6–7
MEDLINE EXPRESS, 295–297
Melokinetic apraxia, 140
Memory, *see also* Memory dysfunction
age-related changes in, 382–385
assessment of, 246
automatic versus effortful processing, 98
changes in normal aging, 90, 96–99, 103,
    111–112, 219
declarative (explicit), 380, 383
episodic, 393
importance of contextual information to,
    96–98
medication effects on, 247–248
meta-, 219
name retrieval, 98
in patients with epilepsy, 405
primary, 381
procedural (implicit), 383, 385
prospective, 385
semantic, 161–162, 175, 393, *see also*
    Language
sensorial, 383
terminology of, 381–382
types of, 383
verbal, 90
visual, 158
working, 93–94, 101, 156, 383
Memory Curve test, 254–255
Memory deficits, psychogenic, 381
Memory disorder, age-associated, *see* Mild
    cognitive impairment
Memory impairment, *see also* Memory
age-related, 327
interventions for, 116–117
language and, 155–156
neuropsychology of, 111–113
    in Alzheimer's disease (AD), 112–113
    in normal aging, 111–112
in traumatic brain injury, 116
treatment of, 379–401
    advances in prevention, 387–388
    assessment instruments for, 390

behavioral training, 381–393
cultural considerations, 380
pathophysiological considerations,
    380–381
pharmacological, 393–397
principles and goals of rehabilitation,
    385–387
terminology of memory, 381–382
Memory maintenance strategy, 387
Memory processes assessment, 254–256
    Functional Organic Memory
        Questionnaire (FOM), 255–256
    verbal memory and learning, 254–255
    Wechsler Memory Scales–Revised, 256
Meningitis vs. chronic dementia, 332
Mental status examination, 331–332
Mental walk technique, 392
Mercury, 250
Meta-memory, 219
Method of loci, 117, 392
MicroCog software, 89, 90–91
Midazolam, 314, *see also* Benzodiazepines
Mild cognitive disorder (MCD), 217–218
Mild cognitive impairment (MCI), 217–218,
    279–286
    criteria for, 280
    diagnosis of, 280–282
    early detection of, 284
    economic impact of early AD diagnosis,
        283
    neuroimaging in, 283
    neuropathologic correlation, 282–283
Mind/body dichotomy, 187–188
Mini-Mental State Examination, 332, 359
Mira y Lopez, E. (1896–1964), 19–20
Mitoxantrone, in multiple sclerosis, 418
Mixed dementia, 351
MLA International Bibliography, 295–297
MMPI findings, in narcolepsy–cataplexy
    syndrome, 229–231
Mnemonics, in memory impairment,
    17, 392
Modafinil, in multiple sclerosis, 419
Modern views on aging, 8–20
Motor activity, cerebral atrophy and, 78
Motor cortex, 127–129
    premotor cortex, 127, 128–129
    primary motor area, 127
    supplementary motor area (SMA),
        127–128, 132

Motor function, 125–150
  age-related functional changes,
      133–140
    decremental theory of aging, 134
    gait, 136
    manual skills, 137–139
    motor learning, 139–140
    oral praxis, 137
    upper and lower limbs, 135
  anatomy of, 127–130
    cortical areas, 127–129
    noncortical structures, 129–130
  brain lesion paradigms vs. age-related,
      126
  limb praxis in healthy elderly,
      140–145
    qualitative analysis, 143–145
    quantitative analysis, 140–143
  lower vs. upper limb decline, 135
  summary and conclusions, 145–146
  theories of motor programs, 130–133
    functional system theory, 131–132
    neural network model, 133
Motor learning, age-related functional
      changes, 139–140
Motor skills, language and, 157
Motor skills assessment, 283–285
Mount Sinai Medical Center Geriatric
      Evaluation and Treatment Unit,
      26, 289
Movement, voluntary vs. involuntary,
      126
Multi-infarction dementia, 344, see also
      Cerebrovascular disease
Multiple sclerosis, 411–423
  clinical manifestations, 416
  clinical types, 413–415
  diagnosis, 416–417
  disease course therapy, 417–418
  pathogenesis, 412–433
  risk factors, 415–416
  special considerations in elderly persons,
      422
  symptom management, 418–421
  treatment, 417–421
Multiple Sleep Latency Test, 227
Multivitamin preparations, 430, see also
      Dietary supplements
Muscles, degeneration of, 28–29
Mutism, akinetic, 345

N

Name retrieval, 98
Naming problems, 164–166, see also
      Language
Narcolepsy–catalepsy syndrome, 229–231
Nascher, Ignatz Leo (American physician),
      24
National Institute of Mental Health (NIMH),
      20, 24–26
National Institute of Neurological and
      Communicative Disorders and
      Stroke (NINCDS) classification,
      338, 340
National Institute on Aging (NIA), 25
National Technical Information Service
      (NTIS), 295–297
Neoplasia, dementia in CNS, 325
Network-based theory of cognitive aging,
      100–101
Neural network model, of motor programs,
      133
Neuroanatomy
  of functional aging brain, 67–81, see also
      under Brain
  of motor functions, 127–130
    cortical areas, 127–129
    noncortical structures, 129–130
Neurobehavioral epidemiology, 35–65,
      see also Demographics;
      Epidemiology
Neurocognitive interference (Stroop effect)
      assessment, 259–260
Neurofibrillary tangles, 282–283, 358
Neurogenic pain, in multiple sclerosis,
      420
Neuroimaging, in mild cognitive
      impairment (MCI), 282
Neuroleptics
  in aggressive conduct, 343
  aging and pharmacology of, 42
  in confusion and agitation, 312–313
  in vascular dementia, 360
Neurological disease, sleep disorders
      associated with, 213–215
Neurological-related changes of emotions
      and personality inventory
      (NECHAPI), 265–267
Neuropathology, in mild cognitive
      impairment (MCI), 282–283

Neuropharmacology, aging and, 41–42, *see also* Pharmacologic treatment
Neuropsychiatric syndromes
  in cerebrovascular disease
    aggressive behavior, 342–344
    apathy, 345–347
    depression, 347–350
    emotional incontinence, 344–345
    fatigue, 347
  interventions for, 119
Neuropsychological assessment, 243–277, *see also* Assessment
Neurotoxicities, 250
Nimodipine, 318
NINDS-AIREN criteria for vascular dementia, 351–353
Nocturnal agitation (delirium), 214
Nonequivalent outcome variables, 301
Nootropic drugs, in cognition enhancement, 318, 391
Norepinephrine reuptake inhibitors, 367
Normal pressure hydrocephalus, idiopathic, 71
NREM/REM sleep, *see under* Sleep; Sleep disorders
Nurse Education Link to the Aged (NELA) Wellness Center, 289
Nursing homes, sleep disorders in, 232

O
Obsessive–compulsive disorder, 190–191
"Occam's Razor," 26–27
Occipital lobe lesions, 272
Off Target Verbosity/Off Topic Speech, 170
Olfactory processing, decline in, 383
On the Origin of Species (Darwin), 13
Oral administration, 311
Oral praxis, age-related functional changes, 137
Organic diseases, sleep disorders associated with, 213
Orthographic lexical retrieval, 167–169, *see also* Language
Outcome variables, 298–299, 301–302, *see also* Statistical issues
Oxfordshire Community Project classification, 340–341

P
Pain, in multiple sclerosis, 420
Paralysis
  pseudobulbar, 344
  supranuclear bulbar, 344
Parasomnias, 212
Parkinson's disease, 192, *see also* Anti-Parkinsonism medications
  depression and, 185
  executive dysfunction in, 114–115
  family response case study, 196
  memory and, 385
  sleep disorders in, 213–214
  sleep-related drug side effects in, 209
  social functioning in, 193–194
  vs. cerebrovascular disease, 346
Paroxetine, 366–367, *see also* Antidepressants; Selective serotonin reuptake inhibitors
Paroxysmal disorders, in multiple sclerosis, 420
Pathoclisis, 67
Pathological crying, 344
Patients, idiosyncratic differences and treatment strategies, 387
Pegboard techniques, 393
Pentoxifylline, 359
Periodic leg movements syndrome ("restless legs"), 210–211
Perserveration, 194
  front lobe atrophy and, 77
  versus mania, 186
Personality changes, in executive dysfunction, 118
Personality characteristics, in sleep disorders, 225, 227
Personality disorders, 345
Pharmacologic treatment, 311–321, *see also* specific medications
  antidepresssants, 315–317
  antiparkinsonian agents : movement control, 313–314
  benzodiazepines: anxiety and sleep disorders, 314–315
  cognitive and behavioral side effects, 318–319
  concluding remarks, 319
  in memory disorders, 393–397
  mode of administration, 311–312

neuroleptics: confusion and agitation, 312–313
nootropic drugs, 318, 391
special considerations in elderly persons, 393–394
Phenothiazines, 312–313, *see also* Neutoleptics
in aggressive conduct, 343
Phenytoin, cognitive effects of, 248, 407
Phonological retrieval, 163–167, *see also* Language
Pick's disease
executive dysfunction in, 114
neuropsychiatric symptoms in, 119
Piquer, Andres (18th century Spanish physician), 10
Plasticity, brain, 26
Plato's *Republic,* 5
Polysomnography, 227
Population, world, 39–40
Positron emission tomography (PET), 333, 340
Post-traumatic amnesia, 380
Post-traumatic parenchymatous hematoma, 358
Postural response, 135, *see also* Motor functions
Practice hypothesis, 168–169
Pragmatic change hypothesis, of language, 171
Praxias
constructive, 268
ideatory, 268
ideomotor, 268
types of, 268
Praxis, 125–150, *see also* Motor function
Prefrontal cortex, 78, *see also* Frontal lobe
Premorbid intellectual functioning assessment, 248–249
Premotor cortex, 127, 128–129
Prevalence, *see* Epidemiology
Prevention, of memory disorders, 387–388
Primary memory, 381
Primary Mental Abilities Test (PMA), 158
Primary motor area, of cortex, 127
Primary progressive multiple sclerosis, 413, 414
Procedural (implicit) memory, 383, 385
Processing operations, *see* Information processing

Profiles in Cognitive Aging (Powell), 89–92
Prosody, 163, *see also* Language
Prospective memory, 385
Pseudobulbar behavior, 246
Pseudobulbar paralysis, 344
Pseudodementia, depressive, 233, 329
Psychiatric disease, *see also* specific disorders
sleep disorders associated with, 212–213
Psychoanalytic views of aging, 15–16
Psychodynamic psychotherapy, 370–372
Psychoeducation, 374–376
life satisfaction course, 376
program for confronting depression, 376–377
Psychogenic memory deficits, 381
Psychological and health biography, 245–248
Psychology
aging as focus of, 18–20
emergence as science, 3–4
Psychosocial problems, in sleep apnea syndrome, 228–229
Psychotherapy
behavioral, 372
cognitive–behavioral, 372–374
in depression, 369–376
interpersonal, 376–377
psychodynamic, 370–372
psychoeducational, 374–376
life satisfaction course, 376
program for confronting depression, 376–377
support, 370
in vascular dementia, 360
Psychotic symptoms, in vascular dementia, 359–360
Psychotropic drugs, sleep-related side effects, 208
Psychotropic medication, aging and pharmacology of, 41–42
PsycINFO®, 295–297
Pteroylglutamic acid (folate), 431–432

Q

Quadrantopsia, 272
Quality of life, 27
Quinidine, cognitive side effects, 319

R

Raven's Progressive Matrices, 77, 158, 253
Reaction time, 95
Reagan, President Ronald, 30
Reality orientation, in memory loss, 117
Reasoning
    changes with normal aging, 90
    frontal aging hypothesis and, 100–102,
        103
    recall and recognition and, 98–99
Recall vs. recognition task performance,
    96–97
Recognition (comparison) cycle, 93–94
Rehabilitation, see Treatment
Relapsing–remitting multiple sclerosis,
    413–414
Reliability and validity issues, see also
        Statistical issues; Validity
    in assessment, 251
REM behavior disorder (REM sleep without
    atonia), 212
REM/NREM sleep, see under Sleep;
    Sleep disorders
Removed treatment method, 301
Repeated treatments method, 301
Repetition tasks, in memory dysfunction,
    116–117
Restless legs (periodic leg movements
    syndrome), 210–211
Retrieval, see Language; Lexical retrieval
Retrograde amnesia, 381
Reversible and selective MAO-A inhibitors
    (RIMA), 366
Rey Auditory–Verbal Learning Test, 216
Risk factors, see also Epidemiology
    for Alzheimer's disease (AD), 45–46
    for dementia, 45–46
    for depression, 46
    for multiple sclerosis, 415–416
    for vascular dementia, 45–46
Roman views on aging, 5–6

S

Salt restriction, 388
Sarcopenia, 28–29
Schizophrenia, 73, 345
Seashore Rhythm Test, 264
Seattle Longitudinal Study, 90

Secondary progressive multiple sclerosis,
    413, 414
Selective attention, 102
Selective serotonin reuptake inhibitors
    (SSRIs), 349–350
    drug interactions, 350
    in multiple sclerosis, 419
Selegiline
    in Parkinson's disease, 314
    sleep-related side effects, 209
Self-awareness, alterations in, 118–119
Semantic memory, 161–162, 175, 393, see
        also Language
Seneca's *Letters to Lucilius,* 6
Senescence (Hall), 14–15
Senility, see also Dementia
    as term, 25
Senso-Perceptive Examination, 264
Sensorial memory, 383
Sensory and motor skills assessment,
    283–285
Sensory changes, with normal aging, 86–88,
    103
Sensory deficits, apathy and, 346
Serotoninergic factors, in emotional
    incontinence, 345
Seville Neuropsychological Test Battery
    (BNS), 253–254, see also
        Assessment and specific test
        instruments
Sex differences
    in amyloid angiopathy, 358
    in brain aging, 68
    in corpus callosum atrophy, 74–75
    in depression, 46–47, 231
    in gait characteristics, 136
    intrahemispheric fissure enlargement and,
        73
    in manual skills decline, 138
    in multiple sclerosis, 415
    in nutritional study designs, 429
    in perceptual speed as predictor of task
        performance, 99
    in recall and recognition, 98–99
    in REM behavior disorder (REM sleep
        without atonia), 212
    in sleep disorders, 207
    in tardive dyskinesia, 313
Sexual dysfunction, in multiple sclerosis,
    421

Shakespeare, William, 8
Silent cerebral infarction, 338–339
Simultagnosia, 272
Single-photon emission positron emission
        tomography (SPECT), 340
Skinner, B. F. (1904–1993), 19
Sleep, *see also* Sleep disorders
  in circadian sleep–wake rhythms,
        205–206
    physiological changes of aging, 204–206
      in cerebral bioelectric activity, 205
      in NREM/REM stages and cycles, 205
    shiftwork and, 211
Sleep apnea syndrome (SAS), 210,
        227–229, *see also* Hypersomnia
Sleep disorders, 42, 206–215
  affective disorders and, 231–233
  assessment of, 227
  benzodiazepines in, 314–315
  cognitive functioning and, 223–233
    hypersomnia (excessive daytime
        sleepiness, EDS), 226–227
    insomnias, 210–211, 224–226
    narcolepsy–catalepsy syndrome,
        229–231
    sleep apnea syndrome (SAS), 227–229
  conclusions, 233–234
  disease-associated, 212–215
    with neurological disease, 213–215
    with organic diseases, 213
    with psychiatric disease, 212–213
  dyssomnias, 207–212
    of circadian rhythms, 211
    of excessive daytime sleepiness (EDS,
        hypersomnia), 210–211, 226–227
    of sleep initiation or maintenance
        (insomnias), 207–209, 210–211,
        224–226
  hypoxemia in, 227, 228
  in institutionalized elderly persons, 232
  MMPI findings in, 225, 227
  parasomnias, 212
  sleep fragmentation, 228
Sleep-related respiratory disturbances
        (SRRDs), 224, *see also* Sleep
        apnea syndrome (SAS)
Slowing down, 160–161
Social and work history, 249–250
Social deficits, in executive dysfunction,
        118–119

Social isolation, 193–194
Social support, loss of, 194–196
Sociocultural attitudes toward aging,
        133–134, 172, 187–188, 197, 380
Sociocultural bias, *see* Cultural bias
Socioeconomic background, 245
Sociological Abstracts, 295–297
Sodium valproate, cognitive effects of, 248,
        407
Solvent exposure, 250
Spasticity, in multiple sclerosis, 419
Spatiovisual integration, 158
Specific domain model, of slowing down,
        160
Specific process model, of slowing down,
        160–161
Speech, *see* Language
Speech production, 137
Speech Sound Perception Test, 264
Speed of processing, 92–96
Speed of retrieval, 96–99, *see also*
        Memory
St. Isidore, 7
Standard Progressive Matrices, 253
Stanford Sleepiness Scale, 227
Statistical conclusion validity, 290
Statistical issues, 287–307
  as applied to evaluation of interventions,
        294
  concepts of validity, 290–294
    construct validity, 291
    external validity, 291–293
    global validity, 293–294
    internal validity, 291
    statistical conclusion validity, 290
  of evaluation design, 294–295
  need for program evaluation, 289–290
  in reform of intervention programs,
        288–289
  UTOST concept of intervention and,
        290–293
Stenosis, asymptomatic carotid, 338
Stimulants, see also specific agents
  in multiple sclerosis, 419
Stress
  multiple sclerosis and, 416
  as risk factor, 389
Stroke, *see* Cerebrovascular disease;
        Vascular dementia
Stroop effect, 259–260

Stroop's Words and Colors Test, 216, 259–260

Subcutaneous administration, 311

Substance abuse, 246–247
  in aggressive conduct, 343
  dementia in, 330

Subsyndromal depression, 231

Suicide, in cerebrovascular disease, 349

Sundowning syndrome, 214–215

"Super aged" concept, 24–25

Supplementary motor area (SMA), of cortex, 127–128, 132

Support psychotherapy, 370

Supranuclear bulbar paralysis, 344

Sur l'homme et le devéloppement de ses facultes, ou essai physique sociale (Quételet), 12–13

Swallowing, 137

Switching replication method, 301

Synaptic plasticity, 26

Syncope, vasovagal, 340

Syndrome athymhormique, 346

Syntax, 162–163, *see also* Language

T

Tacrine, 318

Tactual Performance Test, 263

Tardive dyskinesia, 313

Task performance
  changes with normal aging, 95
  learning of motor tasks, 139
  visuospatial, 99–100

Terminology of memory, 381–382

Thalamic infarction, 355

Thalamic syndromes, apathy and, 346

Thalamo-subthalamic artery infarctions, 346

Thalamus, in motor function, 129

Theophylline, sleep-related side effects, 209

TIAs, 339–340

Tip-of-the-tongue phenomenon, 166–167, *see also* Language; Memory entries

Titanium as carcinogen, 430

Topical anesthetics, cognitive side effects, 319

Topical application, 311

TOT (tip-of-the-tongue) phenomenon, 166–167

Tower of Hanoi/Seville, 260–261

Tower of Hanoi task, prefrontal zone atrophy and, 78

Toxic dementias, 325, 330

Toxic encephalopathy syndromes, 250

Tragicomedia de Calixto y Melibea (de Rojas), 7

Trail Making Test, 216, 261

Transient global amnesia, 381

Transient ischemic attacks (TIAs), 339–340, *see also* Cerebrovascular disease; Vascular dementia

Transitive vs. intransitive gestures, 142–143

Traumatic brain injury
  assessment, 272
  emotional disorders in, 195
  executive dysfunction in, 115–116, 118–119
  self-awareness alterations in, 118–119

Treatment, see also Interventions
  of dementia in primary care, 323–336, *see also* Dementia
  of depression, 363–378
    electroconvulsive therapy (ECT), 350, 368–369
    pharmacological, 364–368, *see also* Antidepressants
    psychotherapy, 369–376, *see also* Psychotherapy
  of memory dysfunction, 379–401
    advances in prevention, 387–388
    assessment instruments for, 390
    behavioral training, 381–393
    cultural considerations, 380
    pathophysiological considerations, 380–381
    pharmacological, 393–397
    principles and goals of rehabilitation, 385–387
    terminology of memory, 381–382
  pharmacologic, 311–321, *see also* Medication side effects and specific medications
    antidepressants, 315–317
    antiparkinsonian agents, 313–314
    benzodiazepines, 314–315
    cognitive and behavioral side effects, 318–319
    concluding remarks, 319
    mode of administration, 311–312

neuroleptics, 312–313
nootropic drugs, 318, 391
Tricyclic antidepressants, 349–350,
  365–366

U

Upper and lower limbs, motor function
  changes, 135
UTOST (units, treatments, outcomes,
  settings, and time) evaluation
  framework, 290–293, *see also*
  Statistical issues
Uvulopalatoplasty, in sleep apnea syndrome,
  229

V

Validity, 290–294, *see also* Statistical issues
  approximation to, 292
  construct, 291
  external, 291–293
  global, 293–294
  internal, 291
  statistical conclusion, 290
Valproic acid, cognitive effects of, 248, 407
Vanishing cues technique, 393
Variables, in statistical evaluation, 298–299,
  301–302
Vascular dementia, 351–360, *see also*
  Cerebrovascular disease; Dementia
  arteriosclerosis and, 353–356
  Binswanger's disease, 357
  CADASIL (cerebral autosomic dominant
    angiopathy with subcortical
    infarctions and leukoencelopathy),
    357–358
  CDP-choline in, 394–395
  classification of, 354
  diagnosis, 358–359
  diagnostic criteria for, 351–353
    DSM-IV, 351
    Hachinski Ischemia Scale, 352
    NIND–AIREN, 351, 352–353
  epidemiology, 43–46
  hematoma-related, 358
  ischemic–hypoxic, 358
  lacunar state, 355–346
  main characteristics of, 351
  pathophysiology of, 354–356

psychotic symptoms in, 359–360
  secondary to intracranial hemorrhage, 358
  treatment of, 359
Vasovagal syncope, 340
Ventricles, cerebral, aging and, 71–74
Verbal fluency assessment, 165, 257–258
Verbal fluency problems, 164–166, *see also*
    Language; Lexical retrieval
Verbal memory and learning assessment,
    254–255
Vigabatrin, cognitive effects of, 407
Vinpocetine, 359, 391
Vision
  changes in normal aging, 86–87
  visuospatial task performance and, 100
Visual attention, 100, 101
Visual impairment, language and, 154–155
Visual/manual integration, 157
Visual memory, 158
Visual Retention test, Benton's, 158
Visual stimulation, therapeutic reduction of,
    119
Visuomotor deficits, in Parkinson's disease,
    115
Visuoperceptive and visuoconstructive
    processes assessment, 262–263
Visuospatial deficits
  of normal aging, 90
  in Parkinson's disease, 115
Visuospatial processing, changes in normal
    aging, 99–100, 103
Vitamin A, 428
Vitamin B, cognitive performance and,
    220
Vitamin B_{12} deficiency, 431–433
Vitamin C (ascorbic acid), 31, 429
  destruction of vitamin B_{12} by, 433
  hemochromatosis and, 429
Vitamin D, 428–429
Vitamin E, 31, 427–428
  in vascular dementia, 359
Vitamins, multiple, 430
Vocabulary, recall and recognition and,
    98–99
Voluntary vs. involuntary movement, 126

W

Walking velocity, 136
Warren, Marjorie (British physician), 24

Wechsler Adult Intelligence Scale (WAIS),
  251–253
  changes with normal aging, 89–90,
    216–217
  language and, 157–158
Wechsler Memory Scale, 282
Wechsler Memory Scale–Revised, 216, 256
Weight lifting, 28–29
Wernicke's aphasia, 271
White matter hyperintensity (leukoaraiosis),
    69, 70, 338
Wisconsin Card Sorting Test, 216
Wisconsin Card Sorting Test (WCST), 77

Word retrieval, 163–169, *see also* Lexical
    retrieval
Work history, 250
Working memory, 93–94, 156, 383
World Health Organization (WHO)
  definition of aggressive behavior, 342
  definition of health, 288
World population, 38–40
Writing problems, 157

Y

Yesavage's Geriatric Depression Scale, 270